Manual of Medical Therapeutics

27th Edition

Department of Medicine
Washington University
School of Medicine
St. Louis, Missouri

Michele Woodley, M.D.
Alison Whelan, M.D.
Editors

Little, Brown and Company
Boston / Toronto / London

To David M. Kipnis, M.D., fifth chairman of the Department of Medicine at Washington University. His remarkable abilities as a clinician, teacher, scientist, and administrator coupled with his vision, judgment, and humanity make him one of the great academic physicians of our time.

Contents

Preface

The Washington University *Manual of Medical Therapeutics* has been updated every three years since it was first prepared in 1944. Each new edition has been extensively revised or rewritten to reflect important advances in medical therapy. This twenty-seventh edition has been expanded to include two chapters on infectious diseases and a new chapter on lipid disorders. Evaluation and management of disorders seen mainly in the outpatient clinics, especially endocrine diseases, have received special attention. Most of the treatment options presented here were not available when the first edition of the manual was written. At that time, the average length of hospital stay for a patient with a myocardial infarction was seven and a half weeks. Today, with new diagnostic and therapeutic modalities, this stay has been reduced to one week. The acuity of illness in the hospitalized patient has increased dramatically even as the length of stay has decreased, increasing the burden on the practicing physician and house officer to expedite diagnosis and management.

This manual is not designed to be a definitive text on internal medicine. Its purpose is to clearly and succinctly present a rational therapeutic approach to medical problems encountered by house officers, practitioners, and students of internal medicine. While there may be several effective therapies for any disease process, the protocols presented here reflect the current approach relied on by the physicians at the Washington University School of Medicine. Selection of the appropriate therapy is the responsibility and privilege of the treating physician. In medicine as in all things, the art of being effective is knowing what to do and when to do it. Use this manual wisely in your practice.

As in the past, the manual has been written by subspecialty fellows and assistant professors at the Washington University School of Medicine with significant input from senior faculty members. We are grateful for the assistance offered by Robyn Burns Schaiff, Pharm.D., and the rest of the Barnes Hospital Pharmacy Department. We also thank Matthew J. Orland, M.D., Mark Frisse, M.D., and William Claiborne Dunagan, M.D., for their encouragement. We are especially thankful for the support and guidance given by William Hartel, D.M.D., and John Wallis, Ph.D., without which this manual and our current careers would not be possible. We also give special thanks to Alyssa, Julia, and Tyler for showing us the importance of learning every day. David M. Kipnis, M.D., Chairman of the Department of Medicine at Washington University School of Medicine, has been a dynamic force at this institution for two decades. His insight and foresight have guided an entire generation of clinicians and investigators. Those of us who have been taught by him have an advantage few others can boast.

M. C. W.
A. J. W.

Manual of
Medical
Therapeutics

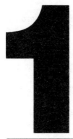

Patient Care in Internal Medicine

Anne M. Pittman

General Care of the Patient

This chapter reviews principles of general patient care, particularly those subjects not covered in any subsequent chapter. Although a general approach to common problems is outlined, it is essential to recognize that therapy must be individualized. All diagnostic and therapeutic procedures should be carefully explained to the patient, including the potential risks, benefits, and alternatives. This will minimize anxiety and provide for appropriate expectations on the part of both the patient and physician.

I. **Hospital orders**

   A. **Initial orders** should be written as soon as possible following admission and evaluation of the patient. Each set of orders should bear the **date and time** written and the legible signature of the physician. All orders should be clear, concise, organized, and legible.

   B. **The content and organization of admission orders** should follow a routine (e.g., the mnemonic ADC VAAN DISML) to ensure that no important therapeutic measures are overlooked.

      1. **A**dmitting diagnosis, location, and physician responsible for the patient.
      2. **D**iagnosis pertinent to nursing care.
      3. **C**ondition of the patient.
      4. **V**ital signs: type (T, HR, RR, BP), frequency, and parameters for notification of the physician (e.g., systolic BP < 90) should be specified.
      5. **A**ctivity limitations.
      6. **A**llergies, sensitivities, and previous reactions.
      7. **N**ursing instructions (e.g., Foley catheter to gravity drainage, wound care, daily weights).
      8. **D**iet.
      9. **I**ntravenous fluids including composition and rate.
      10. **S**edatives, analgesics, and other prn medications.
      11. **M**edications, including dose, frequency, and route of administration.
      12. **L**aboratory tests and radiographic studies.

   C. **Orders should be frequently reevaluated** and altered as the patient status dictates. **When changing an order,** the old order must be specifically canceled before a new one is written.

   D. **Orders for medications to be taken as needed (prn)** require careful consideration to avoid adverse drug interactions. The minimum dosing interval should be specified (e.g., q4h).

II. **Drug therapy**

   A. **Prescriptions** should be written legibly in terms that the patient can understand. Each prescription should include the name of the patient, date, name of the drug, dosage, route of administration, amount dispensed, dosage schedule instructions, and signature of the physician. The number of refills should be limited, especially in patients who appear to be self-injurious. **For narcotics,** write out all numbers in parentheses [e.g., disp. #30 (thirty), refills 2 (two)].

   B. **Adverse drug reactions** occur frequently and the rate increases in proportion to the number of drugs taken. Adverse reactions may be allergic, idiosyncratic, or dose-related extensions of known effects.

1. Take a careful history of previous drug reactions and record them conspicuously on the chart.
2. Use as few drugs as possible.
3. Consider the metabolism, route of excretion, and major adverse effects associated with each drug used. Individualize dosages according to the patient's age, weight, and kidney and liver function.
4. Report unusual drug reactions to the United States Food and Drug Administration.

C. **Drug interactions.** The addition of a new medication should follow careful consideration of the patient's current medical regimen. See Appendix B for a list of commonly used medications and their interactions.

III. **Fever** accompanies many illnesses and is a valuable marker of disease activity. The cause should be ascertained as quickly as possible. In general, fever should not be treated if the cause is not clear. A drug fever or tumor fever (e.g., lymphoma) is always a possibility but is a diagnosis of exclusion.

A. **Fever may cause** increased tissue catabolism, dehydration, exacerbation of heart failure, delirium, and convulsions. Treatment of fever is indicated when these harmful effects ensue or when patient discomfort is extreme. Heat stroke and malignant hyperthermia are medical emergencies requiring prompt recognition and treatment (see Chap. 26).

B. **Treatment**
1. **Antipyretic drugs,** such as aspirin and acetaminophen, are the drugs of choice. They should be given regularly (325–650 mg q4h) until the underlying disease process has been controlled. Acetaminophen should be used cautiously in patients with hepatic insufficiency.
2. **Hypothermic (cooling) blankets** may be effective but require careful monitoring of rectal temperatures and may produce excessive shivering. The blanket should be discontinued when the temperature falls below 39°C.
3. **Ice baths** are reserved for extreme cases of hyperthermia, such as heat stroke (see Chap. 26).

IV. **Relief of pain**
A. **General comments**
1. **Pain** is always subjective and therefore therapy should be individualized. **Objective measurements** such as tachycardia are not reliable. A placebo response does not distinguish organic from psychogenic pain.
2. **Acute pain** usually requires only temporary relief aimed at the presumed cause. **Chronic pain** may occur in many situations. Nonnarcotic preparations should be used when possible. Occasionally, pain is refractory to conventional therapy. Nonpharmacologic modalities, such as nerve blocks, sympathectomy, and relaxation therapy, may be appropriate.

B. **Acetaminophen** has antipyretic and analgesic actions but does not have anti-inflammatory or antiplatelet properties.
1. **Preparations and dosage.** Acetaminophen, 325 mg q6h to 650 mg q4h in tablet, caplet, elixir, or rectal suppository form, is available.
2. **Adverse effects.** The principal advantage of acetaminophen is the lack of gastric toxicity. Hepatic toxicity may be serious, however, and acute overdosage with 10–15 g may cause fatal hepatic necrosis (see Chap. 26).

C. **Aspirin (ASA)** has analgesic, antipyretic, and anti-inflammatory effects.
1. **Pharmacology.** The analgesic and anti-inflammatory activities of aspirin are probably due to its ability to inhibit prostaglandin synthesis. After hepatic metabolism, the drug is cleared by the kidneys.
2. **Preparations and dosages.** Aspirin is used in a dose of 0.3–1.0 g PO q6h for relief of pain. Rectal suppositories (0.3–0.6 g q3–4h) may be irritating to the mucosa and variably absorbed. Enteric coated tablets and nonacetylated salicylates (choline magnesium trisalicylate) may cause less injury to the gastric mucosa than buffered or plain aspirin. The nonacetylated salicylates lack antiplatelet effects.
3. **Adverse effects**
a. **Dose-related side effects** include tinnitus, dizziness, and hearing loss.

   b. **Dyspepsia and bleeding** are often encountered and may be severe.
   c. **Hypersensitivity reactions,** including bronchospasm, laryngeal edema, and urticaria are uncommon, but patients with asthma and nasal polyps are susceptible. (These patients may also react to nonsteroidal anti-inflammatory drugs.)
   d. **Platelet effects** may last for up to 1 week after a single dose. **Aspirin should be avoided** in patients with known bleeding disorders, in those receiving anticoagulant therapy, and during pregnancy.
   e. **Chronic excessive use** may result in interstitial nephritis and papillary necrosis. Aspirin should be used with caution in patients with severe liver or renal disease.
4. **Nonsteroidal anti-inflammatory medications (NSAIDs)** are increasingly prescribed for nonrheumatologic pain such as dental pain, menstrual cramping, headache, and postoperative and musculoskeletal pain.
   a. **Pharmacology.** The analgesic and anti-inflammatory effects are related to the inhibition of cyclooxygenase. Other anti-inflammatory effects have been demonstrated as well. **NSAIDs should be** used with caution in patients with impaired renal and hepatic function.
   b. **Preparations.** Many oral preparations are available (diflunisal, fenoprofen, ibuprofen, indomethacin, ketoprofen, meclofenamic acid, naproxen, phenylbutazone, piroxicam, salsalate, sulindac, tolmetin). They vary in lipid solubility, delivery to synovial tissue, half-lives, and dosing schedules. Ketorolac tromethamine, 30–60 mg IM, is administered as a loading dose, followed by 15–30 mg IM q6h for short-term use. Analgesia peaks at 30–45 minutes.
   c. **Adverse effects.** The most common adverse effects are gastrointestinal and renal. All of these agents cause dyspepsia. **Gastric** erosion, peptic ulceration, and major gastrointestinal bleeding may occur (see Chap. 14). NSAIDs alter the autoregulation of renal blood flow and may cause reversible impairment of glomerular filtration, acute renal failure, interstitial nephritis, and papillary necrosis. **Renal function** should be monitored in patients who are receiving chronic NSAID therapy.
D. **Opioid analgesics**
   1. **Opioid** refers to drugs that are pharmacologically similar to opium or morphine. They are the drugs of choice when analgesia without antipyretic action is desired and should be used with caution in patients with impaired hepatic function.
   2. **Dosing and administration** (see Table 1-1)
      a. **Constant pain** requires continuous analgesia (around-the-clock) with a supplementary (prn) dose for breakthrough pain. Each patient should be maintained at the lowest dosage that provides adequate analgesia. The amount of analgesia needed is frequently underestimated and the duration of action overestimated. If frequent prn doses are being requested, the regular dosage should be increased or the interval decreased.
      b. **If adequate analgesia** cannot be achieved at the maximum recommended dose of one narcotic, or if the side effects are intolerable, the patient should be changed to another preparation beginning at one-half of the equianalgesic dose (see Table 1-1).
      c. **Oral medications** should be used when possible. Parenteral administration is useful in the setting of dysphagia, emesis, and decreased gastrointestinal absorption. The lowest initial dose should be given with a gradual increase in the amount of drug given until maximal analgesia is obtained.
      d. **Continuous intravenous administration** provides steady blood levels and allows rapid dose adjustment. Agents with short half-lives, such as morphine, should be used. **Patient-controlled analgesia (PCA)** is used increasingly for postoperative pain and for pain control in the terminally ill patient. PCA often improves pain relief, decreases anxiety, and allows less total drug to be given.

Table 1-1. Analgesic potency of selected opioid drugs

Drug	Oral-parenteral potency ratio	Potency relative to equivalent parenteral dose of morphine	Usual analgesic dose range and dosing interval (hr)
Morphine	1:6	1.0	5–15 mg IM/SQ (q4–5)
Hydromorphone	1:5	6.0	2–4 mg PO (q4–6) 1–2 mg IM/IV/SQ (q4–6)
Meperidine	1:3	0.15	50–150 mg PO/SQ/IM (q2–3)
Methadone	1:2	1.0	5–15 mg PO (q4–6)
Oxycodone With acet With asa	1:2	1.0	5 mg PO (q6) 5 mg/325 mg acet (q6) 4.5 mg/325 mg asa (q6)
Codeine	1:1.5	0.1	30–60 mg PO/IM/SQ (q4–6)
Propoxyphene With acet	*	<0.1	50 mg/325 mg acet (q4) 100 mg 650 mg acet (q4)

* Not available in parenteral form.
Key: acet = acetaminophen; asa = aspirin.

   3. Selected drugs
     a. Morphine IV is used in the setting of acute myocardial infarction or acute pulmonary edema at doses of 2–4 mg IV over 5 minutes. For severe, chronic pain, a sustained-release preparation (MSIR 5–30 mg PO q4–8h, MS Contin 15–120 mg PO q12h, or a rectal suppository) may be used. MS elixir may be useful in patients with dysphagia.
     b. Hydromorphone is a potent morphine derivative. It can be given cautiously intravenously. It is available as a 3-mg rectal suppository.
     c. Meperidine causes less biliary spasm or constipation than morphine. **It is contraindicated in patients taking monoamine oxidase (MAO) inhibitors and in patients with renal failure** (accumulation of active metabolites causes CNS excitement and seizures). Repetitive dosing is more likely to cause seizures. **Coadministration of hydroxyzine** (25–100 mg IM q4–6h) may decrease nausea and potentiate the analgesic effect of meperidine.
     d. Methadone is very effective when administered orally and suppresses the symptoms of withdrawal from other opioids (due to its extended half-life). Despite its long elimination half-life, its analgesic duration of action is much shorter.
     e. Oxycodone and propoxyphene are usually prescribed orally in combination with aspirin and acetaminophen.
     f. Codeine can also be given in combination with aspirin or acetaminophen. It is an effective cough suppressant at 10–15 mg PO q4-6h.
     g. Mixed agonist–antagonist agents (butorphanol, nalbuphine, oxymorphone, pentazocine) offer few advantages and more adverse effects than the other agents.
   4. Precautions
     a. Opioids are contraindicated in acute disease states in which the pattern and degree of pain are important diagnostic signs (head injuries, abdominal pain). They may also increase intracranial pressure.
     b. Opioids should be used with caution in patient's with hypothyroidism, Addison's disease, hypopituitarism, anemia, respiratory disease (chronic

obstructive pulmonary disease, asthma, kyphoscoliosis, severe obesity), severe malnutrition or debilitation, or chronic cor pulmonale.

c. Dosage should be adjusted for patients with impaired hepatic function.

d. Drugs that potentiate the adverse effects of opioids include phenothiazines, antidepressants, benzodiazepines, and alcohol.

e. Tolerance develops with chronic use and coincides with the development of physical dependence.

f. Physical dependence is characterized by a withdrawal syndrome (anxiety, irritability, diaphoresis, tachycardia, gastrointestinal distress, and temperature instability) when the drug is abruptly stopped. It may occur after only 2 weeks of therapy. Administration of an opioid antagonist may precipitate withdrawal after only 3 days of therapy. The syndrome can be minimized by slowly tapering the medication over several days.

5. **Adverse and toxic effects.** While individuals may tolerate some preparations better than others, at equianalgesic doses, there are few differences.

   a. CNS effects include sedation, euphoria, and pupillary constriction.

   b. Respiratory depression is dose related and is especially pronounced after intravenous administration. Opioids should be used cautiously and at decreased doses in patients with respiratory impairment.

   c. Cardiovascular effects include peripheral vasodilatation and hypotension, especially after intravenous administration.

   d. The most common gastrointestinal effect is constipation. Patients should be provided with stool softeners. Opioids may precipitate toxic megacolon in patients with inflammatory bowel disease. **Nausea and vomiting** may be limited by keeping the patient recumbent.

   e. Opioids increase bladder, ureter, and sphincter tone and may cause **urinary retention.**

   f. Allergic reactions (urticaria, rash, and anaphylaxis) are uncommon.

Sedative and Psychoactive Drug Therapy

I. **Sedative–hypnotic and anxiolytic drugs** are among the most widely prescribed medications in the United States, primarily due to the popularity of benzodiazepines in the treatment of insomnia and anxiety.

A. **Principles of management**

   1. **Insomnia** may be attributed to a variety of underlying medical or psychiatric disorders (e.g., depression). Behavioral and relaxation techniques should be attempted before drug therapy is initiated.

   2. **Anxiety** may be part of the symptom complex seen in major depression, panic disorder, drug toxicity or withdrawal, and metabolic disturbances. These underlying causes require specific therapy. The use of sedative–hypnotic medications in the setting of transient anxiety-provoking situations should be brief. Patients with chronic, nonspecific anxiety generally do not experience sustained improvement in symptoms with pharmacotherapy.

   3. **Physical dependence** develops with regular use of these medications. Abrupt termination of prolonged treatment at usual therapeutic doses can result in a withdrawal syndrome consisting of agitation, irritability, insomnia, tremor, headache, gastrointestinal distress, and perceptual disturbance. Seizures and delirium may occur with discontinuation of barbiturates or high-dose benzodiazepines.

      a. Benzodiazepine dependence may develop after only 4 weeks of therapy. The **withdrawal syndrome** begins 1 to 10 days after abrupt cessation of therapy and may last for several weeks. The probability and intensity of the withdrawal effects are greatest with short-acting drugs. Intermediate-acting drugs should be decreased by 5–10% every 5 days. Patients who have been taking long-acting preparations can be tapered more quickly.

Table 1-2. Selected benzodiazepines

Drug	Route	Dosage	Half-life (hr)
Alprazolam	PO	0.75–4 mg/24 h (in 3 doses)	11–15
Chlordiazepoxide	PO	15–100 mg/24h (in divided doses)	6–30
Clorazepate	PO	7.5–60 mg/24h (in 1–4 doses)	30–100
Diazepam	PO	6–40 mg/24h (in 1–4 doses)	20–50
	IV	2.5–20 mg (slowly)	
Flurazepam	PO	15–30 mg qhs	50–100
Lorazepam*	PO	1–10 mg/24h (in 2–3 doses)	10–20
	IV/IM	0.05 mg/kg (4 mg max)	
Midazolam	IV	0.035–0.1 mg/kg	1–12
	IM	0.08 mg/kg	
Prazepam	PO	20–60 mg/24h (in divided doses or qhs)	36–70
Oxazepam*	PO	30–120 mg/24h (in 3–4 doses)	5–10
Temazepam*	PO	15–30 mg qhs	9–12
Triazolam*	PO	0.125–0.25 mg qhs	2–3

* Metabolites are inactive.

       b. The dose of barbiturates can be decreased by the equivalent of 3 mg phenobarbital per day.
    4. Sedative–hypnotic medications interact additively with other CNS depressants such as alcohol.
B. Benzodiazepines are effective as anxiolytics, hypnotics, anticonvulsants, and muscle relaxants. They are relatively safe in combination with most other medications and in patients with many medical illnesses. They are generally not lethal when taken alone in overdoses. Use should be short term since they produce tolerance and dependence, and the potential for abuse is considerable. Table 1-2 provides a list of selected benzodiazepines and doses.
    1. Pharmacology. Most benzodiazepines undergo oxidation to active metabolites in the liver. However, the metabolites of lorazepam, oxazepam, triazolam, and temazepam are inactive. **Benzodiazepine toxicity** is increased by advanced age, hepatic disease, and concomitant use of alcohol and other CNS depressants, disulfiram, and cimetidine.
       a. Benzodiazepines with long half-lives accumulate during repeated dosage intervals of less than 24 hours. This is of particular concern in the elderly, in whom the half-life may be increased two- to fourfold.
       b. Benzodiazepines with short half-lives are less likely to accumulate after multiple doses, minimizing the likelihood of daytime sedation and performance impairment.
    2. Indications and doses

a. **Relief of anxiety and insomnia** is achieved at the doses outlined in Table 1-2.

b. **The acute treatment of status epilepticus** includes diazepam. It is used to abort prolonged seizure episodes while other longer-acting anticonvulsants are being administered. Diazepam, 1–2 mg per minute IV, is given to a total dose of 5–10 mg. **Extreme caution** should be used to avoid cardiac or respiratory compromise.

c. **Skeletal muscle spasm** is relieved by benzodiazepines. Diazepam, 2–10 mg PO tid–qid, is a useful adjunct to bed rest in the management of sciatica.

d. **Before procedures** such as cardioversion, diazepam, 2–5 mg IV, or midazolam, 1–3 mg IV, over 2–5 minutes will relieve anxiety and reduce the patient's memory of the procedure.

e. **Delirium tremens** and early signs of alcohol withdrawal may require large doses of chlordiazepoxide. Oxazepam has been used because of the lack of active metabolites. The usual starting dose of chlordiazepoxide is 50 mg PO q4–6h (see Chap. 25). Doses should be held for sedation. The drug should be slowly tapered over several days. These patients often have impaired hepatic function and the drug half-lives are prolonged (see Chap. 25).

3. **Toxicity**

a. **Side effects** include drowsiness, dizziness, fatigue, and incoordination. Clinicians are obligated to warn patients about the psychomotor impairment and the hazard of driving after even a single dose of these agents. Patients should also be warned about the possibility of the development of anterograde amnesia.

b. **The elderly** are more susceptible to these effects and may experience paradoxical agitation and delirium.

c. **Respiratory depression** may occur with oral doses in patients with respiratory compromise. This rarely occurs in otherwise healthy patients when these are the only drugs ingested. **Intravenous administration of diazepam and midazolam,** on the other hand, have been associated with hypotension and respiratory or cardiac arrest.

d. **Tolerance** develops to the benzodiazepines and physiologic addiction leads to severe withdrawal if the drug is stopped abruptly (see sec. **I.A.3**).

C. **Buspirone** is an anxiolytic agent with few side effects. There is limited psychomotor impairment or interaction with ethanol and no tolerance or withdrawal. The usual starting dose is 5 mg PO tid, titrating to 10 mg tid as needed. It requires chronic administration to exert its anxiolytic effect. Buspirone has no sedative or hypnotic effect.

D. **Barbiturates** have a poor therapeutic index and have generally been supplanted by the safer benzodiazepines for the treatment of anxiety and insomnia. Elimination requires hepatic and renal metabolism and clearance, and caution should be used in patients with impaired hepatic and renal function.

1. **Preparations.** Long-acting (phenobarbital) and short-acting (amobarbital, pentobarbital, secobarbital) preparations are available. They should be given parenterally only in emergency situations. The usual dose of phenobarbital is 100 mg PO qhs.

2. **Adverse effects.** Barbiturates are CNS depressants that cause drowsiness and mental depression. These effects are additive with the effects of other CNS depressants including alcohol. They cause respiratory depression and are contraindicated in patients with severe pulmonary disease. Barbiturates interact with many other medications (see Appendix B).

3. **Tolerance** to the effects of barbiturates occurs with continued use, and physiologic addiction leads to **severe withdrawal** with abrupt discontinuation of the drug.

4. **Acute barbiturate overdose** or poisoning is a medical emergency (see Chap. 26).

E. **Chloral hydrate** is a rapidly effective hypnotic that seldom produces excitement

Table 1-3. Selected antipsychotic medications

Drug	Daily dose range, oral (mg)
Chlorpromazine	300–800
Clozapine	250–450
Thioridazine	200–600
Thiothixene	6–30
Molindone	50–150
Perphenazine	8–32
Haloperidol	6–40
Fluphenazine	1–20
Trifluoperazine	6–20

or hangover. Elimination requires hepatic metabolism and renal clearance. It should be avoided in patients with hepatic, renal, or cardiac disease. **Common side effects** include gastric irritation and skin reactions. Toxic doses cause both CNS and respiratory depression. Tolerance, addiction, and withdrawal syndromes can be seen with chronic ingestion. A fatal interaction with ethanol and a short-term increase in the effect of warfarin have been reported. The usual hypnotic dose is 0.5–1.0 g PO qhs.

   F. Some antihistamines have sedative effects.

II. Antipsychotic drugs are used in the treatment of psychotic disorders and to control nausea, vomiting, and intractable hiccups. These agents vary widely in their potency and side effects. Addiction does not occur and overdosage rarely results in death.

   A. Pharmacologic properties. These drugs have anticholinergic and anti–alpha-adrenergic effects. Both oral and parenteral administration are effective. The plasma half-life is 10–20 hours for most drugs in this class. These agents should be used cautiously in patients with impaired liver function due to the hepatic metabolism.

   B. Clinical use, preparations, and dosage (Table 1-3)

   1. **Acute psychotic reactions.** The usual drug of choice is haloperidol, 1–5 mg PO, IV (slowly), or IM. This dose can be repeated hourly until the desired effect is achieved.

   2. **Chronic antipsychotic therapy.** These medications are used in the treatment of schizophrenia, schizoaffective disorder, psychotic depression, mania, and organic brain syndrome with psychotic manifestations. Doses vary tremendously depending on the clinical setting, response, and side effects. Furthermore, individuals differ widely in their metabolism of these drugs.

   3. **Nausea and vomiting. Prochlorperazine** is usually given in a dosage of 5–10 mg PO, IM, or IV qid, or as rectal suppository, 25 mg bid. Dystonic reactions may occur.

   4. **Intractable hiccups** may be controlled with **chlorpromazine** in the lowest effective dosage (i.e., 10–25 mg PO q4–6h, 25–50 mg IM q3–4h, 25–100 mg rectal suppository q6–8h).

   5. **Delirium and dementia**

      a. **In the management** of agitation and psychosis in patients with organic brain syndrome, high-potency antipsychotic agents are useful, in conjunction with behavioral interventions. Benzodiazepines and barbiturates produce CNS depression, contributing to behavioral problems and clouding etiologic assessment. **Haloperidol** is the treatment of choice, using the lowest effective dose. Begin using 0.25 mg PO or IM and titrate up as needed. Haloperidol rarely causes hypotension, cardiovascular compromise, or excessive sedation in these dosages, and it can be given to elderly patients. Gradual withdrawal of the medication should be attempted once the target symptoms respond and the patient's condition is stable.

   b. **Sundown syndrome** refers to the appearance of worsening confusion in the evening. Sundowning has been associated with dementia and other organic brain disease, unfamiliar environments, low environmental lighting, and old age. If behavioral intervention such as increased lighting and attention and maintenance of a familiar environment are ineffective, short-term antipsychotic therapy may be beneficial.

C. **Adverse reactions.** For lower-potency and strongly anticholinergic preparations such as chlorpromazine and thioridazine, autonomic and sedative effects outweigh the extrapyramidal reactions. The reverse is true of the high-potency drugs such as haloperidol.

   1. **Postural hypotension** may occasionally be acute and severe after intramuscular administration. If significant hypotension occurs, intravenous fluids and placing the patient in a Trendelenburg position for 1–2 hours are usually sufficient. **If vasopressors** are required, norepinephrine or phenylephrine should be used. Dopamine may exacerbate the psychotic state.

   2. **Anticholinergic effects** include dry mouth, blurred vision, urinary retention, constipation, and tachycardia.

   3. **Extrapyramidal reactions**

      a. **Acute dystonic reactions** may occur soon after therapy is initiated. They are characterized by torticollis, opisthotonos, tics, grimacing, dysarthria, or oculogyric crisis. **Diphenhydramine,** 25–50 mg PO, IM, or IV, is effective treatment. Repeat dosages of diphenhydramine may be required.

      b. **Parkinsonian reactions** occur early in therapy and include tremor, bradykinesia, rigidity, and abnormalities of gait and posture. Treatment with antiparkinsonian drugs such as benztropine (1–2 mg PO or IM) may be required.

      c. **Akathisia** is a sense of motor restlessness in which the patient feels a constant need to move about. It occurs early in therapy and may be managed with benztropine, 1–2 mg PO qd–bid, or trihexyphenidyl, 2–5 mg PO bid–tid.

      d. **Tardive dyskinesia** is a late adverse effect that occurs months to years after therapy is started. It is characterized by involuntary movement of the lips, tongue, jaw, and extremities. The syndrome is frequently unmasked as the dosage of antipsychotic medication is reduced and may persist indefinitely after the drug is stopped. Antidopaminergic drugs may suppress these movements.

   4. **Neuroleptic malignant syndrome** is an infrequent, potentially lethal complication of antipsychotic drug therapy. Clinical manifestations include rigidity, akinesia, altered sensorium, fever, tachycardia, and alteration in blood pressure. Severe muscle rigidity can cause rhabdomyolysis and acute renal failure. Laboratory abnormalities include elevations in CK, liver function tests, and white blood cell count.

   5. **Photosensitivity, urticaria, and maculopapular rashes** may occur. These usually resolve after the offending agent is discontinued.

   6. **Cholestatic jaundice** occurs most commonly with chlorpromazine and is often accompanied by eosinophilia during the first month of therapy. It generally subsides after withdrawal of the drug.

   7. **Transient leukopenia** may develop; however, agranulocytosis is rare during the first 3 months of therapy. Leukocyte counts should be obtained when infections develop in patients who are taking these medications.

   8. **Galactorrhea,** pigmentary retinopathy, keratopathy, and lowering of the seizure threshold have also been reported.

III. **Antidepressants**

A. **Tricyclic antidepressants**

   1. **Pharmacologic properties.** These drugs block the uptake of norepinephrine and serotonin. They are potent antihistamines and anticholinergics and should be used with caution in patients with glaucoma and prostatic hypertrophy. These compounds undergo hepatic metabolism. Individuals differ greatly in their metabolism of these agents.

Table1-4. Selected antidepressant medications

Drug	Usual first-day dose (mg)	Daily dose range (mg)
Amitriptyline	50	100–300
Doxepin	50	100–300
Imipramine	50	100–300
Nortriptyline	25	75–150
Trazodone	150	150–400
Amoxapine	150	200–400
Maprotiline	75	150–225
Protriptyline	15	15–60
Desipramine	50	100–300
Fluoxetine	20	20–80

2. **Indications and dose**
   a. **Amitriptyline** is useful for depressed patients who may benefit from sedation. Desipramine is far less sedating. However, these agents should not be used to treat insomnia unless the symptom is a manifestation of depression. Maprotiline has been associated with a higher incidence of seizures than the other tricyclic antidepressants. Table 1-4 lists selected antidepressant medications from most (amitriptyline) to least (fluoxetine) sedating.
   b. **The usual starting dose** of amitriptyline should be given as a single bedtime dose. This can be increased by 25–50 mg every 2–3 days to a daily dose in the therapeutic range. Patients usually require 2–4 weeks to achieve a significant clinical response. The drug can be increased as tolerated to the maximum therapeutic dose.
   c. **Tricyclic antidepressants are now the leading cause of death by drug overdose** in the United States. Because they are given to patients at high risk of suicide, prescriptions should be limited to a total of 1 g, without any refills, in the early stages of therapy and when the patient appears to be suicidal.
   d. **Elderly patients** generally require approximately one half of the usual dose to achieve a therapeutic response. Nortriptyline and desipramine are rational choices for these patients because they have few cardiovascular or anticholinergic side effects. Nortriptyline infrequently causes postural hypotension. A reasonable approach would be to begin nortriptyline at 10 mg PO qhs, increasing by 10 mg every 3 days to a total of 30–40 mg PO qhs. A plasma drug level should be checked after 1 week to ascertain that a concentration within the therapeutic window has been achieved.
3. **Side effects and toxicities**
   a. **Anticholinergic effects** include blurred vision, constipation, dry mouth, tachycardia, and urinary retention. These effects are increased by drugs that impair hepatic metabolism.
   b. **Cardiovascular effects** include postural hypotension and myocardial depression. Arrhythmias, tachycardia, and electrocardiographic changes such as prolongation of the QRS or QT intervals and ST–T wave changes occur. **These drugs should be used with caution in patients with cardiovascular disease.** The routine use of tricyclic antidepressants in patients with left bundle branch block is contraindicated.
   c. **Tricyclic antidepressants** interact with many drugs (see Appendix B). Norepinephrine, alcohol, and barbiturates may potentiate toxicity of the tricyclic agents.
   d. **Hypersensitivity reactions** include rashes, leukopenia, and cholestatic jaundice.

  e. Sedation occurs in varying degrees depending on the specific preparation. Other CNS effects include anxiety, confusion, tremor, and lowering of the seizure threshold.

B. Fluoxetine is chemically unrelated to other antidepressants. It interacts minimally with alpha-adrenergic, histaminic, and cholinergic receptors.

 1. Indications and dosages. Fluoxetine is as effective as the tricyclic antidepressants in the treatment of depression. It may also be useful in the treatment of obsessive–compulsive disorder. The initial dosage is 20 mg PO in the morning. This can be increased to a maximum of 80 mg/day, although dosages of greater than 40 mg/day may not be more effective. Dosages higher than 20 mg/day should be divided and given in the morning and at noon. The onset of action occurs 2–4 weeks after initiation of therapy.

 2. Side effects include anxiety, headache, insomnia, nausea, and weight loss. Urticaria and rashes require discontinuation of the drug. Fluoxetine may precipitate hypomania and may rarely result in seizures in patients with known seizure disorders. **Manifestations of toxicity** include agitation, seizures, and vomiting. Death has not been associated with fluoxetine alone.

C. Trazodone may be useful for the treatment of severe anxiety or severe insomnia. It is generally not used for severe depression. It is highly sedating, causes postural hypotension, and is associated with ventricular ectopic activity. No deaths or cardiovascular complications have been reported in patients taking trazodone alone. There are a number of drug interactions (see Appendix B).

D. Psychostimulants (methylphenidate, dextroamphetamine) do not exert a primary effect on mood. They are reportedly useful for short-term management of social withdrawal or psychomotor retardation in the depressed elderly patient.

E. Other agents

 1. Monoamine oxidase inhibitors (phenelzine, tranylcypromine, isocarboxazid) may interact with tyramine-containing foods and other drugs to produce a **hypertensive crisis.** Drugs that precipitate this reaction include sympathomimetic amines (e.g., those in decongestants and anorectal preparations), meperidine, methyldopa, and levodopa. Foods include beer, broad beans, canned figs, certain cheeses, chicken livers, chocolate, herring, processed meats, red wines, and yeast. **Treatment** requires immediate administration of an alpha-adrenergic antagonist such as phentolamine, 5 mg IV, given slowly, q4–6h, until the blood pressure is stabilized. Norepinephrine should be available in case of an exaggerated hypotensive response. MAO inhibitors should not be used in combination with CNS depressants. **Seizures,** hyperpyrexia, circulatory collapse, and death have been reported after a single dose of **meperidine** in patients receiving MAO inhibitors.

 2. Lithium has a low therapeutic index, mandating cautious monitoring of serum levels throughout therapy. It is cleared by the kidney; therefore, renal function must be monitored and the dose must be reduced in patients with impaired renal function. The therapeutic range is 0.6–1.2 mEq/liter. At therapeutic levels, **common side effects** include tremor, polydipsia, polyuria, weight gain, gastrointestinal discomfort, and benign reversible T-wave depression on ECG. **Adverse reactions** include goiter, nephrogenic diabetes insipidus, leukocytosis, hypercalcemia, and multiple drug interactions (see Appendix B). Serum levels above 1.5 mEq/liter are accompanied by ataxia, CNS depression, seizures, gastrointestinal disturbance, arrhythmias, and hypotension. Treatment of toxicity is supportive. If renal function is adequate, excretion can be accelerated with osmotic diuresis and sodium bicarbonate infusion. Dialysis is the most effective means of removing the ions and should be reserved for severe toxicity.

IV. Electroconvulsive therapy (ECT) is the most effective treatment for major depression, catatonia, and mania, although its use is generally reserved until pharmacologic therapy has failed. It can be safely administered to all age groups and in the presence of most medical illnesses. The only absolute contraindication is increased intracranial pressure. Recent myocardial infarction, severe pulmonary disease, severe congestive heart failure, severe hypertension, and venous thrombosis are considered to be relative contraindications, and the risks must be weighed against those of suicide, starvation, and immobility. ECT is performed under anesthesia. **Adverse effects** include headaches, confusion, memory loss, myalgias, and minor arrhythmias. Death occurs in approximately 1 in 10,000 patients and is generally associated with cardiac disease, advanced age, and hypertension (*Anesthesiology* 67:367, 1987).

Pregnancy and Medical Therapeutics

Appendix G is a partial list of drugs used during pregnancy at Barnes Hospital, St. Louis, Missouri. **All drugs should be avoided during the first trimester of pregnancy (and, if possible, during the last half of the menstrual cycle in any sexually active fertile female) unless absolutely necessary. As few drugs as possible should be used throughout pregnancy** (G. G. Briggs, R. K. Freeman, and S. J. Yaffe. *Drugs in Pregnancy and Lactation.* Baltimore: Williams & Wilkins, 1986; L. M. Hill and F. Kleinberg. *Mayo Clin. Proc.* 59:707, 755, 1984).

Dermatologic Therapy

I. **Principles of management**
Skin disorders are characterized by pruritus, inflammation, alterations in hydration, and susceptibility to irritation. Some require cleansing and debridement. While these conditions can be treated, attention should be paid to identification of the specific underlying condition and specific therapy.
  A. **Restoration of proper hydration**
    1. **Dry skin** is a common problem in older patients and in many dermatoses.
      a. **Bathing** should be kept to a minimum, followed by application of a bath oil before towel drying. Extrafatted soaps such as Basis should be used. Soap should be used only on the face, axillae, crural areas, feet, and obviously dirty areas.
      b. **Lubricating emollients** should be applied frequently and should be thoroughly rubbed into the skin. Available products include Aquaphor, Eucerin, lanolin, Nivea, white petrolatum, and urea-containing products.
    2. **Excessive moisture** is a problem in intertriginous areas requiring drying and ventilation. In severe cases with maceration, exudation, and erosion, wet compresses should be applied. These should be followed by blotting the area dry. The skin surfaces should be kept separated (see sec. **II.E**).
  B. **Pruritus** and burning can lead to uncontrolled scratching and perpetuate an underlying condition.
    1. **Topical agents** can be used to control symptoms.
      a. **Camphor** 1–3% and **menthol** provide a cooling sensation and can be used up to four times/day.
      b. **Phenol** 0.25–2% causes local hypoesthesia. It should not be used on raw or ulcerated skin.
      c. **Calamine** lotion may be helpful.
    2. **Systemic antihistamines** (H_1 receptor antagonists) are most useful in the treatment of urticaria, but are also useful adjuncts in other skin disorders characterized by pruritus. Commonly used drugs include diphenhydramine, 25–50 mg PO q6–8h, and hydroxyzine, 10–50 mg PO q6–8h. While these agents are effective and inexpensive, the major drawback is sedation. Terfenadine (Seldane), 60 mg PO bid, is not sedating and can be used for daytime dosing with one of the other agents used at night.
  C. **Control of inflammation.** Table 1-5 categorizes commonly used topical steroid preparations by the type of base and strength of preparation.
    1. **Base.** Ointments and creams are more lubricating than gels, lotions, and solutions. A lubricating ointment is best for dry eczema, whereas a lotion

Table 1-5. Commonly used topical corticosteroids

Ointments and creams	Lotions and solutions
Low strength	
Hydrocortisone 1%	Hydrocortisone lotion 1%
Desonide 0.05%	
Medium strength	
Triamcinolone acetonide 0.1%	Triamcinolone acetonide lotion 0.1%
Flurandrenolide 0.05%	Fluocinolone acetonide solution 0.01%
Fluocinolone acetonide 0.025%	Betamethasone valerate lotion 0.1%
Betamethasone valerate 0.1%	
Betamethasone dipropionate 0.05%	
High strength	
Halcinonide 0.1%	
Fluocinonide 0.01% and 0.025%	
Desoximetasone 0.25%	
Highest strength*	
Clobetasol propionate 0.05%	
Betamethasone dipropionate 0.05%	
in optimized vehicle (e.g., Diprolene)	

* May produce adrenal suppression.

    would be more appropriate for a weeping, eczematous dermatitis. Lotions, gels, and solutions are easy to use in hairy areas, including the scalp.

2. **Strength.** Lower-strength preparations are indicated for facial use. Highest-strength preparations are used for hand or foot involvement or for severe and resistant lesions not responsive to lower-strength products. **Fluorinated steroids** are significantly more potent than hydrocortisone or nonfluorinated preparations and **should never be used on the face.** The most potent topical steroids can cause suppression of the pituitary–adrenal axis.

3. **Dosage** of topical steroids depends on the clinical situation. In general, application should be made bid–qid. When cream or ointment is used, roughly 25–40 g is needed to cover the entire body of an adult.

4. **Occlusion.** The potency of the products may be further increased by occlusion with plastic wrap. This is reserved for severe, resistant lesions. Steroid-impregnated tape can be used for occlusion therapy of limited areas of chronic dermatitis. Occlusion can cause sweat retention, atrophy, maceration, folliculitis, and suppression of the pituitary–adrenal axis if extensive areas of skin are involved. Occlusion should be used cautiously.

D. Protection

1. **Cotton and rubber gloves** can be used to avoid excessive contact with water or chemical irritants. The cotton absorbs palmar sweat and should be cleaned or changed frequently.

2. **Barrier creams and ointments** containing silicone may prevent contact of irritating chemicals with sensitive skin but are not substitutes for mechanical barriers.

3. **Sunscreens** are useful adjuncts to long sleeves and wide-brimmed hats for fair-skinned people or patients with dermatoses activated by exposure to ultraviolet light. UVB (280–320 nm) is the principal ultraviolet wavelength responsible for sunburn. Sunscreens for UVB are sufficient for routine use. Certain light-sensitive disorders and photosensitizing drugs respond to UVA (320–400 nm), and combination sunscreens (UVA and UVB) are necessary for these dermatoses (systemic lupus erythematosus, tetracycline, sulfonamides, thiazides, norfloxacin). All sunscreens are most effective if applied 30–60 minutes before exposure and should be reapplied after bathing or excessive sweating.

   a. **Para–aminobenzoic acid (PABA)** and its esters absorb UVB and are ideal for preventing sunburn. Allergic and photosensitivity reactions occur, especially in patients sensitive to benzocaine, procaine, thiazides, and sulfonamides.
   b. **Benzophenone derivatives** (oxybenzone, dioxybenzone) absorb UVB and some UVA.
   c. **Titanium dioxide and zinc oxide** are opaque sunscreens that shield against both UVA and UVB. They are particularly useful on the nose and lips.

II. Specific therapy of selected disorders

A. Acne vulgaris.
Routine treatment includes topical medications and oral antibiotics. Refractory cases should be referred to a dermatologist for isoretinoin and acne surgery. Routine dietary restrictions are not justified.

   1. **Benzoyl peroxide,** 5–10% qhs–bid, has antibacterial and drying effects. Therapy should begin with 5% aqueous base to minimize irritation. More potent alcohol-based gels can be used.
   2. **Retinoic acid,** 0.05–0.1% cream or 0.01–0.025% gel, inhibits comedone formation. Mild facial erythema should be expected. It is applied once daily (e.g., one-half hour after cleansing) and can be alternated cautiously with benzoyl peroxide in patients who do not respond sufficiently to either medication alone.
   3. **Topical antibiotic preparations** include clindamycin, erythromycin, and tetracycline. They can be used alone (e.g., in patients who experience excessive irritation with benzoyl peroxide) or in combination with other topical agents.
   4. **Systemic antibiotics** are used for moderate or severe inflammatory acne, usually in combination with topical therapy. Tetracycline or erythromycin, 500 mg PO bid, should be given until improvement occurs, then gradually reduced as tolerated. Tetracycline should not be given to children or pregnant women.
   5. **Isotretinoin** is a vitamin A derivative effective for refractory nodulocystic acne. It should be given only in consultation with a dermatologist.
       a. **The usual dose** is 1 mg/kg/day in two doses with meals. Therapy is continued for 15–20 weeks. Improvement occurs within 1 month and long remissions may occur.
       b. **Cheilitis,** dry skin, dry nose and mouth, and pruritus are commonly observed.
       c. **Serious complications** include arthralgias, diffuse idiopathic skeletal hyperostosis, pseudotumor cerebri, hyperkalemia, and corneal opacification. **Major fetal abnormalities have been reported.** A pregnancy test should be performed before therapy is initiated, and contraception should be used during therapy and for one month after discontinuation. Liver function test abnormalities and serum lipoprotein levels should be monitored monthly.
   6. **Other therapies** include regular drainage of cysts, nodules, and pustules and removal of closed comedones. Intralesional steriods are used for severe cases.

B. Eczematous dermatitis.
Contact dermatitis, atopic dermatitis, and dyshidrotic eczema are common disorders.

   1. **Acute dermatitis (e.g., poison ivy dermatitis)** is characterized by erythematous, edematous papules and plaques. Vesicle and bulla formation is common. The rash from poison ivy will begin 24–48 hours after exposure. However, new areas may erupt for up to 4 days. Washing with soap and water will remove unbound antigen and prevent further spread. Contact dermatitis cannot be spread by contact with the rash or blister fluid after the skin has been washed. While mild dermatitis will respond to high-potency topical steroids, more extensive cases and those involving the face should be treated with prednisone, 40–80 mg/day for the first 3 days and tapered over 10 days.
   2. **Chronic dermatitis (e.g., atopic or stasis dermatitis, dyshidrotic eczema)** is characterized by lichenification, scaling, intense pruritus, and hyperpigmentation. It is often worsened by scratching. Effective therapy requires hydration, reduction of pruritus, and control of inflammation. The frequent

use of emollients, systemic antihistamines, and topical steroid ointments is beneficial. Successful treatment of stasis dermatitis requires reduction of lower-extremity edema. Stasis ulcers form as a result of trauma in the area of the dermatitis. The utility of topical and systemic antibiotics is controversial.

   3. Seborrheic dermatitis is an erythematous, scaly, frequently oily and yellow eruption that most often involves the scalp, face, and intertriginous areas. It is less pruritic than contact or atopic dermatitis. The scalp is most effectively treated by vigorous washing with 2.5% selenium sulfide shampoo 3 times/week. A keratolytic gel can be used for thick scales. Hydrocortisone 1% cream applied qd–bid is effective for lesions of the face, intertriginous areas, and more inflamed scalp lesions.

C. Psoriasis is a common disorder. Treatment is guided by the extent of skin involvement and location of the lesions.

   1. Mild to moderate psoriasis

   a. Topical corticosteroid creams and ointments (of medium–high strength) should be applied to affected areas tid–qid (see Table 1-5). Overnight occlusion of the steroid-treated areas with plastic wrap will hasten the resolution of the lesions.

   b. Ultraviolet light (UVL), including sunlight, is very effective therapy. Lamps and boxes that deliver UVB light are available for home use.

   c. Tar compounds may be beneficial when alternated with corticosteroids. Tar gels (e.g., Estar, PsoriGel) are cosmetically more acceptable than other preparations. Tar bath preparations can be used for widespread involvement.

   d. Keratolytic agents can initially be alternated with topical steroids when marked hyperkeratosis is present. Salicylic acid 6% gel with overnight occlusion is effective.

   e. Corticosteroid solutions and tar shampoos can be used for scalp lesions. If scaling is prominent, treatment can be continued during the night with a keratolytic preparation or anthralin 0.1–0.4% ointment. In the morning, these are washed out with a tar shampoo.

   2. Severe psoriasis. Chemotherapeutic agents and long-wave UVL should be administered only by a dermatologist.

   a. Chemotherapeutic agents such as methotrexate can be used for patients with severe, generalized eruptions or psoriatic arthritis who are incapacitated by their disease and who are resistant to the above treatments.

   b. Systemic psoralens and high-intensity UVA exposure (PUVA) are effective in the treatment of extensive psoriasis.

   c. Etretinate, a vitamin A derivative, is effective in patients with pustular and erythrodermic forms of the disease. Traces of this agent have been found 2 years after its discontinuation, and it is **teratogenic.** Therefore, the risk-benefit ratio must be considered in women of childbearing age.

D. Urticaria is characterized by raised erythematous, pruritic plaques that are transient in nature. Individual lesions appear, change shape, and disappear within hours. Urticaria accompanied by anaphylaxis (wheezing, stridor, hypotension, abdominal or uterine cramping) is a medical emergency.

   1. Recognition of the precipitating factor is an important step toward eliminating the rash. Urticaria is commonly a reaction to a medication, but may represent an allergic reaction to a food, cosmetic, insect sting, or physical factor (pressure or cold). Urticaria may accompany a connective tissue disease, malignancy, or viral infection. Suspected etiologies should be eliminated. All unnecessary medications (including over-the-counter) should be stopped. Frequently implicated medications (beta-lactam antibiotics, sulfonamides, nonsteroidal anti-inflammatory agents) should be stopped.

   2. Antihistamines are the mainstay of therapy in the absence of systemic symptoms. Hydroxyzine, 10–25 mg PO q6–8h, should be increased to the maximum tolerated dose. If the lesions persist, an H_2 antagonist should be added. Corticosteroids should be used for facial involvement and for lesions refractory to H_1 and H_2 antagonists. Medications should be used around-the-clock for the first 48 hours.

3. **Chronic urticaria and angioedema** persisting for greater than 3 weeks warrant a thorough evaluation to identify and eliminate the causative agent. Tricyclic antidepressants are potent antihistamines and in low doses tend to cause less sedation than hydroxyzine and other traditional antihistamines. Doxepin (Sinequan), 10–25 mg tid, is well tolerated. The evening dose can be increased to 30–50 mg, as tolerated. A combination of traditional and nonsedating antihistamines (terfenadine and astemizole) can be used to maximize control of hives and minimize daytime sedation.

E. **Intertrigo** is an eruption in the body folds that results from skin rubbing on skin. Intertrigo may be colonized by yeast or bacteria. The skin surfaces must be kept separated, cool, and dry. Topical steroids are helpful. The lesions should be cultured. Combination preparations (corticosteroid with iodochlorhydroxyquin, nystatin, or antibiotics) are available.

F. **Fungal skin infections.** Clinical diagnosis should be confirmed by culture or by visualization of fungal forms with 10% potassium hydroxide (KOH).

1. **Candidiasis**
   a. **Intertriginous.** Nystatin cream, 100,000 units/g; miconazole 2% cream or lotion; or clotrimazole 1% cream or solution should be applied bid. Ketoconazole cream can be used once a day.
   b. **Periungual.** Thymol 2–4% in absolute alcohol applied bid–tid is useful.

2. **Dermatophyte infections** of small areas of glabrous skin and feet (tinea corpora, tinea cruris, tinea pedis) respond to miconazole, clotrimazole, haloprogin, and tolnaftate cream or ointment applied bid. Ketoconazole cream can be used once a day. Nystatin is not effective.

3. **Tinea capitis,** onychomycosis, and widespread dermatophyte infections respond to micronized griseofulvin, 0.5–1 g PO daily in divided doses. Therapy is continued until the infection is culture-negative and clinically resolved (4–6 weeks for tinea capitis, 4 weeks for tinea corporis, 6–8 months for fingernail infections). Toenail infections are often resistant to all therapy, but a trial of griseofulvin and topical medication (1–2 years) may be effective. Headache, nausea, and vomiting are the most common side effects of griseofulvin. The complete blood count and liver function tests should be monitored during therapy. Oral ketoconazole, a broad-spectrum antifungal agent, may be effective in resistant cases or in patients not tolerating griseofulvin.

4. **Tinea versicolor.** Regardless of the mode of therapy, this condition recurs.
   a. **Selenium sulfide** 2.5% suspension, applied with scrubbing for 15 minutes daily for 1–2 weeks, will clear scaling. Pigmentary changes are slow to resolve. Further applications (several times monthly) may prevent relapse.
   b. **Clotrimazole,** econazole, haloprogin, ketoconazole, miconazole, and tolnaftate are effective but more expensive.

G. **Scabies**
1. **Lindane** (1% gamma benzene hexachloride) cream or lotion should be applied to the entire body, except the face, with attention to the intertriginous areas, skin folds, and finger webs. It is left on overnight, after which the patient should shower and dress in clothes that are known to be uncontaminated. The procedure should be repeated the following evening. Treatment can be repeated in one week if necessary. **Lindane is contraindicated in young children and pregnant women.** Crotamiton 10% cream can be substituted.
2. **To avoid reinfestation,** all household contacts should be inspected and treated if indicated. All clothes and bed linens should be washed in very hot water or dry-cleaned.

H. **Warts**
1. **Common warts** are most reliably treated with liquid nitrogen cryotherapy. It can be repeated in several weeks if necessary. Daily treatment with a

preparation containing 16.7% salicylic acid and 16.7% lactic acid in a flexible collodion is often effective and painless but produces a slower response.

2. **Plantar warts** can be treated with salicylic acid 40% plaster, cut to fit the lesion. It should be applied daily under adhesive tape occlusion followed by debridement of the macerated skin. Daily application of 16.7% salicylic acid and 16.7% lactic acid in a flexible collodion is also effective.

3. **Condylomata acuminata** require application by the physician of podophyllin 20–25% in tincture of benzoin, avoiding normal skin. It should be washed off after 4 hours. Repeat applications on a weekly basis may be necessary. Liquid nitrogen cryotherapy is also effective.

Therapy of Surgical Patients

Elective surgery has less risk of postoperative complications than emergency surgery, since the patient's general medical condition can be improved by treating malnutrition, metabolic and electrolyte abnormalities, hypoxemia, and anemia. However, in emergency situations, the disadvantages of delaying surgery may offset the benefit of stabilizing the patient.

I. **Cardiovascular considerations** (*Med. Clin. North Am.* 71:413, 1987). The risk of **perioperative myocardial infarction or cardiac death** is greatly increased in patients with the following characteristics: (1) heart failure, (2) myocardial infarction within the last 6 months, (3) unstable angina, (4) more than five ventricular premature contractions (VPCs)/minute, (5) frequent atrial premature contractions (APCs) or more complex atrial arrhythmias, (6) age greater than 70 years, (7) illnesses requiring emergency procedures, (8) evidence of hemodynamically significant aortic stenosis, or those in (9) poor general medical condition. The presence of any three of the first six characteristics listed results in a 50% chance of perioperative myocardial infarction, pulmonary edema, nonfatal ventricular tachycardia, or death. The presence of one of the last three characteristics carries only a 1% risk of such events, whereas any combination of the last three characteristics increases the risk to 5–15% (Tables 1-6 and 1-7). Preoperative evaluation and intraoperative management should be aimed at eliminating these factors and reducing the risk of such an event.

A. **General measures**

1. **Digoxin** is indicated preoperatively to treat patients with symptoms and signs of congestive heart failure who will eventually require long-term treatment. Patients with APCs or a history of paroxysmal supraventricular tachycardia, and patients who might otherwise tolerate these arrhythmias poorly (due to advanced age, subcritical valvular stenosis, or chronic lung disease), may also benefit from perioperative digoxin treatment.

2. **Hemodynamic monitoring** with pulmonary artery or intra-arterial catheters aids in the management of high-risk patients with a history of or presence of congestive heart failure (including S3 gallop or jugular venous distention), aortic stenosis, recent angina, or myocardial infarction. It is prudent to invasively monitor elderly patients and those at risk to develop intraoperative hypotension (i.e., vascular procedures) as well. Monitoring should be continued for 48 hours postoperatively until fluids have been mobilized into the vascular space.

3. **Common postoperative complications**

   a. **Hypertension. Sedation, analgesia, and oxygen** are most effective for the treatment of hypertension in the immediate postoperative period. Marked hypertension should be controlled with nitroprusside or nitroglycerin intravenously (see Chap. 4). Labetalol, 20–40 mg IV; hydralazine, 5–10 mg IV or IM; or methyldopa, 250 mg IV, may also be effective. Diuretics may be used 24–48 hours postoperatively after mobilization into the vascular space has occurred.

   b. **VPCs** are best treated by correcting fluid and electrolyte abnormalities

Table 1-6. Cardiac risk assessment in the preoperative evaluation of noncardiac surgery candidates*

Item	Points
History	
Age greater than 70 years	5
Myocardial infarction within 6 months	10
Physical	
S3 gallop or JVD	11
Important aortic valvular stenosis	3
Electrocardiogram	
Rhythm other than sinus or APCs on preoperative ECG	7
>5 VPCs per minute at any time before surgery	7
Poor general medical status	3
$PO_2 < 60$ or $PCO_2 > 50$	
$K^+ < 3.0$ or $HCO_3 < 20$ mEq/liter	
BUN>50 or creatinine>3 mg/dl	
Abnormal SGOT	
Chronic liver disease	
Bedridden due to noncardiac cause	
Operation	
Intraperitoneal, intrathoracic, aortic surgery	3
Emergency surgery	4
Total points	53

Key: JVD = jugular venous distention.
* Once point total of risk is assessed, see Table 1-7 to characterize the percentage risks of different possible complications (e.g., from minor to life-threatening complication).
Source: Modified from H.H. Weitz and L. Goldman. *Med. Clin. North Am.* 71:416, 1987.

Table 1-7. Risks of cardiac complications in unselected patients older than 40 years who underwent major noncardiac surgery

Class by cardiac risk index	Point total	No or only minor complication (n = 2048) (%)	Life-threatening complication* (n = 60) (%)	Cardiac deaths (n = 33) (%)
I (n = 1127)	0–5	1118 (99)	7 (0.6)	2 (0.2)
II (n = 769)	6–12	735 (96)	25 (3)	9 (1)
III (n = 204)	13–25	175 (86)	23 (11)	6 (3)
IV (n = 41)	≥26	20 (49)	5 (12)	16 (39)

* Life-threatening complications were perioperative myocardial infarction, pulmonary edema, or ventricular tachycardia without progression to cardiac death.
Source: Compiled from numerous sources and modified from H.H. Weitz and L. Goldman. *Med. Clin. North Am.* 71:416, 1987.

(see Chap. 3). Specific antiarrhythmic therapy is reserved for patients with hemodynamic compromise or life-threatening arrhythmias. Lidocaine or procainamide is the drug of choice (see Chap. 7).
  c. **Supraventricular tachycardias** are best treated by correcting the specific precipitating causes such as medications, fever, hypoxemia, and electrolyte abnormalities. In patients with no underlying heart disease who require perioperative therapy with digoxin or verapamil, medications can usually be discontinued before hospital discharge.

   d. Heart failure is usually caused by exogenous fluid administration, and diuretics are the treatment of choice.

   e. Myocardial infarctions tend to occur within 6 days of the procedure. Painless infarctions are common. ECGs should be monitored on days 1, 3, and 6, particularly in patients at high risk for infarctions.

B. Specific conditions

1. **Angina pectoris** confers a high risk, and stabilization of symptoms should precede all elective surgery (see Chap. 5). If emergency surgery is needed, hemodynamic monitoring is indicated.

2. **Cardiac arrhythmias.** Patients with a history of arrhythmias should receive their usual dose of antiarrhythmic medication on the morning of surgery. Prophylactic lidocaine should be reserved for patients with a history of sudden death or symptomatic ventricular arrhythmias. The half-life of lidocaine is prolonged by most general anesthetics, and toxicity may occur. Serum levels of lidocaine should be followed in most cases.

3. **Aortic stenosis.** Patients with suspected aortic stenosis should have preoperative echocardiographic evaluation. In cases of significant stenosis, aortic valve replacement should precede elective surgery.

4. **Permanent transvenous pacemakers** should be placed when indicated, before elective surgery (see Chap. 7). **Temporary transvenous pacemakers** should be used preoperatively in patients at transient risk for bradyarrhythmias or in those who will require a permanent pacemaker but in whom intraoperative bacteremia is likely to develop.

5. **Stable hypertension** with diastolic blood pressures less than 110 mm Hg does not increase the risk of cardiovascular complications (L. Goldman and D. L. Caldera. *Anesthesiology* 50:285, 1979). Antihypertensive medication, especially beta antagonists, should be continued through the morning of surgery. Acute withdrawal is generally not a problem if oral medications can be resumed shortly after surgery.

6. **Patients with prosthetic valves** are at risk for complications of chronic anticoagulation (see Chap. 17) and bacterial endocarditis (see Chap. 13).

II. Pulmonary complications

A. The risk of pulmonary complications is greatest in the setting of acute or chronic lung disease, cigarette smoking, obesity, abdominal or thoracic surgery, and anesthesia time greater than 3 hours. Patients should be advised to quit smoking 3–4 weeks before an elective procedure.

B. Preoperative evaluation of patients with pulmonary disease or symptoms should include spirometry, arterial blood gas analysis, and occasionally radioisotope determination of regional lung function. General anesthesia may induce bronchospasm. Therefore patients with reactive airway disease should be treated preoperatively with aggressive bronchodilator therapy to maximize lung function.

C. Postoperative management should include frequent monitoring of oxygen saturation, arterial blood gases, and incentive spirometry in patients with asthma and chronic obstructive pulmonary disease. **Sedative and narcotic medications should be used cautiously** to minimize respiratory depression. Chest physical therapy, postural drainage, deep breathing exercises, and encouragement of coughing are useful in the management of atelectasis. Antibiotics and bronchodilators may be required to treat infection and bronchospasm.

III. Anticoagulation.
The incidence of venous thrombosis is greatest in patients undergoing major orthopedic procedures. Perioperative anticoagulation is effective in preventing deep venous thrombosis. The risk of clinically important bleeding with moderate-intensity regimens is relatively low, and recent reports indicate that low molecular weight heparin may minimize this complication (*Ann. Intern. Med.* 114:545, 1991).

A. Guidelines differ according to the procedure planned. Regimens begin preoperatively or on the first postoperative day and include warfarin (Coumadin) to a target international normalized ratio (INR) of 2.0–3.0, low-dose heparin

(5000–7500 U SQ bid), or low molecular weight heparin (7500 U SQ bid) (*N. Engl. J. Med.* 324:1865, 1991).

B. Early postoperative ambulation reduces the risk of thromboembolic complications.

C. In patients who require prolonged bed rest, pressure gradient stockings, pneumatic compression, and SQ heparin are effective alternatives.

D. Patients receiving long-term anticoagulation. Oral agents can generally be discontinued 48 hours before surgery. Alternatively, oral anticoagulants can be discontinued 3–5 days before surgery, with initiation of full-dose heparin until 4–6 hours before surgery. Heparin is resumed 12–24 hours postoperatively and oral anticoagulation is restarted when oral intake resumes.

IV. Patients receiving chronic corticosteroid therapy require stress doses of hydrocortisone perioperatively (see Chap. 21).

General Eye Care

I. Ophthalmologic assessment

A. A complete physical examination should include assessment of the external eye and eyelid; pupillary size, shape, and reactivity; extraocular muscle function; and visual fields and visual acuity. A direct fundoscopic examination should be performed.

B. Disturbances of vision should be evaluated by an ophthalmologist. **Sudden, severe, painless loss of vision requires ophthalmologic evaluation in the first few hours.**

C. Burning and itching are usually caused by relatively minor eye disorders. A foreign body sensation, unrelieved by patching the eye, requires referral.

D. Ocular trauma requires urgent ophthalmologic evaluation (see sec. **IV**).

II. Red eye is a common problem. The differential diagnosis includes conjunctivitis, corneal injury or ulceration, foreign body, acute glaucoma, intraocular infections, iritis, scleritis, and episcleritis. If alterations in visual acuity are present, the patient should be referred to an ophthalmologist. Patients with corneal injury or ulceration, acute glaucoma, intraocular infections, iritis, or scleritis also require referral.

A. Conjunctivitis refers to inflammation and infection of the ocular mucosa manifested by itching, burning, and discharge without pain or decreased vision. It may present unilaterally but is usually bilateral after 1–2 days due to self-inoculation.

1. Viral conjunctivitis is often characterized by watery discharge, preauricular adenopathy, coexisting upper-respiratory symptoms, or previous exposure to other infected individuals. **The disease** is limited to 7–10 days in most patients. Individuals should be cautioned to avoid contact with other people, their contralateral uninfected eye, and the ophthalmic solution container until they are asymptomatic. Prolonged cases should be referred to an ophthalmologist.

a. Cold compresses provide symptomatic relief.

b. Artificial tears can provide some symptomatic relief.

c. Ocular decongestants such as naphazoline (e.g., Clear Eyes, 1–2 gtts qid) or tetrahydrazoline (e.g., Visine or Murine Plus, 1–2 gtts qid) are effective but are not generally recommended because side effects of rebound hyperemia and hypersensitivity are common.

2. Bacterial conjunctivitis presents with purulent discharge.

a. Smears and cultures should be taken before treatment.

b. Sulfacetamide, 10% ophthalmic (e.g., sodium sulamyd) drops q3h, while awake, or ointment qid, are usually successful. Tobramycin or gentamicin should be reserved for more serious infections.

c. Gonococcal conjunctivitis requires parenteral antibiotics.

d. Any severe or poorly responsive process should be referred.

3. Allergic conjunctivitis presents with itching, whitish mucus discharge, and boggy conjunctival edema. Patients frequently complain of copious nasal discharge, sneezing, nasal itching, and a history of seasonal upper-respiratory symptoms.

   a. Naphazoline combined with an antihistamine (e.g., pheniramine) can relieve some of the itching.

   b. Intraocular steroid drops or systemic steroids should not be used.

   c. Systemic antihistamines may decrease pruritus.

4. Toxic or hypersensitive conjunctivitis mimics viral and allergic inflammations. Antibiotics, ocular decongestants, contact lens solutions, and eye makeup are common causes. Treatment involves stopping the offending agent.

B. Corneal injury may be caused by trauma or infection.

1. Corneal and conjunctival abrasions should be assessed with fluorescein stain.

   a. A sterile fluorescein strip is placed under the lower lid. The fluorescein will spread across the eye in the tears. After a minute, the strip is removed and the eye rinsed with sterile saline or eyewash. Defects in the conjunctiva or corneal layer will stain bright green.

   b. Minor defects should be irrigated, treated with ophthalmic ointment, and covered with an eye patch. **Referral should take place within 24 hours.**

   c. Abrasions from vegetable matter or contaminated material take longer to heal and must be evaluated daily by an ophthalmologist for signs of infection until healing occurs.

   d. Topical steroids or anesthetic drops should never be used for treatment of abrasions.

2. Corneal ulcerations and extensive abrasions require urgent evaluation.

   a. Bacterial ulceration is actually a corneal abscess characterized by a ground glass haziness or whitish opacification of the cornea. **Decreased vision** is present, but pain can be variable. A predisposing cause, such as an untreated abrasion, inappropriate use of steroid-containing medication, contact lens wear, poor eyelid function, or diabetes mellitus is almost always present. **The patient should be referred immediately.** A culture might be helpful, but antibiotics should be withheld until ophthalmic evaluation. **Under no circumstances should steroid drops be prescribed.**

   b. Herpes simplex keratitis is caused by reactivation of latent virus from the trigeminal nerve. Patients present with a red eye, blurred vision, and a dendritic ulcer on the cornea. Topical antiviral therapy is effective; however, the lesion may be difficult to detect without ophthalmic instrumentation, and any patient with suspected herpetic keratitis should be referred.

III. External eye and eyelid problems

A. Blepharitis refers to inflammation, and occasionally infection, of the eyelid margin. The patient has normal vision but complains of itching, burning, scratchiness, and mattering of the eyelids. Scales, crusting, and sticking together of the lids are noted clinically. **Treatment** relies on warm compresses qid, lid hygiene with dilute shampoo scrubs of the lid margin, and application of ophthalmic sulfacetamide ointment bid. Referral is indicated only if the patient's condition fails to improve.

B. Sties are acute purulent infections of the marginal eye glands. **Chalazion** is a chronic granulomatous inflammation of the eyelid sebaceous glands. Treatment is the same as for blepharitis. Failure to improve requires referral.

C. Exposure keratopathy, such as corneal drying and secondary infection, results from failure of eyelid closure in several disease states. The eyelid can be patched or taped closed, and ocular lubricants (e.g., Lacri-Lube ointment) or ophthalmic antibiotic ointments can be prescribed as frequently as q2h. If this proves inadequate, ophthalmic evaluation should be obtained for the use of a moisture chamber or tarsorrhaphy.

D. Dry eye states are exacerbated by wind, cold air, and smoke in patients with keratoconjunctivitis sicca (e.g., Sjögren's syndrome, atrophy of the accessory tear glands in the elderly). **Artificial tear replacements** (i.e., Hypotears, Tears Naturale) given qid or more frequently often provide symptomatic relief. Referral is necessary only in refractory cases.

- **E. Contact lens care**
  1. **Soft lenses** can be temporarily stored in normal saline. The patient must not replace the soft lenses until they have been properly sterilized.
  2. **Hard lenses** can be stored dry or in saline and can be replaced after careful rinsing.
- **F. Prosthetic eye care** includes removal (at least weekly), cleansing with a mild soap (e.g., Enuclene, baby shampoo), and rinsing before replacement. Prolonged removal of the prosthesis (i.e., weeks) can lead to contracture of the socket and failure of proper fit.

IV. Ocular trauma
- **A. Major injury.** Chemical injury, ruptured globe (corneal laceration), and hyphema threaten vision and require immediate recognition and emergent ophthalmic evaluation (*N. Engl. J. Med.* 325:408, 1991).
  1. **Chemical injuries** (especially after alkali exposure) require immediate profuse irrigation with saline or water, followed by ophthalmic evaluation.
  2. **A ruptured globe** may not be readily apparent on physical examination. Vision may remain intact. Patients who were hammering or using power tools at the time of the injury should be carefully evaluated. Intraocular foreign body should be ruled out with CT scan or plain orbital radiograph. Broad-spectrum antibiotic coverage should be given. The eye should be protected with a metal shield until ophthalmologic evaluation.
  3. **Blunt trauma to the globe** may result in hyphema (blood in the anterior chamber), iritis, retinal detachment, disruption of intraocular tissues, or glaucoma. Hyphema or visual loss necessitates emergent ophthalmologic evaluation.
- **B. Minor trauma**
  1. **Superficial foreign bodies** can be safely removed with a soft cotton swab. Topical anesthesia may be necessary.
  2. **Corneal abrasions** (see sec. **II.B**).

V. Glaucoma can be generally subdivided into two categories.
- **A. Open-angle glaucoma** is usually treated with drops, but occasionally laser therapy or surgery is required.
- **B. Closed (or narrow)-angle glaucoma** can be cured by laser iridectomy, but patients often require medications.
- **C. Acute angle-closure attacks** can rarely be induced by pupillary dilation and usually occur several hours after instillation of the mydriatic drops.
  1. **This problem can be avoided** by using weak agents such as one drop of neosynephrine 2.5% or tropicamide 0.5%.
  2. **An acute angle-closure attack should be treated promptly** with acetazolamide, 250 mg orally, and miotic drops such as pilocarpine 4% ophthalmic solution (2 gtts every 15 minutes).
  3. **Ophthalmologic referral** is necessary within 12 hours.
- **D. Many glaucoma medications** can have systemic side effects (see sec. **X**). Since alternatives are often available, an ophthalmologist should be consulted before any medication is discontinued.

VI. Diabetic eye care (see Chap. 20).

VII. The immunocompromised host frequently has eye problems.
- **A. Retinitis** presents as vague visual symptoms that predate visual loss.
  1. **Candida retinitis** occurs in high-risk patients; 40% of patients with at least one positive fungal blood culture may develop candida retinitis. Early cases can be treated with intravenous amphotericin. Advanced cases require vitrectomy and injection of intraocular antifungal agents. **Any immunocompromised patient with visual symptoms or with a positive blood culture for *Candida* should have an ophthalmologic examination.**
  2. **Cytomegalovirus retinitis** requires intravenous, and occasionally intraocular, gancyclovir for effective control.

3. **Other causes,** especially toxoplasmosis, syphilis, bacterial emboli, and fungi, have been implicated in rare cases and are potentially treatable.

B. **Herpes zoster ophthalmitis** includes keratitis, uveitis, retinitis, optic neuropathy, or orbital inflammation.

   1. **Acyclovir,** 200 mg PO 5 times a day for 10 days, reduces the ocular complications in nonimmunocompromised patients when it is started within 7 days of eruption of the skin lesions.

   2. **Ophthalmic antibiotic ointment** applied to eyelid vesicles can prevent bacterial superinfection.

   3. **Topical and systemic steroids** are occasionally required to control inflammatory complications.

VIII. **Optic nerve swelling** is caused by a variety of entities that are differentiated by vision, visual field, and afferent pupillary defects.

   A. **Papilledema** is a bilateral phenomenon, with normal vision and pupils.

   B. **Optic neuropathy** is usually unilateral, with decreased vision and an afferent pupillary defect.

      1. **Ischemic optic neuropathy,** after ischemic infarction of the optic nerve, has two forms.

         a. **Arteritic optic neuropathy** (e.g., giant cell arteritis) is caused by a granulomatous vasculitis. It is associated with catastrophic visual loss and is suggested by an elevated erythrocyte sedimentation rate (ESR) and confirmed by a positive temporal artery biopsy. **Polymyalgia rheumatica** is closely related to this disorder, and any patient with such visual symptoms, jaw claudication, or scalp or jaw tenderness should be urgently referred to an ophthalmologist. **Treatment with prednisone,** 100 mg PO qd, can protect the contralateral eye and should be initiated immediately on suspicion of the diagnosis (i.e., after the ESR is obtained and before the biopsy). Treatment can be stopped 7–10 days later if the temporal biopsy is normal. High-dose steroids (e.g., methylprednisolone, 1–2 g/day) can rarely restore vision in the involved eye.

         b. **Nonarteritic optic neuropathy** is associated with hypertension. It is analogous to cerebral lacunar infarction and does not require treatment.

      2. **Optic neuritis** is usually idiopathic and strongly associated with multiple sclerosis. There is no effective treatment.

      3. **Other causes** include malignant hypertension, compressive orbital lesions, intraocular diseases, toxic neuropathies, and infiltrative lesions; all require ophthalmologic evaluation.

IX. **Prescribing ophthalmic medications**

   A. **Ophthalmic antibiotics** are available as drops or ointments. Topical ophthalmic sodium sulfacetamide 10% drops (e.g., sodium sulamyd), 2 drops q3h while awake, or ointment qid is usually sufficient. Polysporin ointment (polymyxin and bacitracin) is a good alternative. Tobramycin and gentamicin drops should be reserved for specific indications. Neosporin ointment causes ocular hypersensitivity and should be avoided. Steroid–antibiotic combinations should also be avoided.

   B. **Ophthalmic steroids should only be prescribed by an ophthalmologist.** They can cause cataracts, glaucoma, ocular perforation, and exacerbation of infections.

   C. **Dilating drops** include a single drop of tropicamide 0.5%, which is usually adequate for bedside direct ophthalmoscopy. Ophthalmologists generally use three drops of tropicamide 1% and phenylephrine 2.5%.

   D. **Artificial tear substitutes.** Tear replacement drops provide symptomatic relief and are nonirritating. They are available in a variety of over-the-counter preparations.

   E. **Ocular decongestants.** Tetrahydrazoline and naphazoline are commonly used mild adrenergic agents and are available in combination with an ocular antihistamine (pheniramine) or with phenylephrine. They relieve minor irritation and vasoconstrict surface blood vessels. Overuse may result in hypersensitivity reactions or rebound hyperemia. Pupillary dilation may precipitate an acute angle-closure glaucoma attack.

X. Systemic side effects from ocular medication. Ophthalmic medications are often an unsuspected cause of patient complaints. The following are common toxicities encountered by the internist.

A. Cholinergic agonists for glaucoma (pilocarpine, carbachol, pilogel, pilocerts) usually cause a dull aching in the brow. Rarely, cholinergic toxicity can cause rhinorrhea, salivation, diaphoresis, cramping and other gastrointestinal complaints, and rarely CNS effects.

B. Anticholinesterases for glaucoma and strabismus (echothiophate, iso-flurophate) can cause the same side effects as the cholinergics. In fact, the symptoms can be identical to those of organophosphate poisoning. Many patients experience mild side effects, especially paresthesias. **Toxicity** is much more likely to occur in farmers and others who are exposed to insecticides. Echo-thiophate inhibits serum pseudocholinesterase. Therefore, **it must be discontinued several weeks before surgery,** to avoid possible succinylcholine toxicity. RBC pseudocholinesterase levels can be measured if necessary.

C. Adrenergic agonists for glaucoma (epinephrine, dipivefrin) can cause adrenergic activation with cardiovascular side effects, especially arrhythmias. Dipivefrin is a prodrug that is activated mostly in the eye and therefore produces fewer of these complications.

D. Beta-adrenergic antagonists for glaucoma (timolol, levo-bunolol, betaxolol) are absorbed through the mucosa, and many patients achieve significant plasma levels after a topical dose. Typical **side effects** include bronchospasm, bradycardia, congestive heart failure, mood alterations, and neurologic findings. Betaxolol is cardioselective and has fewer systemic side effects.

E. Carbonic anhydrase inhibitors for glaucoma (acetazolamide, methazolamide) almost always cause a metabolic acidosis and paresthesias. Mood disturbances, fatigue, anorexia, gastrointestinal upset, and diarrhea are common. Occasionally, renal calculi can occur, and these agents should not be used in patients with a history of nephrolithiasis. Rarely, idiosyncratic aplastic anemia has been reported. Methazolamide causes less of a metabolic acidosis than acetazolamide.

F. Cycloplegics for uveitis (atropine, scopolamine, cyclopentolate) are parasympathetic antagonists that can produce systemic toxicity. Facial flushing, disorientation, gastrointestinal upset, and tachycardia are rarely encountered. Small children are more likely to absorb a toxic dose of atropine when it is used to cycloplege the lens and ciliary body before refraction.

G. Adrenergics used for dilating the pupil (phenylephrine) can have a high level of systemic absorption. Hypertension after dilation of the pupil occurs in a small percentage of patients who had been dilated with the 10% solution. Rarely, hemorrhagic complications from a hypertensive crisis have been associated with phenylephrine.

XI. Presurgical evaluation of eye patients. Most eye surgery is done under local retrobulbar anesthesia. Since retinal procedures and orbital surgery can require 2–6 hours and are often done under general anesthesia, cardiac risk assessment is important (see Tables 1-6 and 1-7). **Complications of the local anesthetic agent** include seizures, hypotension, bradycardia, cardiovascular collapse, and respiratory depression or arrest. Coagulopathies can result in retrobulbar hemorrhage, a potentially disastrous complication.

2

Nutritional Therapy

Marc S. Levin

Basic Concepts

I. **Nutrients** must be provided by the diet in adequate amounts; otherwise deficiency syndromes will appear. Suggested daily dietary provisions of nutrients as well as symptoms of deficiency are listed in Table 2-1. Prolonged support of patients on defined parenteral nutrition formulas is allowing continued identification of nutrients required in very small amounts. Oral nutrient requirements and the corresponding recommended dietary allowance (RDA) are frequently higher than parenteral requirements because of variable bioavailability in food and inefficiency in intestinal absorption.

II. **Nutrient stores.** A portion of the daily requirement for some nutrients may come from a storage depot. Depletion of the storage depot depends on the fractional clearance rate of the nutrient (determined by nutrient balance and size of the depot). Depletion is indicative of persistent negative balance and at times will suggest certain pathologic processes (e.g., iron deficiency suggests chronic gastrointestinal blood loss). Urgency of nutrient delivery depends on the actual or anticipated degree of depletion of the storage compartment. For example, some vitamins and minerals have small daily requirements but relatively large body stores (e.g., cobalamin), and supplementation is unnecessary during an average hospitalization.

III. **Energy and protein requirements** are fulfilled by proteins, carbohydrates, and fats.
   A. **Energy (calorie) requirements** must be met in some way every day. Some calories may come from exogenous sources (enteral and parenteral), whereas others may be provided by metabolism of endogenous energy stores. Ideally, the energy intake equals the energy requirement unless weight loss or gain is desired. Daily energy requirements can be estimated from the sum of the basal metabolic rate and the energy expenditure of activity plus an additional 10%.
      1. **The basal metabolic rate (BMR)** is the energy requirement at rest and correlates with body surface area (see Appendix I).
      2. **The energy expenditure of activity (EEA)** can vary greatly and represents a major component of the daily energy requirement in active subjects. Sedentary activity may expend 400–800 kcal/day; light work, 800–1200 kcal/day; moderate mechanical work, 1200–1800 kcal/day; and prolonged heavy labor or exercise, 1800–4500 kcal/day.
      3. **Additional calories are required** to metabolize and utilize delivered foods. A safe addition of 10% of the sum of the BMR and the EEA will satisfy this extra requirement.
      4. **Estimating energy requirements in illness.** The metabolic rate is altered by illness. For example, an increase of 13% occurs for each degree centigrade temperature elevation. EEA is very low in the hospitalized patient. Thus, the total daily energy requirement can generally be estimated by adjusting the BMR for the degree of metabolic stress (Table 2–2). Most nonsurgical hospitalized patients have mild metabolic stress. More accurate estimates in critically ill patients can be made using indirect calorimetry or by calculating oxygen consumption using a thermodilution pulmonary artery catheter if one is in place (see Chap. 9).
   B. **Protein requirements.** There are no body stores for protein; all body proteins

Table 2-1. Nutrients and deficiency syndromes

Nutrient	Recommended daily oral intake in health[a]	Indications of deficiency (syndromes)
Calories	See Basic Concepts, sec. **III.A**	Weight loss (marasmus)
Protein	0.75–0.80 g/kg	Weakness, nail and hair changes, edema (kwashiorkor)
Vitamins		
Thiamine (B_1)	1.1 (1.5) mg	Anorexia, weakness, paresthesias, cardiac failure, cerebellar signs, Wernicke's encephalopathy (beriberi)
Riboflavin (B_2)	1.3 (1.7) mg	Sore lips and tongue, angular stomatitis, skin desquamation and seborrheic dermatitis, anemia
Pantothenic acid	4–7 mg	Fatigue, paresthesias, weakness, "burning feet"
Niacin	15 (19) mg	Dermatitis, painful tongue, angular stomatitis, diarrhea, headache, neuropsychiatric symptoms (pellagra)
Pyridoxine (B_6)	1.6 (2.0) mg	Seborrhea-like facies, cheilosis, glossitis, anemia, peripheral neuritis
Biotin	30–100 µg	Alopecia, dermatitis
Folacin	180 (200) µg	Fatigue, sore tongue, anemia, mouth ulcers, nausea
Cobalamin (B_{12})	2 µg	Insidious weakness, fatigue, sore tongue, paresthesias, lower-extremity numbness, anorexia, diarrhea, hair loss, depression (pernicious anemia)
Ascorbic acid (C)	60 mg	Weakness, irritability, gingivitis, joint pain, loose teeth, easy bleeding (scurvy)
A	800 (1000 R.E.)	Night blindness
D	5 mg[d]	Tetany, muscle weakness, bone growth disorders (rickets), osteopenia (osteomalacia, osteoporosis)
E	8 (10) IU	Areflexia, gait disturbance, paresis of gaze, other neurologic signs, hemolytic anemia
K	65 (80) µg	Easy bruisability
Minerals[b]		
Sodium	500 mg	
Potassium	2000 mg	
Calcium	800 mg	See Chaps. 3 and 23
Phosphorus	800 mg	
Magnesium	350 mg	
Iodine	150 µg	Symptoms of hypothyroidism
Chromium	50–200 µg	Glucose intolerance and impaired release of fatty acids noted in some patients on long-term TPN

Table 2-1. (continued)

Nutrient	Recommended daily oral intake in health[a]	Indications of deficiency (syndromes)
Iron	10 (15) mg	Symptoms of anemia, angular stomatitis, atrophic tongue, koilonychia
Manganese	2–5 mg	Ataxia, retarded skeletal growth, and decreased reproductive function observed in laboratory animals
Copper	1.5–3.0 mg	Neutropenia, anemia, diarrhea, scurvy-like bone changes
Zinc	15 (12) mg	Facial and extremity rash, skin ulcers, alopecia, confusion, apathy, depression, loss of taste
Fluoride	1.5–4 mg	Not recognized
Selenium	70 (55) μg	Muscle weakness, symptoms of cardiac failure
Molybdenum	75–250 μg[c]	Neurologic abnormalities, hypermethioninemia, hypouricemia, hyperuricosuria
Fatty acids		
Linoleic acid	2–4% of daily calories	Dry scaling dermatitis, coarse hair, alopecia, diarrhea
Linolenic acid	0.5% of daily calories	Numbness, paresthesias, weakness, blurred vision

Key: R.E. = retinol equivalents = 1 μg retinol; TPN = total parenteral nutrition.
[a] Listed recommendations are a composite of the Recommended Daily Dietary Allowances (RDA) and minimal requirements when specific recommendations are not available. Some values vary with sex, body size, activity, and caloric requirements. The values given refer to average adults (aged 25–50). Larger doses are needed for replacement of identified deficiencies. Values in parentheses represent the RDA for women when it differs.
[b] Other trace minerals (cobalt, cadmium, arsenic, silicon, vanadium, nickel) have been identified as necessary for normal laboratory animal nutrition, but their roles in human nutrition remain unknown.
[c] Recommended intravenous dosage. Recommended daily oral intake is unknown, and the essentiality of this nutrient is still debated.
[d] As cholecalciferol, 5 μg = 200 IU of vitamin D.

Table 2-2. Estimated adult energy requirements related to degree of metabolic stress

Degree of metabolic stress	Disease examples	Estimated daily requirement	
		Energy (kcal/kg)	Protein (g/kg)
Mild	Elective hospitalization, mild infection	25	0.6–0.8
Moderate	Fracture, severe infection, hyperthyroidism	35	0.8–1.0
Severe	Severe burn, combined stresses	45	1.0–1.5

Table 2-3. Screening assessment of protein-calorie nutritional status

Measurement	Result suggestive of significant malnutrition
Weight status in adults	
Weight loss (%) in past 1 mo	$\geq$5%
Weight loss (%) in past 6 mo	$\geq$10%
Serum albumin	$\leq$2.8 g/dl
Serum transferrin from TIBC	$\leq$150 mg/dl
Total lymphocyte count	$\leq$1200 cells/μl

Key: TIBC = total iron-binding capacity.
Source: Adapted from D.H. Alpers, R.E. Clouse, and W.F. Stenson. *Manual of Nutritional Therapeutics* (2nd ed.). Boston: Little, Brown, 1988. P. 176.

serve a structural or functional role. Consequently, negative protein balance is detrimental in a short period of time. Protein requirements are often stated in terms of nitrogen requirement. The two figures can be interconverted by multiplying the nitrogen requirement (in grams) by 6.25, a factor that approximates the nitrogen weight in average dietary proteins.

1. An **estimate** of the protein requirement for the average healthy adult without excessive losses is 0.75 g/kg body weight.
2. **Increased requirements** occur with excessive losses from the gastrointestinal tract (diarrhea, nasogastric suction, exudation), skin (exfoliative diseases, burns), and draining wounds. Some of these can be measured. **Illness**, in general, increases protein requirements. The increase can be estimated by categorizing the degree of metabolic stress (see Table 2-2).
3. **Positive energy balance** is required for delivered protein substrates to be most effectively utilized for new protein synthesis. See Table 2-2 for energy requirements associated with metabolic stress.

IV. **Nutritional assessments**
   A. **Micronutrients.** Commonly assessed micronutrients include major minerals (Na, K, Ca, P, Mg), iron, zinc, vitamin B_{12}, and folacin (folic acid). Laboratory assessment of other micronutrients is possible. (See D. H. Alpers, R. E. Clouse, and W. F. Stenson. *Manual of Nutritional Therapeutics* (2nd ed.). Boston: Little, Brown, 1988, for interpretation of the tests.) With the exception of iron, plasma levels of minerals do not necessarily correlate with body stores. Thus, the diagnosis of mineral deficiency requires recognition of the corresponding signs and symptoms (see Table 2-1).
   B. **Macronutrients. Protein-calorie assessment** focuses on energy stores (fat) and protein (visceral and skeletal tissue) adequacy. Fat stores (triceps skinfold thickness, body weight in comparison to usual or ideal), skeletal muscle proteins (midarm muscle circumference, creatinine excretion for height), and other proteins or protein-related functions (albumin, transferrin, tests of immune competency) are used to evaluate protein-calorie nutrition. Assessment can help determine if intensive nutritional support should be initiated. Occasionally, elective surgery may be postponed due to protein-calorie malnutrition. See Table 2-3 for screening of nutritional status. Equivocal results on the screening assessment may indicate the need for more comprehensive assessment.

Specialized Nutrient Delivery

I. **Oral protein and calorie supplements**
   A. **Indications.** Because of the variety of supplements available and the specialized characteristics of these products, oral supplements are useful in many circumstances.

1. **As nutritionally balanced dietary supplements** for patients with negative balance (e.g., from anorexia) or increased requirements (e.g., athletes).
2. **To enhance the nutritive value of restricted diets** (e.g., modified consistency diets, including clear liquid, mechanically soft, and very low residue diets).

B. **Commercial products** are available that supplement daily intake with protein, calories, or both. Nutritional features of several of the many available products are listed in Tables 2-4 and 2-5. The supplement that best fits the needs of the patient should be selected.

1. **Features of commercial supplements** that should be considered in selection include the following:
   a. **Lactose content.** Most supplements today are lactose free to avoid inadvertent complications in the lactose-intolerant patient.
   b. **Fat content** varies considerably. Supplements with higher calorie content usually contain more fat. Fat also lowers overall product osmolality. Fat restriction is unnecessary for most patients.
   c. **Osmolality** is lowest in products with fat and complex carbohydrates as calorie sources. Higher osmolality may be associated with more gastrointestinal side effects if large amounts of the supplement are used.
   d. **Residue.** Products that do not utilize blenderized foods are low in vegetable fiber and consequently have low residue compared with the normal balanced diet. Lowest-residue supplements do not contain complete proteins (to further enhance absorption) and are also low in fat. High-fiber supplements (e.g., Jevity, Enrich) are available for patients in whom high-residue diets are more desirable (e.g., patients with irritable bowel syndrome).
   e. **A nutritionally complete** supplement includes micronutrients (vitamins and minerals) as well as protein and calorie sources. The RDA for all nutrients is contained in 1500–2000 ml of the product.

2. **Medium-chain triglyceride oil** (MCT oil) contains triglycerides with 8–10 carbon fatty acid residues that can be absorbed without pancreatic hydrolysis or bile salts. Patients with pancreatic insufficiency or fat malabsorption from cholestasis may benefit from the additional calories provided by this supplement. The **caloric value** of this oil is approximately 8.3 kcal/g (yielding 115 kcal/tbs). Typically, only 3 to 4 tablespoons are tolerated per day, limiting the daily caloric maximum to about 400 kcal.

3. **Supplements with modified amino acid profiles** are available for patients with hepatic or renal failure.
   a. **Liver failure** formulas (e.g., Hepatic-Aid, Travasorb Hepatic) favor branched-chain amino acids over aromatic amino acids. These modifications improve subjective and objective indicators of encephalopathy but probably do not alter outcome of the liver disease. Supplements vary in content of other nutrients; nutritional information labels or inserts should be read if the product is being used as a major nutrient source for any patient. The usual prescribed amount is 2–4 prepared packages daily.
   b. **Renal failure** supplements (Amin-Aid, Travasorb Renal) have increased amounts of essential amino acids with a relatively low total protein content (high calorie-protein ratio) and restricted electrolyte content. Addition of an essential amino acid supplement to a protein-restricted diet can prolong the period of conservative treatment in patients with chronic renal failure (*Am. J. Clin. Nutr.* 33:1654, 1980). The usual prescribed amount is 2–3 prepared packages daily.

C. **Complications** from oral protein-calorie supplementation are uncommon.

II. **Enteral feeding** (tube feeding). This form of intensive nutritional therapy is preferred over parenteral feeding unless bowel rest is indicated. Use of the intestinal tract is attended by less serious side effects and allows for intestinal regulation of absorption.

A. **Commercial products.** Nutritionally complete products listed in Table 2-4 are suitable as complete diets for forced enteral feeding. Many other products are

Table 2-4. Nutritional characteristics of representative lactose-free protein-calorie supplements

Product	Description	kcal/dl	mOsm/kgH$_2$O	Protein (g/dl)	Volume (ml) to meet U.S. RDA of vitamins and minerals
Standard					
Ensure	Low residue, flavored	106	470	3.7	1887
Isocal	Isotonic, low residue	106	270	3.4	2000
Osmolite	Isotonic, low residue	106	300	3.7	1887
Osmolite HN	Isotonic, low residue	106	300	4.4	1321
Precision* LR (powder)	Low residue	110	510	2.6	1710
Sustacal	Low residue	100	650	6.1	1080
Enrich	High dietary fiber	110	480	4.0	1391
Jevity	Isotonic, high dietary fiber	106	310	4.4	1321
Volume-restricted					
Ensure Plus	Low residue, flavored	150	690	5.5	1420
Magnacal	Low residue, flavored	200	590	7.0	1000
Specialty Formulas					
Pulmocare (volume-restricted)	Low residue, higher fat content, flavored	150	490	6.3	947
Vital HN	Elemental, partially hydrolyzed protein, low fat, low residue, flavored	100	500	4.2	1500
Isotein HN	Isotonic, low residue, high nitrogen content, flavored	120	300	6.8	1770
Travasorb Hepatic	Low residue, high branched-chain amino acids	110	600	2.9	2000
Travasorb* Renal (powder)	Low residue, electrolyte free, no fat-soluble vitamins	135	590	2.3	2100

* Values for powders assume the product is used at full strength.

Table 2-5. Representative modules for enteral formulas

Product	Description	kcal/ml or kcal/g	Protein (g/dl or g/100 g)
Polycose liquid	Carbohydrate supplement	2.0	—
Casec powder	Protein supplement	3.7	88
ProMod	Protein supplement, powder	4.2	75
Propac	Protein supplement, powder	4.0	75
Microlipid	Fat supplement, liquid	4.5	—
MCT oil	Medium-chain triglyceride fat supplement, liquid	7.7–8.3	—

available. Blenderized foods are not recommended for use in very small caliber tubes (e.g., <8F) because of the likelihood of tube clogging.

1. **Additional vitamins and minerals** may be necessary for patients with identified micronutrient deficiencies. Nutritionally complete products in general provide only the RDA of individual nutrients.

2. **Elemental diets** (e.g., Vivonex) contain hydrolyzed protein or amino acids as protein sources and little fat. Because of this, the osmolality of the formulas is higher and the oral palatability is poor. Although these "predigested" formulas have been promoted for use in various gastrointestinal disorders, evidence that they are superior to other nutritionally complete formulas is lacking.

3. **Specialized formulas for organ failure** include those with modified amino acid profiles for liver and kidney failure (see sec. **I.B.3**) and those with proportionately higher fat content for respiratory failure (e.g., Pulmocare); the ratio of CO_2 production to O_2 consumption is lower for these formulas compared with predominantly carbohydrate calorie sources.

B. **Tube placement.** Appropriate position of the feeding tube should be documented radiographically before feeding is initiated, especially for obtunded patients.

1. **Nasoduodenal tube placement** may require the use of a stylet that is provided by the manufacturer. Care must be taken to avoid allowing the stiffener to penetrate the side holes at the distal end of the tube. Fluoroscopic guidance is recommended if any device is being used to advance the tube through the pylorus or if a stiffener is being used in an obtunded patient. Metoclopramide, 10 mg IM or IV, may induce sufficient gastric motor activity to advance the tube into the duodenum within minutes if the patient is in the right lateral decubitus position. Endoscopic guidance is occasionally necessary. The tube should pass spontaneously within several hours of placement if feeding is not initiated.

2. **Gastrostomy and jejunostomy** feeding tubes. Percutaneous placement techniques for these tubes using endoscopic or radiographic guidance have expanded and simplified tube feeding possibilities when nasogastric or nasoduodenal placement fails or is impractical (*Surg. Annu.* 18:327, 1986; *A.J.R.* 141:793, 1983).

C. **Techniques of enteral feeding** vary with the type of tube utilized. Large-bore tubes, such as standard gastrostomy tubes, will readily allow bolus feeding (gavage feeding). This type of feeding is recommended only when the tube is in the stomach, since rapid distention of the small intestine is poorly tolerated.

Continuous feeding is utilized for small-intestinal tubes (e.g., nasoduodenal or jejunostomy tubes).

1. **Bolus feeding.** Elevate the head of the bed during the feeding and for at least 2 hours after completion. Aspirate from the tube to check for retained food from a prior feeding. Delay the feeding by at least 1 hour if more than 100 ml of residual food is present. Give 50–100 ml of an isotonic or slightly hypotonic diet every 3 hours to start a feeding schedule. (Low-osmolality formulas listed in Table 2-4 may not need initial dilution.) Increase the amount in 50-ml steps to a maximum of 250–300 ml every 3–4 hours. Increase the concentration to full strength and adjust the final schedule to meet the patient's daily requirements.

2. **Continuous infusion** is used for tubes with feeding ports in the small intestine. A feeding pump is useful to maintain a constant infusion rate.

   a. **Start-up regimen.** Initiate feeding with an appropriate formula diluted to one-half or one-quarter strength with water at a rate of 25–50 ml/hr. (Low-osmolality formulas listed in Table 2-4 may not need initial dilution.) Increase the rate by 25–50 ml/hr at 24-hour intervals as tolerated until a final rate that meets the patient's needs is reached. Increase the formula concentration at any point to test patient tolerance. Some patients may need the additional water provided by the dilute solutions to prevent the hyperosmolarity syndrome (see sec. II.D.3).

   b. **No start-up regimen.** Stepwise advancement of the feeding regimen is frequently unnecessary and may delay achievement of positive nitrogen balance in some patients (*J.P.E.N. J. Parenter. Eternal Nutr.* 10:258, 1986). Individualize the initiation steps for each patient.

D. **Metabolic complications** of enteral feeding may result from using commercially available products with fixed nutrient content.

   1. **Electrolyte disturbances** are detected by periodic monitoring of serum electrolytes, calcium, phosphorus, and magnesium. If deficiencies are detected, supplementation with electrolytes is appropriate. **Trace mineral deficiencies** (e.g., selenium, zinc) have also occurred from long-term use of defined formulas.

   2. **Volume overload** may result from excessive sodium delivery in the feeding formula. A sodium-restricted formula or a concentrated calorie formula may be appropriate depending on the perceived cause of fluid overload. (See D. H. Alpers, R. E. Clouse, and W. F. Stenson. *Manual of Nutritional Therapeutics* (2nd ed.). Boston: Little, Brown, 1988, for a comprehensive list of formulas and their contents.)

   3. **The hyperosmolarity syndrome** (lethargy, obtundation, dehydration, fever) may result from enteral feeding. Laboratory tests reveal hypernatremia and hyperosmolarity. Treatment involves increasing daily free water (supplement or dilute formula) or temporarily providing 5% dextrose in water (D/W) intravenously while adjusting the formula.

E. **Nonmetabolic complications**

   1. **Diarrhea and intestinal discomfort** are often related to feeding technique or formula. The following steps should be undertaken if diarrhea occurs during enteral feeding:

      a. **Review the feeding schedule** to determine whether advancement has occurred too rapidly and consider use of a start-up regimen (see sec. II.C.2.a).

      b. **Check the formula** for characteristics that might not be tolerated by the patient (e.g., lactose, high fat, high osmolality).

      c. **Review medications** to determine whether a diarrhea-causing agent has been added. Concomitant antibiotic use appears to be strongly associated with diarrhea from tube-feeding formulas (*Br. Med. J.* 288:678, 1984).

      d. **Evaluate for usual causes of acute diarrhea** if diarrhea occurs during a stable regimen of enteral feeding.

      e. **Treat diarrhea** from enteral feeding by reducing formula strength or infusion as a first step. A change to another formula may be useful, even if specific nutrient offenders are not identified. Judicious use of antidiar-

Table 2-6. Caloric value and osmolarity of parenteral nutrition fluids

Parenteral fluid	Caloric value (kcal/dl)	Osmolarity (mOsm/liter)
Dextrose solutions (%)		
5	17	250
10	34	500
20	68	1000
50	170	2500
70	237	3500
Lipid emulsions (%)		
10	110	280
20	200	330–340

rheal agents should be a last resort (codeine sulfate, 30 mg q6h, or deodorized tincture of opium, 6–10 drops q6–12h).

2. **Gastric retention.** Mechanical obstruction and motility disturbances are possible causes. Common examples include duodenal ulcer, pyloric channel ulcer, ileus, anticholinergic medications, opiates, CNS disturbances, metabolic derangements, and severe protein deficiency. Treatment must be directed at the cause; use of a small intestine feeding tube (nasoduodenal or jejunostomy) may overcome the problem.

3. **Tracheobronchial aspiration.** The likelihood of aspiration is reduced by maintaining a 30-degree elevation of the head of the bed at all times for patients on continuous infusion schedules and for at least 2 hours after a feeding for patients receiving bolus feedings. Duodenogastric reflux is also less likely if feeding ports are located beyond the ligament of Treitz but may still occur, even with jejunostomy feeding. Aspiration of enteral feedings may be detected by examining pulmonary secretions with glucose-measurement strips.

4. **Esophagitis** may result from nasogastric or nasoduodenal tubes. Treatment is directed at reducing reflux potential (reduce size of bolus feedings; tilt the entire bed, as for any refluxing patient) and neutralizing acid (cimetidine, 300 mg PO qid; ranitidine, 150 mg PO bid; or famotidine, 40 mg PO qd; omeprazole, 20–40 mg PO qd may be effective for refractory cases). Resolution of esophagitis may be difficult with the tube left in place.

5. **Tube clogging** may be prevented by using highly dispersed commercial products in the small-caliber tubes. All medications should be provided in liquid form, and the use of crushed tablets should be avoided when possible. Aluminum-containing antacids may interact with some nutritional formulas to produce plugs. Once a clog occurs, it may not be possible to dislodge it. Perforation and transection of tubes may occur if excessive injection pressure is applied. A stylet may perforate the tube and cause gastrointestinal damage. Full-strength cranberry juice or papain solution (meat tenderizer in water) has been gently instilled with some success in restoring tube patency.

III. **Parenteral supplements of protein and calories** are utilized in many hospitalized patients to reduce the degree of negative nitrogen (protein) balance. Parenteral supplements can be used in combination with oral nutrition to further improve daily intake.

A. **Nutritional values of parenteral solutions**

1. **Dextrose** in parenteral solutions provides 3.4 kcal/g. This is reduced from the 4 kcal/g provided by carbohydrate because parenteral dextrose is weighed as the monohydrate. Thus, 1000 ml of 5% dextrose provides only 170 kcal (Table 2-6).

2. **Lipid emulsions** are calorie sources derived from soybean oil (e.g., Intralipid, Soyacal) or soybean and safflower oils (e.g., Liposyn II). The emulsions are available in 10% or 20% concentrations and provide 1.1 or 2.0 kcal/ml,

respectively (see Table 2-6). These products can also be used to provide essential fatty acids (see sec. **IV.B.4**) and up to 65% of the total daily calories (≤2.5 g/kg maximum).

  a. Administration of the lipid emulsion can be accomplished by running the emulsion in parallel with dextrose-electrolyte solutions. The emulsion should be piggy-backed to the base solution as close to the venous access site as possible. Therapy is begun with a **test dose** of 1 ml/minute for 15 minutes at the initiation of the first bottle, and the patient is observed for adverse effects (see sec. **III.A.2.d**). A **maximum** of 5 ml/kg (10% emulsion) should be delivered on the first day; satisfactory **lipid clearance** should then be determined by (1) drawing a citrated sample on the morning following the first day's infusion (>6 hours after termination), (2) examining the serum for opalescence, and (3) sending the specimen for triglyceride determination. Triglyceride levels should normalize within several hours of termination of the infusion. Lipid clearance must be documented between intermittent lipid infusions at the start of therapy; continuous lipid infusion should not be used if lipid clearance is abnormal. Methods of providing lipid emulsion intermixed with dextrose–amino acid solutions (**3-in-1 solutions**) are also now available for patients receiving stable courses of parenteral nutrition (see sec. **IV.E**).

  b. Advantages of lipid emulsions as calorie sources are (1) concentration of calories in a small volume, (2) reduction of overall infusate osmolarity (and likelihood of thrombophlebitis) if co-infused with hyperosmolar dextrose-electrolyte solutions, (3) lesser CO_2 production compared with equicaloric quantities of dextrose, and (4) reduced blood glucose levels in diabetic patients compared with infusion of equicaloric quantities of glucose alone.

  c. Disadvantages of lipid emulsions include (1) more cumbersome setup and (2) additional side effects and complications not seen with dextrose alone.

  d. Complications of lipid emulsions

    (1) Early or immediate reactions occur in fewer than 1% of patients and include dyspnea, cyanosis, cutaneous allergic phenomena, nausea, vomiting, headache, back pain, flushing, sweating, fever, dizziness, and local inflammation at the infusion site. Hypercoagulability and thrombocytopenia have been reported.

    (2) Delayed adverse reactions include hepatomegaly, jaundice (with centrilobular cholestasis), splenomegaly, thrombocytopenia, leukopenia, and mild elevations in liver enzymes. Decreased pulmonary diffusing capacity has been observed in some patients.

3. Amino acid solutions contain crystalline amino acid profiles that estimate human needs. Although proteins and amino acids have caloric value (4 kcal/g), they are not routinely used in calculating the daily energy provision. This omission is based on the assumption that delivered amino acids will be used for new protein synthesis if other calorie sources are provided in quantities sufficient to meet the daily requirement.

  a. Standard amino acid solutions contain essential and some nonessential amino acids in total concentrations ranging from 3–15% depending on the product.

  b. Modified amino acid formulas for renal failure (Aminess 5.2%, NephrAmine II 5.4%, Aminosyn RF 5.2%, RenAmin 6.5%) and for hepatic failure or marked metabolic stress (HepatAmine 8%, Aminosyn HBC 7%, FreAmine HBC 6.9%) favor essential or branched-chain amino acids, respectively. The rationale for their use in organ failure is similar to that for oral supplements with similar modifications (see sec. **I.B.3**). **Branched-chain amino acids** are directly metabolized by skeletal muscle and can act as an energy source in the presence of metabolic stress. These amino acids also have a regulatory role in protein catabolism and may, by reducing catabolism, improve nitrogen balance during stress.

B. **Prevention of thrombophlebitis**
   1. **Osmolarity should be maintained as low as possible.** Phlebitis is very likely when infusate osmolarity reaches 800–900 mOsm/liter. All additives increase osmolarity (e.g., 40 mEq Na as NaCl will add 80 mOsm).
   2. **A lipid emulsion (isotonic) can be co-infused** with the dextrose–amino acid base solution.
   3. **The IV site should be changed regularly** (e.g., every 3 days).
   4. The addition of small amounts of **heparin** (1000–3000 units/liter) or **hydrocortisone** (50–100 mg/liter) to the base solution may be helpful in some cases.
C. **Addition of usual daily electrolytes** (major minerals: Na, K, Cl) to the base solution is necessary if this is the only IV fluid the patient is receiving. Commercially available amino acid solutions often contain modest amounts of these electrolytes, but the final concentrations will be reduced if the solution is mixed with dextrose in water. The exact formulation of the product used should be confirmed with the supplier, or the final desired concentrations of individual electrolytes can be designated on the order sheet.

IV. **Total parenteral nutrition (TPN)**
   A. **Indications.** Providing all nutrients by parenteral means will maintain nutrient balance, restore depleted nutrients, and allow bowel rest.
      1. **TPN for nutritional repletion** is usually reserved for patients with severe protein and calorie depletion or in whom the course of illness predicts the development of severe depletion. Consultation with a nutritionist is recommended to help in the selection of patients with this indication for TPN.
      2. **Bowel rest** will help in the management of a variety of gastrointestinal disorders. If severe malnutrition is present or if the course of bowel rest is expected to exceed 5–7 days, nutritional support with TPN is recommended.
         a. **Crohn's disease** of the small intestine will undergo in-hospital symptomatic remission in the majority of patients treated with bowel rest and TPN. Remission rates of 80% can be expected (60% long term) in patients without intestinal fistulas. A 30–40% likelihood of fistula closure can be expected, and many fistulas remain healed in follow-up (*Med. Clin. North Am.* 62:185, 1978).
         b. **Inflammatory colitis** (ulcerative colitis and Crohn's colitis) is less responsive to this approach. A randomized, controlled trial suggested that bowel rest with TPN had no advantage over oral feedings in ultimately preventing colectomy (*Gastroenterology* 79:1199, 1980). However, the technique is still utilized for patient comfort (reducing stool) and to prevent nutritional deterioration while observing the response to corticosteroids.
         c. **Short-bowel syndrome.** Bowel rest with TPN is usually required following intestinal resection. Small enteral feedings should be initiated as soon as possible to promote intestinal adaptation to resection.
         d. **Severe pancreatitis.** TPN should prevent nutritional deterioration while bowel rest will prevent intestinal symptoms (e.g., from ileus or obstruction). There are no data to indicate that this approach actually alters the course of the pancreatitis.
   B. **Parenteral nutrient requirements** vary from the RDAs, because RDAs take into account the inefficiency of intestinal absorption and variability of nutrient availability in foods. Exact parenteral requirements for many nutrients are not known. Ranges of usual nutrient requirements and recommended parenteral micronutrient provisions are listed in Table 2-7. Larger provisions are necessary for nutrient deficiencies.
      1. **Usual starting ranges** for major minerals are: Na, 60–80 mEq/d; K, 30–60 mEq/d; Cl, 80–100 mEq/d; Ca, 4.6–9.2 mEq/d; Mg, 8.1–20 mEq/d; and PO_4, 12–24 mmol/d. Acetate is used by the pharmacy to balance the cations in solution. In patients with normal electrolytes, chloride should comprise two thirds of the sum of Na + K. Too little chloride may result in excessive acetate and a metabolic alkalosis.
      2. **Nutrients with small fractional losses and requirements** (e.g., linolenic acid,

Table 2-7. Guidelines for parenteral nutrient delivery for adults[a]

Nutrient	Daily parenteral supplement	Nutrient	Daily parenteral supplement
Water (ml/kg)	30 (1 ml/kcal)	Vitamins[c]	
Calories[b]	25–45 kcal/kg	A	800–1000 R.E.
Protein	0.6–1.5 g/kg	D	200 IU
Linoleic acid	4% of calories	E	10 IU
Linolenic acid	0.5% of calories	C	100 mg
		Thiamine (B_1)	3 mg
Major minerals		Riboflavin (B_2)	3.6 mg
Na	50–250 mEq	Pantothenic acid	15 mg
K	30–200 mEq	Niacin	40 mg
Cl	50–250 mEq	Pyridoxine (B_6)	4 mg
Ca	10–20 mEq	Biotin	60 μg
Mg	10–30 mEq	Folacin	400 μg
P	10–40 mmol	Cobalamin (B_{12})	5 μg
Other minerals			
Zn	2–8 mg		
Cu	0.3–1.5 mg		
Cr	10–15 μg		
Mn	0.15–0.8 mg		
Fe	50 mg/month		
I	50–75 μg		
Se	40–120 μg		
Molybdenum	20 μg		

Key: R.E. = retinol equivalent = 1 μg retinol.

[a] Estimates are based on the RDA for these nutrients and attempt to account for differences in bioavailability between oral and parenteral routes.

[b] Calories may be provided by dextrose alone or by dextrose-lipid combinations (see Specialized Nutrient Delivery, sec. **III.A**).

[c] Source of data: American Medical Association/Nutrition Advisory Group Guidelines (*J.P.E.N. J. Parenter. Enteral Nutr.* 3:258, 1979). Vitamin K supplementation is not included in these guidelines since some patients are receiving anticoagulants. The amount of vitamin D recommended by this group may be too much for long-term TPN therapy (see Specialized Nutrient Delivery, sec. **IV.H.1.k**).

  selenium, iodine) may not need to be delivered in all cases of TPN because of the rarity of the corresponding deficiency states.

3. **Nutrient values of parenteral protein and calorie solutions** have been described in sec. **III.A**.

4. **Essential fatty acid deficiency** can be prevented by providing 4–5% of the caloric provision as linoleic acid. This requirement can usually be met with 1000 ml of 10% lipid emulsion per week or 3–5 oz. of corn or safflower oil per week by mouth (for patients who can tolerate small amounts of oral liquid). **Linolenic acid** deficiency may occur during a long course of TPN but will also be prevented by lipid emulsion (soybean oil) supplementation.

C. **Example formulas.** The TPN prescription will include the following components: water, calories (dextrose, lipid), protein (amino acids), vitamins, major minerals, other minerals, and essential fatty acids.

1. **Examples of dextrose–amino acid combinations** for use in TPN are provided in Table 2-8. These examples include major minerals. Trace minerals, vitamins, and essential fatty acids must also be provided. Many modifications of these formulas will still provide adequate nutritional support.

2. **Lipid emulsions** can be co-infused with the dextrose–amino acid solution to increase daily nonprotein calories (see sec. **III.A.2**).

Table 2-8. Sample formulation of standardized central-vein TPN base solutions for the average patient and for patients requiring base solution modification

Additives	Standard solution: From additives	Standard solution: Provided by amino acid solution[a]	Standard solution: Final content	Heart failure solution (low volume–low Na⁺): From additives	Heart failure: Provided by amino acid solution[a]	Heart failure: Final content	Low K⁺–low Na⁺ solution: From additives	Low K⁺–low Na⁺: Provided by amino acid solution[a]	Low K⁺–low Na⁺: Final content	Renal failure solution: From additives	Renal failure: Provided by amino acid solution[a]	Renal failure: Final content
Crystalline amino acids 8.5%	500 ml		4.25%	300 ml		3.18%	500 ml		4.25%			
Dextrose 50%	500 ml		25%				500 ml		25%			
Dextrose 70%				500 ml		44%				300 ml		26%
Sodium (mEq)	35	5	40		3	3		5	5[b]	[c]	3	3
Potassium (mEq)	40		40	40		40	9		9	[c]		
Chloride (mEq)	35		35			0			0	[c]		
Calcium[d] (mEq)	4.6		4.6	4.6		4.6	4.6		4.6	[c]		
Phosphorus[e] (mmol)	7	5	12	7	3	10	6	5	11	[c]		
Magnesium[f] (mEq)	8.1		8.1	8.1		8.1	8.1		8.1	[c]		
Sulfate[g] (mEq)	8.1		8.1	8.1		8.1	8.1		8.1	[c]		
Gluconate[g] (mEq)	4.6		4.6	4.6		4.6	4.6		4.6	[c]		
Acetate[g] (mEq)	30	37	67	30	22.2	52.2		37	37		22	22
Approx. total vol.			1050 ml			830 ml			1015 ml			800 ml
Amino acids (g)			42.5			25.4			42.5			25.5
Nitrogen (g)			6.5			3.9			6.5			3.2
Nonprotein calories (kcal)[h]			850			1190			850			714
Caloric concentration (kcal/ml)			0.81			1.4			0.84			0.89

[a] Based on electrolyte content of FreAmine III 8.5%.
[b] Additional sodium can be added as NaCl.
[c] Additional only as indicated by serum levels.
[d] Added as calcium gluconate, 0.46 mEq/ml.
[e] Added as potassium phosphate: K^+, 4.4 mEq/ml; phosphorus, 3 mmol/ml.
[f] Added as magnesium sulfate, 4.06 mEq/ml.
[g] Not ordered by the physician; these anions balance the ordered cations.
[h] Dextrose monohydrate provides 3.4 kcal/g.

Source: Adapted from D. H. Alpers, R. E. Clouse, and W. F. Stenson. *Manual of Nutritional Therapeutics* (2nd ed.). Boston: Little, Brown, 1988. P. 252.

3. **Major minerals** should be provided in the range of daily requirements described in Table 2-7. Potassium requirements may be greatest early in the course of TPN.

4. **Trace minerals** should be added to one TPN bottle daily. Commercially available combinations are available that contain zinc (0.8–4 mg/ml), copper (0.2–1 mg/ml), manganese (0.1–0.5 mg/ml), and chromium (2–10 μg/ml). One milliliter per day of a combination solution is satisfactory for most patients. Additional zinc (5–15 mg/day) is recommended if large intestinal fluid losses are occurring. Iodine (1.0 μg/kg/day), selenium (40 μg/day as selenious acid), and molybdenum (20 μg/day) are usually provided only for patients receiving very long courses of TPN.

5. **Iron** requirements can be met by monthly parenteral administration (IM or IV) of 1 ml iron dextran (Imferon; 50 mg elemental iron). Iron dextran (up to 2 ml) can be added to the base solution. Iron may not be added to 3-in-1 admixtures (see sec. **IV.E**). Iron deficiency requires more frequent doses.

6. **Vitamins** are provided by adding a multivitamin preparation to the dextrose–amino acid base solution.
   a. **Multivitamin preparations.** One vial (10 ml) per day of a fat- and water-soluble vitamin combination (e.g., MVI-12) provides recognized vitamins (except vitamin K) in the recommended parenteral maintenance dosages.
   b. **Cobalamin (B_{12}).** Most multivitamin combinations also contain 5 μg of cobalamin (B_{12}). However, if cobalamin (B_{12}) is not included, 200–500 μg/month IM should be provided.
   c. **Additional vitamins** should be given for identified deficiencies.
   d. **Vitamin K**, 5–10 mg/week SQ or IV, must be given separately.

7. **Essential fatty acids** are provided by administration of at least 1000 ml of 10% lipid emulsion per week (see sec. **IV.B.4**).

8. **Regular insulin** added directly to the TPN solution is the preferred method for **reducing hyperglycemia.** The initial dose is 5–10 units regular insulin per liter of 25% dextrose. The dose is then adjusted based on serum glucose levels.

9. **H_2 antagonists.** Ranitidine (150 mg/day) or famotidine (20–40 mg/day) can be added if indicated. Cimetidine is not approved for use in 3-in-1 solutions, but 300 mg/day can be added to conventional TPN base solutions if needed.

D. **Initiation of TPN.** Solutions are usually administered through a central vein, since overall solution osmolarity exceeds the tolerance of peripheral veins (see sec. **III.B.1**). Co-infusion of a base solution that contains all additives with a lipid emulsion will reduce osmolarity such that total nutritional support can be accomplished via a peripheral vein. The examples given in the remainder of this chapter refer to TPN via central vein, where more concentrated solutions may be delivered. The following practices should be observed when TPN is initiated.

1. **A central venous catheter** should be used, with position in the superior vena cava verified by chest radiograph before initiation of TPN. Sterile or strict aseptic technique should be employed.

2. **Occlusive dressings** should be applied to the catheter site and changed every 48 hours.

3. **The TPN port** should not be used to obtain blood. Infusion of blood products or medications into the TPN port should be avoided if possible.

4. **Multiple-lumen catheters.** Whenever possible, single-lumen catheters should be used. The distal port of triple-lumen catheters is acceptable for short-term TPN.

5. **TPN infusion tubing** should be changed every 24 hours. The use of stopcocks should be discouraged.

6. Infuse no more than 1000 ml amino acid–dextrose base solution **in the first 24 hours** using a controlled infusion pump, and increase the daily total by up to 1000 ml/day until the desired daily infusion is reached.

7. **Monitor carefully for hyperglycemia** in the first few days.

8. If continuously infused TPN fluid (base solution) is temporarily interrupted or accidentally discontinued, begin a peripheral intravenous line with 10% dex-

trose in water to prevent hypoglycemia. Blood glucose should be monitored.

E. **3-in-1 admixtures** combine lipids, amino acids, dextrose, and other additives in a single daily bag. Advantages of 3-in-1 admixtures include decreased risk of contamination of the central catheter, increased stability of light-sensitive nutrients, improved lipid clearance, and decreased preparation time and cost. Standard formulations of 3-in-1 admixtures are recommended because the stability of the system may be adversely affected by additives (see Appendix H). Vitamins and minerals should be added as needed.

1. **The total daily solution** can be mixed in a single 3-liter bag.

2. **Initiate** TPN with one half to one third the total daily caloric requirement.

3. **Albumin and iron** should not be added directly to 3-in-1 admixtures.

4. **Additives.** Some other additives that are stable in standard TPN solutions may not be stable in 3-in-1 solutions.

F. **Cyclic TPN.** Patients receiving long, stable courses of TPN or those who are preparing to go home on TPN may benefit from cyclic infusion of parenteral feeding solutions. 3-in-1 solutions are ideal for cyclic TPN. A volumetric pump should be used. The stable patient can be converted to a 12-hour schedule by gradually increasing the rate and decreasing the total time of infusion of 2000 ml solution as follows:

1. Initially, taper the continuous infusion in the morning by reducing the rate to one half of the original rate for 1 hour. Further reduce the rate by one half for an additional hour, and then discontinue the infusion.

2. Observe for **hypoglycemia**. This is unlikely if the patient was not receiving insulin by injection. Glucose levels should be monitored every 30 minutes for several hours for the first few days of cyclic TPN.

3. Reinstitute TPN later in the afternoon by reversing the above steps.

4. Each day, increase the final rate of infusion so that the patient receives the entire 2000 ml in a total of 12 hours. Tapering at the beginning and end of the cycle can be reduced to 1 hour each (30 minutes for each step) within several days of conversion. A final rate of 185 ml/hour for 10 hours with 1 hour of tapering at each end will correctly utilize the 2000 ml. Conversion to cyclic TPN can be accomplished in 3–4 days.

5. Monitoring for **hyperglycemia** during the period of rapid infusion is necessary for the first few days. Patients with poorly controlled blood sugars on continuous TPN are not good candidates for cyclic therapy.

G. **Monitoring during stable TPN**

1. Monitor vital signs (including temperature) 4 times daily, weight daily, and intake and output daily.

2. Check urine for glucose (dipsticks) or blood glucose (fingersticks) 4 times daily in patients with hyperglycemia.

3. Measure electrolytes, BUN, and blood glucose daily for the first week, then twice weekly. Patients with an unstable metabolic status may require more frequent blood determinations.

4. Monitor serum calcium, magnesium, and phosphorus weekly once levels stabilize.

5. Obtain liver enzymes and serum bilirubin weekly.

6. Follow blood counts, serum albumin, prothrombin time, and other desired indicators of nutritional adequacy periodically during the course of TPN.

7. Review requirements for macronutrients and consult appropriate support services (see sec. **V**) to ensure the adequacy of the nutrition regimen.

H. **Complications of TPN**

1. **Metabolic complications**

a. **Hyperglycemia and hyperosmolarity** are more likely to occur in the first few days of therapy. They may also indicate the development of catheter-related sepsis. Hyperglycemia can be treated with regular insulin, 5–10 units per liter of 25% dextrose.

b. **Hypoglycemia** is possible if TPN is discontinued abruptly, especially if insulin is being given. This is treated with IV 10% D/W. When hypoglycemia occurs during tapering of TPN, the infusion rate may be temporarily increased. Gradual discontinuation of continuous-infusion TPN over 48 hours prevents this complication.

c. **Electrolyte abnormalities** should be corrected in subsequent prescriptions. Additional electrolytes may need to be given through a peripheral intravenous line if rapid correction is necessary.

d. **Elevation of BUN** commonly occurs with initiation of TPN. Increases in excess of 75 mg/dl indicate the need to modify the regimen. Free water delivery should be increased if evidence of hyperosmolar dehydration is apparent. If dehydration is not present, a reduction in the base solution rate should lower the BUN.

e. **Hypercapnia** may result from refeeding a malnourished patient who cannot adequately increase minute ventilation. Carbon dioxide production may be reduced by either decreasing the daily calorie provision or by replacing some of the daily dextrose calories with fat calories from a lipid emulsion.

f. **Vitamin deficiency.** The most common deficiency arises from omission of vitamin K, which is not contained in multivitamin preparations. Folacin and vitamin B_{12} are now present in most preparations for IV use. Identified deficiencies are **treated** initially with replacement doses followed by maintenance doses in the regular prescription.

g. **Trace mineral deficiencies.** Delayed appearance of copper, manganese, iodine, molybdenum, and selenium deficiencies may occur.

h. **Reactions to lipid emulsion** (see sec. III.A.2.d).

i. **Liver dysfunction.** Initial elevations in transaminases are common but should not persist for more than 20 days (*J.A.M.A.* 241:2398, 1979). Prolonged elevations of alkaline phosphatase (up to 2 times normal) are noted in many patients. Delayed elevations in transaminases or bilirubin suggest another cause of liver dysfunction. Hepatomegaly, at times painful, may indicate **fatty liver.** CT scan can confirm this suspicion. Treatment consists of reducing total daily calories or providing a mixture of fat and dextrose calories rather than dextrose calories alone.

j. **Gallbladder disease.** Cholelithiasis or gallbladder sludge is detected with unexpectedly high frequency in patients receiving long-term TPN. Changes in bile composition as well as decreased frequency of gallbladder contractions may be responsible. Cholecystectomy may be required in symptomatic patients. Prevention with cholecystokinin injections has been reported (*Surg. Gynecol. Obstet.* 170: 25, 1990).

k. **Metabolic bone disease.** Severe periarticular, lower-extremity, and back pain have occurred several months into TPN therapy. Altered vitamin D metabolism has been incriminated in the pathogenesis of the syndrome (*Ann. Intern. Med.* 94:638, 1981). Temporary discontinuation of TPN will improve symptoms.

2. **Nonmetabolic complications**

a. **Complications related to central catheter placement** include undesirable catheter direction, pneumothorax, arterial puncture, hematoma, thoracic duct puncture, air embolus, and others. Catheter placement should be confirmed with a chest x-ray before beginning TPN infusion.

b. **Venous thrombosis.** This complication may occur insidiously in nearly one third of patients with indwelling central catheters (*J.P.E.N. J. Parenter. Enteral Nutr.* 5:240, 1981). Clinically significant thrombosis often requires removal of the catheter and systemic heparinization. The presence and extent of thrombosis are usually easily determined by injection of radiopaque material directly into the catheter with fluoroscopic observation. Some catheters used for home TPN have been salvaged with the use of streptokinase, but this approach is generally reserved for patients with no other feasible access. A dosage of 250,000 units IV followed by 100,000 units/hour for 48 hours keeping the thrombin time at 1.5–2.5 times control is used (*J.P.E.N. J. Parenter. Enteral Nutr.* 9:55, 1985; *Arch. Intern. Med.* 140:1370, 1980). Addition of 3000 units of heparin to each liter of TPN fluid may reduce the incidence of thrombosis (*Surg. Gynecol. Obstet.* 155:238, 1982).

c. Catheter infection may be heralded by glycosuria or hyperglycemia. Treatment of bacteremia is simplified by removing the infected catheter. Prolonged ($\geq$6 weeks) antibiotic courses can sterilize catheters in patients with limited access alternatives. Injection of **urokinase** (2.5 ml of 2500 IU/ml) into thrombosed, infected central catheters has been reported to assist in sterilizing indwelling catheters (*J.P.E.N. J. Parenter. Enteral Nutr.* 4:387, 1980). Fungemia may be detected in nearly 20% of home-TPN patients with documented catheter-related systemic infection and should be particularly suspected in this group of patients receiving TPN.

V. Support services for nutritional therapy

A. Department of Food and Nutrition (or equivalent dietetics service). The knowledge of dietitians should be utilized to help assess severity of malnutrition, plan optimal nutritional therapeutic programs, assess balance of macronutrients, and monitor progress of intensive nutritional support.

B. Speech pathologists have special training in the mechanics of the oropharyngeal region and can help increase oral intake in the patient with oropharyngeal dysphagia.

C. Pharmacists who supervise the preparation of parenteral nutrition fluids can be consulted regarding electrolyte incompatibilities and acceptability of other additives.

D. Enterostomal therapists should be enlisted to assist patients in adjusting to percutaneous feeding tubes and to help with skin care problems related to feeding tubes or at catheter entry sites.

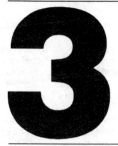

Fluid and Electrolyte Management

Michael H. O'Shea

The fluid, electrolyte, and acid–base composition of the body is tightly regulated by the integrated contributions of the pulmonary, renal, and endocrine organ systems. Cellular function is critically dependent on this stable internal milieu. The importance of this tight regulation is borne out by the myriad of effects that any one fluid or electrolyte disturbance can produce. Similarly, a variety of disease states may produce any given fluid or electrolyte disturbance. Accordingly, the proper diagnosis and therefore treatment of these disorders depends not so much on the superficial interpretation of a particular constellation of signs and symptoms (i.e., pattern recognition) but rather on an understanding of normal physiology and of the predictable response of these organ systems to a pathologic stress.

General Management of Fluids

I. **Salts and solutions**

IV solutions	Osmolality (mOsm/kg)	Glucose (g/liter)	Na (mEq/liter)	Cl (mEq/liter)
5% D/W	252	50		
10% D/W	505	100		
50% D/W	2520	500		
0.45% NaCl[a]	154	b	77	77
0.9%NaCl[a]	308	b	154	154
3% NaCl[a]	1026		513	513
Ringer's lactate[c]	272	b	130	109

[a] 1 g Na$^+$ = 43 mEq. A 4-g sodium diet is approximately equal to a 10-g NaCl diet.
[b] Also available with 5% dextrose.
[c] Also contains K (4 mEq/liter), Ca (3 mEq/liter), and lactate (28 mEq/liter).

Parenteral additives	Volume (ml/ampule)	Total (mEq/ampule)
7.5% sodium bicarbonate	50	44.6
42% sodium phosphate	15	a
15% potassium chloride	30	60
46% potassium phosphate	15	b
10% CaCl·2H$_2$O	10	13.6
10% calcium gluconate	10	4.6
50% magnesium sulfate	10	40.6
27% ammonium chloride	20	100
25% mannitol	50	12.5 (g/ampule)
50% glucose	50	25 (g/ampule)

[a] 42% sodium phosphate contains phosphate (3 mmol/liter) and sodium (4 mEq/liter).
[b] 46% potassium phosphate contains phosphate (3 mmol/liter) and potassium (4.4 mEq/liter).

II. **Maintenance therapy.** Minimum daily water and electrolyte requirements can be provided intravenously to a patient who is temporarily unable to ingest food and fluids. This assumes that normal renal function is present and does not address any preexisting water or electrolyte imbalance. When long-term maintenance is necessary, the enteral route by nasogastric tube or Dobhoff is preferred to IV fluid administration.

   A. **Minimum water requirements** for fluid balance can be estimated from the sum of the urine output necessary to excrete the daily solute load (500 ml/day) and the insensible water losses from the skin and respiratory tract (500–1000 ml/day), minus the amount of water produced from endogenous metabolism (300 ml/day). It is customary to administer 2000–3000 ml of water daily to produce a urine volume of 1000–1500 ml/day since there is no advantage to minimizing urine output. **Weighing the patient daily** is the best means of assessing net gain or loss of fluid, since the gastrointestinal, renal, and insensible fluid losses of the hospitalized patient are unpredictable.

   B. **The electrolytes** that are usually administered during maintenance fluid therapy are sodium and potassium. The kidneys are normally capable of compensating for wide variations in sodium intake; for example, in the absence of sodium intake, urinary sodium excretion can be reduced to less than 5 mEq/day. It is customary to supply 50–150 mEq of sodium daily. Some potassium supplementation is also given, due to continued obligatory renal potassium excretion. Usually, 20–60 mEq/day is given if renal function is adequate. **Carbohydrate** (100–150 g/day) is necessary to minimize protein catabolism and prevent ketosis.

   C. **An adequate maintenance IV fluid regimen** can be accomplished with the administration of 2000 ml of 0.45% NaCl with 5% dextrose and 20 mEq KCl/liter. Calcium, magnesium, phosphorus, vitamins, and protein replacement may be necessary after 1 week of parenteral therapy.

III. **Replacement of abnormal water and electrolyte losses**

   A. **Insensible water losses** average 500–1000 ml/day and depend on respiratory rate, ambient temperature, humidity, and body temperature. Water losses increase by 100–150 ml/day for each degree of body temperature over 37°C. Fluid losses from sweating can vary enormously (0–2000 ml/hour) and depend on physical activity and body and ambient temperature. Replacement of insensible water losses should be with 5% D/W or hypotonic saline.

   B. **Gastrointestinal losses** vary in composition and volume depending on the source. To accurately replace the net electrolyte losses, laboratory measurement of fluid composition can be performed. Approximate electrolyte losses are provided in Table 3-1.

   C. **Urinary losses** of sodium may be significant, particularly in the setting of diuretic use, the recovery phase of acute tubular necrosis, postobstructive diuresis, renal medullary cystic disease, or adrenal insufficiency. Urinary loss of potassium may occur during the recovery phase of acute tubular necrosis, with renal tubular acidosis, diuretic use, and hyperaldosteronism. If prolonged losses occur, measurement of urinary sodium and potassium may help guide replacement.

   D. **Rapid internal fluid shifts** may occur with peritonitis, pancreatitis, portal vein thrombosis, extensive burns, fulminant nephrotic syndrome, ileus, bacterial enteritis, and crush injuries, as well as during the postoperative period. Replacement of sequestered fluid with isotonic saline may be necessary in these situations.

Table 3-1. Electrolyte content of sweat and gastrointestinal secretions

Sweat or gastrointestinal secretion	Electrolyte concentration (mEq/liter)					Replacement amount for each liter lost			
	Na^+	K^+	H^+	Cl^-	HCO_3^-	Isotonic saline (ml)	5% D/W (ml)	KCl[a] (mEq)	$NaHCO_3$[b] (mEq)
Sweat	30–50	5		45–55		300	700	5	
Gastric secretions	40–65	10	90[c]	100–140		300	700	20[d]	
Pancreatic fistula	135–155	5		55–75	70–90	250	750	5	90
Biliary fistula	135–155	5		80–110	35–50	750	250	5	45
Ileostomy fluid	120–130	10		50–60	50–70	300	700	10	67.6
Diarrhea fluid	25–50	35–60		20–40	30–45		1000	35	45

[a] Caution should be used in administering potassium faster than 10 mEq/hour.
[b] One ampule of 7.5% $NaHCO_3^-$ contains 45 mEq HCO_3^-.
[c] Variable (e.g., achlorhydria).
[d] Administration of more than the observed gastric loss of potassium is often required because of enhanced urinary potassium excretion in alkalosis.

Salt and Water

I. **Total body water (TBW)** constitutes about 60% of the body weight. Its distribution is illustrated in the following diagram (ICF = intracellular fluid; ECF = extracellular fluid; IF = interstitial fluid).

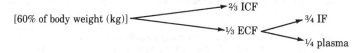

[60% of body weight (kg)] → ⅔ ICF
→ ⅓ ECF → ¾ IF
→ ¼ plasma

The most important determinant of ECF volume is the sodium content. Changes in ECF volume are dictated by net gain or loss of sodium with an accompanying gain or loss of water.

II. **Extracellular fluid volume depletion** occurs with losses of both sodium and water. The character of the fluid lost (see Table 3-1) will dictate the clinical picture. If the loss is isonatremic (e.g., blood loss), the osmolality of the ECF is unaffected and intracellular volume will change minimally. However, loss of hypotonic fluid, which may occur with sweating, hyperventilation, nasogastric suction, vomiting, or severe diarrhea, will lead to hypernatremia. As plasma osmolality rises under these circumstances, intracellular water moves to the ECF as a result of osmotic equilibration across cell membranes. Thus, larger volumes of hypotonic fluid loss may occur before clinical manifestations of ECF volume depletion present themselves. The serum sodium concentration will depend on the volume of fluid lost, its electrolyte composition, and the kidney's ability to maintain homeostasis. (Disorders of serum sodium are discussed in secs. **IV** and **V**.)

A. **Manifestations of ECF volume depletion** depend on its magnitude and on the plasma osmolality. Symptoms include anorexia, nausea, vomiting, apathy, weakness, orthostatic lightheadedness, and syncope. **Weight loss** is not only an important sign of volume contraction but also provides an estimate of the magnitude of the volume deficit. Other physical findings include orthostatic hypotension, poor skin turgor, sunken eyes, absence of axillary sweat, oliguria, and tachycardia. With severe volume depletion, shock and coma may occur. If hyponatremia or hypernatremia is present, symptoms referable to the change in plasma osmolality may also be found (see secs. **IV and V**). There are no laboratory tests that will accurately predict the degree of volume depletion; measurement of urinary sodium, fractional excretion of sodium, and the BUN-creatinine ratio may, however, provide additional diagnostic information (see Chap. 11). A rise in hematocrit and serum protein concentration may also be seen.

B. **Causes of ECF volume depletion** include gastrointestinal losses (vomiting, diarrhea, fistula drainage, nasogastric suction), diuretics, renal or adrenal disease (renal sodium wasting), blood loss, and sequestration of fluid (ileus, burns, peritonitis, pancreatitis).

C. **Treatment** should be directed at restoration of the ECF volume with solutions containing the lost water and electrolytes. During replacement, daily assessments of weight, ongoing fluid losses, and serum electrolyte concentrations are necessary to evaluate the progress of therapy. Mild degrees of volume depletion can be corrected orally (10- to 20-g NaCl diet and 2–4 liters of water/day). Sodium can also be given as sodium bicarbonate if acidosis is present. If more severe deficits accompanied by circulatory compromise are present, the initial treatment should be aggressive isotonic fluid replacement (0.9% saline) until hemodynamic stability has been attained.

III. **Extracellular fluid volume excess**

A. **Manifestations.** Weight gain is the most sensitive and consistent sign of ECF volume excess. Edema, another important manifestation, is usually not apparent until 2–4 kg of fluid have been retained. Other clinical findings include dyspnea, tachycardia, jugular venous distention, hepatojugular reflux, the presence of rales on pulmonary examination, and auscultation of an S3.

B. Causes of ECF volume excess have in common excessive renal sodium and water retention as in heart failure (HF), nephrotic syndrome, renal failure, and cirrhosis. The problem can be further aggravated by unnecessary salt administration (e.g., IV line flushes, parenteral drug solutions, dietary excess).

C. Treatment must address not only the ECF volume excess but also the underlying pathologic process. Treatment of the nephrotic syndrome and the cardiovascular overload associated with renal failure is discussed in Chap. 11. Treatment of HF and cirrhosis is discussed in Chaps. 6 and 16, respectively.

IV. Hyponatremia can result from (1) primary sodium loss and/or primary water gain; (2) an altered distribution of body water due to osmotic effect; or (3) a vagary of laboratory measurement (pseudohyponatremia). As sodium and its attendant anions are the primary determinants of ECF osmolality, hyponatremia is usually accompanied by hypo-osmolality. However, hyponatremia may be associated with a normal or even elevated plasma osmolality. Therefore, initial evaluation should include a clinical estimate of the ECF volume status and both a measured and a calculated plasma osmolality. The calculated plasma osmolality accounts for the contributions of the most prevalent osmotically active solutes:

$$\text{Osmolality (mOsm/kg)} = 2[\text{Na}^+ \text{ (mEq/liter)} + \text{K}^+ \text{ (mEq/liter)}] + [\text{BUN (mg/dl)}/2.8] + [\text{glucose (mg/dl)}/18]$$

If the measured plasma osmolality exceeds the calculated plasma osmolality by more than 10 mOsm/kg, significant quantities of unmeasured osmotically active solutes (e.g., mannitol, ethanol, methanol) are present (increased osmolar gap). In addition, the plasma osmolality provides a means for categorization of the hyponatremic disorders (Fig. 3-1).

A. Hyponatremia with an increase in osmotically active solutes occurs when there is an accumulation of large amounts of solutes restricted primarily to the ECF space. The measured plasma osmolality may be normal or elevated. The increase in ECF osmolality results in a shift of water from the ICF to the ECF, thereby diluting the ECF sodium. **Hyperglycemia** is the most common cause, resulting in a 1.6 mEq/liter decrement in plasma sodium for each 100 mg/dl increment in glucose concentration. The treatment is reduction of the ECF hypertonicity by correction of the underlying disorder.

B. Hyponatremia associated with a normal plasma osmolality, or pseudohyponatremia, is caused by severe hyperlipidemia and hyperproteinemia (>10 g/dl). These two disorders increase the nonaqueous, nonsodium-containing fraction of plasma (normally, 5–7% of plasma volume). The sodium concentration and osmolality of plasma water are normal despite a reduced whole plasma sodium concentration. Treatment of the hyponatremia is not required.

C. Hyponatremia associated with decreased plasma osmolality (hypotonic hyponatremia). This category of hyponatremia results in intracellular volume expansion with consequent derangement of cellular functions, particularly those of the central nervous system. **Manifestations** of hyponatremia generally do not occur until the plasma sodium falls below 120 mEq/liter but may occur at higher concentrations if the rate of fall is rapid. Initial findings include nausea, malaise, lethargy, and cramps, which can progress to psychosis, seizures, and coma. Permanent neurologic damage may occur if severe hyponatremia persists; hence, acute therapy is indicated. **Caution should be exercised when treating hyponatremia** because too rapid a rate of correction may cause central pontine myelinolysis and permanent neurologic damage (*N. Engl. J. Med.* 317:1190, 1987). Because both the hyponatremic state and its overly aggressive correction may have disastrous neurologic consequences, the presence or absence of symptoms and the acuity of the process should influence the treatment decision. In general, the rate of correction should not exceed 2.5 mEq/liter/hour and the total daily increment in serum sodium should not exceed 20 mEq/liter. (*Kidney Int.* 37:1006, 1990).This category can be further subdivided on the basis of the

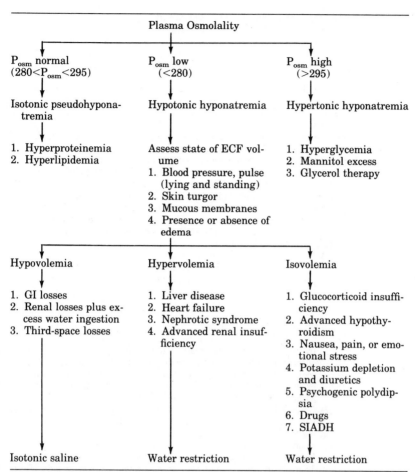

Fig. 3-1. An approach to the assessment and treatment of hyponatremic states. (SIADH = syndrome of inappropriate antidiuretic hormone secretion.) (From H. D. Hume. Disorders of Water Metabolism. In J. P. Kokko and R. L. Tannen [eds.], *Fluids and Electrolytes*. Philadelphia: Saunders, 1986. P. 136.)

clinical assessment of ECF volume status and the urinary sodium (assuming the absence of recent diuretic therapy).

1. **Hypotonic hyponatremia with ECF volume excess** and a urine sodium greater than 20 mEq/liter can occur with renal failure, whereas a urine sodium less than 20 mEq/liter is characteristic of the nephrotic syndrome, HF, or cirrhosis. In these conditions, renal excretion of both sodium and water is impaired but the rise in total body water exceeds that of sodium. The **treatment** of hyponatremia under these conditions is treatment of the underlying disorder coupled with judicious **salt and water restriction,** usually in conjunction with diuretics. **Administration of hypertonic saline is hazardous** and will only exacerbate the volume excess in this form of hyponatremia.

2. **Hypotonic hyponatremia with decreased ECF volume** occurs when total ody sodium is depleted disproportionately to water losses or when a sodium deficit is replaced with hypotonic fluids. This condition can arise from **extrarenal loss** of sodium and water (e.g., vomiting, diarrhea, and third-space sequestration); urinary sodium in this setting is less than 20 mEq/liter. It may also be due to **renal losses** (osmotic diuresis, salt-losing nephropathy, diuretic therapy, proximal renal tubular acidosis, adrenal insufficiency, and vomiting with bicarbonaturia and obligate urinary sodium loss); in this situation, a urinary sodium greater than 20 mEq/liter is typical. The clinical manifestations are usually due to the volume depletion rather than to the hyponatremia. The **treatment** is re-expansion of the ECF volume with isotonic saline and correction of the underlying disorder.

3. **Hypotonic hyponatremia with clinically normal ECF volume**

   a. **The syndrome of inappropriate antidiuretic hormone (SIADH)** secretion is characterized by (1) hypotonic hyponatremia, (2) inappropriately elevated urinary osmolality (usually >200 mOsm/kg) relative to plasma osmolality, (3) elevated urinary sodium (typically >20 mEq/liter), (4) clinical euvolemia, and (5) normal renal, adrenal, and thyroid function. Conditions associated with SIADH include malignant tumors, pulmonary disease, and CNS disorders.

      (1) **Acute treatment** of SIADH should be reserved for those patients with severe, symptomatic hyponatremia (serum sodium <110–115 mEq/liter). This may be accomplished by initiating and maintaining a rapid diuresis with IV furosemide followed by intravenous replacement of urinary sodium and potassium losses (*Ann. Intern. Med.* 78:870, 1973). Replacement of these electrolyte losses can be accomplished with 0.9% saline (rarely, 3% saline is required), to which potassium has been added. Since the urine is inappropriately concentrated in SIADH, administration of isotonic or hypertonic NaCl without diuretics will not ultimately be effective in raising the serum sodium concentration. Acute correction of hyponatremia should not exceed a 20 mEq/liter rise in serum sodium concentration in the first 24 hours of therapy, as mentioned previously.

      (2) **Chronic treatment** of SIADH. **Water restriction** to 500–1000 ml daily is the mainstay of chronic management. **Demeclocycline** (300–600 mg PO bid) may be effective when water restriction alone is unsuccessful; its onset of action may be delayed longer than 1 week. Demeclocycline should not be used in the presence of liver disease, as drug accumulation may lead to nephrotoxicity. Other side effects include photosensitivity and nausea. Furosemide and increased salt intake (*N. Engl. J. Med.* 304:329, 1981) and oral urea (*Am. J. Med.* 69:99, 1980) may also be effective.

   b. **Hypothyroidism** may produce hyponatremia. The impaired free water excretion may be due to increased antidiuretic hormone (ADH) levels or to a reduction in glomerular filtration rate (GFR) and effective renal plasma flow. The treatment is thyroxine replacement and water restriction.

   c. **A variety of drugs** may cause hyponatremia either through stimulation of central ADH release, through a potentiation of its peripheral actions, or through a combination of these mechanisms. Examples include amitriptyline, carbamazepine, clofibrate, cyclophosphamide, morphine, and vincristine. Treatment consists of water restriction and removal of the putative etiologic agent.

   d. **Water intoxication** may result from psychogenic polydipsia, lesions in the thirst center, or administration of hypotonic IV solutions to patients who are unable to dilute their urine normally (e.g., postoperatively or in the presence of renal insufficiency). The acute **treatment** of severe, symptomatic hyponatremia in these situations is identical to that of SIADH. An underlying CNS lesion must be excluded. Treatment of psychogenic polydipsia consists of reassurance and psychiatric counseling. Whatever the cause of water intoxication, water restriction and discontinuation of hypotonic solutions is necessary until the serum sodium concentration normalizes.

  e. Pain, nausea, and emotional stress may stimulate ADH secretion.

  f. Selective glucocorticoid deficiency due to anterior hypopituitarism may cause hyponatremia, as it appears that glucocorticoids are required to completely suppress ADH secretion.

V. Hypernatremia. All hypernatremic states are hyperosmolar. As plasma osmolality exceeds 280–285 mOsm/kg H_2O, there is a linear increase in ADH release by the posterior pituitary. Extracellular fluid volume depletion potentiates this response, whereas ECF volume expansion may blunt it. The renal response to ADH is conservation of free water, characterized by low urine volumes (<500 ml/day) and a high urine osmolality (>1000 mOsm/kg H_2O). In addition, a 2% increase in plasma osmolality should stimulate thirst and thereby an increase in free water intake.

  A. Manifestations. The most common symptoms in hypernatremia can often be attributed to the underlying cause. Signs of volume overload or volume depletion may be prominent and provide a clue to diagnosis. Clinical manifestations attributable to the hypernatremia per se include tremulousness, irritability, ataxia, spasticity, mental confusion, seizures, and coma. Symptoms are more likely to occur with acute rises in plasma sodium concentration. Chronic hypernatremia is characterized by increased CNS intracellular osmolality (accumulation of idiogenic osmoles) beginning about 4 hours after the onset of hypernatremia and stabilizing in 4–7 days. This increase in CNS osmolality prevents cellular dehydration; however, it must also be accounted for when considering the therapy of hypernatremia (see sec. **V.B.2**).

  B. Causes. Hypernatremic states arise from net sodium gain, net water loss, or failure to replace obligate water losses, as in the case of patients unable to obtain water due to an altered mental status or severe debilitating disease. The diagnostic approach is based on an assessment of ECF volume, urine volume, and urine osmolality (U_{osm}).

  1. Hypernatremia with ECF volume expansion signifies net sodium gain. It is usually seen in patients receiving hypertonic saline or $NaHCO_3$. Mild hypernatremia of this sort can also be seen with primary hyperaldosteronism and Cushing's syndrome. **Therapy** must be directed at removal of the excess sodium with diuretics or dialysis (if renal failure is present) followed by replacement of fluid losses with 5% D/W.

  2. Hypernatremia with ECF volume depletion occurs with hypotonic fluid loss, typically in patients who are unable to obtain water in the face of ongoing **extrarenal losses** (e.g., gastrointestinal and insensible losses). Urine volume is decreased and U_{osm} is high. **Renal losses** due to the presence of a diuretic or an osmotic diuresis (e.g., glucose) should be suspected if both urine volume and osmolality are high. Finally, if urine volume is high but U_{osm} is low, diabetes insipidus is the most likely diagnosis (see below).

  The **acute treatment** of hypovolemic hypernatremia depends on the degree of volume depletion. If there is evidence of hemodynamic compromise (e.g., orthostatic hypotension, marked oliguria), salt and water deficits should be corrected initially with isotonic saline. Once hemodynamic stability is achieved, the remaining free water deficit should be corrected with 5% D/W or 0.45% NaCl. The net free water deficit can be estimated as follows:

  Current TBW (liters) = 0.6 × current body weight (kg)

  $$\text{Desired TBW} = \frac{\text{Measured serum } Na^+ \text{ (mEq/liter)} \times \text{current TBW}}{\text{Normal serum } Na^+ \text{ (mEq/liter)}}$$

  Body water deficit (liters) = Desired TBW − current TBW

  In female or cachectic patients, TBW may be only 40–50% of total body weight, and this calculation of water deficit represents a maximum amount.

The serum sodium concentration and ECF volume status should be evaluated every 6 hours. The plasma osmolality should not be corrected at a rate greater than 1 mOsm/kg/hour or the change in sodium concentration should not exceed 1 mEq/liter/hour. Roughly one half of the calculated water deficit can be administered in the first 24 hours, followed by correction of the remaining deficit over the next 1–2 days. Excessively rapid correction is dangerous, particularly in patients with hypernatremia for more than 24 hours, as it may lead to lethargy and seizures secondary to cerebral edema (due to the increased CNS intracellular osmolality).

3. **Hypernatremia with ECF volume depletion secondary to water shift** from the ECF to the ICF can occur with rhabdomyolysis.

4. **Diabetes insipidus (DI)** is due either to an absolute or partial ADH deficiency (central DI) or to renal resistance to ADH (nephrogenic DI). The causes of central DI include hypothalamic or pituitary damage from tumors, granulomas, trauma, surgery, or idiopathic causes. Nephrogenic DI may occur with severe hypokalemia, hypercalcemia, chronic renal failure, medullary or interstitial kidney diseases, or drugs (e.g., lithium, demeclocycline, amphotericin, propoxyphene, methoxyflurane). Diabetes insipidus is characterized by polydipsia and polyuria (urine outputs of 3–10 liters/day), without diurnal variation. Urine osmolality is typically less than 100 mOsm/kg H_2O in the face of an elevated plasma osmolality. Patients who are denied access to water may become severely ill within 24 hours. Initial testing involves water deprivation under direct physician supervision. Failure to appropriately concentrate the urine suggests the diagnosis. A subsequent rise in urinary concentrating ability after SQ injection of aqueous arginine vasopressin (AVP) confirms the diagnosis of central DI. Lack of a response to AVP indicates nephrogenic DI.

The **treatment** of DI depends on the cause. Central DI requires vasopressin administration. It should be given cautiously in patients with coronary artery disease. The preparation of choice is DDAVP, a long-acting vasopressin analog given intranasally at a dose of 5–10 µg once or twice a day. Aqueous vasopressin (duration of action, 4–6h), given parenterally, can also be used. Nephrogenic DI is unresponsive to vasopressin and should be treated by correcting hypokalemia or hypercalcemia and by discontinuation of causative drugs, if possible. Thiazide diuretics combined with a program of modest salt restriction may also be effective by virtue of a reduction of delivery of filtrate to diluting segments of the nephron coupled with an increase in papillary osmolality.

Potassium

The total body potassium of a normal adult is approximately 40–50 mEq/kg body weight. Only about 1.5% is found in the ECF. A typical daily potassium intake is 1.0–1.5 mEq/kg body weight; about 10% of this is excreted in the stool and sweat, the remainder by the kidney. The normal kidney can excrete up to 6 mEq potassium/kg/day. The serum potassium concentration is a general indicator of total body potassium, but various factors can affect its transcellular distribution (acid-–base abnormalities, increased extracellular osmolality, insulin deficiency). For example, one may expect an inverse change of variable magnitude (0.1–0.7 mEq/liter) in serum potassium concentration for each 0.1 unit change in serum pH.

I. **Hypokalemia.** Assuming a normal pH, a normal serum potassium concentration may actually belie a total body deficit of up to 200 mEq. In general, however, each 1 mEq/dl decrease in serum potassium concentration reflects a deficit of approximately 350 mEq. Serum potassium concentrations less than 2 mEq/dl reflect total body potassium deficits of greater than 1000 mEq.

A. **Manifestations of hypokalemia** usually occur at potassium concentrations below 2.5 mEq/liter. A rapid decrease in the serum concentration may induce symptoms at a higher potassium level. Signs and symptoms include malaise, fatigue, neuromuscular disturbances (e.g., weakness, hyporeflexia, paresthesias, cramps, restless legs syndrome, rhabdomyolysis, paralysis), gastrointestinal disorders (e.g., constipation, ileus), and worsening of hepatic encephalopathy. Cardiovascular abnormalities, such as orthostatic hypotension, worsening of hypertension, arrhythmias (particularly with digitalis therapy), and ECG changes (T wave flattening, prominent U waves, and ST segment depression), may occur. Renal and electrolyte abnormalities include metabolic alkalosis, urinary concentrating defects with polyuria and consequent polydipsia, decreased GFR, and glucose intolerance.

B. Causes

1. **Hypokalemia secondary to transcellular shifts** can occur in the presence of beta-agonists, alkalemia, insulin excess, acute glucose loads, delirium tremens, hypokalemic periodic paralysis, and anabolic states.

2. **Hypokalemia with normal acid–base balance** can be due to osmotic diuretics, chronic diarrhea, acute leukemias, aminoglycosides, high doses of some penicillins (poorly reabsorbable anions may result in a more negatively charged distal tubule thereby enhancing potassium secretion), or magnesium deficiency. Prolonged inadequate potassium intake (less than 10–20 mEq/day) can produce a significant deficit because of continued renal and gastrointestinal losses.

3. **Hypokalemia with metabolic acidosis** is usually due to diarrhea, renal tubular acidosis (proximal and distal), amphotericin, diabetic ketoacidosis, laxative abuse, intestinal or biliary fistulas, ureteroenterostomy, or toluene.

4. **Hypokalemia with metabolic alkalosis** can result from gastrointestinal losses (vomiting or nasogastric suction) or renal losses (primary hyperaldosteronism, glucocorticoid excess, Liddle's syndrome, diuretic therapy, or Bartter's syndrome). The alkalosis and volume contraction associated with these disorders further contribute to the potassium deficit by increasing renal losses.

C. Treatment. Potassium can be administered to replace chronic losses or to address decreased serum levels. Patients with ongoing potassium losses should have levels monitored to direct therapy. Prevention of hypokalemia (potassium <3.5 mEq/liter) is most important in patients with cardiac disease and those taking digitalis (to minimize the risk of arrhythmias and conduction disturbances).

1. **Oral therapy.** If a patient consumes a diet that is deficient in potassium-rich foods (e.g., fruit, vegetables), dietary alterations, which can increase potassium intake by 40–60 mEq/day, may be sufficient therapy. **Salt substitutes** provide another economical alternative to prescription potassium supplements; they contain 7–14 mEq potassium/g (5 g equals approximately 1 tsp). **Potassium supplements** are usually given as potassium chloride, although other forms are available. **Chloride** is generally required in cases in which the hypokalemia is associated with ECF volume contraction. **Slow-release KCl tablets or capsules** are useful in patients who are unable to tolerate liquid forms of potassium supplementation. The rare occurrence of gastrointestinal tract ulcers has been reported with these preparations, particularly in the setting of intestinal dysmotility. The nonchloride-containing potassium supplements may be more palatable for those patients who are unable to tolerate the KCl preparations. Severe hyperkalemia can occur during oral potassium supplementation; hence, serum potassium levels should always be monitored during therapy. The potassium-sparing diuretics (spironolactone, triamterene, or amiloride) may be an alternative for patients in whom hypokalemia develops secondary to renal losses. These drugs should not be used in patients with renal insufficiency, in conjunction with potassium supplements, or with other agents that impair potassium secretion (e.g., angiotensin-converting enzyme inhibitors); they should also be used with caution in diabetics (see sec. **II.B.**).

2. **IV therapy.** The IV administration of potassium is appropriate in patients with severe hypokalemia and in those with hypokalemia who are unable to take oral supplements. An approximation of the potassium deficit can be

obtained as discussed previously, but frequent serum potassium determinations are necessary to guide therapy. If the serum potassium is greater than 2.5 mEq/liter and ECG changes are not present, potassium can be given at a rate of up to 10 mEq/hour and in concentrations up to 30 mEq/liter. If the serum potassium is less than 2.5 mEq/liter or accompanied by ECG abnormalities or severe neuromuscular complications, emergency treatment is required. In this setting, potassium can be given through a peripheral IV line at rates up to 40 mEq/hour and in concentrations up to 60 mEq/liter. Continuous ECG monitoring and measurement of the serum potassium concentration every 4 hours should be performed. Once the indications for emergency treatment have resolved, less aggressive replacement should be undertaken as already described. In severe life-threatening hypokalemia, initial potassium replacement should be administered in glucose-free solutions since glucose may cause the serum potassium level to fall further.

II. Hyperkalemia

A. Manifestations of hyperkalemia usually occur when the serum potassium concentration is >6.5 mEq/liter. Neuromuscular manifestations include weakness, paresthesias, areflexia, ascending paralysis, and respiratory failure. **Cardiac manifestations** include bradycardia that can progress to asystole, prolongation of atrioventricular (AV) conduction leading to complete heart block, and ventricular fibrillation. As the serum potassium increases, the ECG manifests progressive changes. Initially, peaked or tented T waves appear. Subsequently, ST segment depression, first-degree AV block, and QRS widening occur. Finally, a biphasic wave (sine wave) representing fusion of the widened QRS and T wave develops, signaling imminent ventricular standstill. The rate of progression is not predictable, and patients may progress from initial ECG changes to dangerous conduction disturbances or arrhythmias within minutes. The ECG changes are exacerbated by coexisting hyponatremia, hypocalcemia, hypermagnesemia, and acidosis.

B. Causes

1. **Decreased renal excretion** can result from (1) hyporeninemic hypoaldosteronism due to intrinsic renal disease (e.g., diabetes and interstitial nephritis) or prostaglandin synthetase inhibitors, (2) hypoaldosteronism (either primary or secondary to heparin, cyclosporine, or angiotensin-converting enzyme inhibitors) or adrenal insufficiency (usually with volume depletion or diminished GFR), (3) acute or chronic renal failure, (4) type IV renal tubular acidosis, (5) decreased distal nephron sodium delivery as in HF, and (6) potassium-sparing diuretics.

2. **Redistribution of potassium from ICF to ECF** can result from acidosis. Because cell membranes are more permeable to organic acids (e.g., ketoacids, lactic acid), organic acids are less likely to cause hyperkalemia than are mineral acids (NH_4Cl, HCl). Other causes of potassium redistribution include hyperkalemic periodic paralysis, digitalis intoxication, insulin deficiency, and a rapid rise of ECF osmolality (hypertonic glucose or mannitol administration). Succinylcholine causes a leakage of potassium from muscle cells that lasts about 10 minutes and is usually inconsequential; however, in patients with extensive tissue destruction, the serum potassium concentration may rise markedly. Beta antagonists, which can block cellular potassium uptake, may cause hyperkalemia in patients with diabetes mellitus, those on dialysis, and those undergoing cardiopulmonary bypass.

3. **A potassium load** can result from **exogenous** sources such as IV potassium administration, blood transfusions, high-dose penicillin therapy (1.7 mEq potassium/1 million units), and oral potassium supplements or salt substitutes. **Endogenous** potassium loads arise from tissue destruction as seen with tumor lysis, burns, crush injuries, massive hemolysis, major surgery, or gastrointestinal bleeding.

4. **Pseudohyperkalemia** describes an artifactually elevated serum potassium. This can occur when potassium is released from cells either during blood sample clotting in the presence of leukocytosis (>70,000/microliter) or

thrombocytosis (>1 million/microliter), or with red blood cell hemolysis due to drawing through a small needle, delay in analysis, or prolonged, excessively tight tourniquet placement. A normal plasma (unclotted sample) potassium level will eliminate leukocytosis and thrombocytosis as causes.

C. Acute treatment. The goals in the treatment of hyperkalemia are (1) to protect the heart from the effects of potassium by antagonizing the effect on cardiac conduction (calcium administration), (2) to shift potassium from the ECF to the ICF (sodium bicarbonate, insulin, and glucose), and (3) to reduce total body potassium (cation-exchange resins, diuretics, dialysis). The need for treatment is urgent if the serum potassium is greater than 7 mEq/liter or if the ECG shows changes of hyperkalemia. Life-threatening arrhythmias may occur at any time during therapy; hence, continuous ECG monitoring is required. The serum potassium should be followed closely during therapy. In patients with hyperkalemia due to tissue destruction or increased total body potassium, therapy directed at net removal of potassium from the body should be initiated simultaneously with acute measures.

1. Calcium administration will temporarily antagonize the cardiac and neuromuscular effects of hyperkalemia. Calcium gluconate (10 ml of a 10% solution) should be given intravenously over 2–5 minutes. A second dose can be given after 5 minutes if no response occurs. Slower infusion rates should be considered in patients receiving digitalis because of the danger of hypercalcemia-induced digitalis toxicity. Unless hypocalcemia is present, further calcium therapy is unlikely to be of benefit. The effect of calcium occurs within minutes and lasts for 1 hour; hence, other modalities should be initiated as soon as possible.

2. Sodium bicarbonate administration causes a shift of potassium from the ECF to the ICF. Treatment with bicarbonate is particularly important in patients with acidosis, since further therapy for hyperkalemia may not be required after correction of the acidosis. One ampule of 7.5% $NaHCO_3$ (44.6 mEq HCO_3) can be given IV over 5 minutes and repeated at 10- to 15-minute intervals if ECG changes persist. The onset of action occurs within 30 minutes and the effect lasts for 1–2 hours. Circulatory overload and hypernatremia can occur when large volumes of hypertonic $NaHCO_3$ are given. Sodium bicarbonate can also be added to glucose infusions (see below). If hypocalcemia is present, seizures and tetany may occur as blood pH rises; hence, calcium should be given first.

3. Glucose and insulin infusions act to shift potassium from the ECF into cells. Regular insulin (10 units) should be given IV at the same time as 1 ampule of 50% glucose (25 g) is given IV over 5 minutes. A response should be seen within 30–60 minutes and the effect typically lasts for several hours. Spot blood glucoses should be followed over this time. An alternative method is to mix 89 mEq $NaHCO_3$ (2 ampules) with 1000 ml of 10% D/W. The first 300 ml can be given over 30 minutes and the remainder over the next 3 hours; 25 units of regular insulin should be given SQ at the time the infusion begins (*Med. Clin. North Am.* 65:165, 1981). The combination of nebulized **albuterol** with insulin and glucose has been shown to be very effective in treating hyperkalemia in dialysis patients; in addition, the co-administration of albuterol may attenuate the hypoglycemic effect of insulin (*Kidney Int.* 38:869, 1990).

4. Cation-exchange resins bind potassium in exchange for another cation (usually sodium) in the intestinal tract, thereby removing potassium from the body. This method of therapy should be given as soon as possible if hyperkalemia results from decreased potassium excretion or an increased potassium load. Each gram of **sodium polystyrene sulfonate** (Kayexalate) binds approximately 1 mEq K^+. This drug also exchanges about 1.5 mEq Na^+ for each 1 mEq potassium removed and should therefore be used with caution in patients who are unable to tolerate sodium loads (HF or severe hypertension); hypernatremia may also occur.

a. Oral administration is the preferred route. Since this drug is constipating, it should be given with a poorly absorbed carrier (osmotic agent) such as sorbitol. The initial dose is 15–30 g of sodium polystyrene sulfonate mixed in 50–100 ml of 20% sorbitol. This dose can be repeated q3–4h up to 4–5 doses/day until the hyperkalemia has resolved.

    b. Rectal administration can be utilized if the oral route is not tolerated or if an ileus is present. An enema will remove K^+ more rapidly than the oral route. A retention enema can be given as a mixture of 50–100 g sodium polystyrene sulfonate in 200 ml of 20% sorbitol or 20% D/W (if sorbitol is not available). Retention of the enema for the desired 30–60 minutes may be facilitated by using an inflated rectal catheter. Enemas can be repeated q4–6h up to 4 doses/day.

  5. Dialysis can remove potassium from the body very effectively but should be reserved for those clinical situations in which more conservative methods have failed or are inappropriate. Of importance, significant hyperkalemic rebound can occur after dialysis as potassium is mobilized from intracellular stores.

D. Chronic treatment. Treatment of the underlying disorder may obviate the need for specific therapy for hyperkalemia. Patients with renal failure (GFR <10 ml/minute) require restriction of dietary potassium to 40–60 mEq/day. Loop diuretics (furosemide, bumetanide) may be efficacious in treating the hyperkalemia as well as the volume overload in renal failure. Sodium polystyrene sulfonate can also be given orally as chronic therapy.

Acid–Base Disturbances

Acid–base homeostasis consists of the regulation of the hydrogen ion concentration. This involves the interdigitation of three physiologic systems: the chemical buffers of the body, the lungs, and the kidneys. The acid generated from the metabolism of most carbon-containing compounds is excreted by the lungs as CO_2 and H_2O. This constitutes the **volatile** acid load and is without major impact on acid–base balance. However, a daily **fixed** acid load is generated from the incomplete metabolism of organic compounds, the metabolism of sulfur-containing amino acids, and the hydrolysis of dietary phosphoproteins. **Chemical buffers,** principally the bicarbonate–carbonic acid buffer pair, serve as the vanguard against this load. The CO_2 and H_2O generated from this system ($H^+ + HCO_3^- \rightleftharpoons H_2CO_3 \rightleftharpoons CO_2 + H_2O$) are then eliminated by **the lungs.** Lastly, **the kidney** serves the critical functions of reabsorbing filtered bicarbonate and of regenerating new bicarbonate via the titration of urinary buffers and the excretion of ammonium. Perturbations of this physiologic framework characterize the clinical acid–base disorders.

I. The approach to the analysis of acid–base disorders involves the sequential consideration of the following questions. (1) Is acidemia or alkalemia present and is its origin respiratory or metabolic? (2) If respiratory, is the disturbance acute or chronic? (3) If a metabolic acidosis is present, what is the anion gap? (4) If a metabolic alkalosis is present, what is the urinary chloride? (5) Is there appropriate compensation for the primary disorder and, if not, what is the mixed disturbance? The information to answer these questions is obtained from a careful history, the arterial blood gases, serum and urine electrolytes, and the rules of compensation (Table 3-2).

II. The arterial blood gases (ABGs). Normal ABG values are pH, 7.36–7.44; PCO_2, 35–45 mm Hg; total CO_2, 24–32 mEq/liter. When obtaining an ABG, the syringe should be coated with 1 ml heparin (1000 units/ml) for anticoagulation. The excess heparin should be expelled to prevent factitious lowering of the pH. The sample should be measured immediately to avoid the effects of cell metabolism. If the sample is cooled with ice, the results will remain accurate up to 1–2 hours after the blood was obtained.

Table 3-2. Summary of expected compensation for simple acid–base disorders

Primary disorder	Initial chemical change	Compensatory response	Equations for expected range of compensation
Metabolic acidosis	HCO_3^- decrease	PCO_2 decrease	$PCO_2 = 1.5\ [HCO_3^-] + 8 \pm 2$ $PCO_2 =$ last 2 digits of pH $\times 100$ $\Delta PCO_2 = 1\text{–}1.3\ (\Delta[HCO_3^-])$ $PCO_2 = [HCO_3^-] + 15$
Metabolic alkalosis	HCO_3^- increase	PCO_2 increase	PCO_2: variable increase $PCO_2 = 0.9\ [HCO_3^-] + 9$ PCO_2 : increases 0.6 mm Hg for each mEq/liter increase in $[HCO_3^-]$
Respiratory acidosis	PCO_2 increase	HCO_3^- increase	Acute $[HCO_3^-]$ increases 1 mEq/liter for every 10 mm Hg increase in PCO_2 Chronic $[HCO_3^-]$ increases 3.5 mEq/liter for every 10 mm Hg increase in PCO_2
Respiratory alkalosis	PCO_2 decrease	HCO_3^- decrease	Acute $[HCO_3^-]$ falls 2 mEq/liter for each 10 mm Hg fall in PCO_2 Chronic $[HCO_3^-]$ falls 5 mEq/liter for each 10 mm Hg fall in PCO_2

Source: M. Emmett and D. W. Seldin. Evaluation of Acid-Base Disorders from Plasma Composition. In D. W. Seldin and G. Giebisch (eds.), *The Regulation of Acid-Base Balance.* New York: Raven, 1989. P. 237.

The Henderson-Hasselbalch equation defines the relationship between pH, PCO_2, and HCO_3^- in blood:

$$pH = 6.1 + \log \frac{[HCO_3^-]}{0.0301 \times PCO_2}$$

The following equation relates the same factors in a more practical way:

$$[H^+] = 24 \times \frac{PCO_2}{[HCO_3^-]}$$

The H^+ concentration in nEq/liter can easily be obtained:

pH	6.90	7.00	7.10	7.20	7.30	7.40	7.50	7.60	7.70
$[H^+]$	125	100	80	64	51	40	32	25	20

Note that the $[H^+]$ falls by 20% for each 0.1 pH unit increment over the entire range. Intermediate values can be interpolated with accuracy.

III. The primary acid–base disturbances result from conditions that initially affect either the $[HCO_3^-]$ (metabolic acidosis and alkalosis) or the PCO_2 (respiratory acidosis and alkalosis). Each of these primary disturbances causes the blood pH to shift away from normal and evokes compensatory responses that return pH toward, but not completely to, normal (see Table 3-2).

A. Metabolic acidosis is a reduction in $[HCO_3^-]$ that reflects either the accumulation of fixed acids or the loss of alkali. The compensatory response is increased ventilation, leading to a fall in PCO_2.

B. Metabolic alkalosis is defined by a primary increase in $[HCO_3^-]$ arising either from a loss of acid or, less commonly, from a gain of bicarbonate. The compensatory response is hypoventilation, leading to a rise in PCO_2.

C. Respiratory acidosis is characterized by a primary increase in PCO_2 due to processes that interfere with the pulmonary excretion of CO_2. The compensatory response is an increase in renal reabsorption and generation of bicarbonate, leading to a rise in serum $[HCO_3^-]$.

D. Respiratory alkalosis is characterized by a decreased PCO_2 due to primary hyperventilation. The compensatory response is increased renal bicarbonate excretion leading to a fall in serum $[HCO_3^-]$.

IV. Metabolic acidosis

A. The causes of metabolic acidosis can be categorized according to **the anion gap (AG).** The anion gap is an indirect measurement of those serum anions not measured by routine laboratory screening. It accounts for the difference between the serum sodium concentration and the sum of the serum chloride and bicarbonate concentrations:

$$AG = [Na^+] - ([Cl^-] + [HCO_3^-])$$

Normal AG $= 12 \pm 4$ mEq/liter

Metabolic acidoses other than hydrochloric acidosis result in a decreased serum bicarbonate without a concomitant rise in serum chloride, thereby increasing the anion gap.

1. Increased AG acidosis occurs with renal insufficiency (GFR <20 ml/min), ketoacidosis (diabetic or alcoholic), lactic acidosis, and drug intoxications (methanol, salicylates, ethylene glycol, paraldehyde).

2. The causes of a **normal AG acidosis** can be grouped according to the serum potassium. Those associated with a **normal to high serum potassium** include hypoaldosteronism, type IV renal tubular acidosis (RTA), moderate renal insufficiency (GFR >20 ml/min), the administration of HCl, and posthypocapnia. Those generally associated with a **low serum potassium** include GI losses of bicarbonate (diarrhea, ureteral diversions, biliary or pancreatic fistulas), carbonic anhydrase inhibitors, and proximal and distal renal tubular acidosis. Impaired renal tubular acid excretion (e.g., versus GI bicarbonate losses) can be discerned with the use of the **urinary anion gap** ($[Na^+ + K^+] - [Cl]$) when urine electrolytes are available. A negative gap signifies normal renal NH_4^+ excretion and, therefore, a nonrenal cause for the acidosis. This assumes a urine pH of less than 6.1 and euvolemia (hypovolemia may impair renal acid excretion as a result of decreased distal tubular flow and sodium delivery).

B. Treatment

1. Acute metabolic acidosis. Parenteral bicarbonate therapy should be considered in patients with a pH below 7.2. Acidosis to this degree can result in myocardial depression, hypotension, and resistance to vasopressor administration. Bicarbonate must be administered cautiously, however, because overalkalinization can induce tetany, seizures, cardiac arrhythmias, and increased lactate production. In addition, bicarbonate given during cardiorespiratory arrest before gas exchange is established can paradoxically lower pH as a result of complete retention of the CO_2 generated. Since the distribution of bicarbonate is about 40% of the body weight, an approximation of the amount of bicarbonate necessary to return the serum concentration to normal can be estimated as follows:

$$HCO_3^- \text{ deficit} = (\text{kg body weight}) \times (0.4) \times (\text{desired } [HCO_3^-] - \text{measured } [HCO_3^-])$$

Since the degree of respiratory compensation, ECF volume status, and progression of the underlying disease may vary from patient to patient, alkali therapy must be guided by frequent assessment of acid–base status and electrolyte levels. Usually, 2–3 ampules of 7.5% $NaHCO_3$ (44.6 mEq/ampule) are added to 1000 ml of 5% D/W. One half the calculated deficit may be replaced in 3–4 hours if severe HF is not present. **No further bicarbonate therapy should be given once the pH reaches 7.2.** Because correction of acidosis without correction of a potassium deficit may lead to profound hypokalemia (due to intracellular shift of potassium), potassium supplementation should be undertaken if the serum potassium concentration begins to fall during correction of the acidosis. Serum calcium should also be monitored and hypocalcemia treated because a relative alkalosis may decrease the ionized calcium concentration.

2. **Chronic metabolic acidosis** is often found in association with chronic renal failure. When the bicarbonate concentration is less than 15 mEq/liter, bicarbonate replacement is necessary to prevent osteomalacia. **Sodium bicarbonate** (available in 325- and 650-mg tablets) containing approximately 12 mEq of alkali per gram may be given in divided doses for a total of 2–4 g/day. Caution must be used in those patients who are unable to tolerate a volume load. **Shohl's solution** (1 mEq $NaHCO_3$/ml solution) may be more palatable for some patients and may cause less abdominal bloating.

C. Specific considerations

1. **AG metabolic acidosis.** Patients frequently present to the emergency room with an AG metabolic acidosis of uncertain cause; an adequate history is often unavailable. Blood tests for toxins can be time consuming and should not be relied on for initial treatment. Serum electrolytes and ABGs can be determined rapidly and the anion gap and osmolar gap (see Salt and Water, sec. **IV**) can be calculated.

   a. **Normal osmolal gap**

      (1) **Diabetic ketoacidosis.** See Chap. 20.

      (2) **Alcoholic ketoacidosis** occurs after the abrupt discontinuation of ethanol consumption and is usually due to vomiting, malnutrition, and volume depletion. Beta-hydroxybutyrate initially predominates in the serum; hence, the nitroprusside ketone reaction (Acetest), which detects acetoacetic acid, can underestimate severity. As beta-hydroxybutyrate is metabolized to acetoacetate, the Acetest becomes increasingly positive, giving the false impression of worsening ketosis. Lactic acidosis may coexist. Serum glucose is typically normal or low. Treatment is directed at replacement of volume and glucose with 5%D/NS; the acidosis, unless severe, usually corrects with these measures. Hypokalemia, hypophosphatemia, and hypomagnesemia may occur, especially after 12–24 hours of therapy.

      (3) **Lactic acidosis** occurs with serum lactic acid levels of > 2–4 mEq/liter. As the level increases, prognosis worsens. Hyperphosphatemia, hyperuricemia, and moderate hyperkalemia can accompany the acidosis. **Type A** lactic acidosis results from inadequate tissue oxygenation as seen in shock, hypoxemia, severe anemia, and carbon monoxide poisoning. **Type B** lactic acidosis is seen in conditions without clinically apparent reduced tissue oxygenation, such as diabetes mellitus, liver or renal failure, neoplasms, sepsis, and drug intoxications (methanol, ethanol, ethylene glycol, salicylates, phenformin). Treatment should address the underlying cause of the lactic acidosis. The use of vasoconstrictor agents may exacerbate lactic acidosis and should be limited, if possible. Correction of serum pH to greater than 7.2 is unwise and can result in "overshoot alkalosis" since oxidation of lactate and endogenous regeneration of bicarbonate occurs once the cause of the lactic acidosis has been corrected. Therapy can be initiated by the administration of 50–100 mEq of sodium bicarbonate over 30–60 minutes as hypertonic $NaHCO_3$ or as an isotonic infusion. The hypernatremia and volume overload that can occur with sodium bicarbonate administration can be pre-

vented by aggressive diuresis. Dialysis may be required in patients with renal failure.

(4) Renal failure results in an AG acidosis only when the GFR falls below 20 ml/minute. Alkali replacement is administered to maintain a serum bicarbonate concentration of approximately 20 mEq/liter to prevent osteomalacia. Oral alkali of 1–2 mEq/kg/day is usually sufficient.

b. Increased osmolal gap. An increased osmolal gap (>10 mOsm/kg) is due to the presence of unmeasured osmotically active substances such as paraldehyde, ethylene glycol, ethanol, and methanol.

(1) Alcoholic acidosis. If enough ethanol remains in the blood, an increased osmolal gap will be present.

(2) Salicylate intoxication can result in respiratory alkalosis and lactic acidosis, in addition to an AG metabolic acidosis. Diagnosis and treatment are described in Chap. 26.

(3) Paraldehyde overdose has manifestations similar to those of ethanol intoxication (see Chap. 26). Treatment is also discussed in Chap. 26.

(4) Methanol ingestion results in symptoms in 12–24 hours. Methanol is metabolized to formic acid, causing optic nerve damage (with symptoms ranging from blurred vision to permanent blindness), nausea, vomiting, CNS depression, and respiratory failure. Treatment is aimed at preventing the formation of toxic levels of formic acid and correcting the acidosis. Details are provided in Chap. 26.

(5) Ethylene glycol is metabolized to aldehydes and oxalate, resulting in symptoms similar to those of ethanol intoxication. Acute tubular necrosis may occur. The diagnosis is suggested by oxalate crystals in the urine in the setting of a serum anion and osmolal gap. Treatment is discussed in Chap. 26.

2. Non-AG metabolic acidosis. The majority of these disorders can be treated with therapy directed at the underlying cause; attention should also be given to alkali therapy, potassium replacement, and volume status. Specific discussion of the RTAs follows (*Med. Clin. North Am.* 67:859, 1983).

a. Hypokalemic RTA

(1) Proximal, type II RTA is due to a reduction in the capacity of the proximal tubule to reclaim filtered bicarbonate. Causes include ingestion of heavy metals, certain inherited disorders, dysproteinemias, hyperparathyroidism, acetazolamide, and interstitial renal diseases. The bicarbonate wasting may occur as part of a generalized defect in proximal tubular transport (Fanconi syndrome) with associated glucosuria, aminoaciduria, hypophosphatemia, hypokalemia, and hypouricemia. Initially, the urine pH is greater than 5.5, but as the serum bicarbonate concentration falls, proximal tubular bicarbonate reabsorption becomes complete and the urine pH becomes normally acidic. **Treatment** should include attempts to correct the underlying cause. Large amounts of **alkali** (5–10 mEq/kg/day) are required. Of concern, alkali therapy can produce severe hypokalemia; aggressive **potassium** replacement may be needed. **Thiazide** diuretics can be used to increase proximal tubule bicarbonate reabsorption by inducing a mild ECF volume depletion.

(2) Distal, type I RTA is due to a defect in distal nephron acidification and is associated with potassium wasting, sodium wasting, hypercalciuria, osteomalacia, and nephrocalcinosis. Urine pH is greater than 5.5. It can occur as a congenital disorder; secondary causes include autoimmune disorders, nephrocalcinosis, amphotericin B, chronic pyelonephritis, and obstructive uropathy. **Treatment** consists of **bicarbonate** replacement (1–2 mEq/kg/day), which can also correct calcium wasting and osteomalacia. As with proximal RTA, potassium replacement may also be necessary.

b. Hyperkalemic distal RTA (type IV). Usually associated with some degree of renal insufficiency, this disorder is characterized by impaired distal nephron excretion of both hydrogen ions and potassium. Patients with this disorder have either mineralocorticoid deficiency or exhibit a renal resistance to mineralocorticoids.

(1) **Mineralocorticoid-sensitive hyperkalemic RTA** results from either primary aldosterone deficiency (primary hypoaldosteronism, Addison's disease, heparin sulfate) or from hyporeninemic hypoaldosteronism (diabetes mellitus, hypertensive nephrosclerosis, tubulointerstitial disease). Urine pH is less than 5.5. Dietary **potassium restriction** to 40–60 mEq/day and **bicarbonate supplementation**, 1.5–2.0 mEq/kg/day, are usually required. Chronic Kayexalate therapy may also be necessary. In patients with normal blood pressure, no edema, and an elevated serum potassium, **fludrocortisone** (Florinef), 0.1–0.2 mg PO qd, can be considered. In the setting of hypertension or edema, **furosemide** may be effective; if furosemide is ineffective and the serum potassium is greater than 6.0 mEq/liter, a cautious trial of fludrocortisone should be considered (with continued diuretics).

(2) **Mineralocorticoid-resistant hyperkalemic RTA** results from renal insensitivity to mineralocorticoids. Two categories of patients have been described. Those patients with **renal sodium wasting and ECF volume depletion** typically have normal–high serum aldosterone levels and are categorically unable to lower the urine pH. These patients can be managed with sodium chloride and bicarbonate supplementation, and with dietary potassium restriction. Conversely, those patients with **ECF volume expansion and hypertension** typically have suppressed renin and aldosterone levels; urine pH may be low. These patients are better managed with dietary NaCl and potassium restriction and with diuretic therapy.

V. **Metabolic alkalosis** occurs with either HCl losses (renal, GI), addition of bicarbonate to the blood, or ECF volume contraction around a fixed blood content of bicarbonate. Because the kidneys are normally capable of excreting a bicarbonate load, there must also be renal mechanisms in effect that maintain the elevated serum bicarbonate. This latter generally occurs as a result of ECF volume contraction, hypokalemia, and/or hypochloremia. Accordingly, both the underlying cause of the alkalosis and the cause of its renal perpetuation must be addressed when considering treatment. **Clinically,** metabolic alkalosis may produce impaired mentation, hypotension, cardiac arrhythmias, hypoventilation, hypokalemia, and a decreased ionized calcium. **Diagnostically,** it is useful to divide the causes of metabolic alkalosis according to the urinary chloride concentration. This in turn has therapeutic implications, as it dictates whether or not the alkalosis can be corrected by the administration of chloride (chloride-responsive vs. chloride-resistant alkalosis).

A. **Chloride-responsive alkalosis** with a urine chloride less than 10 mEq/liter is the more common variety of metabolic alkalosis; it is usually accompanied by ECF volume depletion. It may occur with gastrointestinal HCl losses (vomiting, nasogastric suction, villous adenoma, and congenital chloridorrhea), or with diuretic use (because of the associated ECF volume contraction and hypokalemia). Of note, acute diuretic therapy may actually raise the urinary chloride; this must be accounted for when evaluating a metabolic alkalosis. Posthypercapneic states due to persistent renal bicarbonate retention, excessive alkali administration, or multiple blood transfusions (citrate load) may also cause a chloride-responsive metabolic alkalosis. **Treatment** should be directed at correction of the underlying disorder. Correction of the chloride depletion can be achieved by administration of NaCl tablets or, if significant volume contraction is present, IV saline. Hypokalemia should be treated with potassium chloride. In the setting of volume overload and adequate renal function, acetazolamide, a carbonic anhydrase inhibitor that increases renal bicarbonate excretion, may be useful. The usual dosage is 250–500 mg PO or IV q8h. **Severe metabolic alkalosis** (pH >7.55) with clinically evident systemic effects should be treated with acid therapy, particularly if a contraindication to NaCl administration exists (e.g., HF, renal failure). The amount of acid that would theoretically correct the alkalosis is given by the following formula:

$$H^+ \text{ deficit (mEq)} = 0.5 \times \text{body wt (kg)} \times (\text{measured } [HCO_3{}^-] \\ - \text{ desired } [HCO_3{}^-])$$

One half of the deficit can be replaced over the first 12 hours and the remainder over the next 24 hours, as the clinical situation dictates. An HCl solution consisting of 150 ml of 1.0 N HCl in 1 liter of sterile water ($[H^+] = 130$ mEq/liter) can be administered via a central line (with the position radiographically confirmed) at a rate no greater than 0.2 mEq/kg/hour. Acid infusion should be accompanied by frequent measurements of ABGs and serum electrolytes (at least q4h). Gastric HCl losses may be attenuated with the use of either IV or PO H_2 antagonists. Lastly, in patients with renal failure, alkalosis can be corrected with hemodialysis.

   B. Chloride-resistant alkalosis with a urine chloride greater than 20 mEq/liter is much less common. Except for Bartter's syndrome and magnesium depletion, these patients are generally hypertensive and are not ECF volume depleted. Other causes include primary aldosteronism, Cushing's syndrome, renal artery stenosis, Liddle's syndrome, hypercalcemia, and severe hypokalemia. **Treatment** is directed at the underlying disorder. Potassium and magnesium deficits should be corrected. In states of mineralocorticoid excess, spironolactone may be helpful. Liddle's syndrome can be treated with triamterene and Bartter's syndrome with indomethacin (100–200 mg/day).

VI. Respiratory acidosis is caused by inadequate pulmonary excretion of CO_2. **Causes** include CNS depression (drugs, infection, brain injury), neuromuscular disorders (myopathy, Guillain-Barré syndrome), or pulmonary diseases (chronic obstructive pulmonary disease, asthma, kyphoscoliosis, pneumothorax). **Manifestations** include agitation, asterixis, papilledema, headache, somnolence, hypertension, tachycardia, HF, and cardiac arrhythmias.

   A. The diagnosis should be made when the ABGs reveal a decreased pH and an elevated PCO_2. It is important to determine whether the change in pH is appropriate for the change in PCO_2 in order to differentiate acute from chronic respiratory disturbances and to detect the presence of a mixed disorder (see Table 3-2). Renal compensation occurs over several days. In general, the compensated serum bicarbonate does not exceed 35 mEq/liter; if this occurs, a concomitant metabolic alkalosis is present.

   B. Treatment of respiratory acidosis is directed at improving ventilation (see Chap. 9). Administration of bicarbonate to correct the acidosis may be harmful, since the low pH is an important stimulus for ventilation.

VII. Respiratory alkalosis is due to excessive pulmonary CO_2 excretion (hyperventilation). **Causes** include CNS disorders (anxiety, brainstem tumors, infection), drugs (salicylates, theophylline, catecholamines, progestational drugs), hypoxemia (e.g., due to high altitudes or severe anemia), pulmonary disease (pneumonia, pulmonary emboli, pulmonary edema, interstitial lung disease), gram-negative sepsis, liver disease, pregnancy, and excessive ventilation from mechanical ventilators. Rapid correction of chronic metabolic acidosis can also produce a respiratory alkalosis because of the persistent and more slowly corrected CNS acidosis causing persistent hyperventilation. **Manifestations** include lightheadedness, paresthesias, tetany, syncope, seizures, and cardiac arrhythmias.

   A. The diagnosis should be made when the ABGs reveal an increased pH and a decreased PCO_2. One should determine whether there has been appropriate renal compensation; if not, a mixed disorder is present (see Table 3-2). The serum bicarbonate does not fall below 15 mEq/liter unless a concomitant metabolic acidosis is present.

   B. Treatment should be directed at the underlying disorder. Acute therapy is usually not necessary, unless the pH is greater than 7.5. If hypoxemia is not present, symptoms of acute hyperventilation may be relieved by reassurance and rebreathing into a paper bag. If PCO_2 is rapidly corrected in chronic respiratory alkalosis (as in readjustment of mechanical ventilator settings or rebreathing), metabolic acidosis will ensue because of the previous compensatory decrease in the serum bicarbonate concentration. If persistent hyperventilation occurs (such as in CNS disease or paradoxical CNS acidosis), the use of a CO_2-rebreathing apparatus may be warranted.

VIII.   Mixed acid–base disturbances (*Medicine* 59:161, 1980) are common in the acutely ill patient and can often be predicted from the clinical situation. Careful evaluation of the compensatory changes of the pH, PCO_2, and HCO_3^- is necessary. Measurement of serum electrolytes and calculation of the anion gap must also be performed. The treatment of mixed acid–base disorders should be directed at the underlying pathologic processes.

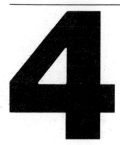

Hypertension

Nancy R. Baird

Definitions and Diagnostic Evaluation

I. **Systemic hypertension (HTN)** affects approximately 20% of white and 30% of black Americans 18 years of age or older. The prevalence of HTN increases with age, affecting greater than 50% of all persons over 65 years of age (*Am. Heart J.* 114:918, 1987). HTN is the most significant risk factor for the development of atherosclerotic coronary artery disease. Of the yearly toll from cardiovascular morbidity and mortality, 35–45% is directly attributable to HTN (*Am. Heart J.* 114:918, 1987). Adult **systolic-diastolic HTN** is arbitrarily defined as a BP of 140/90 mm Hg or greater. More than 90% of hypertensive individuals have **essential HTN,** defined as an elevation of BP in the absence of an identifiable cause. Nearly 80% of adults with essential HTN have **mild HTN,** characterized by a diastolic blood pressure (DBP) of 90–104 mm Hg. The remaining individuals have **moderate HTN** (DBP of 105–114 mm Hg) or **severe HTN** (DBP ≥115 mm Hg). Patients with a recent substantial increase in BP above their baseline value sufficient to cause acute damage to retinal vessels (i.e., hemorrhages, exudates, or papilledema) are considered to have **accelerated-malignant HTN,** irrespective of the absolute level of BP (*Br. Med. J.* 292:235, 1986); the DBP is usually greater than 140 mm Hg. Fewer than 10% of hypertensive patients have **secondary HTN** (e.g., HTN associated with the use of oral contraceptives or corticosteroids, renovascular or renal parenchymal disease, pheochromocytoma, Cushing's syndrome, primary hyperaldosteronism, hyperparathyroidism, or coarctation of the aorta).

II. **Isolated systolic hypertension (ISH),** defined as systolic blood pressure (SBP) greater than 160 mm Hg and DBP less than 90 mm Hg, is an established risk factor for cerebrovascular and ischemic heart disease. It is a distinct pathophysiologic entity that usually begins in the fifth decade and involves up to 11% of the population at age 75 (*Cardiovasc. Clin.* 20:65, 1990). ISH is associated with a progressive reduction in vascular compliance, subsequently causing a gradual rise in systolic pressure with age.

III. **Initial clinical evaluation.** Optimum indirect measurement of BP requires that the size of the sphygmomanometer cuff be appropriate for the circumference of the arm. In addition, BP measurements should be taken with the arm supported at the level of the heart because readings obtained with the arm in a dependent position may result in values that are higher by as much as 10 mm Hg. One should be careful to avoid spuriously low SBP readings due to an auscultatory gap, which is caused by the disappearance and reappearance of Korotkoff sounds in hypertensive patients and may account for up to a 25-mm gap between true BP and measured BP. Elevated BP is usually discovered in asymptomatic individuals during a routine screening examination. To establish the diagnosis of HTN, the physician should average several BP measurements during the initial clinical visit, with the patient as relaxed as possible. A thorough history should be obtained, with careful attention to the use of drugs that might interfere with BP control (e.g., decongestants, oral contraceptives, appetite suppressants, nonsteroidal anti-inflammatory agents, exogenous thyroid hormone, and alcohol consumption). Physical examination should focus on end-organ damage and clues suggestive of secondary causes. Patients with mild BP elevation should have BP measurements repeated within 1–2 months, and individuals with moderate BP elevation should be rechecked within 1–2 weeks of the initial visit. Patients with severe or accelerated-malignant HTN should be treated immediately (see Special Problems, sec. I), as should patients with evidence of end-organ damage (e.g., left ventricular hypertrophy [LVH]).

IV. **Laboratory evaluation** should include urinalysis, hematocrit, plasma glucose, potassium, creatinine, fasting serum cholesterol and triglycerides, calcium, uric acid, chest x-ray, and an ECG. Additional diagnostic testing for the evaluation of secondary causes of HTN may be indicated in the following situations: (1) onset of HTN before 30 years of age and after 60 years of age, (2) HTN that is difficult to control, (3) HTN that no longer responds to therapy, (4) patients with accelerated or malignant HTN, and (5) patients with signs or symptoms of secondary HTN (*Arch. Intern. Med.* 148:1023, 1988). The prevalence of secondary causes of HTN depends on a patient's initial presentation. In one study, 23% of patients with accelerated-malignant HTN had renovascular HTN (*N. Engl. J. Med.* 301:1273, 1979).

Therapeutic Considerations

I. **General considerations.** The treatment goal of hypertension is to prevent the long-term sequelae of the disease. Most patients require lifelong antihypertensive therapy, although a significant percentage of individuals may maintain normal BP after discontinuation of drug treatment. Unless there is an overt need for immediate pharmacologic therapy, most patients should be given the opportunity to achieve a spontaneous reduction of their BP over a closely followed interval of 4–6 months. The primary therapeutic goal is the reduction of BP to less than 140/90 mm Hg in systolic-diastolic HTN and to less than 160/90mm Hg in ISH. In the absence of hypertensive crisis, BP should be reduced gradually to avoid complications such as cerebral ischemia. **Adequate patient education is an essential component of the treatment plan,** as it promotes patient compliance. Physicians should emphasize that (1) lifelong treatment is usually required, (2) symptoms are an unreliable gauge of the severity of HTN, and (3) prognosis improves with adequate management. Cultural and other individual differences among patients must be considered when planning a therapeutic regimen (see below).

A. **Systolic-diastolic HTN.** In the United States, all patients with DBP of 90 mm Hg or greater are considered candidates for drug therapy. Alternatively, the World Health Organization and the International Society of Hypertension recommend that after 3–6 months of observation, a DBP of 95 mm Hg or greater be used as the level at which to begin active drug intervention (*Bull. W.H.O.* 64:31, 1986). The treatment of all degrees of hypertension reduces the morbidity and mortality associated with strokes, renal insufficiency, congestive heart failure (CHF), and progression of HTN (*Cardiovasc. Clin.* 20:49, 1990). The incidence of fatal acute myocardial infarction (MI) is reduced by treatment of moderate to severe HTN (*Lancet* 1:1349, 1985), but there is no prospective evidence that antihypertensive therapy in mild HTN has been effective in reducing the incidence of coronary events (*Br. Med. J.* 291:97, 1985). Concomitant cardiovascular risk factors (e.g., glucose intolerance, smoking, hypercholesterolemia, and left ventricular hypertrophy) should also be evaluated. Caution should precede the use of medications that may adversely affect glucose intolerance, lipid metabolism, or other cardiovascular risk factors. A short trial (2–4 months) of nonpharmacologic therapy may be appropriate for patients with mild HTN who lack evidence of end-organ damage. Drug therapy should be added to nonpharmacologic modalities when the patient profile includes failure of nondrug modalities alone, presence of end-organ damage, or major risk factors for coronary artery disease.

B. **Isolated systolic HTN.** ISH is associated with a two- to fivefold increase in risk of death from all causes and a two- to threefold increase in cardiovascular disease (*Circulation* 61:1179, 1980). A reasonable objective would be to reduce

SBP to less than 160 mm Hg while avoiding side effects; nonpharmacologic therapy should be attempted initially.

II. **Nonpharmacologic therapy** (*Med. Clin. North Am.* 71:921, 1987). Identification and control of other cardiovascular risk factors are strongly indicated for all hypertensive patients. Although smoking has not been shown to cause HTN, physicians should advise their patients who smoke that the most effective measure in reducing their overall cardiovascular risk is to stop smoking. In certain clinical situations, nondrug therapy may be effective in lowering BP.

A. **Weight reduction** should be strongly encouraged in patients who weigh more than 115% of their ideal body weight. A considerable fall in BP may actually occur before ideal body weight is reached. In addition, improvements in cholesterol profile and regression of LVH have been documented in hypertensive patients managed with weight reduction (*N. Engl. J. Med.* 314:334, 1986). Upper-body obesity is an independent risk factor for coronary heart disease (CHD), and the risk is compounded by associated HTN, hypertriglyceridemia, and hyperinsulinemia (*Arch. Intern. Med.* 149:1514, 1989).

B. **Saturated fat intake** should be reduced. A decrease in dietary saturated fat alone or in combination with increased polyunsaturated fat induces a modest reduction in BP (*Prev. Med.* 14:573, 1985).

C. **Alcohol consumption** should be moderated. In large amounts, ethanol clearly has a direct vasopressor effect. Reduction of consumption to less than three drinks per day (30 ml distilled spirits) reduces BP in treated hypertensive patients (*Clin. Exp. Pharmacol. Physiol.* 13:315, 1986). Hypertensive patients should therefore be advised to reduce their ethanol intake.

D. **Regular dynamic exercise** should be advised if the clinical situation permits. Repeated periods of moderately intense dynamic exercise, such as walking, running, or swimming, result in a significant reduction in BP independent of weight loss or altered sodium excretion (*Lancet* 2:473, 1986). Exercise should be performed at least three times per week for at least 30 minutes at a heart rate of 65–70% of a patient's predicted maximal rate. Patients with known coronary artery disease, or a history suggestive of it, and those over 40 years of age with multiple risk factors for coronary disease should undergo exercise stress testing before beginning exercise training.

E. **Sodium restriction** is controversial but appears to be an effective and safe means of lowering BP modestly in some hypertensive patients over 40 years of age (*Br. Med. J.* 293:27, 1986). The efficacy of calcium, magnesium, or potassium supplementation as well as relaxation therapy is unproven but may be helpful in some patients.

III. **Pharmacologic therapy**

A. **Initial drug therapy.** Currently, diuretics, beta-adrenergic antagonists, calcium antagonists, and angiotensin-converting enzyme (ACE) inhibitors are all regarded as initial agents. Unless there is a contraindication to their use, calcium antagonists and ACE inhibitors are good first-choice agents because of their low side effect profile. The majority of patients with mild to moderate hypertension can attain adequate BP control with single-drug therapy. The drug of first choice may be affected by coexistent factors, such as age, race, angina, heart failure (HF), left ventricular hypertrophy (LVH), diabetes, obesity, hyperlipidemia, gout, and bronchospastic or peripheral vascular disease. Blood pressure response is usually consistent within a given class of agents; therefore, if a drug fails to control BP, it is unlikely that another agent from the same class will be effective. At times, however, a change within a drug class may be useful in reducing adverse side effects.

B. **Additional therapy.** More severe cases may require the stepwise addition of drugs from two different classes and, rarely, from a third. If a second drug is needed, it can generally be chosen from among the other first-line agents. Central alpha agonists, minoxidil, hydralazine, and peripherally acting antiadrenergic agents are now generally used as reserve agents.

C. **Adjustment of therapeutic regimen.** When considering a modification of therapy because of inadequate response to the current regimen, the physician should investigate other possible contributing factors. **Poor patient compliance,** use of antagonistic drugs (i.e., sympathomimetics, antidepressants, steroids, nonsteroidal anti-inflammatory agents [NSAIDs]), or increased alcohol intake should be excluded before dosage increases are prescribed. Unacceptable side effects from a particular agent may contribute to poor patient compliance and may require alterations of the antihypertensive regimen. Excessive fluid retention should be evaluated and treated. Continued patient education is imperative. Secondary causes of HTN need to be considered when the aforementioned factors have been carefully excluded.

D. **Individualized approach to therapy based on pathophysiologic profile.** A vast array of effective antihypertensive agents are available. Consideration of an individual's pathogenic derangement of renin secretion, sympathetic tone, and renal sodium secretion as well as the attendant changes in cardiac output, peripheral vascular resistance, and volume status is helpful in making logical therapeutic choices.

1. **The young hypertensive patient** is generally characterized as an active individual with increased sympathetic tone and elevated plasma renin activity; extracellular fluid volume is usually normal or decreased. Thus, ACE inhibitors, combined beta-alpha antagonists, calcium channel antagonists, and alpha$_1$ selective antagonists are preferred. Beta-adrenergic antagonists alone are also effective but may adversely affect high-density lipoprotein (HDL) cholesterol, cause sexual dysfunction, or impede physical-athletic performance by reducing cardiac output.

2. **The elderly hypertensive patient** (60 years and older) often has coexisting medical problems that may modify the selection of initial antihypertensive therapy. Increased vascular resistance is the hallmark of HTN in the elderly, and, in general, these patients have reduced plasma renin activity and greater LVH than younger patients. Diuretics are often chosen as initial therapy and have been shown to decrease the incidence of stroke, HF, and fatal MI in this age group (*Lancet* 1:1349, 1985). Calcium antagonists decrease vascular resistance, have no adverse effects on lipid levels, and are, therefore, good choices for the elderly patient. ACE inhibitors can be used but theoretically are not ideal because of lower serum renin levels in this population. Beta-adrenergic antagonists generally should be avoided because they increase peripheral resistance, decrease cardiac output (CO), and decrease HDL cholesterol (*Ann. Intern. Med.* 110:901, 1989). Agents that produce postural hypotension (i.e., prazosin, guanethidine, guanadrel) should be avoided. Central alpha agonists are generally effective in elderly hypertensive patients. Postural hypotension is rare but sedation occurs commonly. In **elderly patients with ISH,** the data currently support using low doses of diuretics (e.g., chlorthalidone or hydrochlorothiazide) as initial therapy. If a contraindication to diuretics exists, a calcium antagonist, sustained-release nitrate, or ACE inhibitor can be used. Labetalol is well tolerated in low doses, and, because of its alpha$_1$ blocking activity and intrinsic sympathomimetic activity [ISA], it can be used in elderly patients with slow heart rates and arterial insufficiency or mild left ventricular (LV) dysfunction (*Acta Med. Scand.* 212:129, 1983). Therapy should be initiated with smaller than usual doses and adjustments should be made at longer intervals.

3. **Black hypertensive patients** generally have a lower renin level, higher plasma volume, and higher vascular resistance than white patients. Thus, blacks respond well to diuretics alone or in combination with calcium antagonists. ACE inhibitors can also be used in this population. The beta antagonist labetalol has been shown to be particularly effective.

4. **The obese hypertensive patient** is characterized by more modest elevations of vascular resistance, higher cardiac output, expanded intravascular volume, and lower plasma renin activity at any given level of arterial pressure. Even though these patients respond to diuretics, weight reduction is a primary goal of therapy and has been shown to be effective in reducing BP and causing regression of LVH.

5. **The hypertensive diabetic with nephropathy** poses a difficult management problem. Control of blood pressure is the only intervention shown to slow loss of renal function. First-line antihypertensive agents in diabetic patients include ACE inhibitors, calcium antagonists, and alpha antagonists. Although the benefit remains controversial, in hypertensive patients with diabetic nephropathy ACE inhibitors have been shown to increase glomerular filtration rate (GFR) and decrease proteinuria. Therefore, ACE inhibitors should be considered in these patients unless there is a contraindication (*Cardiovasc. Clin.* 6:547, 1988).

6. **The hypertensive patient with LVH** is at increased risk for cardiac arrhythmias and sudden death. Although there is no direct evidence, regression of LVH could be expected to reduce this risk. Agents that have been shown to decrease left ventricular mass in humans are: (1) centrally active adrenergic agonists, (2) ACE inhibitors, and (3) calcium antagonists. Diuretics, alpha-adrenergic antagonists, and direct-acting vasodilators have not been shown to cause a reduction in LVH. Beta antagonists and clonidine have shown conflicting results (*Cardiovasc. Clin.* 20:85, 1990).

IV. Special considerations of therapy

A. **Withdrawal syndrome.** Most patients experience a gradual return of HTN following discontinuation of antihypertensive therapy. Nevertheless, when substituting therapy in patients with moderate to severe HTN, it is reasonable to increase dosages of the new medication in small increments while tapering the previous medication to avoid excessive BP fluctuations. In patients with mild HTN, substitution therapy can be accomplished more quickly. In the case of the **acute withdrawal syndrome (AWS),** HTN develops within 24–72 hours. The rise in BP may occur with or without symptoms and signs of increased sympathetic activity. In a few patients, BP may rise to levels much greater than baseline values (overshoot). The most severe complications of the AWS include encephalopathy, cerebrovascular accident, MI, and sudden death. The AWS is most commonly associated with central-acting agents (clonidine > methyldopa > guanabenz) and beta-adrenergic antagonists (propranolol > metoprolol > pindolol); diuretics may rarely cause this syndrome. These drugs should be tapered over several days to weeks when discontinuing therapy and should be avoided in the noncompliant patient. Management of AWS by reinstitution of the previously administered drug is generally effective. Beta-adrenergic antagonists are contraindicated in AWS caused by clonidine-like drugs because BP may be further increased by unopposed stimulation of alpha-adrenergic receptors. Labetalol, however, has alpha-adrenergic antagonist properties in addition to beta-adrenergic antagonist activity and is therefore useful in the treatment of AWS. Sodium nitroprusside (see Special Problems, sec. **I.A.1**) is the treatment of choice when parenteral administration of an antihypertensive agent is required or the identity of the previously discontinued drug is unknown (*Am. Heart J.* 102:415, 1981).

B. **Secondary serum lipid abnormalities** have been associated with several classes of antihypertensive agents. Thiazide, loop, and potassium-sparing diuretics have been shown to raise serum concentrations of total cholesterol, low-density or very low density lipoprotein (VLDL) cholesterol, and triglyceride levels in short- and long-term studies. The average rise in total cholesterol is 10 mg/dl. Indapamide appears to lack any dyslipidemic properties (*Am J. Cardiol.* 65:11H, 1990). Although there is variation between beta-adrenergic antagonists, most studies indicate that both nonselective and beta$_1$-selective agents increase plasma triglyceride levels and lower HDL. The increase in triglycerides may reach 20–30% above pretreatment levels, whereas HDL cholesterol may decrease by as much as 5-10%. Beta-adrenergic antagonists that possess intrinsic sympathomimetic activity (i.e., oxprenolol, pindolol, and acebutolol) or alpha-antagonist properties (i.e., labetalol) appear to have little or no effect on VLDL and HDL cholesterol. Some antihypertensive agents may favorably affect lipid profiles. Clonidine, guanabenz, guanfacine, and diltiazem have, in limited studies, been shown to have salutary effects on lipid levels. Selective alpha$_1$-adrenergic antagonists (prazosin, doxazosin, terazosin, and trimazosin) have demonstrated neutral or favorable lipid changes. Prazosin has averaged a 12% decrease in the total cholesterol/HDL cholesterol ratio (*Am. Heart J.* 114:998, 1987). ACE inhibitors and nifedipine have caused no significant changes in lipid levels in short-term studies. Although it is not known whether adverse changes in lipid levels induced by pharmacologic antihypertensive therapy alter the risk of coronary artery disease, it is reasonable to consider these effects when selecting antihypertensive agents. These considerations may apply particularly in young patients with mild HTN or in patients with preexisting lipid disorders in whom the benefits of lifelong antihypertensive treatment may be offset by the enhanced cardiovascular risk of prolonged exposure to altered serum lipid levels.

Antihypertensive Agents

I. **Calcium channel antagonists** cause direct arteriolar vasodilation by selective inhibition of slow inward calcium channels in vascular smooth muscle. These agents may also cause an initial natriuresis, obviating the need for concurrent diuretic therapy. Diltiazem and verapamil exhibit negative inotropic, chronotropic, and dromotropic effects on cardiac function. Nifedipine also has cardiodepressant action, but the clinical effect is often negligible, due to concurrent reduction of systemic vascular resistance and reflex increases in adrenergic tone; it can be used safely with beta-adrenergic antagonists. Caution should be exercised in combining therapy with calcium channel antagonists and alpha antagonists (e.g., prazosin), as excessive hypotension may occur. Therapeutic doses of calcium antagonists do not affect glucose tolerance, lipoproteins, uric acid, or serum electrolytes. These drugs are effective when used as single agents in almost all populations, although blood pressure reductions are greater in older patients. Calcium antagonists from the various subclasses have been shown to cause regression of LVH in hypertensive patients. Nifedipine has been used as an alternative agent in the therapy of severe HTN and hypertensive emergencies (see Special Problems). Nifedipine, verapamil, and diltiazem are metabolized by the liver and circulate highly protein bound. The half-life of verapamil and diltiazem is prolonged in patients with cirrhosis and the dosing interval should be adjusted accordingly.

A. **Nifedipine,** 10–40 mg PO tid, may be particularly useful in patients with myocardial ischemia and HTN. A sustained-release preparation, 30–120 mg PO qd, is available and may improve patient compliance. When used for isolated systolic HTN of the elderly, the initial dose should be reduced to 5 mg to avoid possible hypotension. The incidence of palpitations, flushing, or headache due to nifedipine is significantly reduced by the concomitant use of a beta-adrenergic antagonist. Ankle edema may also occur, but does not generally reflect systemic fluid retention. Nifedipine does not appreciably affect serum digoxin levels. This drug should not be used in patients with aortic stenosis, obstructive cardiomyopathy, or severe myocardial depression. Nifedipine can be administered sublingually in patients with hypertensive urgency (see Special Problems, sec. **I.B.1**).

B. **Verapamil,** 120–480 mg PO daily (divided in 3 doses), is not generally used with beta-adrenergic antagonists or other negative inotropic agents (e.g., disopyramide) because of additive cardiodepressant effects. It should be administered judiciously to patients with mild to moderate myocardial dysfunction and avoided in patients with HF. Verapamil may cause digitalis toxicity as a result of a reduction in digoxin clearance. Serum digoxin levels generally increase 50–70% within 1 week of initiating therapy with verapamil (*Am. Heart J.* 108:412, 1984). The maintenance dosage of digoxin should be reduced by 50% when verapamil is given and serum levels should be monitored. Verapamil should not be used in patients with (1) second- or third-degree atrioventricular (AV) block, (2) the sick sinus syndrome (without a pacemaker in place), or (3) atrial flutter/fibrillation who have an accessory bypass tract. The major noncardiovascular side effect of verapamil is constipation, which can be especially problematic in elderly patients. Reversible hepatic dysfunction has been reported; therefore, during therapy with verapamil, it is wise to periodically monitor liver enzymes. Cimetidine may reduce the clearance of verapamil. Sustained-release formulations of verapamil, 120–360 mg qd or bid, are available, are dosage equivalent, and provide a simplified dosing schedule.

C. **Diltiazem,** 120–360 mg PO daily (divided into 3 or 4 doses), has side effects similar to those of verapamil, but the negative inotropic and chronotropic effects are less. Sustained-release preparations are available that allow simplified dosing (60–180 mg PO bid). Serum digoxin levels may increase by as much as 22% over 48 hours when diltiazem is added to a drug regimen. Contraindications are comparable to those for verapamil, although myocardial depression may be less marked. Mild sinoatrial (SA) and AV node depression, resulting in bradycardia and prolongation of the PR interval, often accompany therapy with diltiazem. If asymptomatic, mild bradycardia and PR prolongation do not require discontinuation of diltiazem therapy. Diltiazem and a beta antagonist can be used in combination; however, patients should be carefully observed for excessive bradycardia, AV node blockage, or hypotension. The overall incidence of noncardiac side effects is less with diltiazem and verapamil than with nifedipine.

D. **Nicardipine,** 30–120 mg PO daily (divided in 3 doses), is structurally related to nifedipine but has increased selectivity for coronary and peripheral arteries. Nicardipine has little apparent negative inotropic, chronotropic, or dromotropic effects. It has been shown to have hypotensive effects equal to other calcium channel antagonists. The most common side effects are peripheral edema, flushing, and headache. Studies have shown that nicardipine produces no adverse effect on the lipid profile and does not reduce renal blood flow (*J. Clin. Pharmacol.* 29:481, 1989). Nicardipine would therefore be useful in patients with both cardiac and renal disease.

E. **Isradipine,** 2.5–10.0 mg PO bid, is pharmacologically similar to nicardipine. No detrimental cardiac conduction system abnormalities have been documented. Bioavailability is increased in (1) patients over 65 years of age, (2) patients with mild chronic renal failure, and (3) patients with hepatic insufficiency. Therefore, in these situations smaller doses should probably be used. Adverse reactions include headache, fatigue, edema, and dizziness, and appear to be dose related. Constipation may be less frequent than with verapamil. Clearance of digitalis is not affected by concomitant administration of isradipine.

II. **Angiotensin-converting enzyme inhibitors** lower BP by decreasing peripheral vascular resistance with little change in CO, HR, or GFR. Postulated mechanisms of action include (1) decreases in vasoconstrictor angiotensin-II levels; (2) reduced secretion of aldosterone, which induces a natriuresis; (3) increases in vasodilator bradykinin or prostaglandin levels; and (4) specific renal vasodilation with subsequent enhanced natriuresis. These agents are especially useful in patients with high-renin and renovascular HTN and for severe refractory HTN. Caution should be observed in patients who may have severe HTN secondary to bilateral renal artery stenosis (RAS) or RAS of a solitary kidney. ACE inhibitors are considered the treatment of choice in scleroderma renal crisis. In mild to moderate HTN, these agents can be used as monotherapy even in low-renin hypertensives (i.e., the elderly and blacks [*Clin. Pharmacol. Ther.* 34:297, 1983]). Alternatively, they can be used in combination with beta-adrenergic antagonists, calcium antagonists, or thiazide diuretics. The hypokalemia, hypercholesterolemia, hyperglycemia, and hyperuricemia induced by diuretic therapy can be significantly reduced by the addition of ACE inhibitors (*Med. Clin. North Am.* 71:979, 1987). In patients with **diabetic nephropathy and HTN,** ACE inhibitors may be preferable to beta-adrenergic antagonists or diuretics because glucose regulation is unaltered, renal function is protected, and proteinuria is reduced (*N. Engl. J. Med.* 313:1617, 1985; *Br. Med. J.* 293:467, 471, 1986). A major advantage of ACE inhibitors is their lack of symptomatic side effects. The use of these agents is associated with regression of established LVH in hypertensive patients. A dry cough not associated with asthmatic symptoms is a side effect common to all ACE inhibitors and may be more common with the longer-acting agents.

A. **Captopril,** 25–75 mg PO bid (tid or qid in the presence of HF), produces satisfactory BP responses in smaller doses than originally recommended. Maximum effect is achieved within 60–90 minutes after an oral dose, with the duration of effect being dose dependent. It is excreted primarily by the kidneys; dosage should be regulated carefully in renal insufficiency. Patients who are receiving potent diuretics or who are likely to be volume depleted require careful initiation of therapy with smaller doses (i.e., 6.25–12.5 mg) or temporary discontinuation of diuretic therapy in order to prevent an exaggerated hypotensive response. Diuretics should be added if the BP response to ACE inhibitors is insufficient. **Potassium-sparing diuretics should be avoided** because they may potentiate the hyperkalemic effects of ACE inhibitors. Most side effects are uncommon provided that the total daily dose is 150 mg or less. Adverse reactions include rash, dysgeusia, cough, and proteinuria. Membranous glomerulonephritis has been associated with captopril therapy. Thus, if new-onset proteinuria exceeds 1 g/day, captopril should be discontinued. Reversible neutropenia occurs in fewer than 1% of patients and is common with higher dosages or with preexisting collagen vascular diseases. Urine dipstick protein, WBC counts, and serum potassium should be monitored monthly for several months after initiation of therapy. Hyperkalemia may occur in patients with underlying renal insufficiency. Severe reversible azotemia has been reported in patients with bilateral renal artery stenosis (*N. Engl. J. Med.* 308:373, 1983) or renal artery stenosis in the presence of a single kidney.

B. **Enalapril,** 2.5–40.0 mg PO qd (in 1 or 2 doses), is a prodrug and is metabolized in the liver to form the active drug enalaprilat. Enalaprilat can be administered intravenously (1.25 mg q6h) for patients who are unable to take oral medications. The absence of the sulfhydryl group in its structure differentiates enalapril from captopril, which theoretically lessens the risk of immunologically mediated side effects. Angioedema may occur in 0.2% of patients. Dosage should be adjusted in the presence of renal failure.

C. **Lisinopril,** 10–40 mg PO daily in a single dose, is a long-acting derivative of enalapril that requires no hepatic activation. Dosage should be adjusted in the presence of renal insufficiency. Optimal BP response may require 2–4 weeks of therapy.

D. **Fosinopril,** 10–80 mg PO qd in a single dose, is metabolized similarly to enalapril. It is excreted equally by the liver and kidney. Therefore, dosage adjustments in patients with renal insufficiency are not required because hepatobiliary elimination compensates for reduced renal clearance. Adverse effects are comparable to those of captopril.

E. **Ramipril,** 2.5–20 mg PO qd (in 1 or 2 doses), is metabolized into active metabolites in the liver and subsequently excreted by the kidney. Therefore, dose adjustment is necessary when GFR is less than 40 ml/min. The side effect profile is also similar to that of captopril.

III. **Diuretics** (see Table 4-1 for doses of diuretics)

A. **Thiazide diuretics,** until recently, have been considered the initial drugs advocated for the treatment of mild hypertension. They remain the preferred initial treatment for certain groups of hypertensives (i.e., blacks, the elderly, and the obese). The mechanism of action depends on an initial natriuresis and reduction in plasma volume. A sustained reduction of total vascular resistance is produced with chronic therapy. These drugs are all effective antihypertensive agents, but their full effect may require several weeks to become manifest. Thiazides are not effective diuretics when the GFR is less than 25 ml/min and should be replaced in this situation by a more potent diuretic, such as furosemide or metolazone. In general, little therapeutic advantage is conferred by dosages larger than those listed in Table 4-1, and the risk of adverse metabolic effects is increased. Longer-acting drugs, such as chlorthalidone, may also increase the risk of hypokalemia. Physical side effects may include weakness, muscle cramps, and impotence. Metabolic side effects (e.g., hypokalemia, hypomagnesemia, hyperuricemia, hypercalcemia, hyperglycemia, hyponatremia, hyperlipidemia, and rarely azotemia) are generally mild but may require careful monitoring in

Table 4-1. Antihypertensive doses of diuretics

Diuretic	Daily dosage (mg)
Thiazides	
Bendroflumethiazide (Naturetin)	2.5–5.0
Benzthiazide (Aquatag, Exna)	12.5–50.0
Chlorothiazide (Diuril)	250–500
Cyclothiazide (Anhydron)	1.0–2.0
Hydrochlorothiazide (Esidrix, HydroDiuril, Oretic)	12.5–50.0
Hydroflumethiazide (Saluron)	12.5–50.0
Methyclothiazide (Enduron)	2.5–5.0
Polythiazide (Renese)	1.0–4.0
Trichlormethiazide (Metahydrin, Naqua)	1.0–4.0
Related sulfonamide compounds	
Chlorthalidone (Hygroton)	12.5–50.0
Indapamide (Lozol)	2.5–5.0
Metolazone (Zaroxolyn, Diulo)	1.0–5.0
Quinethazone (Hydromox)	50–100
Loop diuretics	
Bumetanide (Bumex)	0.5–10.0
Ethracrynic acid (Edecrin)	25–200
Furosemide (Lasix)	20–600
Potassium-sparing agents	
Amiloride (Midamor)	5.0–10.0
Spironolactone (Aldactone)	25–400
Triamterene (Dyrenium)	50–100

Source: Modified from N. Kaplan. Systemic Hypertension: Therapy. In N. Kaplan, *Heart Disease* (3rd ed.). Philadelphia: Saunders, 1988. P. 870.

certain patients. Thiazide-induced pancreatitis and an increased risk for lithium toxicity, secondary to reduced renal clearance of lithium, have been reported. Because of a relatively high incidence of side effects, the risk–benefit ratio of these agents is increasingly questioned.

B. **Loop diuretics,** such as **furosemide,** 20–600 mg PO qd (in 1 or 2 doses), have not been shown to be superior to thiazides in the chronic therapy of essential HTN. However, furosemide is the diuretic of choice in patients with impaired renal function (GFR <25 ml/min), in hypertensive emergencies (where it can be used parenterally as adjunctive therapy), and in cases of HTN with fluid retention resistant to thiazides. An oral dose generally initiates diuresis within 30 minutes, with a sustained effect lasting 4–6 hours. Increased venous capacitance is an early beneficial effect of intravenous furosemide in patients with congestive heart failure. Synergism between furosemide and metolazone has been observed in patients with resistant HTN. **Ethacrynic acid,** 25–200 mg PO qd, and **bumetanide,** 0.5–2.0 mg PO qd, have activity similar to furosemide. The most frequent adverse reactions to loop diuretics include volume depletion, hyperuricemia, and hypokalemia. At higher doses, they may be ototoxic, particularly in patients with renal insufficiency. These drugs are contraindicated in states of electrolyte depletion, in women of childbearing potential, and in persons with hypersensitivity. These agents may have adverse effects on serum lipids.

C. **Potassium-sparing diuretics** should be considered when maintenance of normal levels of serum potassium is essential (e.g., in patients with ischemic heart disease, known arrhythmias, poor tolerance of oral potassium supplements, or disease states requiring chronic digitalis therapy). These agents are relatively weak diuretics and are generally used as adjunctive therapy with a more potent diuretic, such as hydrochlorothiazide in the form of a fixed-combination tablet or capsule. These agents are especially useful in refractory edematous conditions due to secondary hyperaldosteronism (congestive heart failure, hepatic cirrhosis, and the nephrotic syndrome). The most serious adverse effect of these drugs is hyperkalemia; thus, they should be avoided in patients with impaired renal function, in those taking potassium supplements or ACE inhibitors, and in diabetics with or without recognized renal insufficiency. Elderly patients and patients with impaired potassium homeostatic mechanisms should have serum potassium, sodium, and creatinine levels monitored frequently, especially during initiation of therapy.

1. **Spironolactone,** 25–400 mg PO qd in single or divided doses, is a competitive antagonist of aldosterone and also inhibits its synthesis. This drug is most useful in conditions associated with hyperaldosteronism. It does not cause hyperglycemia or hyperuricemia; thus, it may be useful in patients who are prone to these adverse effects of thiazides. The drug should be administered for a minimum of 2 weeks before the dosage is adjusted in order to permit adequate assessment of therapeutic response. Adverse effects include prolongation of the half-life of digoxin, gastrointestinal irritation, lethargy, gynecomastia, impotence, and amenorrhea.

2. **Triamterene,** 50–150 mg PO qd (in 1 or 2 doses), directly inhibits Na^+, K^+, and H^+ ion exchange in the distal renal tubule by a mechanism independent of aldosterone. Use of triamterene as a single agent is rarely adequate.

3. **Amiloride,** 5–10 mg PO qd, has a mechanism of action similar to that of triamterene and a rapid onset of action (2–4 hours). However, its maximum effect may not be seen for several days. This drug is useful in patients with hepatic insufficiency who have adequate renal function because it is excreted unchanged into the urine.

D. **Indapamide,** 2.5–5.0 mg PO qd, is a methylindoline diuretic with vasodilatory action. Its effect on blood pressure and edema is similar to that of other diuretics. It reduces peripheral vascular resistance without affecting CO. No adverse effects on serum lipids have been documented. Unlike thiazides, there is little or no effect on renal blood flow. However, its diuretic action decreases with declining renal function. Side effects include hypokalemia, hyperuricemia, hyperglycemia, and volume depletion. It should not be used in renal or hepatic failure.

E. **Potassium supplementation.** Although thiazide-induced hypokalemia has not clearly been shown to influence cardiovascular mortality, increased ventricular ectopic activity has been documented in hypokalemic patients with ischemic heart disease and after an acute MI (*Am. J. Cardiol.* 57:34F, 1986). In addition, hypokalemia may be responsible for the muscle weakness and glucose intolerance observed with diuretic therapy. Prevention of hypokalemia may be accomplished by using a potassium-sparing diuretic. If a second antihypertensive agent is required, adding an ACE inhibitor or beta antagonist to a thiazide diuretic will reduce the risk of hypokalemia by inhibiting diuretic-induced hyperaldosteronism. Potassium supplementation is recommended (1) in symptomatic hypokalemia, (2) in patients with an abnormal resting ECG, (3) when a history of arrhythmias or ischemic heart disease is noted, (4) during concomitant digitalis therapy, and (5) with planned general anesthesia.

IV. **Antiadrenergic agents**

A. **Beta-adrenergic antagonists**

1. **Common properties.** Beta-adrenergic antagonists are effective antihypertensives that can be used as initial therapy in a broad range of patients. These agents may offer advantages in selected populations, including younger white patients with increased adrenergic drive (i.e., wide pulse pressure and tachycardia) or in patients with associated ischemic heart disease (especially with a prior history of MI). Several mechanisms of action have been postulated for the antihypertensive action of these agents, including (1) reduction of HR and CO, (2) reductions of plasma renin level, (3) modulation

of peripheral efferent sympathetic nervous activity, and (4) indirect central effects. Differences among these drugs include cardioselectivity (beta$_1$- versus beta$_2$-adrenergic receptor blocking capacity), lipid solubility, intrinsic sympathomimetic activity (ISA), and mode of excretion. Despite their differences, all of these agents appear to be equally effective antihypertensives.

Major adverse side effects include (1) negative inotropic and chronotropic effects that can precipitate HF or advanced heart block, (2) depression of counterregulatory responses to hypoglycemia in diabetics, (3) exacerbation of bronchospasm, and (4) provocation of Raynaud's phenomenon, claudication, or gangrene. Precipitation of angina or MI with abrupt withdrawal and reductions in HDL cholesterol and elevation of triglyceride levels have also been reported. Agents with ISA have little or no effect on serum cholesterol or lipoprotein levels. Lipophilic agents penetrate the CNS and can cause drowsiness and depression. Less lipophilic agents (i.e., atenolol and nadolol) avoid hepatic metabolism and are excreted unchanged by the kidneys. Therefore, these agents have fewer CNS side effects but require dose reduction in patients with renal insufficiency. In general, beta antagonists appear to induce regression of LVH regardless of their adrenergic receptor specificity (*Am. Heart J.* 114:975, 1987). Beta-adrenergic antagonists should not be used in combination, and caution should be exercised if they are used with other drugs that depress myocardial contractility or AV node conduction (e.g., verapamil). Side effects found with one beta-adrenergic antagonist may be avoided or attenuated by switching to another agent within this class.

2. **Specific agents**
   a. **Cardioselective** (beta$_1$ selective). At low doses, these agents can be given with caution to patients with bronchospastic disease, diabetes, and peripheral vascular disease. At higher doses, these agents lose their beta$_1$ selectivity. Compared with nonselective agents, these drugs may have less of an adverse effect on HDL cholesterol levels. **Atenolol,** 50–200 mg PO qd, is a long-acting, hydrophilic agent with no ISA. **Metoprolol,** 50–100 mg PO bid, is a lipophilic agent with hepatic metabolism and no ISA. Verapamil may elevate blood levels of metoprolol (*Am. J. Cardiol.* 55:1628, 1985). **Acebutolol,** 400–1200 mg PO daily in a qd–bid schedule, possesses ISA and is cleared by the liver and kidney. **Esmolol** (500 µg/kg/min for 1 minute, then 50–200 µg/kg/min IV) is an intravenous cardioselective (with no ISA) agent with a very short duration of action. It is metabolized by red blood cell esterase and has an elimination half-life of about 9 minutes. Esmolol has been used to decrease heart rate and blood pressure in patients with acute MI and unstable angina. It is also used in aortic dissection and hypertensive emergencies (see Special Problems, secs. **I and II**).
   b. **Nonselective. Propranolol,** 40–160 mg PO bid–qid, is the most lipid-soluble drug of this group. A long-acting form is available. Studies show little additional antihypertensive effect with doses above 80 mg/day. Cimetidine, by reducing hepatic blood flow, may increase blood levels of propranolol. Depression, fatigue, and impotence are the most frequent additional side effects. **Timolol,** 10–30 mg PO bid, is a lipid-soluble agent. **Nadolol,** 40–240 mg PO qd, is a hydrophilic, long-acting agent. Dosage should be adjusted with renal insufficiency. **Pindolol,** 5–30 mg PO bid, possesses ISA and is primarily metabolized by the liver. Its partial-agonist activity may ameliorate the peripheral vasoconstriction and resting bradycardia that can occur with other beta-adrenergic antagonists.

3. **Alpha-adrenergic antagonist. Labetalol,** 200–1200 mg PO bid, is a lipophilic agent with beta- and alpha$_1$-adrenergic (postsynaptic) antagonist properties. It also possesses weak ISA and has a neutral or slightly adverse effect on the lipid profile (*Am. Heart J.* 117:911, 1989). Unlike the classical beta antagonists, labetalol has been found to be equally effective in blacks and whites. In contrast to the usual negative inotropic effects of beta antagonists, labetalol produces marked vasodilation and decreased afterload with acute initiation

of therapy and usually maintains CO. An oral dose usually lowers BP within 1–2 hours. The parenteral form can be used to achieve a response within 5 minutes (see Special Problems, sec. **I.A.3**). Severe bradycardia, peripheral vascular symptoms, and HF may occur less frequently with labetalol than with pure beta antagonists. Reflex tachycardia may also occur. Adverse effects include postural hypotension, paresthesias, cholestatic jaundice, tremor, positive antinuclear antibodies, and hypotension when combined with halothane anesthesia.

B. Centrally acting adrenergic agonists. Although the role of the sympathetic nervous system in the genesis and maintenance of essential HTN has not been fully defined, nonselective suppression of adrenergic neural activity provides an effective avenue for BP control. In addition, these agents have been effective in producing regression of LVH. Methyldopa and clonidine stimulate adrenergic receptors within the CNS and elicit a secondary reduction in peripheral sympathetic activity. Guanabenz possesses additional peripheral blocking properties similar to those of guanethidine, guanadrel, and bethanidine. Tricyclic antidepressants may interfere with the hypotensive action of these drugs.

1. **Clonidine,** 0.2–2.4 mg PO daily (divided into a bid schedule, with the larger portion at bedtime), is lipophilic and penetrates the blood–brain barrier. Clonidine binds to and stimulates postsynaptic $alpha_2$-adrenergic receptors in the vasomotor center of the medulla oblongata and the hypothalamus, resulting in a reduction in peripheral sympathetic tone. The drug may also reduce norepinephrine release and increase vagal tone. These combined effects cause a reduction in resting CO and HR, which lower systemic BP. When used as a single agent, clonidine is effective in 50–60% of mildly to moderately hypertensive patients. Clonidine has also been used successfully in hypertensive emergencies (see Special Problems, sec. **I.B.2**). This drug may be suitable for elderly patients, because the occurrence of postural HTN is rare. Dosage should be modified in the presence of renal impairment. The most frequent adverse reactions are dry mouth and drowsiness. Infrequently, sexual dysfunction may occur. To avoid or minimize side effects, one should initiate therapy with 0.1 mg PO bid (once daily for elderly patients) and increase the dosage by 0.1-mg bid increments until the desired effect is achieved. Reduction of dosage over several days to weeks is recommended when discontinuing the drug. Abrupt discontinuation of clonidine may precipitate the **acute withdrawal syndrome.** A transdermal delivery system that is applied once a week may improve patient compliance as well as reduce the incidence of adverse side effects seen with oral drug administration. The patches are available in three sizes (3.5, 7.0, and 10.5 sq cm) and deliver 0.1, 0.2, and 0.3 mg/day, respectively. The patch must be in place for 48–72 hours before its full antihypertensive effect is observed.

2. **Methyldopa,** 500–2000 mg PO daily (in a bid–tid schedule), achieves maximum effect in 4–6 hours and is available for parenteral administration. Methyldopa does not impair renal blood flow or GFR. Since 20–60% is excreted unchanged, the dosing interval should be increased to 12–24 hours in patients with creatinine clearances less than 40 ml/min. The most common side effects are impotence and sodium retention with edema formation. Sedation, depression, xerostomia, and postural hypotension may also occur. Drug fever and galactorrhea (due to prolactin release) occur uncommonly. Methyldopa may cause a positive antinuclear antibody test in about 10% of patients and a **positive direct Coombs' test** in up to 25% of patients (the antibody is directed against the Rh locus of the red blood cell). **Hemolytic anemia** may appear at any time in about 5% of Coombs-positive patients (i.e., <1% of all patients treated with this drug) and is treated by drug withdrawal and observation for 1–2 weeks. Corticosteroids typically are reserved for more severe cases. The Coombs' test usually turns negative within several months but may remain positive for as long as 12–18 months after drug withdrawal. **Hepatic dysfunction,** indistinguishable from viral hepatitis, may occur in approximately 2% of patients and is manifested by elevation of serum

transaminase levels or occasionally by jaundice. It requires termination of the drug and is usually reversible, but fatal hepatic necrosis has been reported. If methyldopa therapy is stopped abruptly, the **acute withdrawal syndrome** may occur (see Therapeutic Considerations, sec. **IV**).

   3. **Guanabenz,** 4–16 mg PO bid, is primarily a central alpha$_2$ agonist like clonidine with peripheral adrenergic neuron antagonist effects like guanethidine. A 10–14% reduction in serum cholesterol concentration has been reported, which may prove advantageous in patients with HTN and hypercholesterolemia. When used as a single agent, this drug has proved effective in 66% of patients with mild to moderate HTN. Unlike other central alpha agonists, long-term treatment does not lead to sodium retention (*J. Cardiovasc. Pharmacol.* 6:S781, 1984). The most frequent side effects are sedation, xerostomia, and weakness. Dizziness and postural HTN occur infrequently. **Acute withdrawal syndrome** may occur following abrupt cessation of therapy (see Therapeutic Considerations, sec. **IV**).

C. Peripherally acting adrenergic antagonists

   1. **Reserpine,** 0.01–0.5 mg PO qd, produces direct inhibition of sympathetic outflow by depleting norepinephrine both peripherally and centrally. The mechanism involves inhibition of dopamine uptake into chromaffin granules, which reduces the production of norepinephrine. Reserpine is most effective when used with a diuretic. Lower doses may limit serious side effects. The most significant side effect is depression. The drug is contraindicated in patients with a history of depression and should be discontinued immediately in individuals in whom signs of depression develop. Drowsiness, nasal congestion, and weight gain occur frequently (5–15%). Gastrointestinal ulceration, impotence, bronchspasm, dysrhythmias, and edema may also occur. **Reserpine should not be used concurrently with monoamine oxidase (MAO) inhibitors or tricyclic antidepressants.**

   2. **Guanethidine,** 25–300 mg PO qd, produces direct peripheral inhibition of sympathetic nerve activity by depleting tissue stores of norepinephrine and by decreasing its release. Treatment should be initiated with 10 mg and gradually increased until BP is controlled or postural hypotension supervenes. The maximum daily dosage is 300 mg. Guanethidine has a long half-life (5 days) and prolonged effects after discontinuation of oral administration. The major side effect is postural hypotension (37%), which is dose related. Other problems include impotence, retrograde ejaculation, diarrhea, weakness, nasal stuffiness, bradycardia, edema, and azotemia. Depression is not produced because of poor CNS penetration. It is contraindicated in the presence of pheochromocytoma because it increases the sensitivity of effector cells to catecholamines. It should also be avoided in patients with HF and should not be used in combination with MAO inhibitors.

   3. **Guanadrel,** 20–30 mg PO bid, is an adrenergic blocking agent that is related to guanethidine. It reaches its maximum effect within 4–6 hours and has a half-life of 12 hours. Therapy should begin with 5–10 mg bid and can be advanced as tolerated (150 mg/day maximum). Pseudotolerance due to fluid retention can generally be prevented by the addition of a diuretic. Side effects are generally the same as for guanethidine but may be less severe.

D. Alpha-adrenergic antagonists

   1. **Prazosin,** 6–15 mg PO daily in divided doses (bid–tid) with an initial dosage of 1 mg PO bid–tid, is a peripheral postsynaptic alpha$_1$-adrenergic receptor antagonist that causes vasodilation of venous capacitance vessels as well as arterioles. The reflex elevation of HR, plasma renin activity, and plasma norepinephrine that may occur with other vasodilators is uncommon with prazosin. This may be secondary to the lack of inhibition of presynaptic alpha$_2$-adrenergic receptors. This agent has been used successfully as a single agent as well as in combination with other antihypertensive drugs, although tachyphylaxis may limit its usefulness. More than 90% of the drug is excreted via the hepatobiliary system; the dosage should be reduced in patients with hepatic insufficiency. It increases renal blood flow and is therefore considered

acceptable in the setting of renal impairment. Prazosin may decrease total cholesterol and serum low-density lipoprotein (LDL) levels as well as increase HDL levels, even in the presence of diuretic therapy (*Am. J. Med.* 76:79, 1984; *Am. J. Med.* 80 [suppl 2A]:71, 1986). The principal side effect is postural hypotension. The **first-dose phenomenon** of sudden syncope occurs in fewer than 1% of patients receiving more than 2 mg during the initiation period and is generally self-limited. This phenomenon can be minimized by giving 1 mg as the first dose at bedtime and by increasing the dose gradually. Thus, the 2- and 5-mg capsules should not be used for initiation of therapy.

2. **Terazosin,** 5–20 mg PO daily, is a long-acting alpha$_1$ selective antagonist that can be given in a single daily dose. Compared with prazosin, terazosin offers a quantitatively similar antihypertensive activity and retains the favorable lipid profile and hemodynamic advantages of alpha$_1$ antagonism (*Int. J. Clin. Pharmacol. Toxicol.* 27:313, 1989).

3. **Doxazosin,** 1–16 mg PO daily, is a long-acting alpha$_1$ selective antagonist similar to terazosin. It is extensively metabolized in the liver and should be used cautiously in patients with hepatic insufficiency. Since approximately 1% is excreted unchanged in the urine, it is suitable for use in patients with renal insufficiency.

4. **Phenoxybenzamine,** 10–40 mg PO tid, and **phentolamine,** 5 mg IV, are both alpha$_1$- and alpha$_2$-adrenergic receptor antagonists that are used almost exclusively for the pre- or intraoperative management of pheochromocytoma. Marked hypotension may occur if these drugs are used in patients with tumors that produce large amounts of epinephrine. The alpha$_2$-adrenergic receptor inhibition permits augmented norepinephrine release, which may uncommonly be accompanied by arrhythmias or MI. Common side effects include tachycardia, hyperperistalsis, and dizziness.

V. **Direct-acting vasodilators**

A. **Hydralazine,** 30–300 mg PO daily in divided doses (bid–qid) with initial dosage of 10 mg PO bid-qid, causes direct arterial vasodilation. Although this drug lowers BP when used as a single agent, sustained antihypertensive action is limited because of reflex Na$^+$ and fluid retention and sympathetic hyperactivity; it should be used in combination with a diuretic and beta-adrenergic antagonist and should be avoided in patients with coronary insufficiency. The most common side effects include headache, nausea, emesis, tachycardia, and postural hypotension. Positive antinuclear antibodies (ANA) may develop in asymptomatic patients. A hydralazine-induced systemic lupus-like syndrome may develop in approximately 10% of patients taking hydralazine. Patients who may be at increased risk for this complication include: (1) those treated with excessive dosages, (2) patients with impaired renal or cardiac function, and (3) patients with the slow hepatic acetylation phenotype. The drug should be discontinued promptly if clinical evidence of a lupus-like syndrome develops and a positive ANA is present. Hydralazine has been reported to enhance clearance of digoxin in patients with preexisting HF.

B. **Minoxidil,** 10–100 mg PO bid with an initial dosage of 5 mg PO qd, is generally used in the management of severe or refractory HTN, especially in patients with renal failure. The precise mechanism of action of this drug is not known. Reflex sympathetic hyperactivity (which may precipitate angina) and fluid retention necessitate concomitant therapy with a diuretic and a beta-adrenergic antagonist. Weight gain is the most common side effect. Hypertrichosis, ECG abnormalities, and pericardial effusion may also occur.

Special Problems

I. **Hypertensive crisis** is defined as a substantial increase in blood pressure, usually with diastolic blood pressure over 120 mm Hg. Hypertensive crises are classified as either emergencies or urgencies (*J.A.M.A.* 255:1607, 1986). Hypertensive **emergencies** include those conditions in which severe end-organ damage is present or progressive. End-organ manifestations include (1) retinal (hemorrhages, exudates, papilledema), (2) cardiac (pulmonary edema, myocardial ischemia or infarcts), (3) CNS (headache, mental status changes, seizure, coma), and (4) renal (hematuria, rising creatinine). Blood pressure control should be accomplished within 1 hour in these situations to reduce the risk of permanent damage or death. Hypertensive **urgencies** include those conditions with minimal or no obvious end-organ damage. Blood pressure control can be accomplished more slowly. The initial goal of therapy should be to achieve a diastolic BP of 100–110 mm Hg; excessive or rapid decreases in BP should be avoided to minimize the risk of cerebral hypoperfusion or coronary insufficiency. Normal BP can be attained gradually over several days as tolerated by the individual patient (*N. Engl. J. Med.* 323:1177, 1990).

A. Parenteral antihypertensive agents are indicated for the immediate reduction of BP in hypertensive patients with intracranial hemorrhage, aortic dissection, rapidly progressive renal failure, eclampsia, or accelerated-malignant HTN complicated by encephalopathy. Judicious administration of these agents to patients with HTN complicated by HF or acute MI may be appropriate. These drugs are also indicated for individuals with uncomplicated accelerated-malignant HTN who are perioperative or in need of emergency surgery. The clinical evaluation of symptoms and signs is more important than absolute BP when assessing a patient with a hypertensive emergency. If possible, an accurate baseline BP should be established before the initiation of therapy. In the setting of a hypertensive emergency, the patient should be admitted to an intensive care unit for close monitoring. An intra-arterial monitor should be used when available (N. Kaplan. *Clinical Hypertension* [5th ed.]. Baltimore: Williams & Wilkins, 1990. P. 274). Although parenteral agents have traditionally been used in patients with uncomplicated accelerated-malignant HTN who are not perioperative or undergoing emergency surgery, oral agents may also be effective in this group (see below); the choice of drug and route of administration must be individualized (*Am. Heart J.* 111:211, 1986). If parenteral agents are used initially, oral medications should be administered shortly thereafter to facilitate rapid weaning from parenteral therapy.

1. Sodium nitroprusside, a direct-acting arterial and venous vasodilator, is the treatment of choice for virtually all hypertensive crises. It reduces BP rapidly, is easily titratable, and its action is short-lived when discontinued (usually within 5 minutes). It is administered intravenously (50 mg in 250 ml of 5% D/W), beginning with an initial dose of 0.5 μg/kg/min (approximately 10 ml/hour). The usual dose is 1–3 μg/kg/min and should not exceed 10 μg/kg/min (see Appendix C). A more pronounced hypotensive effect occurs in those patients taking other antihypertensive agents. Patients should be monitored very closely to avoid an exaggerated hypotensive response with combination therapy. Therapy for more than 24 hours, high doses, or renal insufficiency may cause accumulation of thiocyanate, a toxic metabolite. Thiocyanate toxicity may cause tinnitus, blurred vision, or delirium. Hepatic dysfunction may result in the accumulation of cyanide, which can cause metabolic acidosis, dyspnea, vomiting, dizziness, ataxia, and syncope. Thiocyanate levels should be monitored during prolonged therapy and kept less than 10 mg/dl. Nitrites and thiosulfate can be administered intravenously for cyanide poisoning; hemodialysis should be considered for thiocyanate poisoning.

2. Nitroglycerin given as a continuous intravenous infusion may be appropriate in situations in which sodium nitroprusside is relatively contraindicated, such as in patients with severe coronary artery disease, or advanced renal or hepatic insufficiency. The initial dose is 5–10 μg/min and dosage can be titrated up to 200 μg/min or more depending on the clinical course (see Appendix C). It is the preferred agent in patients with moderate HTN in the setting of acute coronary ischemia or after coronary artery bypass surgery because of its more favorable effects on pulmonary gas exchange and collateral coronary blood flow (*Circulation* 65:1072, 1982). In patients with severely elevated BP, sodium nitroprusside remains the agent of choice.

Because nitroglycerin reduces preload more than afterload, it should be avoided in patients with inferior MI with right ventricular involvement who are highly dependent on preload to maintain cardiac output.

3. **Labetalol** can be administered parenterally in cases of severe HTN or hypertensive crisis, even in patients in the early phase of an acute MI (*Int. J. Cardiol.* 10:149, 1986). Initial IV bolus administration of 20 mg and subsequent doses of 20–80 mg q10min (to a maximum of 300 mg) achieve rapid control of BP; the maximum effect of a single dose occurs within 5 minutes. A continuous infusion can be administered at a rate of 1–2 mg/min with a maximal daily dose of 2400 mg. When given intravenously, the beta-antagonist effect is significantly greater than the alpha-antagonist effect (beta-alpha ratio of 7:1). Symptomatic postural hypotension may occur with IV use, suggesting that patients should be treated in the supine position. Since the half-life of labetalol is 5–8 hours, the IV infusion should be discontinued before one begins oral labetalol. When the supine DBP begins to rise, oral dosing can be initiated at 200 mg PO, followed in 6–12 hours by 200–400 mg PO, depending on the BP response. The usual precautions for beta-adrenergic antagonists should be observed.

4. **Esmolol** is a short-acting cardioselective beta antagonist that can be used parenterally in the treatment of hypertensive emergencies. An initial dose of 500 μg/kg/min for 1 minute is used; then 50–300 μg/kg/min IV is administered. Esmolol is also useful for the treatment of aortic dissection (see Special Problems, sec. II).

5. **Diazoxide, hydralazine, and trimethaphan camsylate** are now rarely used in hypertensive crises and offer little or no advantage to the agents just listed.

B. **Oral antihypertensive agents** have been used successfully in patients with hypertensive crisis when urgent but not immediate reduction of BP is indicated.

1. **Sublingual nifedipine** has an onset of action within 30 minutes and has been used safely in patients with hypertensive urgencies. Reports of clinically important myocardial ischemic events with the use of sublingual nifedipine suggest that it be used with caution in the setting of known coronary artery disease or ECG evidence of LVH (*Ann. Intern. Med.* 107:185, 1987). The capsule (10 mg) can be pierced or chewed and swallowed. The duration of action for the sublingually administered drug is 4–5 hours. During this time, therapy with oral agents that have a longer duration of action should be administered. Side effects include facial flushing and postural hypotension.

2. **Oral clonidine loading** is achieved by using an initial dose of 0.2 mg followed by 0.1 mg/hour to a total dose of 0.7 mg or a reduction in diastolic BP of 20 mm Hg or more. Blood pressure is checked at 15-minute intervals over the first hour, every 30 minutes over the second hour, and then hourly. After 6 hours, a diuretic is added and an 8-hour clonidine dosing interval is begun. Sedative side effects may be significant.

II. **Aortic dissection.** Acute proximal dissection is a surgical emergency, whereas uncomplicated distal dissection can be treated successfully with medical therapy alone. Some authors, however, advocate surgical treatment of all acute dissections (*Circulation* 70 [suppl]:153, 1984). All patients, including those treated surgically, require both acute and chronic antihypertensive therapy in order to provide initial stabilization and to prevent redissection. **Sodium nitroprusside** is considered the initial drug of choice because of predictability of response and absence of tachyphylaxis. The dose should be titrated to achieve a systolic BP of 100–120 mm Hg or to the lowest possible BP that permits adequate organ perfusion. Nitroprusside alone causes an increase in LV dv/dt and subsequent arterial wall shearing forces, which contribute to ongoing intimal dissection. Thus, **when using sodium nitroprusside adequate simultaneous beta-adrenergic antagonist therapy is essential regardless of whether systolic HTN or pain is present.** Traditionally, propranolol has been recommended. The initial dosage is 0.5 mg IV, followed by 1 mg IV q5min until the pulse pressure is reduced to 60 mm Hg or to a total dose of 0.15 mg/kg, followed by a maintenance dose q4–6h. **Esmolol,** a cardioselective IV beta antagonist with a very short duration of action, may be preferable to propranolol, especially in the presence of chronic obstructive pulmonary disease (COPD), asthma, or HF, by allowing closer titration of beta$_1$-receptor antagonism (i.e., target heart rate of 60–80 beats/min) without the liability of concomitant beta$_2$-receptor antagonism. The initial dose is 500 µg/kg/min IV for 4 minutes followed by an IV infusion of 50–300 µg/kg/min. **Intravenous labetalol** (a combined alpha$_1$ selective adrenergic antagonist and nonselective beta antagonist) has been used successfully as a single agent in the treatment of acute aortic dissection (*J.A.M.A.* 258:78, 1987). Labetalol produces a dose-related decrease in BP as well as a lowering of dv/dt. It has the advantage of allowing for oral administration after the acute stage of dissection has been successfully managed. If sodium nitroprusside or beta-adrenergic receptor antagonists cannot be tolerated, the ganglionic-blocking agent trimethaphan camsylate can be used as a single agent. Unlike sodium nitroprusside, trimethaphan reduces LV dv/dt. The dosage is 0.5 g in 500 ml of 5% D/W beginning at 2 mg/min with titration to BP response. Because trimethaphan is associated with rapid tachyphylaxis and sympathoplegia, other drugs are preferable. **Sublingual nifedipine,** because of its combined vasodilator and negative inotropic effects, appears to have a favorable hemodynamic profile in this setting and has been successfully used to treat refractory HTN associated with aortic dissection (*Chest* 88:781, 1985). Hypotension in the setting of aortic dissection may indicate that external rupture has occurred (rupture into the intraperitoneal or intrapleural spaces, or into the pericardium with tamponade). A proximal dissection may occlude the brachial arteries and prevent an accurate determination of BP in one or both arms. Medical therapy of chronic stable aortic dissection should seek to maintain systolic BP at or below a level of 130–140 mm Hg if tolerated. Antihypertensive agents with negative inotropic properties, including calcium channel antagonists, beta antagonists, methyldopa, clonidine, or reserpine, are the preferred agents. Diuretics may need to be added in the acute as well as chronic setting if fluid overload is present.

III. **Hypertension during pregnancy.** The benefit of pharmacologic intervention in the gravid patient with mild HTN and the risk–benefit analysis of nonpharmacologic therapy have not been elucidated. One should be cognizant of the teratogenic and toxic potential of antihypertensive agents to the developing fetus in all hypertensive women of childbearing age (see Appendix G). Drugs that have been shown to be safe during pregnancy include methyldopa, beta antagonists, and hydralazine. Although hydralazine has been used for acute parenteral therapy in severe gestational HTN, it is not recommended for long-term therapy. Captopril, nitroprusside, and diuretics have been associated with adverse effects to the fetus and should not be used in pregnancy. Nifedipine has been used in pregnancy without complications; however, there have been no long-term trials of calcium channel antagonists in pregnancy. In addition, verapamil has been shown to inhibit uterine contractions. Therefore, calcium antagonists should not be used as first-line therapy for gestational hypertension (*Cardiovasc. Clin.* 19:97, 1989).

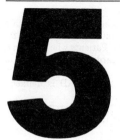

Ischemic Heart Disease

Craig Reiss and Paul Eisenberg

General Considerations

Ischemic heart disease secondary to atherosclerosis of the coronary arteries remains the leading cause of morbidity and mortality in North America. **Risk factors** for the development of coronary artery atherosclerosis include a family history of premature coronary artery disease, cigarette smoking, hypercholesterolemia, hypertension, and diabetes mellitus. Obesity, physical inactivity, and stress may play a lesser role. Coronary artery disease (CAD) may be clinically silent but more commonly is associated with symptoms (e.g., myocardial infarction, angina pectoris, sudden death) (*Am. J. Cardiol.* 37:269, 1976).

Angina Pectoris

I. **Diagnosis.** Angina pectoris is the chest discomfort associated with myocardial ischemia that occurs when myocardial oxygen demand exceeds supply.
   A. **Clinical history.** Angina is typically described as a retrosternal pain, discomfort, heaviness, or pressure radiating to the neck, jaw, shoulders, or arms, lasting 2–5 minutes. It is usually precipitated by exertion and relieved with rest. Dyspnea, nausea and vomiting, diaphoresis, and occasionally palpitations or lightheadedness are common associated symptoms. Factors that increase myocardial oxygen demand or that decrease oxygen supply may precipitate or aggravate angina and should be excluded by history and appropriate laboratory evaluation. In men and older women, a history of typical angina, especially in the presence of other cardiac risk factors, is good evidence of ischemic heart disease (90% probability). In such patients the role of invasive and noninvasive cardiac tests is to assess the severity of CAD to guide therapy and to estimate the risk of myocardial infarction (MI). In patients with chest pain unlikely to be of cardiac origin and without significant cardiac risk factors, the prevalence of ischemic heart disease is low (25%), so that further cardiac evaluation may be necessary to determine whether CAD is present. However, noninvasive tests in this group of patients are often falsely positive (*N. Engl. J. Med* 300:1350, 1979). Noninvasive tests are particularly useful in patients with an intermediate probability of disease.
   B. **Approach to establishing the diagnosis of angina.** When the clinical history suggests the presence of angina, the diagnosis should be confirmed by invasive or noninvasive tests and the need for further medical or invasive intervention should be assessed.
      1. **The resting ECG** may demonstrate the following: (1) significant Q waves (> 0.4 msec) consistent with a prior MI, (2) resting ST segment depression or elevation, and/or (3) T-wave inversion suggestive of myocardial ischemia. Frequently, the resting ECG is entirely normal, even in the presence of significant CAD. However, documentation of ST segment or T-wave abnormalities *during an episode of chest discomfort* can be invaluable for confirming the diagnosis of CAD and may limit the need for further noninvasive testing.
      2. **Exercise electrocardiography** (stress testing) is useful in establishing the

diagnosis of CAD and allows for risk stratification of patients with angina. Exercise sufficient to increase the heart rate to 80% of the predicted maximum is necessary for optimal sensitivity. Patients who have an early or markedly positive test result should undergo cardiac catheterization to define the need for coronary revascularization.

   a. A markedly positive test indicative of severe CAD is defined as the presence of any of the following:

   1. ST segment depression early after the start of exercise.
   2. ≥ 2 mm of new ST segment depression in multiple leads.
   3. New ST segment elevation.
   4. Decreased systolic blood pressure with exercise.
   5. Inability to exercise for more than 2 minutes.
   6. Development of heart failure with exercise.
   7. Prolonged interval to return of ischemic ST segment changes to baseline after exercise.

   In contrast, even in patients with documented CAD, the ability to complete 7 minutes of a standard Bruce protocol without the development of significant ST segment depression is associated with an excellent 4-year survival (*J. Am. Coll. Cardiol.* 3:772, 1984).

3. **Exercise thallium imaging** and **radionuclide ventriculography** improve the sensitivity and specificity of exercise testing and are particularly useful in patients receiving digitalis or with existing ECG abnormalities, such as left ventricular hypertrophy, ST–T changes, left bundle branch block, or preexcitation, which decrease the specificity of ECG exercise testing (*Am. J. Cardiol.* 45:674, 1980). In most centers, addition of an imaging modality to exercise stress testing increases the sensitivity for detection of significant CAD from 70% to 80%, and the specificity from 80% to 90% (*Circulation* 83:363, 1991). The choice of the radionuclide procedure depends on the experience of individual centers.

4. **Exercise two-dimensional echocardiography** performed in experienced centers is useful in the diagnosis of coronary disease, with sensitivity and specificity similar to that of exercise radionuclide ventriculography (*J. Am. Coll. Cardiol.* 2:1085, 1983).

5. **Pharmacologic stress testing.** Dipyridamole thallium stress testing is useful in the evaluation of patients with suspected CAD who are unable to exercise (*N. Engl. J. Med.* 312:389, 1985). Two-dimensional echocardiography has also been used in conjunction with administration of intravenous dipyridamole, adenosine, or infusions of high doses of dobutamine as a means of inducing detectable cardiac ischemia in patients unable to exercise.

6. In patients with suspected CAD in whom the initial assessment suggests left ventricular dysfunction, further evaluation of left ventricular function with **resting two-dimensional echocardiography or radionuclide ventriculography** is warranted. Patients with left ventricular ejection fractions of < 50% and significant CAD have a better prognosis if treated with bypass surgery compared with medical therapy (*N. Engl. J. Med.* 312:1665, 1985). Therefore, in patients in whom CAD is suspected and who have significant left ventricular dysfunction, coronary angiography should be considered to determine the extent of CAD and their suitability for coronary artery bypass grafting (CABG).

7. **Coronary arteriography** remains the definitive test in the diagnosis of CAD and can be performed safely with an incidence of mortality or serious morbidity of 0.1–0.2% This procedure is indicated to document the presence of CAD that cannot be determined with noninvasive methods and is essential in the evaluation of high-risk patients. In addition, this technique provides prognostic information based on the number of significant obstructed coronary arteries and the degree of left ventricular dysfunction. Significant coronary obstruction is usually defined as greater than 70% narrowing of the luminal diameter.

II. Therapy

A. General principles in the management of angina pectoris include the modification of reversible cardiac risk factors. Cessation of cigarette smoking should be emphasized. Elevated serum cholesterol levels should be treated as described in Chap. 22. Recent studies suggest that regression of atherosclerotic plaques is possible, but serum cholesterol must be decreased to 150–180 mg/dl (J.A.M.A. 257:3233, 1987). Specific treatment of angina is directed toward improving myocardial oxygen supply, reducing myocardial oxygen demand, and treating precipitating factors or concurrent disorders that may exacerbate ischemia.

B. Drug therapy. The selection of an effective therapeutic regimen depends on the acuity and severity of symptoms, the presence of associated disease (e.g., pulmonary or renal disease), the patient's age and activity level, and the underlying pathophysiologic mechanism presumed to be responsible for the ischemia (e.g., arterial spasm, fixed stenosis). Because the cause of myocardial ischemia is often multifactorial, a combination of agents with different mechanisms of action is frequently more effective than monotherapy.

1. Nitrates remain important first-line agents for the treatment of angina (*N. Engl. J. Med.* 316:1635, 1987). The primary antianginal effect is an increase in venous capacitance, leading to a reduction in ventricular volume and pressure and improvement in subendocardial perfusion. Coronary vasodilatation, improvement in collateral flow, and afterload reduction augment this primary effect.

a. Sublingual nitroglycerin is available as 0.3-, 0.4-, and 0.6-mg tablets or as a metered-dose spray. Usually, 0.4-mg tablets are prescribed, but occasionally lower doses are required. Peak pharmacologic action occurs within 2 minutes and continues for 15–30 minutes. Nitroglycerin can be repeated at 5-minute intervals if symptoms persist. Patients should be informed of possible side effects (e.g., headache, hypotension), the importance of taking the drug while seated, and the need for airtight storage in the original amber bottle with replacement every 6 months. The patient should be counseled to take nitroglycerin at the first indication of angina and prophylactically before situations that are known to precipitate angina; medical attention should be urgently sought if an anginal attack fails to promptly respond by the third nitroglycerin tablet or if the patient experiences a worsening in the anginal pattern.

b. Long-acting nitrates are indicated in the long-term management of angina pectoris. High doses of oral nitrates must be used because of extensive hepatic degradation after intestinal absorption (first-pass effect). Several preparations of long-acting nitrates are available (Table 5-1). The optimal dosing interval for long-acting oral nitrates has not been established. Administration of isosorbide dinitrate three times a day with meals is convenient and may allow for a sufficient nitrate-free period to prevent the development of tolerance.

c. Topical 2% nitroglycerin ointment is applied to the skin as a 1- to 2-in. measured dose by use of an occlusive dressing every 4–6 hours. The onset of action is approximately 30 minutes. Nitroglycerin ointment is the preferred long-acting nitrate for patients who are unable to take oral medications. Because absorption of topical nitrates may be unpredictable, the intravenous route of administration should always be used when predictable nitrate levels and rapid control of dosage rate are required.

d. The efficacy of **sustained-release nitroglycerin patches** has been limited by the failure of lower-dose patches to induce a high enough concentration of drug to have a therapeutic effect and by the development of tolerance to sustained increased nitroglycerin levels when these concentrations are achieved.

e. Nitrate tolerance and reduction in therapeutic response may occur with all the nitrate preparations, and the imposition of nitrate-free intervals of at least 10–12 hours can enhance treatment efficacy (*N. Engl. J. Med.* 317:805, 1987; *J. Am. Coll. Cardiol.* 16:941, 1990). When nitrates cannot

Table 5-1. Doses and action of commonly used nitroglycerin preparations

Preparation	Dose	Peak action	Duration
Short-acting preparations			
Sublingual nitroglycerin	0.3–0.6 mg	2–5 min	10–30 min
Aerosol nitroglycerin	0.4 mg	2–5 min	10–30 min
Sublingual or chewable isosorbide dinitrate	2.5–10.0 mg	10–30 min	1–2 hr
Longer-acting preparations			
Oral isosorbide dinitrate	5–40 mg	30–60 min	4–6 hr
Sustained-release trinitroglycerin (TNG)	2.5–9.0 mg	30–60 min	4–6 hr
2% nitroglycerin ointment	½–2.0 in.	20–60 min	Depends on dose (3–6 hr)
Nitroglycerin patches	5–15 mg		24 hr

be discontinued, even for a short time, increased doses may be required to overcome tolerance.

2. **Beta-adrenergic antagonists** are also important in the management of stable angina. They reduce the frequency of anginal episodes and raise the anginal threshold (*Am. J. Cardiol.* 77:119, 1984).

a. **Selection.** Beta-adrenergic antagonists are generally classified with respect to their selectivity for cardiac beta$_1$ receptors compared with beta$_2$ receptors. There are no clear differences among the various beta-adrenergic antagonists in their antianginal efficacy (Table 5-2). However, beta$_1$-selective drugs (metoprolol and atenolol) at low doses are less likely to cause bronchospasm or exacerbate peripheral vascular disease. At higher doses, the beta$_1$ selectivity is lost. Agents with intrinsic sympathomimetic action (ISA), such as pindolol, may dilate peripheral vessels and have less effect on resting heart rate. Lipid-insoluble beta antagonists have a longer duration of action and penetrate the CNS to a lesser extent, which may limit CNS side effects. Labetalol has both beta- and alpha-adrenergic antagonist effects. Because of the additional vasodilatation induced by alpha-adrenergic blockade, this agent may be particularly useful in hypertensive patients.

b. **Dosage** should be carefully titrated on an individual basis to achieve a resting heart rate of 55–60 beats/minute and an exercise heart rate that does not exceed 90–100 beats/minute. Resting, asymptomatic bradycardia is not an indication that therapy should be stopped. Resting heart rate cannot be used to evaluate therapy in patients taking agents with intrinsic sympathomimetic activity. Increasing the dose of a beta-adrenergic antagonist may improve antianginal effects in some patients but may also increase the incidence of side effects. The patient should be observed for signs of bronchospasm or congestive heart failure when beta-adrenergic antagonist therapy is initiated and when the dose is being adjusted.

Table 5-2. Doses and action of selected beta-adrenergic antagonists

Agent	Dose (PO)	Actions
Propranolol	20–60 mg qid	β_1, β_2
Long-acting propranolol	80–160 mg qd	β_1, β_2
Nadolol	40–80 mg qd	β_1, β_2
Timolol	20 mg bid	β_1, β_2
Metoprolol	50–100 mg bid	β_1
Atenolol	50–100 mg qd	β_1
Acebutolol	200–600 mg bid	β_1, ISA
Pindolol	5–20 mg tid	β_1, β_2, ISA
Labetalol	100–600 mg bid	β_1, β_2, α-blocker

Key: ISA = intrinsic sympathomimetic activity.

   c. Contraindications to the use of beta-adrenergic antagonists include severe heart failure, history of bronchospasm, atrioventricular (AV) nodal block, severe peripheral vascular disease, and marked resting bradycardia. In patients with heart failure or depressed left ventricular ejection fraction, beta-adrenergic antagonist therapy can be attempted but should be started at a low dose, with gradual increases as tolerated.
   d. Side effects of beta-adrenergic antagonists include bronchospasm, nausea, diarrhea, postural hypotension, claudication, impotence, fatigue, headache, nightmares, depression, hallucinations, deterioration in intellectual capacity, salt retention, and the potential masking of hypoglycemia in insulin-dependent diabetics. Infrequently, abrupt withdrawal of these agents may precipitate arrhythmias, MI, and even sudden death; therefore, when beta-adrenergic antagonists must be stopped, patients should be monitored for sympathetic rebound (see Chap. 4).
 3. Calcium channel antagonists are a heterogeneous group of agents that cause a variable degree of coronary and peripheral artery vasodilation and have negative inotropic effects. Because peripheral vascular resistance is generally reduced by these agents, cardiac afterload decreases, which tends to preserve or increase cardiac output despite the negative inotropic effects of agents such as nifedipine. The antianginal effects of calcium channel antagonists are due to direct coronary vasodilatation and an improvement in the efficiency of myocardial performance. Calcium channel antagonists are indicated in the management of stable and unstable angina, and are the agents of choice in patients unable to tolerate beta-adrenergic antagonists and nitrates. In addition, because these agents are potent coronary vasodilators, they are particularly effective in patients with coronary vasospasm (Prinzmetal's angina). Calcium channel antagonists can be used as first-line single-agent therapy in many patients or in combination with nitrates or beta-adrenergic antagonists in those with angina refractory to single-drug therapy (*Mayo Clin. Proc.* 60:539, 1985; *J. Am. Coll. Cardiol.* 1:492, 1983).
   a. Nifedipine (*Am. J. Cardiol.* 71:645, 1981) has profound arteriolar vasodilating properties but no effect on atrioventricular nodal conduction. Although nifedipine has negative inotropic effects, the decrease in peripheral vascular resistance induced by pharmacologic doses usually results in an increase in cardiac output. Common side effects include dizziness, headache, hypotension, flushing, nausea, and peripheral edema, all of which occur less frequently with the sustained-release preparation. Nifedipine is contraindicated in patients with hypotension. In patients with decreased left ventricular ejection fractions, worsening heart failure often

occurs (*Circulation* 82:1954, 1990). The dosage is 10–30 mg tid or qid or 30–120 mg qd (for the sustained-release preparation).

   b. Nicardipine (*Am. Heart J.* 114:793, 1987) is similar to nifedipine but has been shown in some uncontrolled studies to have fewer negative inotropic effects, with similar vasodilating properties. The drug may therefore be useful in patients with impaired left ventricular function in whom other calcium channel antagonists are thought to be contraindicated. The dosage is 20–40 mg tid.

   c. Verapamil (*Circulation* 65:17, 1982) has arteriolar vasodilating properties and markedly slows atrioventricular conduction. It has a greater negative inotropic effect than nifedipine or diltiazem, limiting its use in patients with significant left ventricular dysfunction. It is a valuable agent in the treatment of supraventricular tachyarrhythmias but may produce bradycardia and advanced atrioventricular block. Sick sinus syndrome, atrioventricular nodal disease, and significant congestive heart failure are contraindications to the use of verapamil. Verapamil should be used cautiously, if at all, in patients treated with other agents that depress AV node function such as beta-blockers, or in the presence of digitalis intoxication. Constipation is the most common troublesome side effect. The dosage is 40–120 mg tid or 180–240 mg qd for the sustained-release preparation.

   d. Diltiazem (*Am. J. Cardiol.* 54:738, 1984) is an arteriolar vasodilator and also prolongs atrioventricular nodal conduction and decreases the heart rate modestly. Concomitant use of beta-adrenergic antagonists may potentiate atrioventricular nodal conduction disturbances as well as excessive sinoatrial nodal depression; therefore, combination therapy is rarely indicated. Despite data suggesting that the negative inotropic effects of diltiazem are modest, one clinical trial found that its use increased mortality in patients with left ventricular dysfunction and recent MI (*N. Engl. J. Med.* 319:385, 1988). The dosage is 30–90 mg qid or 60–120 mg bid for the long-acting preparation.

4. Aspirin prolongs survival in patients with unstable angina (*N. Engl. J. Med.* 309:396, 1983; *N. Engl. J. Med.* 313:1369, 1985) and is effective in the primary prevention of cardiovascular events (*N. Engl. J. Med.* 318:262, 1988). The beneficial effects of aspirin appear to be greater in men than in women in most studies. Inhibition of platelet function is presumed to be the mechanism of aspirin's effect. Most clinicians recommend daily use of aspirin in low doses (80–325 mg qd) for patients with known CAD or multiple risk factors.

C. Invasive therapy. Percutaneous transluminal coronary angioplasty (PTCA) and CABG are invasive procedures designed to improve regional myocardial blood flow by dilating or bypassing stenotic coronary lesions.

   1. CABG is beneficial in patients with angina that is refractory to medical management, even if only single-vessel disease is present. In addition, it appears to prolong life compared with medical therapy in patients with triple-vessel disease, particularly when there is significant left ventricular dysfunction or easily inducible ischemia, and in patients with left main coronary disease (*Circulation* 68:939, 1983).

   a. Results. Improvement of ischemic symptoms is achieved in 80–90% of patients, and 50–75% are symptom free for variable periods after bypass surgery (*Circulation* 65:225, 1982). Angina recurs at a rate of 10–20% each year in patients who initially benefit from CABG and correlates with graft occlusion or progression of native coronary disease. The use of internal mammary artery grafts is associated with 90% graft patency at 10 years compared with 40% for saphenous vein grafts (*J. Thorac. Cardiovasc. Surg.* 89:248, 1985).

   b. Medical versus surgical therapy. The risks of CABG include a 1–3% operative mortality and a 5–10% incidence of perioperative MI. Approximately 15–20% of grafts close in the first year; over the next 5 years, 2%

close per year, and subsequently 4% occlude each year. Some data suggest that three-vessel disease can be successfully managed with medical therapy, with a 2–3% yearly mortality. Because there are constant improvements in both medical and surgical management of CAD, it is difficult to unequivocally recommend one therapy or the other except in patients with left main disease, in whom the mortality associated with medical treatment approaches 30% at 18 months (*Prog. Cardiovasc. Dis.* 22:73, 1979). The best therapy for a given patient will depend on considerations of his or her lifestyle, severity of ischemia, evidence of silent ischemia, and extent of the coronary artery lesions, as well as the amount of myocardium subtended by critical stenoses. At 10 years, excluding patients with left main disease, in patients with mild angina survival advantage for CABG compared with medical therapy is only evident in those with three-vessel disease and a left ventricular ejection fraction of 35–50% (*Circulation* 82:1629, 1990). In patients with more severe angina or easily induced ischemia, CABG may be indicated even in the absence of three-vessel disease (*J. Am. Coll. Cardiol.* 17:543, 1991).

2. **PTCA** is accomplished by positioning a specially designed balloon catheter across the stenotic coronary artery segment and inflating the balloon to increase the luminal diameter via atherosclerotic plaque rupture. Dilatation of multivessel lesions, branch stenoses, and distal lesions is possible in many patients. Successful dilatation is initially achieved in 75–90% of patients. Approximately 15–30% of initially dilated vessels will develop restenosis within 9 months, but repeat angioplasty of these lesions is highly successful (*N. Engl. J. Med.* 318:265, 1988). Patients undergoing PTCA should, in general, be candidates for CABG, since surgery may be necessary if PTCA fails or if complications arise. Potential complications of PTCA include coronary artery dissection, occlusion, and spasm, with a 5–10% incidence of MI and 3–5% requirement for emergency CABG.

Unstable Angina

I. **Definition and diagnosis.** Unstable angina is a clinical syndrome characterized by angina of new onset, angina at rest or with minimal exertion, or a crescendo pattern of angina with episodes of increasing frequency, severity, or duration. Although the pathophysiology is heterogeneous, in most patients, the transition from stable to unstable atherosclerotic disease appears to be due to rupture or fissuring of atherosclerotic plaques, resulting in thrombus formation, increased platelet reactivity, and increased coronary vasomotor tone (*Circulation* 77:1213, 1988). In a small percentage of patients, unstable ischemic symptoms are precipitated by severe anemia, hypertension, or heart failure.

A. **Risk of MI.** The development of unstable symptoms carries a 10–20% risk of progression to acute MI. Patients who are thought to be at a higher risk for progression to acute infarction include those with new onset of pain at rest or a sudden change in anginal pattern, particularly when associated with labile ST–T changes on the ECG. Recurrent or persistent pain after treatment is initiated also is associated with an increased incidence of subsequent infarction. Clinical evidence of left ventricular dysfunction, pulmonary edema, transient mitral regurgitation, or hypotension during episodes of ischemia identifies patients with extensive areas of myocardium at risk. The development of new ST segment depression or elevation or deep T-wave inversions in the anterior precordial leads in the absence of MI are findings that suggest severe underlying CAD (*Am. Heart J.* 103:730, 1982).

II. **Management** includes hospitalization, bed rest, sedation, and the correction of precipitating conditions such as hypertension, anemia, or hypoxemia. The goals of treatment are to aggressively relieve ischemic symptoms with antianginal drugs, by use of intravenous preparations when necessary, and to inhibit thrombosis in high-risk patients.

A. **Treatment of ischemia.** In general, intravenous nitroglycerin is preferred to oral or cutaneous preparations because of the ability to more rapidly achieve predictable blood levels of drug. Patients should also receive a beta-adrenergic antagonist when not contraindicated or a calcium channel antagonist, preferably verapamil or diltiazem. Nifedipine generally should not be used without concomitant beta adrenergic antagonist therapy in such patients (*Circulation* 73:331, 1986; *J. Am. Coll. Cardiol.* 5:717, 1985). The choice of specific agent should be dictated by the underlying pathophysiology and associated hemodynamics.

B. **Narcotic analgesics** such as morphine sulfate are reserved for treatment of pain that is refractory to aggressive medical therapy.

C. **Anticoagulants.** Intravenous heparin appears to decrease the incidence of MI in patients with unstable angina (*N. Engl. J. Med.* 319:1105, 1988; *Lancet* 1:1225, 1981).

D. **Aspirin** has been shown to reduce both mortality and the occurrence of nonfatal infarction in patients with unstable angina when administered either in low (325 mg PO qd) or high (325 mg PO q6h) dosages (*N. Engl. J. Med.* 309:396, 1983; *N. Engl. J. Med.* 313:1369, 1985). The combination of heparin and aspirin has not been shown to provide a greater reduction in risk of infarction and has been associated with increased bleeding complications (*N. Engl. J. Med.* 319:1105, 1988). Increased bleeding complications have been reported in patients treated with aspirin who undergo CABG.

E. **Intra-aortic balloon counterpulsation** is indicated in patients with ischemic symptoms that are refractory to medical therapy. Because this procedure is associated with a 10–15% risk of significant vascular complications, it should only be pursued as a means to stabilize the patient's condition before CABG or PTCA.

III. **Prognosis.** Most patients (75–85%) respond to aggressive medical management and, when stable, should undergo elective coronary angiography to evaluate the severity of CAD and their suitability for PTCA or CABG. Those who continue to experience symptoms despite adequate medical therapy are candidates for emergency coronary angiography and subsequent PTCA or bypass surgery. Although aggressive evaluation is often indicated because of the risk of progression to MI, selected patients can be evaluated with noninvasive tests to assess their prognosis (see sec. I.B).

Coronary Vasospasm and Variant Angina

I. **Definition.** Prinzmetal's variant angina is characterized by episodes of chest pain at rest associated with transient ST segment elevations on the electrocardiogram due to coronary artery vasospasm without evolution of MI. Symptomatic coronary vasospasm typically occurs in association with a fixed atherosclerotic lesion but may occasionally be seen in normal arteries, in which case it is associated with a better prognosis (*Circulation* 65:825, 1982). Episodes of vasospasm may be accompanied by arrhythmia, such as ventricular tachyarrhythmia or heart block (*Am. J. Cardiol.* 50:203, 1982) and may rarely progress to MI or sudden death. Sustained coronary vasospasm is also thought to play a role in MIs associated with cocaine or amphetamine abuse.

II. **Diagnosis.** Transient ST segment elevation during episodes of chest pain is indicative of coronary vasospasm. Ambulatory ECG monitoring is often useful in detecting such episodes. Coronary arteriography is indicated to evaluate the extent of underlying CAD and the diagnosis can be confirmed by demonstrating coronary artery narrowing during a spontaneous or provoked episode of characteristic chest pain. Intravenous ergonovine maleate is often used to provoke vasospasm during coronary angiography (*Am. J. Cardiol.* 46:335, 1980).

III. **Management.** Acute episodes of coronary vasospasm generally respond to **sublingual nitroglycerin**. **Nifedipine** (10 mg), which is chewed and swallowed for more rapid onset of action, can be used for refractory spasm in the absence of hypotension. Long-acting nitrates or calcium channel antagonists have been demonstrated to reduce the frequency of episodes of chest pain when used for long-term treatment of patients with classic Prinzmetal's angina (*Am. Heart J.* 103:44, 1982). Cigarette smoking appears to predispose to coronary vasospasm, so patients should be strongly advised to stop smoking. CABG or PTCA is of benefit only in the presence of significant fixed obstructions.

Silent Ischemia

I. **Silent ischemia,** or that known to be present on the basis of objective evidence of ischemia but not accompanied by angina or anginal equivalents, occurs in 2.5% of middle-aged men without signs or symptoms of CAD (type 1) and at least 40% of patients with angina (type 3) (*Ann. Intern. Med.* 109:312, 1988). The clinical significance and prognostic implications of silent ischemia are not well established and there are no convincing data showing that reduction of silent ischemia is beneficial. However, in patients with unstable angina and those recovering from an MI the presence of silent ischemia as identified on ambulatory ECG monitoring identifies a high-risk population for development of subsequent cardiac events (*N. Engl. J. Med.* 314:1214, 1986; *J.A.M.A.* 259:1030, 1988). In these subgroups of patients, attempts to identify and treat silent ischemia may be warranted. Twenty-four–hour continuous ambulatory ECG monitoring, thallium perfusion scintigraphy, radionuclide ventriculography, and echocardiography may be used to diagnose silent ischemia.

II. **Therapy** for silent ischemia is similar to that associated with symptoms. In a study of patients with stable angina and a high frequency of silent ischemia, propranolol was more effective than diltiazem or nifedipine (*Circulation* 82:1962, 1990). PTCA or CABG may also be effective. Therapeutic efficacy of various interventions can be assessed by ambulatory ECG monitoring.

Myocardial Infarction

I. **Definition.** MI constitutes a medical emergency requiring prompt hospitalization in an intensive care setting and careful medical management. Mortality from MI is greatest within the first 2 hours after onset of symptoms and can be significantly reduced by expeditious transport to the hospital and intensive care unit and by the prompt treatment of ventricular arrhythmias. Occlusive or near-occlusive thrombus overlying or adjacent to a ruptured atherosclerotic plaque appears to be the cause. Rarely, infarction occurs with normal or minimally diseased coronary arteries as a result of coronary spasm or embolism.

II. **Diagnosis.** Definitive diagnosis of MI requires at least two of the following criteria: (1) a history of prolonged chest discomfort, (2) ECG changes consistent with ischemia or necrosis, or (3) elevated cardiac enzymes.

   A. **History.** The initial diagnosis of acute MI is based on the clinical history, physical examination, and interpretation of the ECG. Chest pain associated with MI resembles that of angina pectoris but is typically more severe and of longer duration and is not relieved by rest or nitroglycerin. Accompanying symptoms include dyspnea, nausea, vomiting, fatigue, diaphoresis, and palpitations. MI may occur without chest pain, especially in postoperative patients, the elderly, and patients with diabetes mellitus or hypertension, in whom symptoms may be isolated dyspnea, exacerbation of heart failure, or acute confusion. Other causes for chest pain should be considered (Table 5–3).

   B. **Physical examination.** The initial examination should be directed at identifying hemodynamic instability or pulmonary congestion, or both. Hypotension, cool extremities, diaphoresis, and confusion are often indicative of cardiogenic shock. Elevation in the jugular venous pulse indicates volume overload or right ventricular failure. Auscultation of heart typically demonstrates an S4, reflecting decreased left ventricular compliance, and less commonly an S3, suggesting

Table 5-3. Selected differential diagnosis of MI

Diagnosis	ECG findings mimicking MI	Diagnostic evaluation
Pericarditis	ST elevation	Echocardiography
Myocarditis	ST elevation Q waves	Echocardiography
Acute aortic dissection	ST elevation or depression or nonspecific	Chest CT or MRI, transesophageal echocardiography, aortography
Pneumothorax	New poor R-wave progression V1–V6 or acute QRS axis shift	Chest x-ray
Pulmonary embolism	Inferior ST elevation or ST shifts V1–V3	Ventilation-perfusion scan
Acute cholecystitis	Inferior ST elevation	Abdominal ultrasound

heart failure. Murmurs of various causes may be apparent, but new systolic murmurs are of particular importance, suggesting the presence of mitral regurgitation or a ventricular septal defect.

1. **Clinical stratification.** Patients with acute MI should be stratified into high- and low-risk subgroups based on findings of the initial examination. Those without evidence of pulmonary congestion or shock (Killip class I) have an excellent prognosis (mortality <5%) and generally require less aggressive management, and the prognosis with only mild pulmonary congestion or an isolated S3 gallop (Killip class II) is also reasonably good. Patients with pulmonary edema (Killip class III) often have extensive left ventricular dysfunction or acute mitral regurgitation and require aggressive management. Patients with hypotension and evidence of shock (Killip class IV) have a mortality approaching 80% unless the cause of shock is potentially treatable. Cardiogenic shock due to right ventricular infarction occurs in patients with inferior wall infarction and is often clinically recognized by the presence of elevated jugular venous pressures without evidence of pulmonary congestion.

C. **Electrocardiography.** Serial ECGs are essential; an ECG should be obtained on admission and daily during hospitalization in the cardiac intensive care unit for evaluation of recurrent chest pain or arrhythmias as well as to aid diagnosis. Although some patients initially have a normal ECG, the majority of patients with MI do not.

1. **ST–T changes.** Convex ST segment elevation with either peaked upright or inverted T waves is usually indicative of acute myocardial injury. ST segment depression, particularly when it persists, may also be indicative of an acute MI.

2. **Q waves.** The development of new Q waves is generally considered diagnostic of MI but may occur in patients with prolonged ischemia (stunned myocardium) and occasionally in patients with myocarditis.

3. **Non–Q-wave infarction.** MI may occur in the absence of evolution of Q waves; this is referred to as a non–Q-wave MI. Although the extent of infarction in patients with non–Q-wave MI is often less than in patients with Q-wave infarction, they are at high risk of recurrent MI and have a similar long-term prognosis.

4. **ECG changes that mimic MI.** ST segment elevation and evolution of Q waves rarely may result from preexcitation syndromes, pericarditis, cardiomyopathy, chronic obstructive pulmonary disease, and pulmonary embolism, among others (see Table 5-3).

Table 5-4. Selected causes of increased plasma MB–CK activity other than MI

I. Myocardial injury other than MI
   a. Myocarditis
   b. Pericarditis (? due to associated myocarditis)
   c. Myocardial contusion/blunt chest trauma
   d. Defibrillation (> 300 joules × 2)
   e. Cardiac surgery

II. Noncardiac muscle injury
   a. Low percentage MB–CK relative to total CK
      1. Extensive muscle trauma
      2. Rhabdomyolysis
   b. High percentage MB–CK to total CK
      1. Polymyositis
      2. Muscular dystrophy
      3. Myopathies
      4. Vigorous exercise in trained athletes (e.g., marathon runners)
      5. Patients with chronic renal insufficiency (? only with myopathy)

III. Nonmuscle sources of MB–CK or BB–CK
      1. Intracerebral hemorrhage (BB–CK)
      2. Extensive intracerebral infarction (BB–CK)
      3. Prostatic carcinoma (BB–CK)
      4. Bronchogenic carcinoma (BB–CK, MB–CK rare)

IV. Delayed clearance of CK
      1. Hypothyroidism (? only with myopathy)

   D. Cardiac enzymes. The levels in plasma of aspartate and aminotransferase, creatine kinase (CK), and lactate dehydrogenase (LDH) progressively increase as myocardial necrosis evolves. Although these enzymes are found in many organs, the MB isoenzyme of creatine kinase (MB–CK) and the LDH_1 isoenzyme are relatively specific for myocardial necrosis.

   1. Creatine kinase (*N. Engl. J. Med.* 313:1050, 1985) exists in three plasma isoenzymes: MM, MB, and BB, found predominantly in muscle, heart, and brain, respectively.

   a. Increased plasma MB–CK activity has a greater than 95% sensitivity and specificity for myocardial injury when measured within 24–36 hours of chest pain. With MI, plasma MB–CK activity increases within 4–6 hours of chest pain, reaches a peak in 12–20 hours, and returns to baseline in 36–48 hours, depending on the extent of myocardial necrosis. Increased plasma concentrations of MB–CK are almost always indicative of myocardial cell death, although not always due to MI (Table 5–4).

   b. Increased MB–CK not due to MI. Infrequently, elevations in MB–CK occur as a result of release from noncardiac sources, delayed clearance in MB–CK, or cross-reactivity of some assays for MB–CK with BB–CK. A cause of increased MB–CK other than MI should be considered when elevations persist without change over serial samples, in contrast to the typical rise and fall that occur with MI.

   2. LDH, which exists as five isoenzymes, is present in most body tissues. With acute MI, elevations in LDH levels become detectable by 12 hours after chest pain, reach a peak in 24–48 hours, and remain elevated for 10–14 days after infarction. An LDH_1-LDH_2 ratio greater than 1.0 is consistent with MI. The diagnostic sensitivity and specificity of LDH isoenzymes are reduced in the presence of hemolysis, megaloblastic anemia, or renal insufficiency or damage, and by various solid tumors that induce elevation of LDH_1. Measurement of plasma LDH isoenzymes is not necessary in all individuals in whom MI is suspected but is a valuable adjunct to CK determinations in patients presenting 24 hours or more after onset of symptoms.

   3. Use of cardiac enzymes. In patients in whom MI is suspected, determinations

of plasma CK and MB–CK should be performed on admission and two to three times thereafter (q12h). In patients presenting 24 hours or more after onset of symptoms, if the MB–CK isoenzyme levels are not diagnostic, plasma LDH should be measured. If the LDH is elevated, LDH isoenzymes should be assayed. The assay should be repeated if the LDH_1-LDH_2 ratio is only slightly less than 1.0 on admission (*Ann. Intern. Med.* 102:221, 1986).

E. Radionuclide studies

1. **Technetium-99m–pyrophosphate scintigraphy** is generally used for the diagnosis of MI in patients hospitalized late after onset of symptoms in whom cardiac enzymes are no longer elevated or are unreliable. Imaging is optimal 2–7 days after MI. Focal increases in technetium pyrophosphate uptake are generally diagnostic of infarction, but diffuse uptake may occur in patients without MI when unstable angina, cardiomyopathy, cardiac amyloidosis, or pericarditis is present and after cardioversion. This technique is highly sensitive (> 90%) in detecting large transmural infarcts but is less reliable in the detection of small non–Q-wave MIs (*Semin. Nucl. Med.* 10:168, 1980).

2. **Antimyosin monoclonal antibodies** bind to the intracellular protein myosin in areas of myocardial necrosis. Some preliminary reports suggest that this method may be more sensitive than technetium pyrophosphate imaging.

3. **Noninvasive assessment of cardiac function** should be a part of the early evaluation of most patients with suspected MI.

   a. **Two-dimensional echocardiography** images the cardiac structures, pericardium, and ascending aorta and allows for identification of regional wall motion abnormalities, valvular abnormalities, and global left and right ventricular function. With Doppler and color flow Doppler techniques, blood flow within the heart can also be characterized. In patients with MI, Doppler imaging is indicated in the evaluation of new or changed murmurs to define the presence or absence of valvular regurgitation or ventricular septal rupture (*Br. Heart J.* 47:461, 1982; *Mayo Clin. Proc.* 62:59, 1987). In patients in whom traditional echocardiographic and Doppler studies are inadequate, **transesophageal echocardiography** may be indicated.

   b. **Radionuclide ventriculography (RVG)** allows for characterization of right and left ventricular ejection fraction and assessment of regional wall motion abnormalities. Because RVG provides less information regarding the cardiac structures, echocardiography is generally preferred in the initial evaluation of patients with MI. However, RVG is useful when echocardiographic studies are inadequate to completely assess regional wall motion, or to quantify left or right ventricular function.

III. Management. Mortality in patients with MI results from both arrhythmias and pump failure. Prompt detection and treatment of potentially lethal ventricular arrhythmias decreases hospital mortality. Most of the in-hospital mortality associated with MI is in patients with extensive left ventricular dysfunction and shock. Because myocardial necrosis evolves over several hours, early restoration of perfusion by thrombolysis or PTCA reduces infarct size and preserves left ventricular function. Large-scale clinical trials have shown that administration of fibrinolytic agents reduces mortality, particularly when therapy is started within 4 hours of the onset of symptoms (*Lancet* 1:398, 1986).

A. Immediate management. Initially, the goals are to relieve ischemic pain, provide supplemental oxygen, and recognize and treat potentially life-threatening complications of infarction such as hypotension, pulmonary edema, or ventricular arrhythmias.

1. **Analgesia.** Adequate control of pain reduces oxygen consumption and decreases levels of circulating catecholamines.

   a. **Sublingual nitroglycerin** (0.4 mg) should be given to most patients with ischemic chest pain in the absence of hypotension and can be repeated every 5 minutes. If symptoms persist after three doses, morphine should be given. Hypotension may occur in patients with volume depletion or inferior MI complicated by right ventricular infarction and should be treated by elevation of the lower extremities and intravenous saline infusion. A vagotonic response may also occur, particularly with intravenous nitroglycerin, and can be treated with atropine (see sec. **IV.A.3**).

  b. Morphine sulfate is the drug of choice for the treatment of the pain of infarction. Morphine also induces modest venodilation, which decreases preload, has a modest arterial vasodilating effect, and has a vagotonic effect that can decrease heart rate. Morphine is given intravenously in doses of 1–4 mg and can be repeated every 5–10 minutes until pain is controlled or side effects develop. Nausea, vomiting, dizziness, hypotension, and respiratory depression are all potential adverse effects of morphine sulfate. Nausea and vomiting can be avoided by concomitant use of an antiemetic agent. Hypotension is prevented by adequate hydration, and the vagotonic effects of morphine can be treated with atropine sulfate in doses of 0.3–0.5 mg given intravenously. **Naloxone hydrochloride,** administered in increments of 0.4 mg IV to a total dose of 1.2 mg, reverses the effects of morphine and can be used for treatment of respiratory depression. Due to the short half-life of naloxone (30–90 min), multiple doses may be required.

  c. Meperidine hydrochloride given in doses of 10–20 mg IV is an alternative to morphine but is not as effective an analgesic and may cause increases in heart rate and blood pressure.

2. **Oxygen therapy,** 2–4 liters/min via nasal cannula, is indicated in most patients with acute MI because mild hypoxemia is common. Patients in respiratory distress should be given oxygen by face mask, preferably at concentrations of 60–100%, until blood gas measurements are available. Arterial blood gas measurements should only be obtained on admission if the patient is in respiratory distress or is not a candidate for thrombolytic therapy. Subsequently, oxygen therapy should be adjusted to maintain the hemoglobin oxygen saturation at greater than 90%. Increasing oxygen tension to supranormal levels is not indicated because it may produce an increase in blood pressure and systemic vascular resistance. **Intubation and mechanical ventilation** are indicated if persistent hypoxemia is documented (arterial O_2 saturation <90%) or there is ventilatory failure (PCO_2 > 45–50 mm Hg) despite administration of 100% oxygen by mask. Prompt institution of mechanical ventilation improves oxygenation and decreases the work of breathing, which can significantly reduce myocardial oxygen demand.

B. Reperfusion

1. **Thrombolytic therapy.** Approximately 90% of patients with acute MI and ST segment elevation have complete thrombotic occlusion of the infarct-related coronary artery (*N. Engl. J. Med.* 303:897, 1980). Administration of fibrinolytic agents will induce clot lysis and restore blood flow in 60–90% of patients, depending on the agent used. In the absence of contraindications, thrombolytic therapy is the treatment of choice for restoring perfusion in patients with acute MI. In specialized centers, emergency PTCA appears to provide similar results, but this approach should generally be reserved for patients with contraindications to thrombolysis or those with cardiogenic shock.

  a. Patient selection. Thrombolytic therapy is indicated in patients with ischemic symptoms persisting more than 30 minutes that are associated with new ST segment elevation of at least 0.1 mV in at least two leads in the inferior, anterior, or lateral location, or ST segment depression in the anterior leads when due to posterior wall infarction. Optimal myocardial salvage generally requires treatment to be initiated within 4–6 hours of the onset of chest pain (*Lancet* 1:398, 1986). Although treatment should also be considered in patients who present later and have persistent ST segment elevation after administration of sublingual nitroglycerin, have not evolved significant Q waves, or have persistent chest pain. **Thrombolysis is contraindicated** in patients with a documented bleeding disorder, recent history of gastrointestinal or genitourinary hemorrhage, recorded blood pressure greater than 200/120 mm Hg, a history of cerebrovascular

Table 5-5. Doses of fibrinolytic agents for MI

Agents without fibrin specificity

Streptokinase
  1.5 million IU IV over 60 minutes (more rapid infusion can cause hypotension)
Urokinase*
  3 million IU IV over 60 minutes
Anistreplase (acylated streptokinase-plasmin complex)
  30 IU IV bolus over 2 minutes

Agents with fibrin specificity

Alteplase (recombinant tissue plasminogen activator [rt-PA])
  100 mg IV over 3 hours, usually with an initial 6-mg bolus followed by continuous infusion for a total of 60 mg the first hour, and then 40 mg over the next 2 hours
  Although not approved by the Food and Drug Administration, a regimen in which the dose of rt-PA is given more rapidly is preferred by many and is administered as a 15-mg IV bolus followed by 0.75 mg/kg (up to 50 mg) IV infusion over 30 minutes, then 0.5 mg/kg (up to 35 mg) IV infusion over 60 minutes (*J. Am. Coll. Cardiol.* 14:1566, 1989)

*Not approved for IV administration by the FDA.

accident, recent head trauma, or major surgery or an invasive procedure in the last 2 weeks, and in those who have undergone prolonged CPR, are pregnant, have suspected aortic dissection, have diabetic hemorrhagic retinopathy, or are suffering from a concurrent serious illness. The age of the patient should not be an absolute contraindication to thrombolysis because the prognosis after MI is worse in the elderly. In general, in patients with relative contraindications the decision to initiate thrombolytic therapy should be individualized based on an assessment of the risk of severe bleeding compared with the risk of complications of MI. For example, an 82-year-old patient with an extensive anterior wall MI should probably be treated in the absence of other contraindications.

   b. **Specific agents.** Fibrinolytic agents can be classified based on the extent to which they have specificity for activating plasminogen bound to fibrin compared with circulating plasminogen. Agents such as streptokinase induce a generalized fibrinolytic state characterized by extensive fibrinogen degradation, high concentration of circulating fibrinogen degradation products (FDPs), and depletion of the inhibitor of plasmin activity, alpha$_2$ antiplasmin (*N. Engl. J. Med.* 317:850, 1987). In comparison, recombinant tissue plasminogen activator (rt-PA) less frequently induces a lytic state and appears to result in a higher rate of early coronary reperfusion (*Circulation* 76:142, 1987). Intravenous doses of the currently available agents are listed in Table 5-5.

   c. **Adjuvant therapy**
      (1) Adjunctive intravenous **heparin** therapy has been shown to increase the rate of late coronary artery patency with t-PA (*N. Engl. J. Med.* 323:1433, 1990). Heparin, 5000 units IV bolus, followed by a 1000-unit/hour continuous infusion titrated to maintain the activated partial thromboplastin time (aPTT) at twice control value should be given when thrombolytic therapy is initiated, particularly with rt-PA. Subcutaneous heparin, 12,500 units q12h, may also be effective in decreasing mortality in patients treated with streptokinase or rt-PA.
      (2) **Aspirin** has been shown to decrease mortality in patients given streptokinase (*Lancet* 2:349, 1988). Chewable aspirin, 160 mg, can be given when therapy is initiated and oral aspirin should be continued as either 160 or 325 mg qd. The optimal dose of aspirin has not been established.

(3) **Beta-adrenergic antagonists** have been shown to decrease the incidence of nonfatal reinfarction and recurrent ischemic events in patients treated with t-PA for acute MI (*N. Engl. J. Med.* 320:618, 1989). Although definitive criteria have not been established, their use should be considered in patients without contraindications (see sec. **C.1**).

(4) **Lidocaine** should be used to treat documented ventricular arrhythmias; however, its efficacy in preventing reperfusion arrhythmias has not been established (see Chap. 7).

d. **Monitoring thrombolytic therapy** with coagulation assays is of value in documenting the effects of fibrinolytic agents on hemostasis and is necessary to titrate the dose of heparin (*Am. J. Med.* 76:879, 1984). With streptokinase or urokinase there is extensive fibrinogen degradation, resulting in increased concentrations of fibrin(ogen) degradation products and increases in the thrombin time and aPTT. Fibrinogen degradation is modest in most patients treated with t-PA, and the aPTT is often not prolonged. Routine assessment of fibrinogen levels is not mandatory; when necessary, it should be recognized that clotting-based methods of determining fibrinogen levels (Clauss assay) may measure lower levels of fibrinogen than are actually present. Although levels less than 100 mg/dl are associated with an increased risk of bleeding, they are not predictive in an individual patient. The aPTT should be monitored in all patients to allow titration of heparin and should be maintained at 1.5–2.0 times control (see Chap. 17). In patients in whom there is systemic lytic activity, the aPTT may be markedly prolonged for 6–8 hours after administration of the fibrinolytic agents because of the effects of fibrinogen degradation and FDPs.

e. **Complications.** Bleeding is the most common adverse effect of thrombolytic therapy. Hematomas develop at sites of vascular access in as many as 45% of patients, and transfusions are required in 10–20% of patients. For this reason, venipuncture should be limited and arterial puncture avoided if thrombolytic therapy is considered. In patients who hemorrhage, fresh frozen plasma can be given to reverse the lytic state. Cryoprecipitate can also be used to replete fibrinogen and factor VIII. Because platelet dysfunction often accompanies the lytic state, platelet transfusions may be useful in patients with markedly prolonged bleeding times (*Ann. Intern. Med* 12:1010, 1989). The incidence of intracranial hemorrhage is approximately 0.4%. Although streptokinase can cause anaphylaxis, no serious allergic reactions have been reported with urokinase or rt-PA.

2. **Coronary angiography with PTCA** has been used as a primary therapy for acute MI and, in addition to opening an occluded vessel, has the advantage of dilating the residual stenosis in the infarct-related vessel (*Circulation* 82:1910, 1990). PTCA should not be performed routinely during the first 48 hours after thrombolytic therapy but may be indicated in patients in whom reperfusion has apparently failed, such as those with persistent chest pain or persistent ST segment elevation. Coronary angiography should be performed promptly in patients with recurrent myocardial ischemia or in those in whom ischemia is provoked during predischarge exercise testing (*N. Engl. J. Med.* 320:618, 1989). In addition, many recommend that selected high-risk patients undergo coronary angiography to determine the extent of CAD and assess vessel patency.

3. **CABG.** Acute surgical revascularization has been performed successfully in the setting of MI (*Ann. Thorac. Surg.* 41:119, 1986), but delays required in preparation for surgery make this approach an unacceptable alternative to thrombolysis or PTCA as primary treatment for acute MI.

C. **Other measures to reduce infarct size**

1. **Beta-adrenergic receptor antagonists** decrease myocardial oxygen consumption by reducing the heart rate, contractility, and blood pressure. Intravenous

beta-adrenergic antagonists have been shown to reduce infarct size and mortality in several clinical trials (*Am. J. Med.* 74:113, 1983; *Lancet* 2:57, 1986). Therefore, intravenous beta-adrenergic antagonists are indicated in most patients with acute MI who present within the first 4–6 hours after the onset of symptoms. Patients with evidence of sympathetic hyperactivity manifested by tachycardia and hypertension in the absence of **heart failure** or the presence of continued ischemic pain may particularly benefit.

a. Contraindications to beta-adrenergic antagonists. Patients with a resting heart rate below 50–55 beats/min, systolic blood pressure less than 95 mm Hg, significant first-degree atrioventricular block (PR > 0.24 sec) or second- or third-degree block, obstructive lung disease by history or wheezes on examination, or evidence of significant heart failure on examination or chest radiograph should not receive beta-blockers.

b. Intravenous doses of beta-adrenergic antagonists. Metoprolol (15 mg IV given in 5-mg doses q5min, followed by 50- to 100-mg q12h oral dose), **propranolol** (0.1 mg/kg IV divided into 3 doses q5–10min, followed in 1 hour by 20- to 40-mg oral dose q6–8h), **atenolol** (5–10 mg IV, followed by 100 mg PO/day), and **timolol** (1 mg repeated after 10 minutes and followed by a 0.6-mg/kg maintenance infusion for 24 hours and then by a 10-mg oral dose q12h) have all been used in the treatment of patients with acute MI (*Eur. Heart J.* 6:199, 1985; *N. Engl. J. Med.* 310:9, 1984). Although there is no evidence that **esmolol hydrochloride** reduces infarct size or decreases mortality, because of its extremely short half-life (10 minutes), it is particularly useful in patients at high risk for complications of beta-blockade. It is administered as an initial 250- to 500-μg/kg bolus over 1 minute, followed by a maintenance infusion beginning at 50 μg/kg/minute and titrated to a heart rate of 55–60 beats/minute (*Circulation* 72:873, 1985). Timolol injection is not available in the United States.

2. Calcium channel–blocking agents have also been investigated as a measure to decrease infarct size, but the results of clinical trials have been disappointing. **Diltiazem** in one trial was found to have no benefit when given prophylactically to patients with MI and increased mortality in patients with left ventricular ejection fractions less than 40% or clinical evidence of heart failure. However, in patients with non–Q-wave MI and good left ventricular function, treatment with diltiazem may help prevent recurrent infarction (*N. Engl. J. Med.* 315:423, 1986).

3. Nitroglycerin (*Circulation* 68:576, 1983) may have a beneficial effect on infarct size in selected subgroups of patients when treatment is started early and hypotension is avoided (*Circulation* 76:906, 1989). Intravenous nitroglycerin is initiated as a 10-μg/minute infusion that is increased in 10-μg/minute increments at 10- to 15-minute intervals. The blood pressure should be closely monitored and the dose should not be increased further without invasive hemodynamic monitoring once there has been a 10–15% reduction in systolic blood pressure, although a greater reduction is usually well tolerated in patients who are initially hypertensive. Hypotension is most likely to occur in patients with MI who have relative volume depletion (low preload) or those with inferior MI complicated by right ventricular dysfunction (see Appendix C and Table 5-6).

D. Anticoagulant and antiplatelet therapy

1. Heparin administered either as a continuous intravenous infusion or a high dose subcutaneously (12,500 units q12h) appears to decrease mortality in patients with MI regardless of whether they receive thrombolytic therapy (*Lancet* 2:182, 1989) and may decrease the incidence of mural thrombi (*J. Am. Coll. Cardiol.* 8:419, 1985; *Am. Heart J.* 109:616, 1985). However, the risk of bleeding complications due to anticoagulation are probably greater than the potential benefits in patients at low risk for complications after MI. Therefore, in the absence of contraindications anticoagulation with intravenous or high-dose subcutaneous heparin should be considered primarily in those patients with large anterior MIs, patients at risk of developing mural thrombosis, and selected patients at risk for recurrent MI. In the absence of more aggressive anticoagulation, all patients admitted to the intensive care unit should be given low-dose heparin, 5000 units subcutaneously q8–12h, until they are fully ambulatory to prevent the development of deep venous thrombosis (*Am. Heart J.* 99:574, 1980).

    a. Long-term anticoagulation. Patients with documented mural thrombus or extensive anterior MI with apical involvement should be treated with **warfarin (Coumadin)** for 3 months. In the absence of these conditions, either **aspirin** or **Coumadin** can be given for secondary prevention (see below).

  2. Aspirin. It is reasonable to give most patients with MI aspirin on admission and to continue aspirin long term for secondary prevention. In patients fully anticoagulated with intravenous heparin or when long-term anticoagulation with Coumadin is anticipated, concurrent aspirin therapy has been associated with an increase in bleeding complications. Aspirin may also increase bleeding in patients who subsequently undergo cardiac surgery.

E. Subsequent management of patients with MI

  1. General measures. Patients with MI should be admitted to the intensive care unit. Intravenous access is mandatory. Continuous ECG monitoring should be established and observed by nursing personnel trained in the recognition of arrhythmias. Visitors should be limited, and visitation periods should be kept brief to allow for patient rest. Oral rather than rectal temperatures should be obtained. Patients with uncomplicated MIs generally spend 2–3 days in the intensive care unit and then can be transferred to a "step down" unit with ambulatory monitoring capability for the remainder of their 7- to 10-day hospital stay. If complications arise during the initial post-MI period, the stay in the intensive care unit should be extended until the patient's condition improves.

  2. Sedation is beneficial during the initial days after MI and can be achieved with low doses of a benzodiazepine or other anxiolytic agent (see Chap. 1).

  3. Diet and bowel care. For the first day after MI, the diet should be liquid or soft followed by a 1200- to 1800-calorie, no added salt, low-cholesterol diet. Caffeinated beverages, as well as very hot or cold liquids, should be avoided. Since constipation is a common problem, stool softeners or mild laxatives are routinely given.

  4. Prophylactic lidocaine is generally unnecessary once the patient has been admitted to the intensive care unit because ventricular arrhythmias can generally be treated promptly. However, if lidocaine has been started before admission it can be continued for at least 24 hours (see sec. **IV.A.1.a**).

IV. Complications

  A. Arrhythmias often occur in the first 24 hours after MI. While life-threatening arrhythmias such as ventricular tachycardia (VT) or fibrillation (VF) are of most concern, any arrhythmia that results in hemodynamic compromise should be vigorously treated, by electrical cardioversion if necessary. Potentially exacerbating conditions should be considered and corrected when possible, including adverse effects of drugs, hypoxemia, acidosis, or electrolyte imbalances (especially potassium, calcium, and magnesium disorders). Left ventricular (LV) failure, recurrent ischemia, or hypotension may also predispose to arrhythmias and should be promptly managed.

  1. Ventricular arrhythmias

    a. Ventricular premature depolarizations (VPDs) occur commonly in the acute MI period and may herald VT or VF. In the majority of patients, VT and VF are not preceded by "warning arrhythmias" (*Circulation* 74:653, 1986). VPDs should be treated if they occur more frequently than 5 per minute, appear in the vulnerable period of the cardiac cycle (R on T phenomenon), occur in salvos of two or more with sufficient frequency to induce hemodynamic compromise, or occur in multiple forms (see Chap. 7).

      (1) Lidocaine is the initial treatment of choice for suppression of VPDs and is administered as an initial intravenous bolus of 1 mg/kg followed by one or more boluses of 0.5 mg/kg 3–5 minutes apart until ectopy resolves or a total dose of 3 mg/kg has been given, followed by a continuous intravenous infusion of 2–4 mg/minute (20–50 μg/kg/min). Since the half-life of lidocaine is prolonged with heart failure, liver disease, and hypotension and in the elderly, the total dose should be decreased by 50% in these situations. Blood levels should be checked in patients in whom lidocaine clearance may be impaired or when high doses or prolonged infusions are used.

(2) Procainamide is used when lidocaine is ineffective and is started as a 500- to 1000-mg loading dose given at a rate no faster than 50 mg/minute followed by a 2- to 5-mg/minute maintenance infusion (see Appendix C). During the infusion QRS duration, QT interval, vital signs, and procainamide and N-acetylprocainamide (NAPA) blood levels should be carefully monitored. In patients with renal failure, accumulation of NAPA may occur.

b. VT and VF. Immediate cardioversion or defibrillation is the treatment of choice for VF or VT with hemodynamic compromise. Specific protocols are outlined in Chap. 8.

c. Accelerated idioventricular rhythm (AIVR) occurs frequently in patients in whom coronary reperfusion is achieved, and occasionally in other patients with MI. AIVR is a wide complex escape rhythm (rate 60–110 beats/min) that occurs when the sinus rate slows below 60 per minute, and is generally unaccompanied by hemodynamic compromise. AIVR is usually benign, with a duration of less than 48 hours, and does not require specific therapy except for close observation. When AIVR is associated with hemodynamic deterioration or it precipitates VT or VF, administration of atropine or overdrive pacing is effective treatment.

2. Supraventricular tachycardias (see Chap. 7)

a. Sinus tachycardia is common in patients with acute MI and is frequently associated with heart failure, hypoxemia, pain, anxiety, fever, hypovolemia, or adverse drug effects. Persistent sinus tachycardia is a poor prognostic indicator and is often an indication for invasive hemodynamic evaluation. Treatment is directed at correcting underlying causes. In the absence of heart failure and after correction of contributing causes, judicious use of beta-blockers is indicated, especially when hypertension accompanies the sinus tachycardia. Intravenous metoprolol, propranolol, or esmolol is usually effective treatment.

b. Paroxysmal supraventricular tachycardia (PSVT) occurs infrequently in patients with MI but should be treated to prevent exacerbation of myocardial ischemia. Cardioversion is the treatment of choice in the presence of hypotension, ischemia, or heart failure. If the patient's condition is stable, vagotonic maneuvers such as careful carotid sinus massage can be attempted. For PSVT that is refractory to vagotonic maneuvers, **adenosine, verapamil, propranolol, or digoxin** can be given as outlined in Chap. 7.

c. Atrial flutter often responds poorly to pharmacologic measures. If the patient's condition is unstable, cardioversion beginning at low energy levels (50 joules) is the treatment of choice. This may convert the rhythm to sinus or to atrial fibrillation. Rapid atrial pacing may also be beneficial and is the treatment of choice in patients with digitalis intoxication. For patients in stable condition, verapamil, propranolol, or digoxin can be used. These drugs will decrease the ventricular response and may convert the rhythm to atrial fibrillation. Because of the risk of 1:1 conduction with atrial flutter, even patients in a stable condition should be electrically cardioverted when there is no response to initial pharmacologic therapy (see Chap. 7).

d. Atrial fibrillation is deleterious to the ischemic myocardium because the ventricular response is usually rapid and the atrial contribution to ventricular filling is lost. Cardioversion starting with 100 joules is the treatment of choice for atrial fibrillation with rapid ventricular response and hemodynamic compromise. If the ventricular rate is slow (less than 100 beats/min) in the absence of treatment with drugs that depress atrioventricular node conduction, placement of a transvenous endocardial pacemaker should be considered before cardioversion to avoid asystole. For patients who are stable hemodynamically, verapamil, propranolol, or digoxin can be used to control ventricular response. Frequently, atrial fibrillation in the acute MI period may be transient and therefore not require long-term treatment.

e. **Accelerated junctional rhythm** is usually a benign escape rhythm in patients with sinus bradycardia and requires no specific therapy. Occasionally in patients with cardiogenic shock or digitalis toxicity **nonparoxysmal junctional tachycardia** (70–130 beats/min) may occur. Treatment is directed toward the underlying condition.

3. **Bradycardias**
   a. **Sinus bradycardia** may occur in patients with acute MI, particularly in patients with inferior MI. Treatment is only indicated in patients with hypotension or decreased cardiac output due to the bradycardia. Atropine sulfate, 0.5–1.0 mg IV repeated at 5-minute intervals to a maximum of 2 mg, is usually effective. Temporary atrial or ventricular pacing is preferred for refractory or recurrent symptomatic bradycardia.
   b. **Atrioventricular conduction disturbances,** including first-degree (prolongation of PR interval), second-degree, or third-degree (complete) AV block, occur frequently in patients with MI.
      (1) **First-degree AV block** should be recognized primarily because it may be a contraindication to the use of verapamil, diltiazem, or beta-adrenergic antagonists. Often, first-degree AV block is caused by treatment with digitalis or other agents that slow AV node conduction.
      (2) **Second-degree block** includes Mobitz type I (Wenckebach), manifested by gradual prolongation of the PR interval and a narrow QRS complex before the nonconducted P wave, and Mobitz type II, in which the dropped beats are not preceded by PR prolongation and the QRS complex is wide. In Mobitz type I the site of block is usually within the AV node, whereas in most instances, the block in Mobitz type II is located below the bundle of His. Mobitz type I (Wenckebach) block does not require specific therapy, but temporary transvenous pacing is indicated in the presence of symptomatic bradycardia. Mobitz type II block may progress to complete AV block and requires pacemaker insertion whether or not the patient is symptomatic.
      (3) **In third-degree heart block** there is atrioventricular dissociation, often with a slow ventricular escape rhythm. In patients with anterior MI, complete AV block may develop abruptly, often being preceded only by first-degree block or some form of intraventricular block, and is associated with a large area of infarction and high mortality. In patients with inferior MI, heart block may be preceded by first- or second-degree AV block, and often the junctional or ventricular escape rhythm is not associated with symptoms. Nonetheless, third-degree block in the setting of an MI generally requires emergency transvenous pacing because of the potential for progression to asystole. The consequences of third-degree AV block are most deleterious in patients in whom maintenance of cardiac output depends on a synchronized atrial contribution to ventricular filling, typically those with large anterior MI or inferior MI complicated by right ventricular infarction. In such patients atrioventricular pacing is indicated.
      (4) **Indications for transvenous pacing in patients with MI** include: (1) asystole, (2) third-degree heart block, (3) new right bundle branch block with left anterior or posterior hemiblock (new right bundle branch block alone is considered by many an indication for temporary

pacing), (4) new left bundle branch block, (5) Mobitz type II second-degree heart block, and (6) symptomatic bradycardia not responsive to atropine. Indications for permanent pacing after MI are discussed in Chap. 7.

B. Hypertension in patients with MI is common and should be treated promptly. Increases in afterload and subsequent elevation in myocardial oxygen demand may increase infarct size or produce infarct expansion. In general, patients with MI should be treated initially with short-acting titratable intravenous agents. The following approach to treatment of patients with MI and hypertension is suggested:

1. **Bed rest, analgesia, and sedation** are frequently sufficient in controlling mild to moderate elevations in blood pressure.

2. **Beta-adrenergic antagonists** are often appropriate and should be administered in small parenteral doses, as described in sec. **III.C.1.** If intravenous preparations are tolerated, oral therapy can be initiated (see Table 5-2).

3. Indications for the use of **calcium channel antagonists** in the treatment of hypertension in the acute MI period have not been well defined. However, these agents are effective in reducing blood pressure and may be appropriate if nitrates or beta-blockers are ineffective or contraindicated (see sec. **III.C.2**).

4. **Intravenous nitroprusside** is indicated in the treatment of moderate to severe hypertension and results in a prompt reduction in blood pressure by dilation of the venous and arterial circulation. The initial dose is 10–15 µg/minute administered as a continuous intravenous infusion, with increases in 5- to 10-µg increments q5–10min as required for control of blood pressure (see Appendix C). Doses as high as 400 µg/minute are occasionally necessary. Solutions should be prepared in 5% dextrose and water just before use and shielded from light because the drug is photosensitive. With prolonged therapy, high doses, or renal dysfunction, toxic plasma concentrations of thiocyanate, a metabolite that is excreted by the kidneys, may increase, so that levels should be monitored under these circumstances. Cyanide toxicity may occur with even brief infusion or low infusion rates, and is manifested by the development of lactic acidosis due to inhibition of aerobic metabolism and clinical deterioration. The maximum dose rate of 10 µg/kg/min should never be used for more than 10 minutes (*Clin. Pharmacokinet.* 9:239, 1984).

5. **Intravenous nitroglycerin** induces venodilatation and modest arteriolar dilatation. In patients with elevated left ventricular filling pressures, doses sufficient to decrease modest hypertension can often be given, but with normal left ventricular filling pressures the antihypertensive effects are limited. This drug is often effective in the treatment of hypertension associated with heart failure or when there are continued ischemic symptoms. The initial dose is 10 µg/minute by continuous infusion with increases in 5- to 10-µg/minute increments until blood pressure is controlled.

C. Hemodynamic complications

1. **Left ventricular pump failure** in the setting of MI is associated with both decreased left ventricular systolic function and decreased compliance (e.g., stiff ventricle). The severity of pump failure is related to the extent of infarction, ranging from mild pulmonary congestion to cardiogenic shock. Acute mechanical complications of MI such as acute mitral regurgitation, ventricular septal rupture, or exacerbation of underlying chronic valvular disease may also result in pulmonary edema or shock. Thus, in patients with clinical evidence of pump failure or shock, the initial evaluation should include noninvasive imaging of ventricular function with radionuclide ventriculography or two-dimensional echocardiography and Doppler studies.

   a. **Treatment of mild heart failure.** In patients with mild pulmonary congestion or an S3 gallop, diuretics are generally appropriate but must be used cautiously because most patients with MI are not volume overloaded and overdiuresis may lead to hypovolemia and inappropriately reduce left ventricular filling pressures. Furosemide, beginning with 10 to 20 mg IV, is the treatment of choice. (Diuretic regimens are discussed in detail in Chap. 4.)

  (1) Topical nitrates or low doses of intravenous nitroglycerin in patients who are hemodynamically stable will often be of benefit by decreasing left ventricular filling pressures.

  (2) Digoxin, 0.125–0.25 mg by mouth daily, is often used in the treatment of patients with mild chronic heart failure, but whether it has beneficial effects on long-term survival is controversial. Digoxin should not be used in the acute management of heart failure in patients with MI.

  (3) Angiotensin converting enzyme inhibitors improve symptoms in patients with mild to moderate heart failure (*J.A.M.A.* 259:539, 1988) and improve survival in patients with severe heart failure (*N. Engl. J. Med.* 316:1429, 1987). **Captopril,** 6.5–50.0 mg PO q6h–q8h, or **enalapril,** 2.5–20.0 mg bid, can be used starting with the lower doses to avoid hypotension. In patients with significant congestive heart failure or those with hypotension who do not respond to initial therapy, invasive hemodynamic monitoring with a balloon-tipped pulmonary artery catheter should be considered.

 b. Indications for pulmonary artery catheterization include the following: (1) severe or progressive congestive heart failure; (2) cardiogenic shock or progressive hypotension; (3) clinical signs suggestive of mitral regurgitation, ventricular septal defect, or hemodynamically significant pericardial effusion; (4) hypotension unresponsive to simple conventional measures (i.e., intravenous fluids); (5) unexplained or severe cyanosis, hypoxemia, tachypnea, diaphoresis, or acidosis; (6) unexplained or refractory sinus tachycardia or other tachyarrhythmias; or (7) the need for parenteral vasoactive agents that must be closely monitored to avoid deleterious changes in heart rate or blood pressure (*J. Am. Coll. Cardiol.* 16:249, 1990). Pulmonary arterial and systemic arterial catheters should be inserted only by trained individuals under sterile conditions. Catheter position should be confirmed by chest radiograph. Complications of pulmonary artery catheterization include arrhythmias, hemorrhage, pneumothorax (with subclavian or internal jugular approach), endocarditis, sepsis, catheter knotting, and balloon rupture. In patients with left bundle branch block, consideration should be given to placing a temporary pacemaker because pulmonary artery catheterization can induce complete heart block in such individuals. In addition, in patients undergoing pulmonary artery catheterization, systemic blood pressure should be measured frequently, either noninvasively or by use of a radial or femoral arterial catheter when cuff pressure is unreliable or difficult to obtain; urinary output should be closely monitored with an indwelling catheter if necessary.

 c. Management of hemodynamic subsets of patients with left ventricular dysfunction. Pulmonary artery catheterization allows for measurement of the pressures in the right atrium (RAP), right ventricle, and pulmonary artery and measurement of the pulmonary artery occlusive pressure (PAOP). Pressures should be measured at end inspiration and in general should be determined from a strip-chart recording. In addition, cardiac index (CI = cardiac output/body surface area) can be measured by the thermodilution or Fick methods, and mixed venous blood gases can be obtained. The systemic vascular resistance (SVR = [(mean arterial pressure − RAP)/cardiac output] × 80) should also be calculated (normal range 900–1350 dynes-sec-cm^{-5}). In some circumstances catheters that allow for continuous measurement of mixed venous oxygen saturation or right ventricular ejection fraction may be useful. Patients with MI can be categorized into several hemodynamic subsets that are useful for defining treatment strategies (*J. Am. Coll. Cardiol.* 16:249, 1990). Establishing baseline measurements and subsequent trends is more important than single absolute values. It is also important to recognize that, while guidelines for management of hemodynamic complications are useful, therapy must be based on individual responses to initial therapy. All hemodynamic data should be evaluated in terms of the clinical response and viewed critically if they fail to correlate with other physiologic parameters (such as urine output). Patients should be managed aggressively to minimize the duration of catheterization.

(1) Decreased LV filling pressure (PAOP <15–18 mm Hg) when accompanied by hypotension, decreased cardiac index (< 2.5 liters/min/m^2), oliguria, or persistent sinus tachycardia should be treated by rapid infusion of normal saline. Because LV compliance is decreased in patients with anterior MI, a PAOP of 15–18 mm Hg is generally an appropriate end point for volume resuscitation.

(2) Elevated LV filling pressure (PAOP >18 mm Hg) with normal cardiac index (>2.5 liters/min/m^2) is an indication of volume overload or decreased LV compliance. Often, such patients can be treated with a diuretic alone. Topical nitrates or intravenous nitroglycerin can also be used when increased filling pressures persist despite diuresis.

(3) Elevated LV filling pressure (PAOP >18 mm Hg), decreased cardiac index (<2.5 liters/min/m^2), and systolic arterial pressure >100 mm Hg are indications of significant LV systolic dysfunction. Because the blood pressure is maintained, afterload reduction with nitroglycerin or nitroprusside is the treatment of choice. Nitroglycerin is preferred particularly early after the onset of infarction because it may also induce coronary vasodilatation and increase myocardial blood flow to ischemic regions. Nitroprusside has less favorable effects in terms of coronary blood flow (*N. Engl. J. Med.* 306:1121, 1129, and 1168, 1982) but is a more potent vasodilator and is indicated when marked hypertension is present. If blood pressure falls or cardiac index does not improve, an inotropic agent, such as dobutamine or amrinone, should be added (Table 5-6).

(4) Elevated LV filling pressure (PAOP >18 mm Hg), decreased cardiac index (<2.5 liters/min/m^2), and systolic arterial pressure less than 100 mm Hg are indications of extensive left ventricular dysfunction. Cardiogenic shock is considered present when the systolic blood pressure is less than 90 mm Hg and there is evidence of organ hypoperfusion (such as oliguria and confusion). Thrombolysis is contraindicated in most patients with shock because of unpredictable pharmacokinetics of fibrinolytic agents in this setting and the need for invasive vascular procedures. However, because the mortality of patients with cardiogenic shock is nearly 80% despite aggressive intervention, once stabilized the patient should be aggressively evaluated for the potential for myocardial salvage with emergency PTCA (*Circulation* 78:1345, 1988) and for the presence of treatable mechanical complications of infarction, such as severe mitral regurgitation or ventricular septal rupture (see sec. **IV.D**). Initial support of the circulation with a vasopressor is essential; norepinephrine is preferred in markedly hypotensive patients (systolic blood pressure $<$ 70 mm Hg), but dopamine is usually sufficient in patients with a systolic blood pressure of 70–90 mm Hg. In patients with a systolic blood pressure near 90 mm Hg, dobutamine is often sufficient (see Table 5-6). Patients who do not respond to initial pharmacologic interventions or require high doses of vasopressors and are candidates for aggressive intervention should be supported with an intra-aortic balloon pump.

(5) Right ventricular infarction is characterized by a decreased cardiac index (<2.5 liters/min/m^2), with normal or decreased LV filling pressures and elevated right atrial pressure (>10 mm Hg) in patients with inferior MI (*Chest* 77:220, 1980). In some patients elevation of

Table 5-6. Doses and actions of vasoactive and inotropic agents used in patients with MI

Agent	Dose	Action	Precautions
Dobutamine (see Appendix C)	2.5–15.0 µg/kg-/min; start at lower doses	Positive inotrope, beta-adrenergic agonist	Heart rate and oxygen consumption may increase, may exacerbate arrhythmias
Amrinone (*Am. J. Cardiol.* 56:29B, 1985)	0.75 mg/kg initial dose, followed by 5–10 µg/kg/min infusion	Positive inotrope, phosphodiesterase inhibitor	May exacerbate arrhythmias
Dopamine (see Appendix C)	0.5–2.0 µg/kg/min	Dilates renal and mesenteric arteries	
	2.0–6.0 µg/kg/min	Positive inotrope; beta-adrenergic agonist	Increases heart rate and increases PAOP
	>10 µg/kg/min	Vasopressor alpha-adrenergic agonist	Similar but less potent than norepinephrine at these doses
Intravenous nitroglycerin	10–400 µg/min; start at lower doses	Venodilator with modest arteriolar dilator effects, coronary vasodilator	Hypotension in patients with low PAOP
Nitroprusside (see Appendix C)	0.5–2.0 µg/kg/min	Arteriolar and venodilator	Thiocyanate toxicity in patients with renal failure or with high doses

right atrial pressure may not be evident until fluids are given. Clinical signs include elevation of the jugular venous pulsations, a positive Kussmaul's sign (increase in jugular venous pressures with inspiration), and right-sided third and fourth heart sounds with clear lung fields. The ECG may show right precordial ST segment elevation. Echocardiography is often useful in confirming the diagnosis (*Am. Heart J.* 107:505, 1984). Hemodynamic responses to right ventricular infarction range from asymptomatic elevation of right-sided pressures to severe shock. Patients with a systolic blood pressure of 90–100 mm Hg and depressed cardiac index often respond to fluids, which should be given until the PAOP is 15–18 mm Hg; excessive fluid administration should be avoided. If the cardiac index is still decreased after fluid administration or if hypotension is more severe, dobutamine should be administered. Most often the combination of volume resuscitation and inotropic support with dobutamine will increase the systolic blood pressure to greater than 90 mm Hg. However, patients with refractory severe hypotension should be supported with intraaortic balloon counterpulsation. In patients with heart block causing atrioventricular dysynchrony, AV sequential pacing may have marked beneficial hemodynamic effects.

D. Mechanical complications

    1. Infarct expansion. Thinning and expansion of the infarcted myocardial wall that follow MI may adversely alter ventricular geometry and function. Agents that decrease afterload, particularly angiotensin converting enzyme inhibitors, may limit infarct expansion and ventricular dilatation after infarction (*N. Engl. J. Med.* 319:80, 1988). Use of steroids or nonsteroidal anti-inflammatory drugs should be avoided in patients with MI because they appear to augment myocardial thinning (*Circulation* 53 [suppl I]: I-204, 1976; *Can. J. Cardiol.* 5:211, 1989).

2. **Hemodynamically significant mitral regurgitation** may occur in patients with acute MI and is associated with a poorer prognosis compared with that for patients without mitral regurgitation (*Am. J. Cardiol.* 65:1169, 1990).

   a. **Diagnosis.** Most patients with hemodynamically significant mitral regurgitation have a typical holosystolic murmur. With moderate to severe mitral regurgitation, pulmonary edema is usually present. Papillary muscle rupture or severe disruption of the valve is invariably associated with cardiogenic shock. Although the presence of a large V wave on the pulmonary artery pressure tracing obtained with pulmonary artery catheterization is suggestive of mitral regurgitation, it is neither sensitive nor specific and may occur in patients with ventricular septal rupture. Two-dimensional echocardiography with Doppler imaging is the initial diagnostic test of choice. However, in critically ill patients technical difficulties often limit the sensitivity of conventional echocardiographic imaging; these can be overcome by **transesophageal echocardiography.**

   b. **Initial management** of patients with mitral regurgitation should include pharmacologic afterload reduction with intravenous nitroglycerin or nitroprusside; dobutamine may be of benefit in patients with borderline hypotension. In patients with severe mitral regurgitation intra-aortic balloon counterpulsation is often necessary to stabilize the patient before surgical intervention.

3. **Rupture of the interventricular septum** is suggested by the development of a systolic murmur, the concomitant onset of pulmonary edema, and, almost always, cardiogenic shock. Interventricular septal rupture complicates 1–5% of MIs and generally occurs within 7 days.

   a. **Diagnosis.** Ventricular septal rupture typically produces a holosystolic murmur that is heard best along the lower left sternal border and is most often associated with a systolic thrill. Two-dimensional echocardiography with Doppler imaging is an extremely sensitive and specific technique for detecting these or other intracardiac shunts and valvular regurgitation and therefore should always be part of the initial evaluation of patients with a new murmur or cardiogenic shock after MI. The presence of a ventricular septal rupture can be documented by a greater than 5% increase in hemoglobin oxygen saturation between the right atrium and right ventricle with right heart catheterization.

   b. **Management.** Initial management of patients with ventricular septal rupture is similar to that already outlined for cardiogenic shock and should include invasive hemodynamic monitoring. Vasodilators such as nitroglycerin or nitroprusside are indicated to reduce afterload, but the majority of patients will require intra-aortic balloon counterpulsation before an attempt at surgical repair.

4. **Rupture of the left ventricular free wall (cardiorrhexis)** is a catastrophic complication of MI responsible for 8–15% of all associated mortality. Rupture is more frequent in women, in patients with MI as the first indication of CAD, in patients with hypertension, and in those treated with steroids or nonsteroidal anti-inflammatory drugs (*Am. J. Cardiol.* 40:429, 1977). Rupture typically occurs during the first week after MI and presents as sudden hemodynamic collapse. Bradyarrhythmias, including sinus and junctional bradycardia and idioventricular rhythm, ST segment and T-wave abnormalities, and, eventually, electromechanical dissociation, may accompany left ventricular rupture. Although sudden death is usual, some instances of left ventricular rupture may be preceded by recurrent pericardial pain secondary

to the accumulation of blood in the pericardial space with or without the signs of pericardial effusion or tamponade and hypotension. Echocardiography may be useful in identifying patients with thinned ventricular walls at risk for rupture or those in whom partial rupture has occurred. Prompt recognition at this stage may allow for successful surgical repair. Pericardiocentesis in the event of tamponade and the prompt institution of intra-aortic balloon counterpulsation may prove life sustaining until surgical correction can be performed.

5. **Ventricular aneurysm,** a localized outpouching of the left ventricular cavity related to a region of akinetic or dyskinetic myocardium, may be suspected on the basis of persistent post-MI ST segment elevation, intractable heart failure, or poorly controlled ventricular arrhythmias (*N. Engl. J. Med.* 311:1001, 1984). Patients with aneurysms are at risk for development of mural thrombi and peripheral embolization.

   a. **Diagnosis.** Echocardiography and left ventricular angiography are useful to define the extent of aneurysmal involvement of the left ventricular wall, but two-dimensional echocardiography is the test of choice for determining the presence of mural thrombus.

   b. **Management.** Patients with mural thrombi should be given anticoagulants (see sec. **III.D.1**). Surgical correction of the aneurysm is indicated in some patients with refractory left heart failure, life-threatening ventricular arrhythmias, or recurrent systemic embolization.

   c. True ventricular aneurysm should be distinguished from **pseudoaneurysm,** a form of cardiac rupture in which pericardial extravasation of blood is restricted locally by the pericardium and an aneurysm with a narrow connection to the left ventricular cavity develops. These aneurysms occur after transmural infarctions and, because of their high incidence of rupture, should be surgically corrected (*Thorax* 38:25, 1983).

E. **Recurrent ischemia and infarction**

   1. **Recurrent ischemia.** Patients with signs or symptoms of recurrent ischemia in the post-MI period should be aggressively managed, and prompt coronary angiography should be performed to identify those patients who will benefit from interventional therapy with PTCA or CABG.

   2. **Extension or recurrence of infarction** occurs in 10–20% of patients after MI (*Circulation* 65:918, 1982) and is often preceded by recurrent chest discomfort despite initial therapy. Patients with recurrent chest pain or ECG changes should be reevaluated for new myocardial necrosis with MB–CK isoenzyme measurements. Most infarct extensions occur within 7–10 days of infarction; therefore, discharge from the hospital before this time is not advised in high-risk patients (e.g., patients with recurrent ischemia, extensive infarction, symptomatic heart failure, or arrhythmias).

F. **Pericardial complications after MI**

   1. **Acute pericarditis** generally occurs in patients with large infarctions. Pain due to pericarditis is typically substernal, with radiation to the back, and is exacerbated by deep breathing or movement and relieved by sitting up. A pericardial friction rub may be appreciated on careful examination but is often evanescent, and the classic ECG findings associated with pericarditis may be masked by the infarct (*N. Engl. J. Med.* 311:1211, 1984). Aspirin can be used to relieve the pain. Use of corticosteroids or nonsteroidal antiinflammatory drugs is contraindicated because they retard myocardial scar formation and may increase the incidence of rupture (see sec. **III.D.1**). In patients who are being treated with intravenous heparin, the presence of active pericarditis may increase the risk of hemorrhagic cardiac tamponade. Thus, in such patients this potential risk should be balanced against the need for continued anticoagulation.

   2. **Post-MI or Dressler's syndrome** is an uncommon late complication of MI characterized by pericarditis, pleuritis, pericardial or pleural effusions, fever, leukocytosis, elevated sedimentation rate, and elevated levels of antimyocardial antibodies (*Am. J. Cardiol.* 50:1269, 1982). Patients typically have

malaise, fever, and chest pain, but the syndrome may be mistaken for angina or MI, and the ECG may show diffuse, marked ST segment elevation. Onset of symptoms is usually between the second and tenth weeks after MI, and the course may be lengthy, with frequent remissions and exacerbations. Therapy is aimed at relieving symptoms and consists of **nonsteroidal anti-inflammatory** agents such as aspirin (650 mg orally q6–8h) or indomethacin (25–50 mg orally q6-8h). Corticosteroids such as **prednisone** (1 mg/kg orally qd) may be required for severe symptoms and, when used, should be tapered gradually to minimize exacerbation of symptoms. Anticoagulants should be discontinued if possible since hemorrhagic pericarditis with tamponade can occur. Constrictive pericarditis may complicate the post-MI syndrome but is rare.

V. Rehabilitation. Although tissue repair may not be complete for up to 6 weeks after MI, the length of hospitalization and level of activity should be adjusted to the individual patient. In general the length of hospitalization for patients with uncomplicated MI is 7–10 days, with ECG monitoring in a telemetry unit. Longer hospitalization is often necessary for those with complications. Patients should be kept at bed rest, but movement in bed and dangling of the feet over the side of the bed should be encouraged. Within 24 hours after admission, patients with an uncomplicated course should begin sitting in a chair, may use a bedside commode, and should be encouraged to help themselves with regard to shaving, using the toilet, and feeding. Patients should be encouraged to begin walking in the room on the third day after admission and should be fully ambulatory by 5–7 days. Instructions regarding activity, including sexual activity, should be given before discharge. Depending on the extent of infarction, patients can return to work 4–8 weeks after discharge. Supervised exercise rehabilitation can begin on discharge from the hospital.

VI. Secondary prevention

A. Modification of cardiac risk factors is important after MI. Cessation of tobacco use is recommended to those patients who are smokers, and information regarding hospital or American Heart Association smoking cessation programs should be provided. Patients with hypercholesterolemia, hypertension, or diabetes should be identified and treated appropriately. Regular aerobic exercise, preferably in a structured setting, is recommended for those patients who have had an uncomplicated post-MI course and are at low risk for subsequent cardiac events.

B. Medical therapy. Beta-adrenergic antagonists (such as 10 mg bid timolol, 20–80 mg qid propranolol, or 100 mg bid metoprolol) reduce mortality and reinfarction after MI (*N. Engl. J. Med.* 313:1055, 1985). Beta-adrenergic antagonists with intrinsic sympathomimetic activity do not appear to be as effective. Antiplatelet agents, such as aspirin alone (300–1500 mg/day) may also be valuable in secondary prevention (*N. Engl. J. Med.* 318:245, 1988). Therapeutic anticoagulation with Coumadin has also been shown to be effective (*N. Engl. J. Med.* 323:147, 1990), but whether it is more effective than aspirin has not been determined.

C. Risk stratification with exercise stress testing, with or without the use of thallium perfusion imaging or radionuclide ventriculography, can help identify those patients at high risk for subsequent cardiac events. Submaximal exercise testing can be performed safely 7–10 days after an uncomplicated MI, and patients with a positive test result should undergo cardiac catheterization to further assess coronary anatomy and subsequent prognosis. Those individuals who complete the submaximal protocol without evidence of ischemia are at very low risk for cardiac events during the next year (*N. Engl. J. Med.* 314:161, 1986). Coronary angiography should similarly be performed in patients with non-Q-wave infarctions or post-MI courses complicated by recurrent ischemia, significant heart failure, or ventricular arrhythmias. Maximal exercise testing can be safely performed 4–6 weeks after MI.

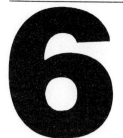

Heart Failure

Daniel P. Kelly and
Edward T.A. Fry

Clinical Diagnosis

I. **Definition.** Heart failure (HF) is the inability of the heart to maintain an output adequate to meet the metabolic demands of the body. It is a common condition associated with extremely high morbidity and mortality.

II. **Pathophysiology.** The clinical syndrome of heart failure manifests as organ hypoperfusion and inadequate tissue oxygen delivery due to a low cardiac output and decreased cardiac reserve ("forward failure") as well as pulmonary and venous congestion ("backward failure"). A variety of compensatory adaptations occur, which include (1) increased left ventricular volume (dilatation) and mass (hypertrophy), (2) increased systemic vascular resistance (SVR) secondary to enhanced activity of the sympathetic nervous system and elevated levels of circulating catecholamines, and (3) activation of the renin-angiotensin and vasopressin (ADH) systems. These secondary mechanisms, in conjunction with actual "pump failure," play a role in the pathophysiology of HF.

III. **The clinical manifestations** of HF vary depending on the rapidity of decompensation, underlying etiology, and age of the patient. Signs and symptoms of **low cardiac output** include fatigue, exercise intolerance, and decreased peripheral perfusion. Extreme deterioration in cardiac output and elevated SVR result in hypoperfusion of organs such as the kidney (decreased urine output) and brain (confusion and lethargy), and ultimately shock. **Chronic pulmonary and systemic venous congestion** results in orthopnea, dyspnea on exertion, peripheral edema, elevated jugular venous pressure, pleural and pericardial effusions, and hepatic congestion. Acute elevations in left ventricular volume and pulmonary venous pressure result in pulmonary edema. Associated laboratory abnormalities include elevation of BUN and creatinine, hyponatremia, and elevation of serum enzymes of hepatic origin.

IV. **The diagnosis** of HF should be suspected by clinical presentation. Radiographic evidence of cardiomegaly and pulmonary vascular redistribution is common. Depressed ventricular function may be confirmed by echocardiography, radionuclide ventriculography, or cardiac catheterization with cineangiography. Abnormalities in the ECG are frequently present and include arrhythmias, conduction delays, and nonspecific ST–T changes, which often reflect the underlying etiology.

V. **Etiology.** Hypertension and coronary artery disease, with attendant myocardial dysfunction, are the most frequent causes of HF in the United States. Additional etiologies include primary abnormalities of myocardial muscle, abnormalities of valvular function, and pericardial disease. "High-output" heart failure may occur in circumstances of severe anemia, arteriovenous shunts, thyrotoxicosis, or beriberi. Depending on the etiology, the heart may be dilated (predominantly systolic dysfunction) or nondilated (predominantly diastolic dysfunction). Table 6-1 contains one of a variety of HF etiology classification schemes.

General Management Considerations

I. **The initial approach** to the patient with HF must be individualized according to severity, acuity of presentation, etiology, presence of coexisting illnesses, and

Table 6-1. Common causes of heart failure

I. Coronary artery disease   *CAD*

II. Hypertensive heart disease   *HT.*
   A. Diastolic dysfunction
   B. Systolic dysfunction

III. Dilated cardiomyopathy
   A. Idiopathic
   B. Toxic (e.g., alcohol, doxorubicin hydrochloride)
   C. Infection (viral, parasitic, and others)
   D. Collagen vascular disease

IV. Valvular heart disease

V. Hypertrophic cardiomyopathy

VI. Restrictive cardiomyopathy
   A. Amyloidosis
   B. Sarcoidosis
   C. Hemochromatosis

VII. Constrictive pericarditis

VIII. High-output heart failure
   A. Chronic anemia
   B. Atrioventricular shunts
   C. Thyrotoxicosis

precipitating factors. Identification of etiology and precipitating factors is essential since the beneficial effect of one type of treatment of HF (e.g., nitrates for ischemia) may be deleterious when applied to another (e.g., aortic stenosis). After careful history-taking, physical examination, and directed diagnostic evaluation, treatment should be based on clinical assessment of the degree of myocardial dysfunction, total body and intravascular volume status, and extent of peripheral vasoconstriction. General principles of treatment include correction of precipitating processes, control of fluid and sodium retention, optimization of myocardial contractile function, minimization of cardiac workload, and reduction of pulmonary and systemic venous congestion. Close attention to simple clinical parameters such as weight, pulse, blood pressure, fluid intake, and urine output is critical to guiding treatment of HF.

II. **Precipitants** of HF include myocardial ischemia or infarction, hypertension, ventricular or supraventricular arrhythmias, infection, anemia, pregnancy, thyroid disease, volume overload, toxins (alcohol, doxorubicin), drugs (beta antagonists, nonsteroidal anti-inflammatory drugs, calcium antagonists), pulmonary embolism, and dietary or medical noncompliance.

III. **Nonpharmacologic** therapeutic measures are generally employed in conjunction with specific pharmacologic measures:
   A. **Restriction of physical activity** and bed rest reduce myocardial workload and oxygen consumption in patients with symptomatic HF. Following stabilization, carefully guided cardiac rehabilitation and exercise may improve functional capacity in selected patients with HF, especially when due to coronary artery disease (*Lancet* 335:63, 1990). Emotional stress contributes to symptoms of HF and should be reduced. Prophylaxis against deep venous thrombosis should be provided with subcutaneous heparin during periods of bed rest.
   B. **Weight loss** in obese patients reduces systemic vascular resistance as well as myocardial demands. However, maintenance of adequate caloric intake in patients with severe heart failure is necessary to prevent or correct cardiac cachexia.
   C. **Dietary sodium restriction** (≤ 2 g Na^+ per day) will facilitate control of congestive signs or symptoms and help minimize diuretic requirements.

D. Fluid and free water restriction (≤ 1.5 liters per day) may improve hyponatremia and volume overload.

E. Dialysis or ultrafiltration may be necessary in patients in severe HF with associated secondary or underlying renal dysfunction who cannot respond adequately to fluid and sodium limitation or to diuretics. Other mechanical methods of fluid removal such as therapeutic thoracentesis, paracentesis, phlebotomy, and rotating tourniquets may provide temporary symptomatic relief of dyspnea and ascites, as well as edema and pulmonary congestion.

F. Discontinuation of negative inotropic medications (e.g., beta-adrenergic antagonists, verapamil, diltiazem, type I_A and I_C antiarrhythmics), if possible, may improve HF symptoms in patients with low left ventricular (LV) ejection fraction and impaired contractility. Nonsteroidal anti-inflammatory drugs (NSAIDs) may attenuate the efficacy of or potentiate the renal toxicity of angiotensin-converting enzyme (ACE) inhibitors.

G. Administration of oxygen may relieve dyspnea, improve oxygen delivery, reduce the work of breathing, and limit pulmonary vasoconstriction in patients with hypoxemia. Complete cessation of cigarette smoking is also important to optimize oxygen-carrying capacity and to reduce the risk of coronary disease.

Specific Pharmacologic Agents

Principles of pharmacologic therapy include control of sodium and fluid retention, vasodilator therapy, and inotropic support.

I. Diuretics (Table 6-2) in conjunction with restriction of dietary sodium and fluids often lead to clinical improvement in patients with mild to moderate HF. Frequent assessment of the patient's weight along with careful observation of fluid intake and output are essential during initiation and maintenance of therapy. When diuretics are initiated for an acute exacerbation of HF, the goal of therapy should be a maximum net loss of 0.5–1.0 liter of fluid per day (0.5–1.0 kg body weight) to prevent intravascular volume depletion. Frequent complications of therapy include hypokalemia, hyponatremia, and volume depletion. Serum electrolytes, BUN, and creatinine should be followed closely after institution of diuretic therapy. Hypokalemia may be life threatening in patients receiving digoxin or in those who have severe left ventricular dysfunction predisposing to ventricular arrhythmias; a potassium-sparing agent or potassium supplementation should be considered in these patients.

A. Thiazide diuretics (hydrochlorothiazide, chlorthalidone) can be used as initial agents in patients with normal renal function in whom only a mild diuresis is desired. Metolazone, unlike other thiazides, exerts its action at the proximal as well as at the distal tubule. When used in combination with a loop diuretic, it may effect a diuresis in patients with low glomerular filtration rate (GFR). Use of thiazides may be complicated by hypercalcemia, hyperuricemia, rash, pancreatitis, vasculitis, and increased low-density lipoprotein levels.

B. Loop diuretics (furosemide, bumetanide, ethacrynic acid) should be used in patients who require significant diuresis and in patients with markedly decreased renal function. Furosemide reduces preload acutely by causing direct venodilatation when administered intravenously. This property renders furosemide particularly useful for the management of severe heart failure or acute pulmonary edema. Chronic HF may become refractory to oral diuretics as a result of diminished GI absorption secondary to bowel edema, but patients respond readily when given an equivalent dose of intravenous diuretic. Use of loop diuretics may be complicated by hyperuricemia, hypocalcemia, ototoxicity, rash, and vasculitis. Furosemide and bumetanide are sulfa derivatives and may cause drug reactions in sulfa-sensitive patients. Ethacrynic acid can generally be used safely in such patients; however, it is the most ototoxic of the loop diuretics.

C. Potassium-sparing diuretics (spironolactone, triamterene, amiloride) are min-

Table 6-2. Diuretic agents used in heart failure

Agent	Site of action	Relative potency	Route of administration[a]	Average daily dose (mg)[b]	Onset of action	Duration of action
Thiazides						
Chlorothiazide	Distal tubule	+ +	PO	250–500	2 hr	6–12 hr
			IV	500	15 min	1 hr
Hydrochlorothiazide	Distal tubule	+ +	PO	25–100	2 hr	12 hr
Chlorthalidone	Distal tubule	+ + +	PO	25–100	2 hr	48 hr
Metolazone	Proximal, distal tubules	+ + +	PO	2.5–20	1 hr	24–48 hr
Indapamide	Distal tubule	+ +	PO	2.5–5	2 hr	24 hr
Loop diuretics	Loop of Henle	+ + + +				
Furosemide			PO	20–80[c]	1 hr	6–8 hr
			IV, IM	10–80[c]	5 min	2–4 hr
Ethacrynic acid			PO	25–100	30 min	6–8 hr
			IV	50	5 min	3 hr
Bumetanide			PO	0.5–2	30 min	2 hr
			IV, IM	0.5–2 (10 max)	5 min	30 min
Potassium-sparing diuretics	Distal tubule, collecting duct	+				
Spironolactone			PO	50–200	1–2 days	2–3 days
Triamterene			PO	100–200	2–4 days	7–9 days
Amiloride			PO	5–10	2 hr	24 hr

[a] IV doses should be given slowly over 1–2 minutes.
[b] Dose and dosing intervals should be determined by the patient's clinical response.
[c] Larger doses may be required in patients with renal insufficiency.

imally effective for the management of HF when used alone. However, when combined with a thiazide or loop diuretic they are often effective in maintaining normal serum potassium levels. The potential for development of life-threatening hyperkalemia exists with the use of these agents. Serum potassium must be monitored closely following their administration; concomitant use of ACE inhibitors increases the risk of hyperkalemia.

II. **Digitalis glycosides** increase myocardial contractility through reversible inhibition of sarcolemmal sodium–potassium adenosine triphosphatase (ATPase) activity. Digoxin is most efficacious in the management of HF (1) accompanied or caused by atrial fibrillation or flutter (or other supraventricular tachycardias that respond to digoxin) or (2) in patients with dilated left ventricles and impaired systolic function manifest by a third heart sound, low ejection fraction, and large cardiothoracic ratio. Several studies have shown an improvement in ejection fraction and exercise tolerance in patients with chronic HF while receiving digoxin (*N. Engl. J. Med.* 320:677, 1989; *N. Engl. J. Med.* 306:699, 1982). The toxic-therapeutic ratio is narrow and mandates careful follow up of patients receiving this drug. Hypokalemia and hypoxemia may exacerbate toxicity; they should be corrected before initiation of therapy and monitored while the patient receives digoxin.

A. **Dosage** and route of administration are dictated by the underlying condition and the severity of illness. Bioavailability is less with oral preparations (approximately 60–75% in tablet form), and onset of action is more rapid with IV therapy (15–30 minutes versus 2 hours with the oral administration). With normal renal function, the serum half-life is 36–38 hours. **Digoxin loading** is accomplished by giving 0.25–0.5 mg PO or IV initially, followed by 0.25 mg q6h to a total dose of 1.0–1.5 mg. Evidence of toxicity (see below) should be sought before each successive dose. **Maintenance therapy** is affected by the patient's age, lean body weight, and renal function. With normal renal function, the usual daily dose is 0.125–0.375 mg. The dosage should be decreased in patients with renal insufficiency. Frequent assessment of serum digoxin levels should ultimately determine optimum dosing in patients with renal insufficiency, those receiving drugs that may interfere with digoxin metabolism, and when noncompliance is suspected. Drug levels should not be drawn within 6 hours of administration of a dose since distribution is incomplete and the result is uninterpretable.

B. **Drug interactions** with digoxin are frequent and include impaired absorption of digoxin by cholestyramine, kaolin-pectin, and antacids, which may decrease bioavailability by up to 25%. Oral antibiotics such as erythromycin and tetracycline may increase digoxin levels by 10–40%. Quinidine may increase serum digoxin levels up to twofold; the maintenance dose of digoxin should therefore be reduced by 50% in patients receiving both drugs. Verapamil and amiodarone also increase digoxin levels significantly.

C. **Contraindications** to use are rare, but additional caution should be exercised in several settings. Since digoxin may increase myocardial oxygen demand, its use in the presence of acute myocardial infarction (MI) should be limited to the treatment of supraventricular tachyarrhythmias. Atrioventricular (AV) conduction disturbances may be exacerbated by digoxin; conversely, conduction through accessory AV pathways may be potentiated. Electrolyte abnormalities, especially hypokalemia and hypomagnesemia, increase the likelihood of digoxin toxicity and should always be corrected before initiation of therapy. **Cardioversion in the presence of digoxin toxicity is contraindicated,** as potentially fatal ventricular arrhythmias may be precipitated; however, with serum levels in the therapeutic range, cardioversion can be attempted with little increased risk.

D. **Digoxin toxicity** remains an important clinical problem, occurring in 5–15% of patients at some time during therapy. The therapeutic range is narrow; toxicity may develop despite serum levels within the normal range. Factors that most frequently contribute to the development of toxicity include drug interactions, hypokalemia, hypoxemia, hypothyroidism, renal insufficiency, and volume depletion.

1. **Clinical manifestations** of digoxin toxicity include virtually all forms of

cardiac arrhythmias. Ventricular premature depolarizations (often in a bigeminal pattern), junctional tachycardia, and varying degrees of second-degree AV block are frequently seen. Bidirectional ventricular tachycardia, paroxysmal atrial tachycardia with AV block, and regularization of atrial fibrillation occur almost exclusively as a result of digoxin toxicity. Noncardiac manifestations of toxicity include gastrointestinal and neuropsychiatric symptoms. Anorexia, nausea, vomiting, and diarrhea are common and may compound toxic effects by worsening hypokalemia. Altered mental status, agitation, lethargy, and visual disturbances (scotomas and color perception changes) are frequent.

2. **Treatment of digoxin toxicity** includes discontinuation of the drug, correction of precipitating factors, and continuous ECG monitoring. The serum potassium should be maintained in the high-normal range. Symptomatic bradycardia can be controlled with atropine or temporary pacing as needed; sympathomimetics should be avoided, as they may precipitate or worsen ventricular arrhythmias. Lidocaine or phenytoin should be used to control ventricular and atrial arrhythmias; quinidine should not be used, because it may elevate serum levels further (see Chap. 7). Cardioversion is contraindicated unless all other measures of controlling toxic arrhythmias have been exhausted.

3. **Digoxin-specific Fab antibody fragments** are effective in rapidly reversing life-threatening digoxin intoxication (*N. Engl. J. Med.* 307:1357, 1982; *J. Am. Coll. Cardiol.* 5:118A, 1985) and should be considered when other modes of therapy are inadequate. Digoxin–Fab fragment complexes are cleared from the circulation via renal excretion. Patients with renal failure could theoretically experience rebound intoxication if the complex dissociated while still in the circulation; this has not been observed clinically in patients with renal dysfunction. Total serum digoxin levels are no longer meaningful following administration of Fab fragments; free (unbound) digoxin can be measured when serum level monitoring is required. Significant adverse effects have not been reported with the use of the antibody fragments. Each 40-mg vial of Fab fragments neutralizes approximately 0.6 mg of digoxin. Dosage is based on the estimated amount of drug ingested or the steady-state serum level and can be calculated as follows:

Acute digoxin ingestion:

$$\text{Dose (no. of vials)} = [\text{ingested dose (mg)} \times 0.8]/0.6$$

Chronic digoxin intoxication:

$$\text{Dose (no. of vials)} = [\text{serum level (ng/ml)} \times \text{weight (kg)}]/100$$

The Fab fragments should be reconstituted in **sterile water** (4 ml/vial) and the total dose is administered over a 30-minute period. **The Fab fragments may precipitate in saline.** The dosage should be repeated if toxicity is not adequately reversed with the initial administration.

III. **Vasodilator therapy.** Arterial and venous vasoconstriction occurs in patients with heart failure due to compensatory activation of the adrenergic and renin-angiotensin systems as well as a result of increased secretion of arginine vasopressin. Arterial vasoconstriction impairs myocardial performance by increasing the impedance (**afterload**) against which the ventricle ejects, raising intracardiac filling pressures, increasing myocardial wall stress, and predisposing to subendocardial ischemia. In addition, reflexive arteriolar vasoconstriction within renal, hepatic, mesenteric, cerebral, and myocardial vascular beds contributes to further hypoperfusion and to vital organ dysfunction in patients with severe heart failure. Venous vasoconstriction limits venous capacitance, resulting in venous congestion and elevated diastolic ventricular filling pressures (**preload**). Pulmonary arterial vasoconstriction may occur as a result of hypoxia or in response to chronically elevated pulmonary blood flow (e.g., left-to-right intracardiac shunts) or chronically elevated left atrial pressure (e.g., mitral stenosis, mitral regurgitation, or left ventricular failure). Vasodilators may selectively reduce afterload, preload, or both (balanced vasodilators). Agents with predominantly venodilatory properties decrease preload and ventricular filling pressures by favoring redistribution of blood from the pulmonary to the systemic venous bed. Arterial dilators reduce afterload in the absence of obstructive or stenotic valvular lesions by decreasing systemic vascular resistance, which results in improved cardiac output, decreased ventricular filling pressure, and decreased wall stress. Patients with valvular regurgitation, severe HF with elevated SVR, or HF with associated hypertension are most likely to benefit from afterload reduction with arterial vasodilators. Efficacy as well as toxicity of vasodilator therapy depends on intravascular volume and preload. Hypotension, orthostasis, and prerenal azotemia may result from treatment with venous or arterial dilators in the setting of low or normal ventricular filling pressures. Particular caution is necessary in patients with fixed cardiac output (e.g., aortic stenosis, idiopathic hypertrophic subaortic stenosis) or with predominantly diastolic dysfunction (restrictive or hypertrophic cardiomyopathy, tamponade).

A. **Parenteral vasodilators** should be reserved for patients with severe heart failure or those unable to take oral medications (e.g., perioperatively). Vasodilator therapy should be guided by continuous central hemodynamic monitoring (pulmonary artery catheterization). Because of rapid onset of action and short half-lives, parenteral agents should be started at low doses to avoid hypotension and increased cautiously to the lowest effective dose, as well as discontinued slowly to avoid rebound vasoconstriction.

1. **Nitroglycerin** is a potent vasodilator with effects on venous and, to a lesser extent, arterial vascular beds. It relieves pulmonary and systemic venous congestion. It is also an effective coronary vasodilator and therefore is the preferred vasodilator for treatment of heart failure in the setting of acute MI or unstable angina. Onset of action is rapid, with a half-life of 1–3 minutes, which allows rapid titration and discontinuation if necessary. Intravenous nitroglycerin is initiated through absorption-resistant tubing at a dose of 10 μg/minute by infusion pump. Dose can be titrated according to hemodynamic effect and is limited by development of hypotension. Doses greater than 300 μg/minute provide little if any additional benefit and may be associated with significant hypotension. In the absence of adequate preload, intravenous nitroglycerin may cause hypotension that is typically responsive to discontinuation of the infusion and volume expansion. Tolerance necessitating increased dose develops in as little as 12 hours. Conversion to intermittent oral or topical nitrate preparations should be accomplished as early as possible to reduce risks of developing tolerance.

2. **Sodium nitroprusside** is a potent arterial vasodilator with less potent venodilatory properties. It appears to be a direct vasodilator with a short half-life of 1–3 minutes. Its predominant effect is to reduce afterload and it is particularly effective in patients with heart failure who are hypertensive or have severe valvular regurgitation. Nitroprusside should be used cautiously in patients with myocardial ischemia due to theoretic concerns of "coronary steal" reducing myocardial blood flow. The initial dose of 10 μg/minute can be titrated (maximal dose is 300–400 μg/min) to desired hemodynamic effect or until hypotension develops. Nitroprusside's 1- to 3- minute half-life is due to its degradation in the bloodstream with release of cyanide, which is hepatically metabolized to thiocyanate and then subsequently renally excreted. Accordingly, toxic levels of thiocyanate (>10 mg/dl) may develop rapidly in patients with renal insufficiency, necessitating close monitoring of serum levels. Thiocyanate toxicity is manifest as nausea, mental status changes, abdominal pain, or seizures. Methemoglobinemia is a rare complication of treatment with nitroprusside.

B. **Oral vasodilators** should be considered in patients with symptomatic chronic HF and in patients being weaned from parenteral agents. When initiating treatment with oral vasodilators, it may be prudent to begin with agents with short half-lives.

1. **Angiotensin-converting enzyme (ACE) inhibitors** antagonize the vasoconstriction, vital organ hypoperfusion, hyponatremia, hypokalemia, and fluid retention attributable to compensatory activation of the renin-angiotensin system in patients with HF. Treatment with ACE inhibitors decreases ventricular filling pressures and systemic vascular resistance while increasing cardiac output, with little or no change in blood pressure or heart rate. Hypotension and renal insufficiency may develop in the setting of reduced preload and may reverse with reduction in diuretic or venodilator doses or cautious volume expansion. Tolerance is unusual. Absence of an initial beneficial response to treatment with an ACE inhibitor does not preclude long-term benefit. Marked renal insufficiency may occur in patients with bilateral renal artery stenosis (*N. Engl. J. Med.* 308:373, 1983). Adverse effects include rash, angioedema, dysgeusia, proteinuria, hyperkalemia, leukopenia, and cough. Renal function, electrolytes, urinalysis, and blood counts must be followed carefully during treatment. Potassium-sparing diuretics should be avoided during treatment with ACE inhibitors. ACE inhibitors are cleared by the kidneys, necessitating careful dose titration in those patients with a creatinine clearance of less than 30 ml/minute.

   a. **Captopril** is a sulfhydryl-containing ACE inhibitor approved for use in HF. It has been shown to significantly reduce symptoms of HF, improve exercise tolerance, and increase functional capacity (*J. Am. Coll. Cardiol.* 2:755, 1983). Treatment is initiated at dosages of 6.25–12.5 mg PO q6–8h. Hemodynamic effect may be seen with the first dose. The dose of captopril can be increased at each subsequent dosage interval, with close attention to blood pressure, urine output, and renal function. Captopril attenuates ventricular enlargement and improves hemodynamics in patients with left ventricular dysfunction due to anterior MI (*N. Engl. J. Med.* 319:80, 1988). Maximal effect in HF generally occurs at a dosage of 50 mg q6–8h. Agranulocytosis may be more common with captopril than with other ACE inhibitors, particularly in patients with associated collagen vascular disease or serum creatinine greater than 1.5 mg/dl.

   b. **Enalapril** is a prodrug that is hepatically hydrolyzed to the active ACE inhibitor enalaprilat. Enalapril improves survival in patients with severe heart failure (*N. Engl. J. Med.* 316:1429, 1987; *N. Engl. J. Med.* 325:293, 1991). Onset of action and duration of effect (12–24 hr) are significantly longer than with captopril (6–8 hr). The initial dose is 2.5–5.0 mg PO qd. Patients with severe heart failure, hyponatremia (sodium <130 mEq/liter), or creatinine greater than 1.6 mg/dl should start treatment at 2.5 mg PO qd under close observation. Higher initial doses may result in prolonged hypotension, renal insufficiency, and hyperkalemia. Doses should be titrated carefully to a maximum of 20 mg PO bid. The incidence of agranulocytosis may be less with enalapril than with captopril.

   c. **Enalaprilat** is a de-esterified active metabolite of enalapril that is available for intravenous administration. Onset of action is more rapid and pharmacologic half-life is shorter than with enalapril. The initial dosage is 1.25 mg IV q6h, administered over 5 minutes, and can be titrated to a maximal dosage of 5.0 mg IV q6h. Patients concurrently taking diuretics or with impaired renal function (serum creatinine >3.0 mg/dl, creatinine clearance <30 ml/min) should initially receive 0.625 mg IV q6h. When converting from intravenous to oral administration, 0.625 mg IV q6h of enalaprilat is approximately equivalent to 2.5 mg PO qd of enalapril.

   d. **Lisinopril** is a long-acting ACE inhibitor approved for use in hypertension. The initial dosage is 10 mg PO qd in patients with creatinine clearance (Cl_{Cr}) greater than 30 ml/minute. Patients with a Cl_{Cr} of 10–30 ml/minute should start at 5.0 mg PO qd. In patients with severe renal insufficiency (Cl_{Cr} <10 ml/min), the initial dose should be 2.5 mg PO qd. The hypotensive effect of lisinopril is potentiated by diuretics. If possible, diuretics should be discontinued or doses reduced while patients are followed carefully before treatment with lisinopril is started.

2. **Nitrates** are predominantly venodilators and are therefore beneficial in relieving symptoms of venous and pulmonary congestion. Nitrates reduce myocardial ischemia by decreasing ventricular filling pressures and by directly dilating coronary arteries. In patients with reduced preload, hypotension may develop that is responsive to volume expansion and reduction in dose. Improved hemodynamics and symptomatic relief may be seen after the first dose in the majority of patients but may be transient due to development of tolerance (see Chap. 5). Nitrates can be administered in oral short-acting or sustained-release forms as well as topically.

3. **Hydralazine** is a pure afterload-reducing agent that acts directly on arterial smooth muscle to produce vasodilatation. Hydralazine is particularly useful in the treatment of chronic mitral regurgitation and aortic insufficiency (see Specific Management Considerations, sec. I). Dosage requirements vary widely but average 25–100 mg PO tid or qid. Hemodynamic tolerance may occur. Reflex tachycardia and increased myocardial oxygen consumption may occur; therefore, use of hydralazine in patients with ischemic heart disease should be undertaken cautiously. Other adverse effects include headache, flushing, nausea, vomiting, and fluid retention. A **drug-induced lupus syndrome** may develop in up to 15% of patients receiving daily doses of 400 mg or more but is generally reversible on discontinuation of the drug.

4. **Adrenergic-receptor antagonists** theoretically may counteract some of the adverse effects attributable to compensatory activation of the sympathetic nervous system in HF. Alpha-adrenergic blockade reduces vasoconstriction, systemic vascular resistance, and afterload by antagonizing the effects of norepinephrine. Beta-adrenergic blockade as a treatment of HF is controversial but may limit the adverse effects of catecholamines on the failing heart, including down-regulation of myocardial beta receptors in the setting of HF.

   a. **Alpha-receptor antagonists**

      (1) **Prazosin** is a balanced vasodilator that significantly reduces right and left ventricular pressures as well as systemic blood pressure. Its efficacy is transient and limited by the rapid development of tolerance or **tachyphylaxis** (within 24–48 hours), and therefore it is generally not recommended for the treatment of HF. Profound reduction in blood pressure may occur after the first dose (1 mg PO), which should therefore be given at bedtime or while the patient is supine. The usual starting dosage is 1 mg PO bid–tid. The maximum dosage is 10 mg PO q6h. Orthostasis and sodium and fluid retention are common side effects. The drug may accumulate as a result of reduced elimination in patients with HF or renal insufficiency.

      (2) **Doxazosin** is a new, potent alpha-receptor antagonist approved for use in hypertension. Onset of action is 2–6 hours. Orthostatic hypotension and reflex tachycardia may occur. Tolerance to the antihypertensive effects of doxazosin generally does not occur. It is metabolized hepatically, potentially necessitating dose reduction in patients with liver disease. Treatment is initiated at a dosage of 1 mg PO qd and can be titrated gradually to 16 mg PO qd.

   b. **Beta-adrenergic antagonists** theoretically may attenuate some of the deleterious effects of increased beta-adrenergic activity in patients with HF, especially in those with associated coronary artery disease and LV dysfunction attributable to ischemia. In carefully selected patients, treatment with beta-antagonists may improve exercise tolerance, LV ejection fraction, and functional class (*Circulation* 72:536, 1985). Patients receiving beta-antagonists should be monitored closely, preferably with documentation of a beneficial hemodynamic response, and should initially receive low doses of short-acting agents. With the exception of patients with hypertrophic cardiomyopathy and dynamic outflow obstruction or diastolic dysfunction, treatment with beta-antagonists is not generally recommended in patients with HF due to their potent negative inotropic and chronotropic effects.

5. **Calcium channel antagonists** directly relax vascular smooth muscle and inhibit entry of calcium into myocardial cells. The main utility of these agents in the treatment of HF is derived from reduction of ischemia in patients with underlying coronary heart disease. In addition, these agents have beneficial effects on diastolic relaxation (see Specific Management Considerations, sec. **IV**) and afterload reduction (particularly nifedipine, nicardipine, and isradipine). All calcium antagonists have intrinsic negative inotropic properties and thus must be used with caution in patients with LV dysfunction.

   a. **Nifedipine** has predominantly arterial vasodilator effects that typically offset its negative inotropic effect. Nifedipine may be useful in patients with HF who also have hypertension or underlying ischemia. However, nifedipine may increase hospital admissions due to HF exacerbations (*Circulation* 18:1954, 1990). Treatment is initiated at a dosage of 10 mg PO q8h and can be increased to 40 mg PO q6h. A sustained-release preparation is available and can be given once a day.

   b. **Nicardipine** is a potent arterial vasodilating calcium channel antagonist that may be effective in treating patients with HF who have associated ischemia or hypertension. The starting dosage of 20 mg PO q8h can be increased up to 40 mg PO q8h.

   c. **Diltiazem** and **verapamil** have significant negative inotropic properties and may precipitate HF in patients with poor ventricular function. However, each may be effective in patients with diastolic dysfunction, particularly those with hypertrophic cardiomyopathy, with or without obstruction. Diltiazem can be started at a dosage of 30 mg PO q6h and increased gradually to 90 mg PO q6h. The initial dosage of verapamil is 40–80 mg PO q8h, which can be increased to 120 mg PO q8h. Both diltiazem and verapamil are available in sustained-release preparations. Common side effects of both agents, in addition to precipitating HF, include hypotension, heart block, constipation, and fatigue.

   d. **Isradipine** is a new dihydropyridine calcium channel antagonist approved for use in hypertension. It directly dilates arterioles, reduces blood pressure and systemic vascular resistance, and results in a small increase in resting heart rate and cardiac output. It also has a direct diuretic effect. There are no significant effects on conduction. Onset of action is rapid (2–3 hr), with a duration of action of 12 hours. The starting dosage is 2.5 mg PO bid and can be titrated up to a dosage of 10 mg PO bid.

IV. **Inotropic agents**

   A. **Sympathomimetic agents** are potent inotropic agents primarily used to treat severe HF. Beneficial and adverse effects are mediated by stimulation of myocardial beta adrenoreceptors. The most important adverse effects are related to the arrhythmogenic nature of these agents and the potential for exacerbation of myocardial ischemia; tachycardia and ventricular irritability may be lessened by decreasing dosage. Treatment should be guided by careful hemodynamic and electrocardiographic monitoring.

   1. **Dopamine** is an endogenous catecholamine with positive inotropic properties due to **beta$_1$-adrenoreceptor stimulation** at doses of approximately 2–5 µg/kg/min. At lower doses (1–3 µg/kg/min), dopamine exerts a selective vasodilating effect on renal and mesenteric arterioles through **dopaminergic-receptor stimulation** and may improve renal blood flow and urine output. At doses above 5–10 µg/kg/min, **alpha-adrenoreceptor** stimulation occurs; the resulting peripheral vasoconstriction increases SVR, which may be deleterious in patients with low cardiac output and HF. For parenteral inotropic support, dopamine should be used primarily for stabilization of the hypotensive patient.

   2. **Dobutamine** is a synthetic agent that selectively stimulates beta$_1$ adrenoreceptors; beta$_2$ and alpha receptors are activated to a much lesser degree. Its predominant hemodynamic effect is direct inotropic stimulation with reflex vasodilatation resulting in afterload reduction and augmentation of cardiac

output. Blood pressure generally remains constant and heart rate may increase minimally. Tachycardia may result from excessive doses or if left ventricular filling pressure falls in response to improved ventricular performance. Dobutamine is administered as a constant infusion that is initiated at a rate of 1–2 µg/kg/min and is gradually increased to obtain the desired hemodynamic effect or until excessive tachycardia or ventricular irritability occurs. In the absence of excessive tachycardia, dobutamine does not increase myocardial oxygen requirements. For refractory chronic HF, intermittent infusion of dobutamine for 2–4 days has been shown to provide clinical improvement that may persist for weeks to months (*Circulation* 69:113, 1984). Such therapy should be undertaken only if patients are closely monitored and infusion rates of 10 µg/kg/min or less are used. Dobutamine should not be used in patients with conditions in which HF results predominantly from diastolic dysfunction (e.g., hypertrophic cardiomyopathy) or in high-output heart failure. Tolerance to the effects of chronically administered dobutamine has been described.

3. **Levodopa,** administered orally in dosages of 1–2 g q6h, is converted peripherally to dopamine and has been shown to produce hemodynamic and clinical improvement in selected patients with severe HF (*N. Engl. J. Med.* 310:1357, 1984). The efficacy and safety of levodopa and other orally active beta-adrenergic agonists for the treatment of HF have not been established. Severe nausea and vomiting may complicate use of levodopa.

B. **Phosphodiesterase inhibitors** increase myocardial contractility and produce vasodilation by increasing intracellular cyclic adenosine monophosphate (AMP). **Amrinone,** a cardiac bipyridine, is the only agent of this class that is available for clinical use. Its net hemodynamic effects are similar to those of dobutamine. It is administered intravenously with an initial bolus of 0.75 µg/kg given over 2–3 minutes, followed by a continuous infusion of 2.5–10 µg/kg/min. Caution should be exercised in patients already receiving vasodilator therapy, as the combined effects with amrinone may produce excessive hypotension. Tachycardia as well as atrial and ventricular arrhythmias may occur. Thrombocytopenia due to decreased platelet survival may occur, especially with prolonged infusions, necessitating reduction in dose or discontinuation if severe or if associated with clinically significant bleeding. Due to its different mechanism of action, the hemodynamic effects of amrinone may be additive to those of digoxin and synergistic with those of dobutamine or dopamine.

Specific Management Considerations

I. **Valvular heart disease**

A. **Mitral stenosis (MS)** impedes blood flow from the lungs and left atrium into the left ventricle. Chronic rheumatic heart disease is the most common etiology; it may also result from calcium deposition in the mitral annulus and leaflets, as a congenital malformation, or, rarely, in association with connective tissue disorders. Mitral stenosis can also occur in prosthetic mitral valves (most commonly bioprosthetic valves) as a result of calcification. Left atrial myxoma and cor triatriatum may mimic MS clinically.

1. **Pathophysiology.** Significant MS results in elevation of left atrial, pulmonary venous, and pulmonary capillary pressures with resultant pulmonary congestion. The degree of pressure elevation depends on the severity of the pressure gradient across the mitral valve, which depends on the severity of obstruction, flow across the valve, time allowed for diastolic filling, and presence of effective atrial contraction. Therefore, factors that augment flow across the stenotic mitral valve, such as tachycardia, exercise, fever, and pregnancy, cause marked increases in left atrial pressure and may exacerbate symptoms. Left atrial enlargement and fibrillation may result in atrial thrombus formation, which probably accounts for the high incidence

(approximately 20%) of systemic embolization in patients with MS who are not anticoagulated.

2. **Diagnosis.** Symptoms of dyspnea and pulmonary congestion are prominent. Physical signs of right heart volume and pressure overload are often present in conjunction with a prominent first heart sound, early diastolic "opening snap," and rumbling diastolic murmur. The diagnosis and severity of MS can be confirmed by two-dimensional and Doppler echocardiography. Cardiac catheterization is indicated in patients with (1) likelihood of concomitant coronary artery disease (CAD) or (2) technically suboptimal or nondiagnostic echocardiographic studies, and (3) to evaluate other suspected valvular lesions such as mitral regurgitation (which may render commissurotomy untenable).

3. **Medical management**
   a. **Factors that increase left atrial pressure** should be identified and alleviated if possible, including tachycardia, fever, and vigorous physical activity.
   b. **Diuretics** (see Table 6–2) are the mainstay of therapy for pulmonary congestion and edema.
   c. **Anticoagulant therapy** is indicated for patients with MS and atrial fibrillation, as they are at high risk for thromboembolic events. Heparin therapy should be instituted at the onset of atrial fibrillation, followed by long-term warfarin therapy. In the absence of prior embolic events, marked left atrial enlargement, or demonstrable atrial thrombi, patients with sinus rhythm probably do not require anticoagulation.
   d. **Atrial fibrillation may be poorly tolerated. Synchronized DC cardioversion** should be used acutely if hemodynamic compromise (hypotension, pulmonary edema) accompanies the onset of atrial fibrillation. In less emergent situations, the ventricular response rate to atrial fibrillation should be controlled with digoxin. If control of ventricular response with digoxin is not adequate, **verapamil,** 2.5–5.0 mg IV, 80 mg PO tid, or **propranolol,** 20 mg PO q6h, can be used to provide greater diastolic filling time. An attempt to restore and maintain sinus rhythm is indicated except in the presence of marked left atrial enlargement (i.e., >6 cm). Following institution of rate control measures, elective cardioversion should be attempted with administration of a type I_a antiarrhythmic agent (quinidine or procainamide) (see Chap. 7). **Elective attempts at chemical or electrical cardioversion should be preceded by anticoagulation therapy for 3 weeks** to minimize the risk of systemic embolization on resumption of normal sinus rhythm. If attempted chemical cardioversion fails to restore sinus rhythm, elective synchronized DC cardioversion should be attempted. Following conversion to sinus rhythm, type I_a antiarrhythmics can be continued in an effort to maintain sinus rhythm.
   e. **Infective endocarditis prophylaxis** is indicated (see Chap. 13).
   f. **Continuous prophylaxis** against recurrent rheumatic fever is indicated in young patients, patients at high risk for streptococcal infection (parents of young children, school teachers, medical and military personnel, and those in crowded living conditions), and those with acute rheumatic fever within the previous 5 years. Continuous antibiotic prophylaxis may be provided through various regimens (see Chap.13).

4. **Surgical considerations**
   a. Patients with severe symptoms and significant MS should undergo commissurotomy or mitral valve replacement (MVR). Those with pulmonary hypertension, even if minimally symptomatic, should also be treated surgically.
   b. Patients with **mild to moderate symptoms** generally show improvement with diuretic therapy and can be followed closely for development of worsening MS.
   c. A systemic thromboembolic event does not by itself mandate MVR.

However, patients with significant MS and recurrent thromboembolic events despite therapeutic anticoagulation may benefit from MVR.

   d. Percutaneous balloon mitral valvuloplasty has been shown to reduce the mitral valve gradient and improve cardiac output in patients with MS. This procedure may be considered an alternative to surgery with acceptable morbidity and mortality in select patients without significant mitral regurgitation or a severely calcified valve.

B. Aortic stenosis (AS) in the adult population may result from (1) calcification and degeneration of a congenitally normal valve, (2) calcification and fibrosis of a congenitally bicuspid aortic valve, or (3) rheumatic valvular disease.

   1. Pathophysiology. Aortic stenosis produces a pressure gradient from the left ventricle to the aorta causing pressure overload of the left ventricle, which leads to concentric hypertrophy. As a result, left ventricular compliance is reduced, left ventricular end-diastolic pressure rises, and myocardial oxygen demand is increased as left ventricular mass and wall stress are increased. Elevated LV end-diastolic pressure decreases the perfusion pressure across the myocardium, leading to subendocardial ischemia.

   2. The diagnosis of significant aortic stenosis is based on clinical suspicion raised by the presence of one or more of the classic symptom triad of **angina, syncope, and heart failure.** The physical findings of AS include a slowly rising carotid pulse, which is sustained (pulsus parvus et tardus), and a mid- to late-peaking systolic murmur, which is usually harsh in quality. The pressure gradient across the stenotic aortic valve is directly related to the severity of obstruction and the cardiac output. Therefore, the intensity of the systolic murmur may diminish as the cardiac output decreases with increasingly severe AS. In general, murmurs of long duration that peak late in systole indicate severe AS. Doppler echocardiography provides a noninvasive estimation of the aortic valve gradient that correlates well with that found at cardiac catheterization. Most patients being considered for aortic valve replacement require preoperative cardiac catheterization with coronary arteriography to determine the presence and extent of concomitant CAD.

   3. Medical management

      a. Infective endocarditis occurs with increased frequency, and prophylaxis is indicated (see Chap. 13).

      b. Vigorous exercise and physical activity should be avoided in patients with severe AS.

      c. Atrial (and ventricular) arrhythmias are poorly tolerated and should be treated aggressively.

      d. Digoxin may be useful in patients with HF in the presence of left ventricular dilatation and impaired systolic function. However, in severe AS, due to the fixed obstruction of left ventricular outflow, inotropic therapy is of little benefit.

      e. Diuretics may be useful in treating congestive symptoms but must be used with extreme caution. Reduction of left ventricular filling pressure in patients with AS may decrease cardiac output and systemic blood pressure.

      f. Nitrates and other vasodilators should be avoided in patients with severe AS if at all possible. These agents reduce left ventricular filling pressure and may lower systemic blood pressure, which may have catastrophic consequences. Patients with AS in whom angina develops may occasionally require treatment with nitroglycerin. Such therapy should be initiated only under strict supervision by a physician at the bedside. Volume expansion with saline may be necessary to avoid excessive preload reduction. If nitroglycerin results in hypotension that does not respond to aggressive volume expansion, parenteral inotropic agents (e.g., dobutamine), vasopressors, or both should be given.

      g. Asymptomatic patients with mild to moderate AS can be followed closely with clinical assessment and Doppler echocardiography performed at 6- to 12-month intervals.

4. Surgical considerations

a. **Symptomatic patients** should undergo evaluation for possible aortic valve replacement, including two-dimensional and Doppler echocardiography. Coronary arteriography should be performed in men older than 40 years and women older than 50 years, as well as in all patients with anginal symptoms; left ventriculography is indicated in patients with coexistent mitral regurgitation. Those found to have severe AS (aortic valve area ≤ 0.8 cm^2) should undergo valve replacement unless co-morbid conditions preclude surgery. Asymptomatic patients with severe AS are rare, and the timing of valve replacement in these patients is controversial. **Impaired left ventricular function** should not be considered an absolute contraindication to aortic valve replacement in severe AS. Many patients with severe depression of left ventricular function show marked improvement on relief of outflow obstruction after aortic valve replacement. Patients with significant **concomitant coronary disease** should undergo surgical revascularization, if indicated, at the time of aortic valve replacement, because the operative morbidity and mortality for the combined procedure is no greater than for aortic valve replacement alone.

b. **Intra-aortic balloon counterpulsation** may stabilize the condition of patients with critical AS and hemodynamic decompensation until aortic valve replacement can be accomplished. It should not be used when significant aortic insufficiency coexists with AS.

c. **Percutaneous balloon aortic valvuloplasty** can reduce the aortic valve gradient and improve symptoms and left ventricular function with acceptably low morbidity and mortality in select patients. Unfortunately, a high rate of restenosis occurs. At present, its use should be limited to patients who either refuse surgery or are poor surgical candidates due to co-morbid conditions.

C. Mitral regurgitation (MR)

1. **Chronic MR,** as an isolated lesion, is most commonly caused by myxomatous degeneration of the mitral valve. Other common etiologies include rheumatic heart disease, calcification of the mitral valve annulus, CAD with associated papillary muscle dysfunction, infective endocarditis, and connective tissue diseases (e.g., Marfan's syndrome, Ehlers-Danlos syndrome).

a. **Pathophysiology.** Chronic MR imposes a volume overload on the left ventricle as a result of regurgitation of a fraction of the blood flow into the left atrium. Normal forward cardiac output is maintained early in the course of the disease, but with progressive MR, compensatory mechanisms no longer accommodate increasing left ventricular end-diastolic volume. Accordingly, ejection fraction falls and symptoms of left heart failure develop. Symptoms of pulmonary venous congestion and dyspnea on exertion are often present.

b. **The diagnosis** is suggested by the characteristic physical findings of well-preserved carotid pulsations, an enlarged apical impulse (point of maximal impulse [PMI]), and an apical holosystolic murmur. Doppler and two-dimensional echocardiography may confirm the diagnosis, estimate the severity of MR, and provide clues as to its etiology. Cardiac catheterization and contrast left ventriculography remain the standard for gauging the severity of MR and are required for assessing the need for mitral valve replacement in most patients.

c. **Medical management**

(1) **Infective endocarditis prophylaxis** should be given (see Chap 13).

(2) **Anticoagulant therapy** should be considered, particularly in the presence of atrial fibrillation, an enlarged left atrium, or a previous embolic event; however, the incidence of thromboembolic events is lower than in MS.

(3) **Atrial fibrillation** should be anticipated in the later stages of MR as the left atrium dilates and should be treated as previously outlined in sec. **I.A.**

(4) **Diuretics** are useful for treating congestive symptoms. **Nitrates** can also be used to reduce preload and ventricular size, which may decrease the severity of MR (*Am. J. Cardiol.* 43:773, 1979).

(5) **Digoxin** may be useful in the presence of impaired left ventricular systolic function.

(6) **Vasodilators** provide hemodynamic improvement in MR by reducing SVR, thus decreasing the mitral regurgitant fraction and augmenting forward cardiac output. Beneficial effects have been demonstrated with **nitroprusside, hydralazine, captopril, and enalapril.** Whether the need for mitral valve replacement can be delayed or precluded by vasodilator therapy remains unknown.

d. **Surgical considerations**

(1) **Moderate to severe symptoms** despite medical therapy should prompt consideration for mitral valve repair or replacement, provided that left ventricular function is adequate (LV ejection fraction >40%).

(2) **Patients with minimal or no symptoms** should be followed closely with noninvasive assessment of left ventricular size and systolic function (by echocardiography or radionuclide ventriculography) every 6–12 months. However, left ventricular ejection fraction does not provide an accurate assessment of intrinsic left ventricular contractility in MR. Generally, by the time a significant decrease in ejection fraction is noted, marked left ventricular dysfunction has occurred and mitral valve replacement with its attendant increase in left ventricular afterload may be poorly tolerated or may fail to improve the patient's symptoms. Patients should be considered for mitral valve repair or replacement when the ejection fraction approaches 50–55%.

2. **Acute mitral regurgitation** can result from papillary muscle dysfunction or rupture due to myocardial ischemia and MI, infective endocarditis with flail or perforated leaflets, severe myxomatous disease with rupture of a chorda resulting in a flail leaflet, or trauma.

a. **The pathophysiology** of acute MR differs from that of chronic MR in that compensatory increases in left atrial and left ventricular compliance do not occur. The result is a sudden increase in pulmonary venous pressure leading to acute pulmonary edema. Acute MR frequently results in acute cardiogenic shock necessitating emergent diagnostic evaluation and treatment.

b. **Medical management**

(1) **Afterload reduction** should be initiated emergently with **sodium nitroprusside,** which allows rapid titration guided by systemic blood pressure and central hemodynamics. Approximately 50% of patients with acute MR can be stabilized in this manner, thereby allowing mitral valve replacement to proceed under more controlled conditions.

(2) **Furosemide,** with or without nitrates, can be used as systemic blood pressure tolerates to relieve pulmonary congestion. However, the direct venodilating effect of nitroprusside may render other preload-reducing maneuvers unnecessary.

(3) **Intra-aortic balloon counterpulsation** is indicated in cases of severe hemodynamic instability to reduce SVR and improve forward cardiac output.

c. **Surgical therapy** is indicated urgently in patients with acute MR and hemodynamic compromise whose condition cannot be stabilized medically. In those with infective endocarditis who are hemodynamically stable, valve replacement should be delayed for several days while antibiotic therapy is initiated. If refractory hemodynamic deterioration develops, surgery should not be delayed.

D. **Aortic insufficiency (AI)** may occur as a result of an abnormality of the aortic valve itself, dilatation and distortion of the aortic root, or both. Causes of valvular aortic insufficiency include rheumatic fever, endocarditis, trauma, connective tissue diseases, and congenital bicuspid aortic valve. Dilatation or distortion of the aortic root producing AI may be due to systemic hypertension, ascending aortic dissection, syphilis, cystic medionecrosis, Marfan's syndrome, ankylosing spondylitis, and osteogenesis imperfecta. Chronic AI typically presents insidiously, while acute AI usually is manifest as severe HF and impending cardiogenic shock.

1. **Pathophysiology.** The diastolic regurgitant flow from the aorta into the left ventricle causes increased LV end-diastolic volume (LVEDV) and pressure (LVEDP). In turn, the left ventricle becomes dilated and hypertrophied, which serves to maintain stroke volume and prevent further increase in LVEDP. In acute AI, the chronic compensatory mechanisms are not active and therefore the increase in LVEDP is marked. In chronic AI, increases in peripheral resistance (e.g., hypertension) lead to increased regurgitant flow and raise diastolic filling pressure and volume.

2. **Diagnosis** of AI may be suspected based on clinical findings, including a wide pulse pressure, bounding pulses, and an aortic diastolic murmur. The presence of AI can be confirmed by two-dimensional and Doppler echocardiography or cardiac catheterization with ascending aortography.

3. **Medical management** is reserved for patients with chronic, stable AI or for stabilization of patients with severe or acute AI before definitive surgical treatment.

   a. **Treatment of underlying or precipitating causes** such as endocarditis, syphilis, and connective tissue diseases should occur concomitantly with treatment of HF.

   b. Patients with AI should receive **prophylaxis for endocarditis** (see Chap 13).

   c. Heavy exertion and vigorous sports should be restricted in patients with AI and associated LV dysfunction and limited cardiac reserve.

   d. **Fluid and salt restriction,** diuretics, and digoxin are the cornerstones of therapy for symptomatic patients with chronic AI.

   e. **Vasodilators** may be beneficial in symptomatic patients with **chronic AI.** In patients with **acute AI,** afterload reduction with sodium nitroprusside as directed by hemodynamic monitoring should be employed to stabilize the patient's condition before urgent valve replacement.

4. **Surgical treatment**

   a. **Aortic valve replacement (AVR)** and repair of associated aortic root abnormalities should be undertaken urgently in patients with **acute AI.** In patients with infective endocarditis who are hemodynamically stable with medical therapy, valve replacement is preferentially deferred for several days while treatment with antibiotics is initiated. Patients in whom hemodynamic instability develops require emergent surgery.

   b. AVR should be considered in patients with **chronic AI** who have severe AI, or in whom symptoms of moderate to severe HF (NYHA class III–IV) or LV dysfunction develop. The clinical outcome and extent of reversibility of LV dysfunction following AVR depend on duration of dysfunction, dilatation of the LV (end-systolic diameter and volume), and degree of systolic dysfunction.

II. **Cardiogenic pulmonary edema**

A. **Pathophysiology. Cardiogenic pulmonary edema (CPE)** occurs when the pulmonary capillary pressure (PCP) exceeds the forces (serum oncotic pressure and interstitial hydrostatic pressure) that maintain fluid within the vascular space. Accumulation of fluid in the pulmonary interstitium is followed by alveolar flooding and disturbance of gas exchange. Increased PCP may be caused by left ventricular failure of any cause, obstruction to transmitral flow (e.g., mitral stenosis, atrial myxoma), or rarely by pulmonary veno-occlusive disease.

B. **Diagnosis**

1. **Clinical manifestations** of CPE usually occur rapidly and include dyspnea, air hunger, anxiety, and restlessness. Physical signs of decreased peripheral perfusion, pulmonary congestion, use of accessory respiratory muscles, and wheezing are often present. The patient may expectorate a pink frothy fluid.

2. **Radiographic abnormalities** include cardiomegaly, interstitial and perihilar

engorgement, Kerley B lines, and pleural effusions. The radiographic abnormalities may lag several hours behind the development of symptoms and their resolution may be out of phase with clinical improvement.

C. Management

1. **Initial supportive treatment** of CPE includes administration of oxygen via nasal cannula or mask in a concentration sufficient to raise PO_2 to greater than 60 mm Hg. Mechanical ventilation is indicated if hypercapnia coexists or if oxygenation is inadequate while using a high-flow, tight-fitting mask at 100% concentration. **A sitting position** improves pulmonary function and assists in venous pooling. Cardiac workload should be decreased by placing the patient at strict bed rest and by reducing pain and anxiety.

2. **Pharmacologic treatment**

   a. **Morphine sulfate** reduces anxiety and dilates pulmonary and systemic veins. Morphine, 2–5 mg IV, can be given safely over several minutes and can be repeated q10–25 min until an effect is seen. An opioid antagonist (naloxone, 0.4–0.8 mg IV) must be available in the event that respiratory depression results from morphine treatment.

   b. **Furosemide** is a potent venodilator and decreases pulmonary congestion within minutes of intravenous infusion, well before its diuretic action begins. An initial dose of 20–40 mg should be given over several minutes and can be increased, based on response, to a maximum of 200 mg on subsequent doses.

   c. **Venodilators** such as nitroglycerin (TNG) augment the effect of furosemide but should be used cautiously. Nitroglycerin, 0.4 mg SL, can be followed with TNG ointment 2%, 1–2 in. topically. Intravenous TNG may be required, particularly if symptoms of cardiac ischemia are present (see Chap. 5).

   d. **Inotropic agents** such as dobutamine or phosphodiesterase inhibitors may be helpful after initial treatment of CPE in patients with cardiogenic shock (see sec. **VII.A.1**).

3. **Mechanical reduction of pulmonary congestion** may be of temporizing benefit in cases of severe pulmonary edema. **Soft rubber tourniquets** or sphygmomanometer cuffs can be applied to all but one extremity, allowing arterial perfusion but restricting venous flow (i.e., inflate cuff to a pressure greater than diastolic, but less than systolic), and should be rotated every 15–20 minutes to the free extremity. **Phlebotomy** and removal of 250–500 ml blood is occasionally helpful in patients with relatively fixed intravascular volume (e.g., those with renal failure) or when pharmacologic therapy is inadequate.

4. **Right heart catheterization** and placement of an indwelling pulmonary artery catheter (e.g., **Swan-Ganz catheter**) may be necessary in cases in which a prompt response to therapy does not occur. The Swan-Ganz catheter will allow differentiation between cardiogenic and noncardiogenic causes of pulmonary edema via measurement of the PCP and will allow hemodynamic monitoring during therapy (see Chaps. 5 and 9).

5. **Precipitating factors** should be identified if possible because several causes are surgically correctable. Common precipitants of pulmonary edema include severe hypertension, myocardial infarction or ischemia (particularly if associated mitral regurgitation exists), acute valvular regurgitation secondary to endocarditis, and volume overload in the setting of severe LV dysfunction. Successful resolution of pulmonary edema can often only be accomplished by correction of the underlying process.

III. Dilated cardiomyopathy is a disease of heart muscle characterized by a reduction in ventricular contractile function. Dilatation may occur secondary to progression of any process that causes HF, although certain etiologies appear to primarily cause an isolated myopathic process (see Table 6–1). In the majority of cases, however, no etiologic or associated condition can be identified.

A. Pathophysiology and clinical features. Dilatation of the cardiac chambers and varying degrees of hypertrophy are anatomic hallmarks. Heart failure is often present. Tricuspid and mitral regurgitation are common due to the effect of chamber dilatation on the valvular apparatus. Atrial and ventricular arrhythmias are seen in as many as half of these patients and are likely responsible for the high incidence of sudden death in these patients.

B. Diagnosis can be confirmed with echocardiography or radionuclide angiography. Two-dimensional and Doppler echocardiography are helpful in differentiating this condition from hypertrophic or restrictive cardiomyopathy, pericardial disease, and valvular disorders. The ECG is almost always abnormal but changes are typically nonspecific. Endomyocardial biopsy may help establish a diagnosis in patients clinically suspected to have a potentially treatable underlying disease such as sarcoidosis, hemochromatosis, or active myocarditis. Transvenous endomyocardial biopsy is a safe procedure in experienced hands.

C. Medical management of symptomatic patients is similar to that for HF from any cause. The therapeutic strategies include control of total body sodium and fluid and appropriate **preload and afterload reduction** using vasodilator therapy. Appropriate immunizations against influenza and pneumococcal pneumonia are recommended. Additional therapeutic considerations are outlined below.

  1. Complex ventricular ectopy, including nonsustained ventricular tachycardia, is frequently seen during ambulatory monitoring of these patients. Patients with complex ventricular ectopy and HF have a high incidence of sudden death. However, the empiric use of antiarrhythmic agents to suppress nonsustained asymptomatic ventricular ectopy has not been shown to improve survival and could result in drug-induced depression of ventricular function, proarrhythmic effects, or both. Invasive electrophysiologic studies employing programmed stimulation should be considered in patients with symptomatic or sustained arrhythmias to guide optimal therapy and to determine which patients are likely to benefit from the placement of an automatic defibrillator (see Chap. 7). Signal-averaged ECG may help select which patients should undergo programmed stimulation.

  2. Chronic oral anticoagulation should be considered because of the high incidence of **mural thrombi** found by echocardiography or autopsy (*Circulation* 78:1388, 1988). Patients with severe left ventricular dysfunction, a prior history of thromboembolic events, or atrial fibrillation are at highest risk for a thromboembolic event.

  3. Immunosuppressive therapy with agents such as prednisone, azathioprine, and cyclosporine for biopsy-proven **active myocarditis** has been advocated by some, but the efficacy has not been definitely established. Large-scale randomized trials designed to determine the efficacy of these agents in patients with myocarditis are ongoing.

D. Surgical management. Primary valvular disease and coronary disease should be evaluated and surgically corrected as indicated (see sec. I and Chap. 5). Revascularization with percutaneous transluminal coronary angioplasty (PTCA) or coronary artery bypass surgery, resulting in improved or stabilized LV function in selected patients with CAD. Intra-aortic balloon pumping and ventricular assist devices may be necessary for stabilization of patients in whom cardiac transplantation is an option or before other definitive surgical therapies.

IV. Hypertrophic cardiomyopathy (HCM) is a myocardial disorder characterized by ventricular hypertrophy, diminished LV cavity dimensions, normal or enhanced contractile function, and impaired ventricular relaxation (diastolic dysfunction). The idiopathic form of HCM has an early onset (as early as the first decade of life) without associated hypertension. Many cases have a **genetic component** with autosomal dominant transmission and a variable phenotypic expressivity and penetrance. An **acquired form** also occurs in elderly patients with a history of hypertension.

  A. Pathophysiology. The hypertrophy is typically predominant in the interventricular septum (asymmetric hypertrophy) but may involve all ventricular segments equally. Hemodynamically, the disease can be classified according to the presence or absence of **left ventricular outflow tract obstruction.** Left ventricular outflow obstruction may occur at rest but is enhanced by factors that increase LV contractility or decrease ventricular volume. **Ventricular diastolic abnormalities** of delayed ventricular relaxation and decreased compliance are common and may lead to pulmonary congestion. Myocardial ischemia occurs and is likely secondary to a myocardial supply-demand mismatch. Systolic anterior motion (SAM) of the anterior leaflet of the mitral valve is often associated with mitral regurgitation and may play a role in LV outflow tract obstruction.

B. **Clinical presentation** varies considerably, but may include angina, syncope, dyspnea, cardiac failure, arrhythmias, or sudden death. Patients of all ages may be affected, but **sudden death** is most common in children and young adults between 10 and 35 years of age and often occurs during periods of strenuous exertion. Physical findings include a bisferiens carotid pulse (in the presence of obstruction); a forceful, double or triple apical impulse; and a coarse systolic outflow murmur localized along the left sternal border that is accentuated by maneuvers that decrease preload (e.g., Valsalva maneuver).

C. **The diagnosis** is suspected on the basis of clinical presentation and/or a family history suggestive of familial HCM and is confirmed by two-dimensional echocardiography. Doppler flow studies may be useful in establishing the presence of a significant LV outflow gradient at rest or with provocation.

D. **Management** is directed toward relief of symptoms and prevention of arrhythmias, sudden death, and infection. The treatment of asymptomatic individuals is controversial. There is no conclusive evidence that medical therapy in asymptomatic patients will prevent sudden death. All individuals with HCM should avoid participation in strenuous physical activities including most competitive sports.

1. **Medical therapy in the symptomatic patient**

   a. **Beta-adrenergic antagonists** may reduce symptoms of HCM by reducing myocardial contractility and heart rate. Unfortunately, symptoms may recur during long-term therapy. Most patients will show improvement with oral doses of propranolol in the range of 160–320 mg/day (or its equivalent). Higher doses of beta-antagonist therapy may be necessary in patients with refractory or recurrent symptoms, although dosages over 480 mg/day are associated with a higher incidence of side effects.

   b. **Verapamil** will improve symptoms in most patients, primarily through its action on augmentation of diastolic ventricular filling. Therapy with verapamil should be initiated at low doses, with careful hemodynamic monitoring in those patients with outflow obstruction. The dose should be increased gradually over several days to weeks if symptoms persist. Experience with other calcium antagonists is limited and their use is not routinely recommended.

   c. **Diuretics** may improve pulmonary congestive symptoms in those patients with elevated pulmonary venous pressures (particularly in the small subset of patients in whom a congestive form of cardiomyopathy develops). These agents should be avoided in patients with severe LV outflow obstruction because excessive preload reduction may worsen the obstruction.

   d. **Nitrates and vasodilators should be avoided** because of the risk of precipitously increasing the LV outflow gradient.

2. **Atrial and ventricular arrhythmias** occur commonly in patients with HCM. Supraventricular tachyarrhythmias are tolerated poorly and should be aggressively treated; DC cardioversion is indicated if hemodynamic compromise develops. Digoxin is relatively contraindicated because of its positive inotropic properties and potential for exacerbating ventricular outflow obstruction. **Atrial fibrillation** is usually extremely poorly tolerated and should be converted to sinus rhythm. Verapamil or beta-antagonists can be used to control the ventricular response before cardioversion. Procainamide or disopyramide (see Chap. 7 for doses) may be efficacious in the chronic suppression of atrial fibrillation. Patients with nonsustained ventricular tachycardia detected on ambulatory monitoring are at increased risk for sudden death.

However, the benefit of suppression of these arrhythmias with medical therapy has not been established and the risk of a proarrhythmic effect of antiarrhythmic therapy exists. The role of invasive electrophysiologic testing in these patients is presently being evaluated. Symptomatic ventricular arrhythmias should be treated as outlined in Chap. 7.

3. Prophylaxis for endocarditis is indicated (see Chap. 13).

4. Anticoagulation is recommended if paroxysmal or chronic atrial fibrillation develops.

5. Surgical therapy is useful in the treatment of symptoms but has not been shown to alter the natural history of HCM. The most frequently used operative procedure involves septal myotomy or myectomy or mitral valve replacement.

V. Restrictive cardiomyopathy results from pathologic infiltration of the myocardium by a variety of processes such as amyloidosis and sarcoidosis. Less common causes include glycogen storage diseases, endomyocardial fibrosis, and hypereosinophilic syndromes.

A. Pathophysiology and diagnosis. Myocardial infiltration results in abnormal diastolic ventricular filling. It is often difficult to differentiate between restrictive cardiomyopathy and constrictive pericarditis because of similar clinical presentations and hemodynamics. In contrast to constrictive pericarditis, restrictive cardiomyopathy may result in varying degrees of left ventricular systolic dysfunction, depending on the duration and nature of the underlying disease. Echocardiography may reveal thickening of the myocardium and varying degrees of systolic ventricular dysfunction. Doppler echocardiographic analysis may demonstrate evidence of abnormal diastolic filling patterns and elevated venous pressure. The ECG may show conduction system disease or low voltage, in contrast to the increased voltage seen with ventricular hypertrophy. Cardiac catheterization reveals elevated right and left ventricular filling pressures and a classic dip-and-plateau pattern in the right and left ventricular pressure tracing. Right ventricular endomyocardial biopsy may be diagnostic and should be considered in patients in whom a diagnosis is not established.

B. Management

1. General measures include judicious use of diuretics for pulmonary and systemic congestion and digoxin if left ventricular dysfunction is present. Digoxin should be avoided in patients with cardiac amyloidosis because they appear to be more susceptible to the development of digoxin toxicity. In some cases, vasodilator therapy may be beneficial but these agents should be used with caution to avoid excessive reduction in preload; elevated filling pressures may be required to maintain adequate cardiac output.

2. Specific therapy aimed at amelioration of the underlying cause should be instituted. Cardiac hemochromatosis may respond to reduction of total body iron stores via phlebotomy or chelation therapy with deferoxamine. Cardiac sarcoidosis may respond to corticosteroid therapy, but prolongation of survival with this approach has not been established. There is no known effective therapy to reverse the progression of cardiac amyloidosis.

VI. Pericardial disease

A. Cardiac tamponade results from increased intrapericardial pressure secondary to fluid accumulation within the pericardial space. Pericarditis of any cause may lead to cardiac tamponade. Idiopathic (or viral) and neoplastic forms are the most frequent causes.

1. The **diagnosis** should be suspected in patients with elevated jugular venous pressure, hypotension, pulsus paradoxus, tachycardia, evidence of poor peripheral perfusion, and distant heart sounds. Echocardiography can confirm the diagnosis. Right heart catheterization may be necessary to determine the hemodynamic significance of a pericardial effusion, especially in patients with a subacute or chronic presentation. Hemodynamic findings of elevated, equalized, diastolic pressures are present in the patient with cardiac tamponade.

2. Definitive treatment consists of emergent drainage of the pericardial space via **pericardiocentesis** or **surgical pericardiotomy.** Emergent pericardiocen-

Table 6-3. Classification of shock

| Type of shock | Hemodynamics | | | Potential etiologies |
	Filling pressures	CO	SVR	
Cardiogenic	↑	↓	↑	Myocardial infarction Cardiomyopathy Valvular heart disease Arrhythmias Acute VSD, MR
Distributive (septic)	↓	↑	↓	Sepsis Anaphylaxis Toxic shock syndrome
Hypovolemic	↓	↑↓	↑	Hemorrhage Volume depletion Hypoadrenal crisis
Obstructive	↑ (proximal) ↓ (distal)	↓	↑	Pulmonary embolism Tamponade Tension pneumothorax

Key: CO = cardiac output; SVR = systemic vascular resistance; VSD = ventricular septal defect; MR = mitral regurgitation.

tesis should be performed with echocardiographic guidance if possible. If pericardial drainage cannot be performed emergently, stabilization with parenteral inotropic support and aggressive administration of intravenous saline to maintain adequate ventricular filling are indicated. Diuretics, nitrates, or any other preload-reducing agents are absolutely contraindicated.

B. Constrictive pericarditis may develop as a late complication of pericardial inflammation. Constrictive pericarditis may occur as a result of mediastinal irradiation or postpericardiotomy syndrome following cardiac surgery. The majority of cases are of unknown etiology, although tuberculous pericarditis is a leading cause in some underdeveloped countries.

    1. Pathophysiology and diagnosis. The noncompliant pericardium causes impairment of ventricular filling and progressive elevation of venous pressure. In contrast to cardiac tamponade, the clinical presentation is characteristically insidious, with gradual development of symptoms of fatigue, exercise intolerance, and venous congestion. Physical findings include jugular venous distention with prominent X and Y descents, inspiratory elevation of the jugular venous pressure (Kussmaul's sign), peripheral edema, ascites, and a pericardial knock during diastole. Echocardiography may reveal pericardial thickening and diminished diastolic filling. In addition, a chest CT scan and MRI may detect pericardial thickening. Cardiac catheterization is usually necessary to demonstrate elevated and equalized diastolic pressures in all four cardiac chambers. The diagnosis of constrictive pericarditis is often difficult to distinguish from restrictive cardiomyopathy (see sec. **V**).

    2. Definitive treatment requires complete pericardiectomy, which is accompanied by significant perioperative mortality (5–10%) but results in clinical improvement in 90% of patients. Patients who are minimally symptomatic can be managed with judicious sodium and fluid restriction and diuretic therapy but must be followed closely to detect hemodynamic deterioration.

VII. Shock is a clinical syndrome of systemic hypotension, acidemia, and impairment of vital organ function resulting from tissue hypoperfusion. Although typically acute, its onset may be gradual and insidious. Shock can be classified based on characteristic pathophysiologic and hemodynamic changes (Table 6–3). Treatment of shock requires hemodynamic stabilization with intravenous fluids and vasopressors to maintain vital organ perfusion with concomitant identification and treatment of underlying pathologic processes.

A. Classification of shock

  1. Cardiogenic shock occurs as a result of inadequate cardiac output, impaired oxygen delivery, and reduced tissue perfusion caused by loss of effective contractile function of myocardium (acute MI, hemodynamically significant tachy- or bradyarrhythmias, cardiomyopathy) or from mechanical processes reducing adequate forward output (acute valvular regurgitation, acute ventricular septal defect, critical aortic stenosis, HCM). Hemodynamically, filling pressures are elevated (pulmonary artery wedge pressure >18 mm Hg), cardiac output is depressed (index <2.0 liters/min/m^2), peripheral vascular resistance is increased, and mean arterial blood pressure is low (MAP <60 mm Hg).

    a. Initial treatment is directed toward maintaining adequate systemic blood pressure, cardiac output, and myocardial perfusion with volume expansion and vasopressors or inotropes. Initial treatment is guided by hemodynamic monitoring while the precipitating cause is identified and treated. Prompt diagnosis is mandatory and may require emergent echocardiography or cardiac catheterization.

    b. Mechanical support with intra-aortic balloon counterpulsation (IABP) may be necessary before and during recovery from definitive surgical treatment.

  2. Distributive shock (septic shock) is manifest as vasodilatation, low central filling pressures and intravascular volume, reduction in peripheral vascular resistance, loss of capillary integrity with extravascular transudation of intravascular fluid (capillary leak), and an initially increased cardiac output.

    a. Treatment includes hemodynamic support with intravenous fluids (saline, colloid) and vasopressors (dopamine, epinephrine, levarterenol [Levophed], phenylephrine [Neo-Synephrine]) as identification of underlying processes is initiated. Adjunctive treatment may include antibiotics, surgical drainage of abscesses, and removal of potential sources of infection (e.g., urethral and intravenous catheters, wound packing, tampons).

    b. Treatment of anaphylaxis is discussed in Chap. 26.

    c. Use of steroids in the treatment of septic shock is not recommended in the absence of adrenal suppression.

  3. Hypovolemic shock results from loss of greater than 20% of the circulating blood volume due to acute hemorrhage, fluid depletion, or dehydration. In the absence of obvious trauma or hemorrhage, occult sources of bleeding and volume loss should be considered (gastrointestinal, intra- or retroperitoneal, femoral compartment, intrathoracic, aortic dissection). Intracardiac filling pressures are decreased, cardiac output is normal or increased, and systemic vascular resistance is elevated due to compensatory vasoconstriction.

    a. Rapid **volume expansion** with fluids, colloid, and blood products is paramount. Coexisting problems such as congestive heart failure, valvular heart disease, myocardial ischemia, or renal insufficiency must be carefully monitored, and invasive hemodynamic monitoring during acute management of hypovolemic shock may be required.

    b. Correction of coagulopathy and electrolyte imbalance as well as utilization of invasive diagnostic and therapeutic procedures (surgery, endoscopy, interventional radiologic procedures) need to be addressed urgently.

    c. Hypoadrenal (addisonian) crisis is a form of hypovolemic shock due to inadequate release of mineralocorticoids and glucocorticoids from the adrenal gland. In addition to hypotension, patients may manifest hyponatremia, hyperkalemia, acidosis, and hypoglycemia. Adrenal insufficiency may occur acutely (adrenal hemorrhage) or insidiously (metastasis, tuberculosis). In patients whose adrenal function has been suppressed by chronic steroid therapy, hypoadrenal crisis may develop if steroid replacement is discontinued abruptly or if metabolic or physical stress (i.e., infection, surgery) develops. Once the diagnosis is suspected on clinical grounds, treatment should be initiated immediately by volume expansion with intravenous saline and steroid replacement with hydrocortisone, 100 mg IV q8h (see Chap. 21).

4. Obstructive shock may result from massive pulmonary embolism, cardiac tamponade, atrial myxoma, acute valvular stenosis (e.g., prosthetic valve thrombosis), or tension pneumothorax. Cardiac output is severely reduced due to impairment of ventricular filling or obstruction to blood flow, despite adequate intravascular volume, contractility, and vascular tone.

    a. Initial treatment is supportive, with volume expansion and vasopressors. However, since the precipitating factors are mechanical, rapid diagnosis is essential to identify the obstructive process and guide emergent therapy.

    b. Specific treatment of mechanical problems may include pericardiocentesis, chest tube placement, thrombolytic therapy (for massive pulmonary embolus or valve thrombosis), embolectomy, or emergent cardiac surgery.

VIII. Cardiac transplantation is an effective therapeutic option for selected patients with severe end-stage heart disease that has become refractory to aggressive medical therapy and for which there are no other conventional surgical or interventional treatment options (e.g., coronary artery bypass grafting, valve surgery, PTCA).

A. Candidates considered for transplantation should be less than 60 years old, have advanced heart disease (NYHA functional class III–IV), have a strong psychosocial support system, have exhausted all other therapeutic options, and be free of irreversible extracardiac organ dysfunction that would limit functional recovery or predispose to posttransplant complications.

B. Survival rates of up to 90% at 1 year and 70% at 5 years have been reported since the introduction of cyclosporine. In general, functional capacity improves significantly after transplantation. Greater than 75% of recipients return to their pre-illness occupation or activity.

C. Immunosuppressive therapy typically includes cyclosporine, azathioprine, and corticosteroids in combination to minimize the risks of rejection and infection as well as the side effects of each agent. Various antilymphocyte antibody preparations (ALG, ATG, OKT-3) have been employed as initial induction therapy or for treatment of severe rejection or rejection refractory to treatment with pulse corticosteroids (methylprednisolone, 0.5–1.0 g IV qd for 3 days). Serial endomyocardial biopsies are performed in all heart transplant recipients to monitor rejection.

D. Posttransplant complications include acute and chronic rejection, infection due to immunosuppression (see Chap. 13), adverse effects of immunosuppressive agents, and the development of posttransplant coronary arteriopathy.

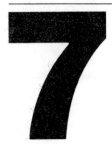

Cardiac Arrhythmias

Mark L. Cohen and
Bruce D. Lindsay

Recognition and Management

Over the past decade improved techniques of intracardiac recording and stimulation have identified mechanisms underlying the pathophysiology of many common arrhythmias and provided a rational basis for their diagnosis and treatment. Some arrhythmias are benign and may not warrant intervention, while others are disabling or life threatening and should be treated aggressively. Appropriate therapy should be determined by the pathophysiology of the arrhythmia, the natural history of the disorder, and the efficacy of treatment. This chapter reviews the recognition and management of specific arrhythmias, use of antiarrhythmic medications, techniques of cardioversion, and general principles of cardiac pacing.

I. **General approach.** Accurate diagnosis and appropriate therapy of disturbances in cardiac rhythm require careful analysis of the patient's history (especially relating to the new use of drugs affecting the heart), physical examination, and ECG, as well as an understanding of the nature of these rhythm disturbances and of the available therapeutic modalities. When possible, one should adhere to this approach in evaluating patients with rhythm disturbances.

A. **History.** The frequency, duration, mode of onset, and mode of cessation of the arrhythmia should be determined. Symptoms or a history of any disease that may directly or indirectly influence the cardiovascular system should be elicited. The patient's medications should be carefully reviewed.

B. **Physical examination.** The blood pressure and both apical and peripheral pulses should be taken. Jugular venous pulsations should be observed for the patterns of atrial activity and atrioventricular (AV) synchrony. The heart should be auscultated for murmurs, gallops, or variations in the first heart sound. Evidence of cardiomegaly, congestive heart failure (CHF), thyroid dysfunction, or respiratory embarrassment should be sought.

C. **Laboratory studies.** Electrolytes (K^+, Ca^{2+}, and Mg^{2+}), arterial blood gases, antiarrhythmic drug levels, and thyroid function should be determined. A chest radiograph should be obtained.

D. **Thorough review of the ECG.** It is especially important to define atrial activity. The following are often helpful.

1. A long **rhythm strip** with evaluation of multiple leads. Leads aVF and V_1 are generally the most valuable in identifying atrial activity. Recording the rhythm strip at 50 mm/sec and 20 mm/mV gain may better discriminate P waves.

2. **Bipolar exploring leads** ("Lewis leads") may accentuate atrial activity. Lead I is monitored with the left arm lead placed posteriorly or over the left ventricular apex and the right arm lead used to explore the precordium.

3. **Carotid sinus massage.** Vagotonic maneuvers often slow the ventricular response and facilitate identification of atrial activity. The patient should be supine with an IV line in place and the ECG monitored. Before massage, the carotid vessels should be auscultated for bruits; carotid massage is rarely so essential that it need be done if bruits are heard. The right carotid sinus should be massaged first, for no more than 10 seconds. If this is ineffective, the left carotid should be massaged. **The left and right carotids should never**

be massaged simultaneously. A concomitant Valsalva maneuver (expiration against a closed glottis) may further augment vagal tone. Adjuncts to carotid sinus massage can be found in sec. **II.E.2.**

4. An **esophageal lead** may be necessary to identify atrial activity. If an esophageal lead is not available, one can be made by passing a pacemaker wire through a nasogastric tube. The electrode tip of the pacemaker wire should not be extended beyond the terminal part of the tube when it is passed into the esophagus. The nasogastric tube should be passed to approximately 50 cm and the proximal end of the pacing wire attached to an exploring (V lead) electrode. The electrode tip should then be extruded from the distal end of the nasogastric tube and the electrogram should be recorded. Identification of atrial activity is facilitated if multiple leads can be monitored simultaneously. P-wave activity is generally of short duration and has a more rapid intrinsic deflection than does QRS activity. The lead should be withdrawn at 1-cm intervals until the P wave and QRS morphologies are determined. Having the patient hold a midinspiration breath reduces respiratory motion.

5. An **intra-atrial** electrogram can be obtained if other methods are inadequate. This procedure should be done under sterile conditions with a **well-grounded ECG machine** or special amplifier.

II. **Specific arrhythmias.** Once the diagnosis has been established, additional therapy should be directed at **correction of underlying abnormalities** (e.g., hypoxia, acid–base or electrolyte imbalance, CHF, hypotension, anxiety). This alone may terminate the arrhythmia and may be necessary if other therapeutic modalities are to be effective.

A. **Sinus tachycardia** is a physiologic response to physical or emotional stress.

1. **ECG recognition.** The rate is 100–160 beats/minute with minimal cyclic variation. In response to carotid sinus massage, the rate slows transiently, then returns to its previous level. In severe hypermetabolic states, in which heart rates may exceed 160 beats/minute, there may be no response to carotid sinus massage.

2. **Therapy.** Treatment of sinus tachycardia itself is rarely required since it is frequently a physiologic response to maintain cardiac output. Primary therapy is correction of the underlying abnormality. When antiarrhythmic therapy is necessary, propranolol, 10–40 mg PO q6h, or 1-mg IV aliquots (repeated q5–10 min, with a total IV dose not to exceed 0.15 mg/kg acutely), is generally effective. Esmolol (see Antiarrhythmic Agents, sec. **II.D**) will be equally effective, and has the advantage of a short half-life in the event of hypotension or bronchial constriction. Digitalis is not useful unless CHF is present.

B. **Sinus bradycardia** is not in itself pathologic. Asymptomatic heart rates below 60 beats/minute (often in the range of 45–50 beats/min) occur as a result of enhanced vagal tone and may be seen in normal persons of all ages; they usually require no therapy. If the sinus bradycardia is inappropriate for the clinical situation (e.g., hypotension, fever) or if symptoms are present, primary sinus node disease (see sec. **IV**) should be considered. Sinus bradycardia may also occur with increased intracranial pressure, hypothyroidism, hypothermia, or inferior myocardial infarction, or in response to drugs, including beta antagonists and verapamil.

1. **ECG recognition.** The sinus rate is less than 60 beats/minute and may demonstrate marked sinus arrhythmia. Patients with heart rates less than 40 beats/minute may manifest angina, hypotension, heart failure, or an impaired level of consciousness.

2. **Therapy**

a. Asymptomatic patients require no treatment.

b. Sinus bradycardia associated with hemodynamic compromise or symptoms can be treated with atropine (0.5–2.0 mg IV), isoproterenol (1–4 µg/min), or ventricular pacing (Table 7–1).

C. **Atrial premature depolarizations (APDs)** occur in patients of all ages but may reflect underlying heart disease. They are exacerbated by myocardial ischemia,

Table 7-1. Drugs used for treatment of bradyarrhythmias

Agent	Treatment
Atropine	IV: 0.5–2.0 mg
	SQ: 0.5–2.0 mg
Isoproterenol	IV: 1 mg in 250 ml and titrate, generally 1–4 μg/min
Epinephrine	IV: 1-mg bolus for asystole
	1 mg in 100 ml D_5W; initiate infusion at 2 μg/min and titrate for bradyarrhythmias
	SQ: 0.2–0.3 ml of 1:1000 q1–2h

pericardial inflammation, a variety of drugs, disturbances in acid–base or electrolyte balance, and pulmonary disease. Emotional stress or the use of caffeine, tobacco, or alcohol also may increase the frequency of APDs.

1. **ECG recognition.** APDs are preceded by a P wave (which may have a different configuration from the normal P morphology). They are followed by a normal QRS complex. Atrioventricular conduction following an APD depends on the inherent function of the AV conduction system. Late-coupled APDs can be conducted normally, but early-coupled APDs are associated with a prolonged PR interval or aberrant conduction (usually right bundle branch block). Very early APDs may block in the AV node or His bundle and result in a pause simulating a sinus pause or exit block. APDs usually reset the sinus node, resulting in an ectopic–P- to sinus–P-wave interval similar to the sinus P–P interval.

2. **Therapy**
   a. **Asymptomatic** individuals without evidence for sustained atrial tachyarrhythmias require no specific therapy acutely other than elimination of underlying or precipitating disorders.
   b. **Symptomatic** APDs may be suppressed with class Ia or Ic drugs. Patients with a history of atrial fibrillation or flutter, however, should not receive these drugs without concomitant therapy with AV nodal depressant drugs (digoxin, beta antagonists, or verapamil) to control the ventricular response. Patients with catecholamine-related APDs can be treated effectively with a beta antagonist alone.
   c. APDs that initiate **atrial fibrillation or flutter** should be treated with a combination of drugs directed at suppressing the APDs (class Ia or Ic) and drugs directed at slowing the ventricular response (digitalis, beta antagonist, or verapamil).
   d. Patients with APDs initiating **recurrent SVT** resistant to therapy with AV nodal depressant drugs should be treated with class Ia or Ic drugs. These drugs can be used as single agents if the patient has no history of atrial fibrillation or flutter.

D. **Ventricular premature depolarizations (VPDs)** are due to intraventricular reentry or disturbances in automaticity and occur in normal subjects and patients with heart disease. They are exacerbated by electrolyte imbalance, hypoxia, acid–base imbalance, endocrine disorders such as thyrotoxicosis, and a variety of medications. Digitalis, phenothiazines, tricyclic antidepressants, and antiarrhythmic agents may increase the frequency of VPDs. In the absence of demonstrable heart disease, VPDs are not generally associated with an increased risk of sudden death. They have greater prognostic significance in the presence of coronary artery disease, cardiomyopathy, and possibly mitral valve prolapse.

1. **ECG recognition.** VPDs are premature QRS complexes, generally different in QRS morphology, and greater than 0.12 seconds in duration. The T wave is usually large and opposite in direction to the major deflection of the QRS. The

QRS is not preceded by a premature P wave, although a sinus P wave occurring at its usual time may be present. A retrograde P wave may follow the QRS, be hidden in the QRS, or not be visible on the surface ECG. Although differentiation of a VPD from a supraventricular beat conducted aberrantly is not always possible, the presence of a compensatory pause, fusion beats, and initial QRS forces different in direction from normal sinus beats favors a ventricular origin.

2. **Indications for treatment.** Reasons for treating patients with VPDs include reducing symptoms accompanying an irregular heart rhythm and preventing sustained ventricular tachycardia (VT) or ventricular fibrillation (VF).

   a. Patients with **symptomatic VPDs** can be treated empirically, with alleviation of symptoms serving as an objective therapeutic end point.

   b. The indications for treating patients with **asymptomatic VPDs** or runs of **nonsustained VT** evoke controversy. The decision to treat patients with complex ventricular ectopy should be made only after considering the potential benefits and risks of administering antiarrhythmic agents to asymptomatic patients. In approximately 30–40% of patients receiving antiarrhythmic medications, adverse reactions develop that necessitate discontinuation of these drugs. Among these risks are proarrhythmic effects, which are observed in 5–15% of patients. Ventricular ectopy that occurs in the absence of organic heart disease is not generally associated with an increased risk of sudden death. Although patients with depressed ventricular function are at greater risk of sustained ventricular arrhythmias, the predictive value of ventricular ectopy for sudden death is very low (*Circulation* 74:653, 1986). Despite several clinical trials, there is no evidence that empiric antiarrhythmic therapy reduces the incidence of sudden death (*Am. J. Cardiol.* 66:451, 1990). In patients with a prior myocardial infarction, effective suppression of ventricular ectopy with either encainide or flecainide was associated with a 3.6-fold **increase in mortality** when compared to placebo (*N. Engl. J. Med.* 321:406, 1989). Based on these considerations **empiric antiarrhythmic therapy is not recommended.**

3. **Therapy**

   a. **Acute** suppression of VPDs is best achieved with IV lidocaine or procainamide.

   b. **Chronic** suppression of VPDs may occur with the use of class I agents. Beta antagonists and calcium channel antagonists rarely suppress VPDs; nonetheless, beta antagonists are the only class of drugs shown to reduce the incidence of sudden death in patients with a prior myocardial infarction. Encainide or flecainide should not be used for the suppression of VPDs in patients who have had a myocardial infarction. Amiodarone should be reserved for sustained ventricular arrhythmias that fail to respond to conventional agents.

E. **Paroxysmal supraventricular tachycardia** (SVT) occurs in patients of all ages, with and without underlying heart disease. SVT is most often due to reentry, generally within the AV node or involving an accessory pathway, although sinus node reentry, intra-atrial reentry, and SVT due to enhanced automaticity can also occur. The response to therapy depends on the mechanism involved (*Ann. Intern. Med.* 87:346, 1977).

   1. **ECG recognition** (Table 7-2). The rate of these arrhythmias ranges from 150–250 beats/minute. The QRS complex is generally normal, but aberration may occur.

      a. **AV nodal reentry** is the most common cause of SVT, accounting for 60% of cases. As shown in Fig. 7-1, the reentrant circuit is localized to the AV node and adjacent atrial tissue. Conceptually, AV node reentry is due to the longitudinal dissociation of this region into two functionally distinct pathways. During SVT, anterograde conduction occurs over one pathway and retrograde conduction over the other, resulting in nearly simultaneous ventricular and atrial activation. As a result, retrograde **P waves**

Table 7-2. Electrocardiographic diagnosis of SVT: Value of P-wave position during SVT

Type	ECG manifestations
AV node reentry	Retrograde P wave most frequently buried in QRS or with short RP (RP <50% RR interval)
Orthodromic SVT utilizing an accessory pathway	Eccentric retrograde P wave with short RP (RP <50% RR interval) and negative P wave lead I
Intra-atrial reentry	Positive P wave in leads II, III, aVF (RP >50% RR interval), with PR related to SVT rate
Sinus node reentry	P-wave morphology identical to sinus rhythm (RP >50% RR interval), with PR related to SVT rate
Automatic atrial tachycardia	Positive or negative P wave in leads II, III, aVF (RP >50% RR interval), with PR related to SVT rate

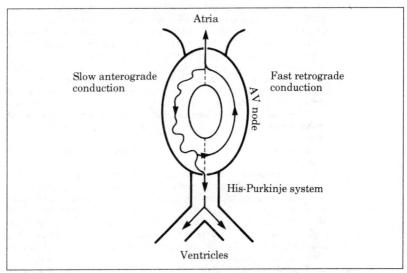

Fig. 7-1. The AV node and adjacent tissue are longitudinally dissociated into slowly conducting and rapidly conducting pathways. During typical AV node reentry, anterograde conduction occurs over the slow pathway and retrograde conduction over the fast pathway. Activation of the atria and ventricles occurs almost simultaneously.

are buried within the QRS complexes and are not visible on the surface ECG or **appear immediately after the QRS complex** (negative in leads II, III, and aVF; RP interval <50% of RR interval). Atrioventricular node reentry cannot exist in the presence of AV node block but can persist if AV block is intra- or infra-His. Since intra-His and infra-His blocks are uncommon, especially in young patients, the presence of AV block during SVT markedly reduces the chance that AV node reentry is the responsible mechanism.

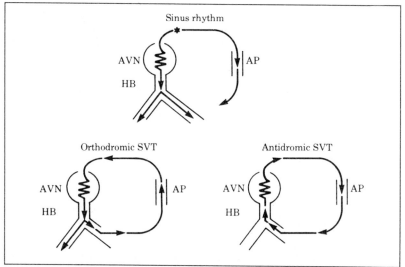

Fig. 7-2. Atrioventricular conduction in WPW syndrome. During sinus rhythm, anterograde conduction occurs over both the atrioventricular node (AVN) and the accessory pathway (AP). During orthodromic supraventricular tachycardia (SVT) the AVN comprises the anterograde limb and the AP comprises the retrograde limb of the reentrant circuit. Activation of the atria follows ventricular activation. During antidromic SVT the AP comprises the anterograde limb and the AVN the retrograde limb of reentry. (HB = His bundle.)

    b. **Wolff-Parkinson-White (WPW) syndrome** is the second most common form of SVT and accounts for 25% of cases. The reentrant circuit involves the atria, AV node, His-Purkinje system, ventricular muscle, and an **accessory pathway (AP).** Reentrant SVT utilizing an AP cannot occur in the presence of AV block. The APs are either manifest or concealed. **Manifest** APs conduct anterogradely during sinus rhythm, and characteristic delta waves and a short (<0.12 sec) PR interval are observed in the ECG, reflecting ventricular preexcitation. **Concealed** APs only conduct retrogradely, and ventricular preexcitation is not present during sinus rhythm. Accordingly, the PR interval and QRS complex are normal. **Orthodromic** SVT occurs with manifest and concealed APs and is the most common type. During orthodromic SVT, shown in Fig. 7-2, anterograde conduction occurs through the AV node to the ventricles and returns retrogradely via the AP to excite the atria, resulting in a **P wave that immediately follows the QRS complex.** In the majority of patients with orthodromic SVT, the AP is left sided. Consequently, during SVT, atrial activation proceeds left to right and the **P wave is generally negative in lead I.** Since the ventricular activation sequence is normal, the delta wave is not present and the QRS complex appears normal unless aberration occurs. **Antidromic** SVT is rare and can only occur in manifest APs. Figure 7-2 demonstrates that anterograde conduction occurs through the AP to the ventricles and returns retrogradely through the AV node to the atria. The resulting P wave immediately follows the QRS complex but may be difficult to detect because of the repolarization abnormality. During antidromic SVT the ventricle is exclusively activated by the AP, so the pronounced delta wave and widened QRS complex resemble ventricular tachycardia.

  c. Sinus node reentry is a rare cause of SVT. The reentrant circuit is localized to the sinus node, and during SVT the **P-wave morphology is identical to that observed during normal sinus rhythm.** The AV node is not part of the reentrant circuit, and the PR interval or presence of AV block depends on the intrinsic properties of the AV node.

  d. Intra-atrial reentry accounts for 5% of SVT. The reentrant circuit is localized to the atria, and during SVT the **P wave precedes the QRS (RP >50% RR), indicating an anterograde atrial activation sequence.** Since the AV node is not part of the reentrant circuit, the atrial tachycardia is not affected by AV block.

  e. Automatic atrial foci account for 5% of SVT. During SVT the **P-wave morphology depends on the location of the ectopic pacemaker.** In automatic SVT the P-wave morphology of the first beat initiating the SVT is identical to subsequent P waves. In contrast, the P-wave morphology of the APD triggering reentrant SVT generally differs from the P-wave morphology during the tachycardia. In automatic SVT, as in SVT due to sinus node or intra-atrial reentry, the AV node is not an integral part of the underlying mechanism. The PR interval or presence of AV block depends on the inherent function of the AV conduction system, independent of the atrial rhythm.

2. Acute therapy

  a. Immediate cardioversion (see Cardioversion) is indicated for prompt termination of reentrant SVT if the patient has angina, hypotension, dyspnea, or heart failure.

  b. Vagal stimulation may terminate some SVTs by increasing parasympathetic tone while inhibiting sympathetic outflow. Vagal stimulation is **particularly useful for reentrant SVTs that utilize either the sinus or AV node as part or all of the reentrant circuit.** Carotid sinus massage (see sec. **I.D.3**) is the preferred method of enhancing vagal tone.

  c. Adenosine (see Table 7-4) causes transient complete AV node block and often transient sinus node arrest. Interruption of AV node conduction terminates AV node reentry and orthodromic SVT or provides brief heart block during which multiple consecutive P waves can be seen in atrial tachycardia or atrial flutter. The dose is 6–12 mg (less if injected into a central line) given as a rapid IV bolus into a peripheral vein. The onset of action is 15–30 seconds and the duration only seconds. The patient is likely to experience a flush or pressure sensation in the chest, lasting less than 1 minute.

  d. Verapamil also prolongs AV nodal refractiveness and terminates AV node reentry and orthodromic SVT. Verapamil may increase AV block and slow the ventricular rate during automatic or intra-atrial reentrant SVT. The dose is 5–10 mg IV administered over 2–3 minutes. It should be used cautiously in elderly patients and is contraindicated in those with hypotension or high-degree AV block (see Antiarrhythmic Agents, sec. **IV**).

  e. Beta antagonists are effective in terminating reentrant SVTs involving the sinus node and AV node. Although the AV node is not critical to the initiation or maintenance of intra-atrial reentrant SVT or automatic SVT, these agents slow the ventricular rate. Propranolol and esmolol have been approved for the treatment of SVT. The dose of propranolol is 0.15 mg/kg given intravenously at a rate of 1 mg/minute. Esmolol is a short-acting $beta_1$ selective antagonist that is less likely to induce bronchospasm (see Antiarrhythmic Agents, sec. **II.D** for dosage and administration).

  f. Digoxin. The initial dose is 0.5–0.75 mg IV or PO, followed by aliquots of 0.25 mg q2h as needed, to a maximum dose of 1.5–2.0 mg. The full effect may require a complete loading dose. Caution should be exercised if carotid sinus massage is repeated since this drug increases carotid baroreceptor sensitivity. As with verapamil and propranolol, digoxin slows AV nodal conduction and is **effective in terminating AV nodal reentrant SVT.** Digoxin is likewise effective in slowing the ventricular response during other types of SVT.

- **g. Quinidine and procainamide** in conventional doses may terminate intra-atrial reentry, atrioventricular reentry incorporating an accessory pathway, AV node reentry, or automatic atrial tachycardias.
- **h. Elective cardioversion** or **rapid atrial pacing** may be required if the preceding techniques prove unsuccessful. The reentrant forms of SVT are almost always responsive, but automatic SVT generally continues unabated.
- **i. Management of patients with WPW** is detailed in sec. **VI.**

3. **Prophylaxis against recurrence** is often more difficult than termination of the acute episode. Decisions regarding prophylactic therapy should be based on the SVT mechanism, frequency of episodes, underlying heart disease, and symptoms. Patients with infrequent episodes that are not associated with disabling symptoms may prefer intermittent acute treatment (single oral or IV administration of an effective antiarrhythmic drug) to chronic therapy. On the other hand, patients with frequent episodes or episodes associated with disabling symptoms should be treated chronically.

- **a. SVT due to AV node reentry** may be difficult to prevent. In 70% of cases, AV node depressant agents including digoxin, beta antagonists, or verapamil are effective and exert their beneficial actions primarily on the anterograde limb of the microreentrant circuit. In 30% of cases, procainamide, quinidine, or disopyramide is effective as a single agent and affects retrograde conduction primarily. Rarely, a combination of both types of agents is effective; generally, however, such combinations offset the salutary effects of each drug. Flecainide is effective in up to 70% of patients and is usually well tolerated. Cryothermal lesions that are applied intraoperatively or applications of radiofrequency electrical current (*N. Engl. J. Med.* 83:827, 1991) delivered by catheters can effectively modify the AV node and eliminate the tachycardia without loss of normal atrioventricular conduction. These curative procedures can be performed with few risks and are an effective alternative to pharmacologic agents.
- **b. WPW syndrome** (see sec. **VI**).
- **c. Sinus node reentry** is often prevented by treatment with beta-adrenergic or calcium channel antagonists.
- **d. Intra-atrial reentry** and **automatic SVT** are prevented best with quinidine or procainamide. Concomitant treatment with an AV node depressant drug is recommended if the ventricular response rate is rapid.
- **e.** Invasive electrophysiologic study may be necessary to determine the mechanism and optimal treatment.

F. **Atrial fibrillation** may be either **chronic** (usually associated with organic heart disease due to coronary artery disease or mitral valve disease, or chronic obstructive pulmonary disease) or **paroxysmal,** which may be seen with preexcitation syndromes, pulmonary embolism, thyrotoxicosis, and alcohol ingestion and, on occasion, without a demonstrable etiology.

1. **ECG recognition.** Discrete atrial activity is not present, and the ventricular response is usually an irregularly irregular rate between 160 and 200 beats/minute in the absence of AV node blocking drugs (digoxin, beta antagonists, verapamil). Carotid sinus massage slows the ventricular rate transiently but generally does not restore sinus rhythm.

- **a.** Atrial fibrillation with a **regular ventricular response** should raise suspicion of an accelerated junctional rhythm due to digitalis excess.
- **b.** A **slow ventricular response** (<120 beats/min) in the untreated patient implies underlying disease in the AV conduction system.
- **c.** Atrial fibrillation in patients with preexcitation syndromes may be associated with an extremely rapid ventricular response. A rapid irregular wide complex tachycardia is observed.

2. Therapy

a. **Emergent cardioversion** (see Cardioversion) is necessary in patients with a rapid ventricular response and those who have angina, hypotension, dyspnea, or heart failure.

b. In **hemodynamically stable** patients, digoxin, verapamil, propranolol, or esmolol can be given intravenously or orally (depending on the clinical situation) to slow the ventricular response. If the blood pressure is measured before each aliquot of propranolol or verapamil is given (every 2–3 min), or frequently during esmolol infusion, the ventricular rate can be controlled safely within 30 minutes in most patients. Propranolol or esmolol may be useful even in the presence of heart failure if a disease that inhibits ventricular filling is present (mitral stenosis or hypertrophic cardiomyopathy). After initial therapy, a maintenance dose of digoxin, verapamil, or propranolol should control the ventricular response between 70 and 90 beats/minute at rest. A combination of these agents is frequently beneficial. Serum digoxin levels considered toxic in other circumstances may be necessary to control the ventricular response. The serum potassium level should be carefully monitored when large doses of digoxin are used.

c. **The decision** to attempt to restore sinus rhythm should be made on the basis of (1) left atrial size (a left atrial size by echocardiogram >4.5 cm is generally not associated with long-term maintenance of sinus rhythm), (2) the duration of the arrhythmia, and (3) the need to reestablish sinus rhythm.

d. **Elective restoration** to sinus rhythm can be attempted pharmacologically and should generally be done in a monitored hospital setting. Administration of a class Ia or Ic drug restores sinus rhythm in approximately 30% of patients. These agents also reduce the energy requirement for DC cardioversion. **The ventricular response should be controlled before the administration of class Ia agents.** Intravenous procainamide is effective in up to 88% of patients with recent onset of atrial fibrillation and normal left atrial size by echocardiogram. If conversion to sinus rhythm is successful, oral therapy with class Ia or Ic agents effectively maintains sinus rhythm in up to 70% of patients who do not have marked atrial enlargement. If atrial fibrillation persists, cardioversion can be attempted electrically.

e. Patients manifesting a **wide complex irregular tachycardia** may have atrial fibrillation with ventricular preexcitation and should be managed as outlined in sec. **VI.B.3.**

3. Indications for anticoagulation

a. **Elective cardioversion** (electrical or pharmacologic). Ideally, the patient should receive a 3-week course of oral **anticoagulation** before conversion and for 2–3 weeks after conversion (*Am. Heart J.* 104:617, 1982).

b. Patients undergoing **emergent cardioversion,** especially those with a history of embolism or evidence of mitral valve disease, should receive anticoagulant therapy for 2–3 weeks after conversion unless there is a contraindication.

c. Oral anticoagulation is advised for patients with concomitant mitral valve disease, left ventricular failure, or cardiomyopathy. It should also be considered for patients older than 60 because the risk of stroke is greater in this population.

G. Atrial flutter.
The spectrum of disease states associated with atrial flutter is similar to that associated with atrial fibrillation.

1. ECG recognition.
The rhythm is characterized by a generally constant atrial rate of 240–350 beats/minute. However, in certain patients, especially those with dilated atria or those receiving class Ia or Ic antiarrhythmic agents, the atrial rate may be slower. The ventricular rate varies with the degree of AV block, which is usually 2:1 in untreated patients. Although 1:1 conduction is relatively uncommon, it is potentially life threatening. It is more likely to occur in patients with preexcitation syndrome or those receiving a class Ia or

Ic antiarrhythmic drug in the absence of an AV nodal depressant. Atrial flutter with 1:1 conduction may be difficult to differentiate from VT because of aberrant conduction. **Vagal maneuvers** usually cause a reduction in the ventricular rate because of an increase in the degree of AV block, which reveals the characteristic flutter waves. This response is often abrupt, with the ventricular response subsequently returning to the original rate. Characteristic **flutter waves** are best seen in leads II, III, aVF, and V_1.

2. **Therapy**
   a. The indications for **emergent cardioversion** are the same as for atrial fibrillation (see sec. **F.2.a**).
   b. If the patient is **hemodynamically stable,** digoxin, verapamil, or beta antagonists (propranolol or esmolol) can be used alone or in combination to control the ventricular response until arrangements are made for elective cardioversion. The patient's heart rate should be monitored and cardioversion should be performed immediately if the rate cannot be adequately controlled or the patient's condition deteriorates.
   c. If atrial flutter is **refractory to medical management,** cardioversion is the therapy of choice. In the majority of patients, **cardioversion** to sinus rhythm succeeds at low energies (≤ 50 joules), and atrial flutter can be converted to the more easily managed atrial fibrillation with even lower energy (5–10 joules). Rapid atrial pacing should be considered if cardioversion is contraindicated because of high-grade AV block or digoxin toxicity, or if the atrial flutter is recurrent and one wishes to assess a variety of drug regimens.
   d. Cardioversion may also be accomplished pharmacologically in patients with atrial flutter who are hemodynamically stable. **Intravenous procainamide** (see Antiarrhythmic Agents, sec. **I.A.4.d.(2)**) may be effective. On occasion, **oral** maintenance doses of class Ia or Ic drugs will be successful. **These agents should not be used until the ventricular response has been controlled.**

H. **Multifocal atrial tachycardia (MAT)** usually occurs in patients with severe pulmonary disease or severe heart disease, often in the context of acute respiratory insufficiency. Exacerbating factors may include digitalis intoxication, theophylline administration, postoperative state, electrolyte or metabolic imbalance, pulmonary edema, septicemia, hypoxemia, and hypercarbia.
   1. **ECG recognition.** Three or more different ectopic P-wave morphologies characterize MAT; frequently, there are varying PR intervals with an atrial rate of 100–200 beats/minute. Nonconducted P waves and an isoelectric baseline are common. A chaotic atrial mechanism has the same morphologic characteristics and differs only in that the atrial rate is less than 100 beats/minute.
   2. **Therapy should be directed at the underlying causes,** with particular attention to the patient's pulmonary status. **Digoxin is rarely beneficial** and may be harmful. Verapamil or quinidine in maintenance dosages may be effective but should never be used as primary therapy until the underlying causes have been corrected. Propranolol may reduce the ventricular response but is usually contraindicated by the underlying cardiopulmonary disease.

I. **Digitalis-induced arrhythmias** (see Chap. 6).

J. **Ventricular tachycardia** occurs most often in the setting of ischemic heart disease, including acute myocardial infarction and classic or variant angina, and following recovery from myocardial infarction particularly when it is complicated by development of a ventricular aneurysm. Other common causes include cardiomyopathy, prolonged QT syndrome, drug toxicity, and metabolic disorders. In addition, VT may occur in otherwise healthy individuals. In most cases it is due to a reentrant mechanism, although in some instances disturbances in automaticity may be responsible.
   1. **ECG recognition.** VT is defined as a series of three or more wide QRS complexes (duration >0.12 sec) of abnormal morphology, occurring at a rate of 100–250 beats/minute and accompanied by ST- and T-wave changes in a

direction opposite to the major QRS deflection. VT is often classified as nonsustained or sustained. Although arbitrary, sustained VT is defined as lasting longer than 30 seconds or associated with immediate hemodynamic collapse. The QRS contours may be uniform, multiform, or vary in a more or less repetitive manner (i.e., torsades de pointes, bidirectional VT). Retrograde atrial activation may be apparent, or the atria may be independent and exhibit atrioventricular dissociation. Differentiation of VT from SVT with aberrancy based on analysis of the surface ECG can be difficult and at times impossible. Intravenous verapamil as a "diagnostic challenge" can cause hypotension and should not be used. Features favoring VT include the following (*Am. J. Med.* 64:27, 1978):

a. QRS duration ≥ 0.14 seconds.

b. Left axis deviation.

c. AV dissociation.

d. Monophasic or biphasic RBBB QRS complexes, with left axis deviation and an R-S ratio of less than 1 in V_6. These criteria are not valid when left axis deviation is present during sinus rhythm.

Additional criteria for left bundle branch block morphology tachycardias are the following (*Am. J. Cardiol.* 61:1279, 1988):

(1) R in V_1 or V_2 >30 msec.

(2) Any Q in V_6.

(3) Onset of QRS to nadir of S in V_1 or V_2 >60 msec.

(4) Notching of the downstroke of the S in V_1 or V_2.

Intracardiac recordings are required occasionally.

2. Acute therapy

a. If sustained VT is associated with hypotension, heart failure, dyspnea or angina, **immediate cardioversion** is indicated. If the patient is without a pulse, defibrillation with 200 joules should be performed, followed by 360 joules if VT continues. In less dire circumstances, cardioversion should be attempted with a synchronized discharge of 50 joules, followed by progressively higher energies if initial attempts are not successful. Intravenous lidocaine (or procainamide or bretylium when appropriate) should be administered concomitantly.

b. If sustained VT is well tolerated by the patient, the following antiarrhythmic agents may be effective in terminating the arrhythmia. If the patient's condition deteriorates, immediate electrical cardioversion is indicated.

(1) Lidocaine should be given with an initial bolus of 1 mg/kg, followed by 0.5-mg/kg bolus injections every 8–10 minutes, if necessary, to a total dose of 3 mg/kg. Concurrent with bolus therapy, a maintenance infusion of 2 mg/minute should be started.

(2) Procainamide is the drug of second choice. The loading dose is 1500 mg in 150 ml D_5W or normal saline given at 50 mg/minute to a maximum of 15 mg/kg. After the loading dose a constant infusion of 2–4 mg/minute should be started. Blood pressure monitoring is imperative, as hypotension may occur. Hypotension usually responds to slowing the rate of infusion.

(3) Bretylium may be of benefit when the rhythm is refractory to the preceding measures. An initial dose of 5–10 mg/kg should be given in a 1:4 dilution with D_5W by infusion over 8–10 minutes, followed by a constant infusion of 1–2 mg/minute. Nausea, vomiting, and hypotension are not infrequent side effects.

(4) These agents can be continued for several days if necessary. Serum drug levels should be monitored and the infusion rate adjusted to maintain therapeutic levels. Attention should be given to conditions that predispose to drug toxicity, such as hepatic or renal insufficiency, heart failure, and metabolic and electrolyte abnormalities.

c. Underdrive or overdrive ventricular pacing can be used to terminate VT but should be performed only by experienced personnel.

3. **Chronic therapy** (Table 7-3). Invasive electrophysiologic (EP) testing is advised to judge the efficacy of these drugs for long-term treatment of sustained VT not occurring within 72 hours of myocardial infarction (see sec. VII).

   a. **Type Ia.** Quinidine, procainamide, or disopyramide, often in relatively high dosages, are the drugs usually used first for prevention of recurrent VT. Unfortunately, trials with these drugs have at best a 35% chance of success of preventing VT. Moricizine is a newer drug with combined class Ia and Ib properties. Patients with VT that is refractory to one of these drugs are unlikely to respond to the others.

   b. **Types Ib and Ic.** Mexiletine, tocainide, flecainide, and propafenone provide alternatives to therapy with type Ia agents. The combination of mexiletine and quinidine may be effective when neither is successful when used alone. Propafenone has beta-antagonist properties that can cause heart failure or bronchospasm.

   c. **Amiodarone** is a potent antiarrhythmic agent with substantial toxicity associated with long-term use. It should be reserved for sustained ventricular arrhythmias that are refractory to conventional agents.

   d. Beta antagonists are generally not effective for reentrant VT but may prevent VT induced by catecholamines or ischemia.

   e. Ventricular pacing may be helpful in preventing bradycardia-dependent VT but is generally not effective if the intrinsic heart rate is over 60 beats/minute.

   f. Several surgical approaches guided by electrophysiologic ventricular mapping are effective in treating some patients with medically refractory VT.

   g. **Implantable cardioverter–defibrillators** effectively reduce mortality in selected patients with life-threatening ventricular arrhythmias (*J. Am. Coll. Cardiol.* 13:1353, 1989). The implantable cardioverter–defibrillator is intended for patients who have survived a cardiac arrest or recurrent sustained VT not associated with acute myocardial infarction in whom conventional medical therapy is ineffective. It is contraindicated for patients whose ventricular arrhythmia may be due to a reversible cause (e.g., hypokalemia) or in whom ventricular arrhythmias occur with unacceptable frequency. Discharges are painful and may not prevent syncope before terminating the arrhythmia. Unwarranted discharges may be induced by nonsustained VT, atrial fibrillation, SVT, or sinus tachycardia when the ventricular rate exceeds the programmed arrhythmia rate detection criterion. Implantation requires a limited thoracotomy. When permanent pacing is indicated, a bipolar pacemaker is required, because the stimulus of a unipolar pacemaker adversely affects arrhythmia recognition by the implantable cardioverter–defibrillator.

4. **Torsades de pointes**

   a. **ECG recognition.** Torsades de pointes (*Prog. Cardiovasc. Dis.* 33:115, 1988) is a rare form of ventricular tachycardia in which the amplitude of the ventricular complexes varies in a sinusoidal pattern, with complexes of low amplitude linking phases of opposite polarity. The rate ranges from 160–280 beats/minute.

   b. **Etiology.** Torsades usually occurs in the setting of bradycardia or ventricular bigeminy having a compensatory pause and is usually initiated by a VPD falling on the T wave, causing a long RR to be followed by a short RR. In general, a long QT_c interval (normal upper limit of QT_c is 0.46 for men and 0.47 for women) is present before the tachycardia; however, random ECGs may exhibit a normal QT_c. The use of antiarrhythmic agents, phenothiazines, and tricyclics may lengthen the QT_c and induce or exacerbate torsades de pointes. Quinidine is the principal offender, but procainamide, disopyramide, amiodarone, and sotalol may also be responsible. Other causes include hypokalemia, hypomagnesemia, hypocalcemia, liquid protein diets, myocardial ischemia, and cardiomyopathies. The

Table 7-3. Dosages of class I antiarrhythmic agents[a]

Drug	Half-life (hr) Normal	ESRD	Route of metabolism	Oral dose	IV dose
Ia					
Procainamide	3–6	6–59	Renal 76–93%; hepatic 7–24%	250–1000 mg q3h; sustained release q6h	100 mg q5min, or 50 mg/min up to 15 mg/kg; maintenance infusion 2–6 mg/min
Quinidine	5–7	5–14	Hepatic 80–90%; renal 10–20%	Sulfate 200–400 mg q6h; polygalacturonate 275–550 mg q8–12h; glucuronate 324–648 mg q8–12h	—
Disopyramide	4–10	10–18	Renal 90%; hepatic 10%	100–200 mg q6–8h	—
Moricizine	1–6	?	Renal 39% (metabolites); hepatic 99%	100–300 mg q8h	—
Ib					
Lidocaine	1–2	1–3	Hepatic 90%; renal 10%	—	1 mg/kg; repeat 0.5 mg/kg q8–10min, if needed, to a total of 3 mg/kg; maintenance infusion of 2 mg/min
Mexiletine	8–10	9–13	Hepatic 85–90%; renal 10–15%	200–400 mg q8h	—
Tocainide	10–14	27	Hepatic 25%; renal 20–40%	300–800 mg q8h	—
Ic					
Flecainide	12–27	26	Renal 35%; hepatic 65%	100–200 mg q12h	—
Propafenone	2–32	?	Hepatic, renal	150–300 mg q8h	—

Key: ESRD = end-stage renal disease.

[a] Dosage adjustment is often indicated in the presence of renal or hepatic dysfunction.

[b] Moderate beta antagonist at usual doses. Long half-life in poor metabolizers (7% of population).

arrhythmia is responsible for syncope and sudden death in the congenital long-QT syndromes. Although intracerebral hemorrhage may prolong the QT_c, it is rarely associated with torsades de pointes.

c. **Therapy.** Torsades de pointes characteristically is a recurrent nonsustained arrhythmia; however, when it becomes sustained it can be fatal. Withdrawal of the offending agent or correction of the underlying electrolyte abnormality is often sufficient treatment. Active measures are required if torsades de pointes is incessant or causes hemodynamic compromise. Conversion and suppression of torsades can be achieved with **magnesium sulfate** administered intravenously (*Circulation* 77:392, 1988), 2g (e.g., 10 ml of a 20% solution) given over 1 minute, repeated in 5 minutes if necessary, followed by 3–20 mg/minute continuous infusion. This is effective even in patients with normal magnesium levels. The serum magnesium level should be followed and patients observed for signs of toxicity. Pause-dependent torsades de pointes is usually associated with drugs that prolong the QT interval or electrolyte abnormalities. If necessary, temporary pacing or an isoproterenol infusion can be used to suppress torsades de pointes by maintaining the heart rate at 90–120 beats/minute; however, these measures should be used cautiously in patients with severe coronary artery disease. Some patients may respond to treatment with lidocaine, phenytoin, or bretylium. Beta antagonists are useful in the management of congential long-QT syndromes but may be deleterious in drug-induced torsades de pointes. The use of class Ia drugs is contraindicated. An implantable cardioverter–defibrillator should be considered for patients in whom the reliability of medical therapy is uncertain.

K. **Ventricular fibrillation** (see Specific Arrest Sequences in Chap. 8)

III. **Stokes-Adams attacks** result from the transient cerebral ischemia that follows a sudden decrease in cardiac output due to a change in cardiac rate or rhythm. They may occur during episodes of VT, VF, complete heart block with an inadequate ventricular rate, or transient asystole. Stokes-Adams attacks may be seen with sick sinus syndrome (see sec. **IV**), carotid sinus hypersensitivity (see sec. **V**), and the subclavian steal syndrome. Symptoms of impaired consciousness begin 3–10 seconds after circulatory arrest. The attacks often begin suddenly, seldom last longer than 1–2 minutes, and are not generally followed by neurologic sequelae. Acute myocardial infarction or a cerebrovascular accident may be the cause or the result of such an attack. When observed the patient suddenly becomes pale and collapses, and on regaining consciousness often appears flushed. Ambulatory monitoring may document the cause of these attacks. If the attacks are due to tachyarrhythmias, appropriate antiarrhythmic drugs should be given. If they are due to bradyarrhythmias, most commonly complete heart block, a pacemaker is indicated.

When Stokes-Adams attacks due to complete heart block with a slow ventricular escape rhythm require **emergency treatment, isoproterenol** or **epinephrine** (see Table 7-1) can be used to increase the ventricular rate. Isoproterenol is preferred because it has a substantial chronotropic effect, is less likely to provoke ventricular arrhythmias, and will not cause excessive blood pressure elevation. **Temporary pacing** may be required for patients with prolonged or recurrent bradyarrhythmias until arrangements can be made to implant a permanent pacemaker.

IV. **Sick sinus syndrome (SSS)** includes a spectrum of disorders of impulse initiation and conduction, including marked sinus bradycardia, sinus arrest, sinoatrial block, AV node dysfunction, and recurrent supraventricular tachyarrhythmias. It is associated with ischemic, rheumatic, hypertensive, or idiopathic heart disease. It should be distinguished from sinus bradycardia due to increased vagal tone, which is commonly recognized in older patients at rest and in physically well-conditioned individuals. Manifestations may include atrial fibrillation with a slow ventricular response, an inappropriately slow heart rate, or prolonged sinus recovery following APDs or paroxysmal supraventricular arrhythmias.

Symptoms (fatigue, lightheadedness, syncope, angina, dyspnea) occur from long pauses caused by sinus node arrest, inappropriate bradyarrhythmias, or periods of

AV block. In symptomatic patients, the diagnosis can often be made from an ambulatory monitor. These patients do not have a markedly increased incidence of sudden death. In the absence of correlated symptoms, therapy is not necessary. In most circumstances, **pacemaker therapy should be utilized only when the arrhythmias diagnosed by ambulatory monitoring correlate with the symptom complex of the patient** and cannot be eliminated by withdrawing a provocative drug.

In patients with the **tachycardia–bradycardia syndrome,** there is alternation of rapid and slow heart rates. Bursts of supraventricular arrhythmias, most frequently atrial fibrillation, may alternate with long periods of sinus node or AV node dysfunction, or both. Therapy aimed at preventing or controlling the rapid atrial arrhythmias may enhance the bradyarrhythmias. In this circumstance, a pacemaker should be employed before therapy of the tachyarrhythmias.

V. **Carotid sinus hypersensitivity (CSH)** is a syndrome of enhanced responsiveness to carotid sinus stimulation. Two subtypes are observed clinically: (1) **cardioinhibitory** hypersensitivity, which is defined as ventricular asystole exceeding 3 seconds in duration during carotid sinus stimulation, and (2) **vasodepressor** hypersensitivity, which is defined as a decrease in systolic blood pressure of at least 50 mm Hg (due to vasodilatation) without associated cardiac slowing, or a decrease in systolic blood pressure exceeding 30 mm Hg associated with reproduction of the patient's clinical symptoms. Some patients have a combination of the two forms. Either subtype may result in presyncope or syncope during direct carotid sinus massage or during such maneuvers as head-turning or neck extension. Since many elderly patients satisfy the above criteria for CSH but do not have associated symptoms, it is essential to reproduce the clinical symptoms during testing (i.e., carotid sinus massage) before initiation of therapy. Asymptomatic patients do not require therapy, and those with infrequent and mild symptoms can often be managed by avoidance of tight collars and rapid neck movements. Therapy for patients with severe symptoms depends on the subtype. **Cardioinhibitory CSH** requires implantation of a permanent pacemaker. **Vasodepressor CSH** is much more difficult to treat. Some patients may respond to mineralocorticoid supplements, and severe cases may require surgical denervation of the carotid sinus. Atropine will acutely abolish the bradycardia response but not prevent vasodilatation. Drugs, including digitalis, beta antagonists, alpha-methyldopa, and clonidine, may enhance CSH and be responsible for symptoms in some patients; these drugs should be avoided if possible.

VI. **Wolff-Parkinson-White syndrome** is the most common form of ventricular preexcitation and is due to an accessory pathway (Kent bundle) connecting the atria and ventricles (*Curr. Probl. Cardiol.* 13(4), 1988). The majority of patients have normal hearts, but WPW has been associated with Ebstein's anomaly, hypertrophic cardiomyopathy, and other congenital abnormalities. An echocardiogram may help to identify associated structural disorders. Approximately 50% of patients with ventricular preexcitation eventually experience tachycardias, which are illustrated schematically in Fig. 7-2. **Orthodromic** atrioventricular reentrant tachycardia is the most common form of SVT, characterized by anterograde conduction through the AV node and retrograde conduction through the AP. Rarely, **antidromic** SVT is observed with anterograde conduction through the AP and retrograde conduction through the AV node. In addition, approximately 15–20% of patients with WPW syndrome experience paroxysmal **atrial fibrillation,** which poses special problems in management. In contrast to AV nodal tissue, APs do not conduct decrementally (prolonged AV conduction with increasing heart rate). Consequently, atrial fibrillation with ventricular rates exceeding 300 beats/minute can occur due to rapid anterograde conduction over the AP. Such patients may suffer hemodynamic collapse with degeneration to VF. **Concealed APs** only conduct in a retrograde fashion. While orthodromic SVT is observed in patients with concealed APs, antidromic SVT and atrial fibrillation with anterograde conduction over the AP cannot occur.

A. **ECG recognition**

1. During **sinus rhythm** patients with manifest APs demonstrate ventricular preexcitation. Ventricular fusion results from anterograde conduction via the normal AV conduction pathway and simultaneous conduction through the

AP (see Fig. 7-2). Each P wave is followed by a QRS complex with a short PR interval (<0.12 seconds). The QRS complex is wide, with a slurred onset known as the delta wave. Secondary ST–T wave changes are present in a direction generally opposite to the major delta and QRS vectors. These patterns may mimic bundle branch block, myocardial infarction, or ventricular hypertrophy (*Am. J. Cardiol.* 59:1093, 1987). Concealed APs are not associated with any ECG abnormalities during sinus rhythm.

2. **Orthodromic and antidromic SVT** (see sec. **II.E.1.b**)
3. **Atrial fibrillation** with anterograde conduction via the AP predominantly appears as a rapid, irregular, wide complex tachycardia simulating VT.

B. **Therapy**
   1. **Asymptomatic patients** do not require empiric therapy. Results of exercise testing provide some basis to assess the risk for development of life-threatening arrhythmias. Sudden loss of preexcitation with increasing heart rate suggests that the accessory pathway has relatively long anterograde refractory properties and that the patient is at low risk of a rapid ventricular rate during atrial fibrillation. Progressive preexcitation with maximal heart rates is observed in patients whose accessory pathways have relatively short refractory properties but does not accurately identify patients in whom atrial fibrillation with a malignant ventricular rate will occur. The decision to initiate therapy in asymptomatic patients with persistent preexcitation should be balanced by recognition that greater risk may attend the treatment than the underlying disorder.
   2. **Orthodromic and antidromic SVT** can be treated **acutely** with drugs that alter AV conduction (adenosine, digoxin, beta antagonists, or verapamil) or with drugs that alter conduction through the AP (procainamide, lidocaine). Since orthodromic and antidromic SVT occasionally convert to atrial fibrillation, a defibrillator should be available for immediate cardioversion. This is particularly important if AV node depressant agents have been administered. **Chronic prophylactic** therapy is best guided by the results of electrophysiologic testing, particularly for patients with a history of hemodynamic intolerance to SVT, syncope, or atrial fibrillation with a rapid ventricular response. If empiric therapy is the only alternative, a class Ia or Ic agent or a beta antagonist is preferred. The addition of an AV node depressant to a class Ia or Ic agent will not necessarily improve efficacy.
   3. Patients with **atrial fibrillation** and a rapid ventricular response are at risk of VF; this represents a medical emergency and should be treated by immediate cardioversion. Atrial fibrillation with a moderate ventricular response can be treated acutely with intravenous procainamide, which slows conduction through the accessory pathway. Other class Ia or Ic agents may be effective for chronic therapy. Digoxin and verapamil may accelerate the ventricular rate and should not be used in patients with WPW syndrome who are at risk of atrial fibrillation. Propranolol generally does not accelerate the ventricular response and can be used with caution.
   4. If a sustained tachyarrhythmia is refractory to drug therapy or if the patient is hemodynamically compromised, cardioversion should be employed. Some episodes of SVT refractory to medical therapy can be managed by underdrive or overdrive pacing.
   5. **Ablation** of accessory pathways by radiofrequency current delivered percutaneously through electrode catheters is now being performed routinely during electrophysiology studies. This technique offers a safe, effective, nonsurgical cure of preexcitation syndromes. Successful interruption of accessory pathways has been accomplished in more than 95% of patients (*N. Engl. J. Med.* 324:1605, 1991). Radiofrequency ablation is indicated in patients who (1) have sustained supraventricular arrhythmias refractory to medical management, (2) are experiencing intolerable side effects to antiarrhythmic agents, and (3) are at risk for sudden death due to atrial fibrillation having a rapid ventricular response. Ablation of the accessory pathway also provides an alternative to life-long medical therapy in young patients.

VII. Programmed electrical stimulation (PES). Electrophysiology studies use percutaneous endocardial catheter electrodes to record intracardiac electrograms and
employ programmed electrical stimuli for the evaluation of complex supraventricular and ventricular arrhythmias. The primary indications for electrophysiology
studies are to (1) identify the mechanism of a tachycardia, (2) select an effective
antiarrhythmic regimen, (3) localize the anatomic substrate of an arrhythmia in
preparation for surgical intervention, (4) evaluate conduction abnormalities, and
(5) effect a cure by ablation of arrhythmogenic lesion. Complications of electrophysiology studies (*Circulation* 73:II–28, 1986) include death (0.06%), cardiac perforation (0.2%), major hemorrhage (0.05%), arterial injury (0.1%), and major venous
thrombosis (0.2%).

Electrophysiology studies are especially accurate in identifying the mechanism of
SVT. PES induces SVT in 90–95% of patients with clinical episodes of AV nodal
reentrant tachycardia or WPW syndrome. Once the mechanism of the tachycardia
has been identified, a curative ablation procedure can be performed. A catheter is
positioned at the site of arrhythmogenic tissue and the tissue is selectively ablated
by applications of radiofrequency current. Because the coagulation necrosis induced
by radiofrequency current is approximately 5 mm in diameter, significant damage
to normal tissue can be avoided.

Electrophysiology studies have been used extensively in the evaluation of ventricular arrhythmias (*Circulation* 72:1, 1985). Programmed ventricular stimulation
reproducibly induces sustained VT or VF in 75% of survivors of sudden cardiac
death and 95% of patients with sustained monomorphic VT. Whether PES identifies
patients with nonsustained VT at risk of sudden death requires further investigation. Patients generally undergo PES during a drug-free period to ascertain that the
arrhythmia can be reliably induced. In patients in whom PES induces VT,
subsequent studies assess the efficacy of antiarrhythmic agents in preventing
induction of ventricular arrhythmias and relate efficacy to plasma levels. In
patients treated with an antiarrhythmic regimen that prevented induction of
sustained VT previously inducible by PES, a recurrence rate of 10% can be expected
in the first 2 years of therapy, compared with a recurrence rate of approximately
50% in patients treated with a regimen that failed to prevent induction of VT (C.
Gottlieb and M. E. Josephson. The Preference of Programmed Stimulation-Guided
Therapy for Sustained Ventricular Arrhythmias. In P. Brugada and J. J. Wellens
(eds.), *Cardiac Arrhythmias: Where To Go From Here?* Mount Kisko: Futura, 1987.
Pp. 421–434). Patients who have survived VT or VF but do not have inducible
arrhythmias are at risk of a recurrence. Empiric antiarrhythmic therapy does not
improve survival and may increase mortality. In such patients an implantable
defibrillator should be strongly considered.

Antiarrhythmic Agents

Selection of the appropriate antiarrhythmic agent may be difficult since no drug is
effective in all patients and each has substantial toxicity. It is preferable to use a
single agent at the lowest effective dose because combinations of antiarrhythmic
agents generally have cumulative toxicities without a predictable increase in
efficacy; however, when a single antiarrhythmic medication fails, the addition of a
second agent may be beneficial. The growing number of antiarrhythmic agents
approved for clinical use have been classified according to their electrophysiologic
effects on isolated myocardial tissue (*J. Clin. Pharmacol.* 24:129, 1984). Class I
drugs are fast sodium channel blockers, class II drugs are beta antagonists, those in
class III prolong repolarization, and class IV is comprised of calcium antagonists.
The class I and class III agents can be effective in suppressing complex ventricular
ectopy. However, they have a significant incidence of proarrhythmia and, as shown
in the Cardiac Arrhythmia Suppression Trial, encainide and flecainide increased
mortality when they were used to treat ventricular ectopy in patients with a prior

myocardial infarction (see Recognition and Management, sec. **II.D.2.b**). Therefore, treating asymptomatic ventricular ectopy with antiarrhythmic agents with the intent of improving prognosis is not recommended. In patients with severely symptomatic ventricular ectopy or sustained VT/VF, the type Ia agents are generally used as the first line of therapy, while other drugs are reserved for arrhythmias resistant to conventional therapy and for patients intolerant of conventional agents. Electrophysiologic testing is recommended to provide a therapeutic end point for most patients with life-threatening ventricular arrhythmias.

I. **Class I agents** (see Table 7-3). These drugs bind to Na^+ channels and impede Na^+ influx during phase 0 of the action potential, which results in depression of conduction velocity. Class I drugs can be further classified by the relative kinetics of dissociation of these effects: Ia, intermediate duration; Ib, relatively brief; and Ic, longest. In addition, quinidine, procainamide, and disopyramide prolong repolarization, while moricizine and the class Ib drugs tend to shorten repolarization.

A. **Class Ia agents: quinidine, procainamide, disopyramide, and moricizine**

1. **Toxicity and precautions.** Several adverse effects are shared by these agents and are additive when they are used in combination.

a. **Proarrhythmic effects** have been reported with each agent. As serum concentrations increase, QRS and QT_c intervals widen, reflecting progressive slowing in conduction velocity and prolongation of cellular repolarization, respectively. Toxic doses may paradoxically enhance Purkinje fiber automaticity, giving rise to bizarre ventricular arrhythmias. QT prolongation and torsades de pointes occur in 1–3% of patients who are treated with quinidine, procainamide, or disopyramide. Type Ia agents should be discontinued if an increase of more than 25% occurs in the QT_c interval ($QT_c = QT$ measured $\div \sqrt{RR}$ interval [sec]) during therapy.

b. **Sinoatrial block, AV block, intraventricular block, or asystole** may occur. Class Ia agents should not be administered to patients with preexisting second- or third-degree AV block without a temporary or permanent pacemaker and should be used with caution in patients with sick sinus syndrome or bundle branch block. They should be discontinued if an increase of 50% or more occurs in the QRS duration (25% in patients with an underlying intraventricular conduction delay).

c. **Myocardial depression** may be observed in patients with severe left ventricular dysfunction, particularly with disopyramide, which should not be administered to patients with heart failure.

d. **Increased ventricular response to atrial fibrillation or flutter** may be observed. These agents slow intra-atrial conduction and have an indirect vagolytic effect on AV node conduction. As a result, the atrial rate may slow, more atrial impulses may penetrate the AV node, and the ventricular response rate may increase. Accordingly, the ventricular rate should be controlled before therapy with class I drugs is initiated.

e. **Hypotension** can occur as a result of decreased peripheral vascular resistance and decreased myocardial contractility. This effect is most pronounced during parenteral administration. Quinidine has alpha-adrenergic blocking properties that accentuate its hypotensive effects and generally preclude its parenteral use. Disopyramide is not available for parenteral administration.

f. **Gastrointestinal reactions** include diarrhea, nausea, and vomiting. They are dose related and occur most commonly with quinidine.

2. **Clinical utility**

a. **Suppression of APDs and VPDs.** Class Ia agents are effective in suppressing symptomatic APDs and complex ventricular ectopy. Suppression of asymptomatic ventricular ectopy to prevent sustained VT or VF is not recommended. Moreover, these agents may facilitate the occurrence of sustained ventricular arrhythmias.

b. **Prevention of sustained VT or VF.** Class Ia agents are effective in preventing recurrences of sustained VT or VF in selected patients who have survived a spontaneous episode of sustained ventricular arrhythmia. Each agent prevents induction of sustained VT or VF during programmed stimulation in approximately 30–35% of patients who were inducible in the drug-free state (see Recognition and Management, sec. **VII**). In addition, intravenous procainamide may be effective in terminating sustained episodes of VT not associated with significant hemodynamic decompensation.

c. **Termination and prevention of atrial fibrillation or flutter.** Class Ia agents have comparable efficacy in converting atrial fibrillation or flutter to sinus rhythm and maintaining sinus rhythm following cardioversion. The rate of success varies and depends on the chronicity of the arrhythmia and atrial size.

d. **Termination and prevention of automatic and reentrant SVT.** Efficacy is most often seen in the treatment of intra-atrial reentry, AV node reentry, and reentry using a manifest or concealed accessory pathway.

3. **Quinidine**

a. **Pharmacokinetics.** Absorption of an oral dose is virtually complete, with peak serum levels achieved in 2 hours. The serum half-life is 5–7 hours, with 50–80% of the drug in the plasma being protein bound. The drug is metabolized primarily in the liver and then excreted in the urine. The serum half-life is not significantly altered in patients with renal dysfunction or congestive heart failure but increases with age and in the presence of hepatic dysfunction. **Serum levels** of 1.3–5.0 µg/ml correlate with clinical efficacy.

b. **Additional toxicities** include cinchonism (salivation, tinnitus, vertigo, headache, visual disturbance, confusion), thrombocytopenia, rash, hepatitis, hemolytic anemia, proteinuria, fever, and angioedema.

c. **Drug interactions.** Serum digoxin levels increase about twofold with therapeutic doses of quinidine. Antacids delay drug absorption. Warfarin (Coumadin) effects may be potentiated by quinidine. Phenobarbital and phenytoin reduce the serum half-life significantly.

d. **Preparation and dosage**

(1) Quinidine sulfate is available in tablets or capsules of 200 and 300 mg. The usual dosage is 200 mg q6h, with a maximum dose of 2.4 g/day. Extended release tablets (300 mg) are given q8–12h.

(2) Quinidine polygalacturonate is available in 275-mg tablets. This form causes less gastric irritation and can be given q8–12h.

(3) Quinidine gluconate is available in sustained-release tablets of 324 mg. The drug can be administered q8–12h.

(4) For **intravenous** use quinidine gluconate is provided in 10-ml vials containing 80 mg/ml. A solution of 10 ml (800 mg) diluted in D_5W to a final volume of 50 ml can be infused at a rate of 16 mg (1 ml) per minute to achieve therapeutic plasma concentrations. A total dose ranging from 300–700 mg may be required. Because of quinidine's propensity to cause **hypotension,** intravenous administration should be avoided when possible. The electrocardiogram and blood pressure must be monitored continuously. Maintenance therapy with intravenous infusion is not recommended.

4. **Procainamide**

a. **Pharmacokinetics.** Absorption of an oral dose is rapid. Initial effects are seen within 20–30 minutes following oral ingestion and immediately after IV administration. The peak serum concentration is reached 1 hour after an oral dose. At therapeutic concentrations, 15% of the drug is protein bound. Procainamide is eliminated by both hepatic metabolism and renal excretion. Normally, 75–95% is eliminated in the urine; 30–60% appears as unchanged drug and the remainder as metabolites. The major metabolic pathway is hepatic acylation to N-acetylprocainamide (NAPA), the metabolite that accounts for the prolongation of repolarization. The serum half-life of procainamide is approximately 3 hours, but in patients with heart failure or severe renal dysfunction, it may be as long as 5 and 59 hours, respectively. NAPA has a serum half-life of 6–8 hours, but it may be as long as 70 hours in patients with severe renal dysfunction. **Serum procainamide levels** of 8–12 µg/ml correlate with clinical efficacy. Combined procainamide and NAPA levels greater than 30 µg/ml are associated with increased toxicity.

b. Additional toxicity and precautions

    (1) A lupus-like syndrome (fever, serositis, arthritis) may be seen in 33% of patients during chronic therapy. This syndrome usually spares the kidneys and abates when the drug is stopped. Positive antinuclear antibodies, frequently in high titer, may develop in 75% of patients during chronic administration but are not an indication to discontinue the drug if no other signs or symptoms of drug-induced lupus erythematosus are present.

    (2) Other reactions include fever, rash, nausea, vomiting, diarrhea, confusion, and agranulocytosis.

    (3) Due to the additive toxicity of the pharmacologically active metabolite NAPA, both NAPA and procainamide serum levels should be monitored routinely during therapy. Toxicity is more common in patients with renal dysfunction.

c. Drug interactions. Warfarin and digoxin preparations do not interact with procainamide.

d. Preparation and dosage

    (1) Oral. Capsules of 250, 375, and 500 mg are available. A total oral daily dosage of 50 mg/kg body weight administered in six to eight divided doses results in therapeutic serum levels. To obtain a therapeutic level initially, a loading dose of 750–1000 mg is frequently necessary. The suggested maintenance dosage is 0.5–1.0 g q4–6h. In general, the sustained-release preparation is preferred, and permits q6h dosing intervals. Tablets are available as 250, 500, and 750 mg. The wax matrix of the tablet is passed in the stool.

    (2) Intravenous. Procainamide is available in 10-ml vials providing 100 mg/ml or as a 2-ml vial providing 500 mg/ml. To avoid hypotension, the drug should be infused continuously at a rate not exceeding 50 mg/minute until the arrhythmia is suppressed or a maximum loading dose of 15 mg/kg has been administered. Vital signs should be checked q5min during the infusion. A maintenance infusion of 2–5 mg/minute can then be used (2 g procainamide diluted in 500 ml D_5W will give a mixture in which 1 ml/min = 4 mg/min).

5. Disopyramide

a. Pharmacokinetics. Oral doses of disopyramide are 50–80% absorbed and reach a peak plasma concentration in 2 hours. Protein binding is concentration dependent and is 55–65% in the therapeutic range. With an oral dose of disopyramide, 50% is excreted unchanged in the urine. The remainder undergoes hepatic degradation, and some metabolites are excreted in the urine. In healthy subjects, the serum half-life ranges from 4–10 hours, with a mean of 7 hours. The half-life increases in patients with acute myocardial infarction and with reductions in creatinine clearance. **Serum levels** of 2–4 µg/ml correlate with clinical efficacy.

b. Additional toxicity and precautions

    (1) Disopyramide should not be used in patients with heart failure or shock.

    (2) Anticholinergic effects include dry mouth, urinary retention, constipation, blurred vision, abdominal pain, exacerbation of glaucoma, and drying of bronchial secretions. It should be used with caution in patients with myasthenia gravis because its anticholinergic properties may precipitate a crisis.

    (3) Toxicity is more common in patients with renal or hepatic dysfunction.

    c. Drug interactions. Phenytoin or other hepatic enzyme inducers may lower plasma levels of disopyramide. Digoxin levels are not affected by disopyramide.

    d. Preparations and dosage. Available formulations include 100- and 150-mg capsules. The usual maintenance dosage is 100–300 mg PO q6–8h. In patients with hepatic dysfunction, heart failure, or moderate renal insufficiency (creatinine clearance >40 ml/min), dosage should not exceed 100 mg q6h. In patients with marked renal impairment, the recommended dosage regimen is a 200-mg loading dose, followed by 100 mg q12h for creatinine clearances of 15–40 ml/min; or 100 mg q24h for creatinine clearances less than 15 ml/min. A sustained-release preparation is available in 100- and 150-mg capsules and permits a q12h dosing interval.

6. Moricizine is classified as a Ia agent because of its inhibition of the rapid rise of the action potential (phase 0). The repolarization effects, however, are more similar to those of the Ib agents. The effects on the ECG are mild increases in the PR and QRS duration. The QT interval is not changed substantially. Although moricizine is structurally similar to the phenothiazines, no central or peripheral autonomic effects occur. The efficacy of moricizine for the treatment of sustained ventricular arrhythmias is low and the incidence of proarrhythmic effect is high. Its utility in the management of atrial arrhythmias requires further study.

    a. Pharmacokinetics. Absorption of an oral dose is complete, but extensive first-pass metabolism results in a bioavailability of 38%. The half-life is 1–6 hours initially but then decreases as the drug induces its own metabolism. Sixty percent of the drug is excreted through the GI tract, with the remaining 40% eliminated as metabolites in the urine. Only 1% is excreted as parent drug in the urine. Patients with hepatic or renal insufficiency should be treated with a low dose and the ECG should be carefully monitored.

    b. Toxicity is mild, with dizziness, postural hypotension, nausea and vomiting, and headache occurring in 10–15% of patients. Symptoms are dose related and worse with q12h dosing. Myocardial depression has been observed in patients with severe ventricular dysfunction. Genitourinary, hematologic, and hepatic toxicity is reversible and infrequent.

    c. Drug interactions are infrequent. Digoxin and warfarin levels are not affected. Theophylline clearance is increased, with a resultant decrease in levels. Cimetidine decreases moricizine metabolism, with a 40% increase in serum levels.

    d. Preparation and dosage. The starting dosage is 200 mg PO q8h, which can be increased every 3 days by 150 mg/day to a maximum of 900 mg/day. Twice-daily dosing may provide effective therapy but may increase side effects. Tablets are available in 200-, 250-, and 300-mg sizes.

B. Class Ib agents. Lidocaine, mexiletine, tocainide, and phenytoin (see Table 7–3) are effective in treating both automatic and reentrant ventricular arrhythmias, but not supraventricular arrhythmias. Lidocaine and phenytoin are also the antiarrhythmic drugs most effective in treating digitalis-induced arrhythmias. At therapeutic concentrations, class Ib agents do not have significant electrophysiologic effects on sinus, atrial, or AV nodal tissue. However, in higher doses they can produce sinus arrest and heart block in patients with underlying abnormalities of impulse generation and propagation. They are myocardial depressants and should be used with caution in patients with severe left ventricular dysfunction.

1. Lidocaine

    a. Pharmacokinetics. The onset of action is immediate following IV administration. The distribution half-life of a single IV dose is 8–17 minutes. After tissue loading has occurred, the half-life is 87–108 minutes. When lidocaine is given intramuscularly, antiarrhythmic blood levels are usually obtained within 5–15 minutes and persist for 60–90 minutes. About 70% of the drug is protein bound, and 90% is metabolized by the liver, with less than 10% excreted unchanged in the urine. The serum half-life is prolonged in patients with hepatic dysfunction, heart failure, and shock, and in patients over 70 years of age. **Therapeutic serum levels** are 2–6 µg/ml (achievable with an infusion rate of 3–5 mg/min), but adverse reactions have been observed at lower levels.

b. **Clinical utility**

(1) Lidocaine is the drug of choice for **emergency treatment of VT** or hemodynamically significant ventricular ectopy, particularly in the setting of acute myocardial infarction (see Chap. 5).

(2) The drug can be used on a **prophylactic basis** if ventricular arrhythmias are anticipated during cardioversion or in the setting of an acute myocardial infarction.

(3) Lidocaine may be effective in slowing the rapid ventricular response in patients with atrial fibrillation or flutter who have anterograde conduction over an accessory pathway.

c. **Toxicity and precautions**

(1) Central nervous system effects include convulsions, confusion, stupor, and, rarely, respiratory arrest. These generally resolve when the drug is stopped, but seizures may require treatment with IV diazepam.

(2) Significant negative inotropic effects are usually seen only with high levels.

(3) Induction of arrhythmias may occur occasionally, including sinus arrest, AV block, and augmentation in AV conduction or atrial rate in patients with atrial flutter or fibrillation.

d. **Drug interactions.** Decreased metabolism occurs with propranolol and cimetidine.

e. **Preparations and dosage.** Lidocaine is supplied as a 1% or 2% solution or in ampules for IV bolus therapy (50 or 100 mg/ampule). It is also available in single-use vials of 1–2 g for preparing IV infusions. **Initial therapy** should consist of an IV bolus of 1 mg/kg; to obtain and maintain therapeutic levels, the initial bolus is followed by 0.5 mg/kg bolus injections every 8–10 minutes, if necessary, to a total of 3 mg/kg. At the time of the initial bolus, **maintenance therapy** should also begin with an IV infusion at a rate of 2–4 mg/minute (30–50 µg/kg/min). This can be done by adding 2 g lidocaine to 250 ml D_5W; at this dilution, 1 ml solution contains 8 mg lidocaine. The initial bolus and maintenance dose should be reduced by 50% in patients with heart failure, shock, and hepatic dysfunction, and in patients over 70 years of age. In such instances plasma levels should be monitored during prolonged infusions. Endotracheal or IM administration should be used only when IV administration is impossible. The recommended dose is 300 mg, although in the early hours of acute myocardial infarction, higher doses may be necessary.

2. **Mexiletine.** Mexiletine is similar to lidocaine in its chemical structure, electrophysiologic properties, clinical spectrum of antiarrhythmic activity, and toxicities.

a. **Pharmacokinetics.** Approximately 90% of mexiletine is absorbed after ingestion, with peak plasma concentrations observed within 2–4 hours; however, absorption may be delayed and less complete in patients with acute myocardial infarction. Approximately 55% of mexiletine in serum is protein bound. It is eliminated primarily by the liver, but 10% is excreted unchanged by the kidneys. The half-life in normal subjects is 8–10 hours, but a variable increase may be observed in patients with acute myocardial infarction, in whom the half-life may exceed 20 hours. Hepatic congestion and liver disease may be expected to delay clearance of mexiletine. The margin between **therapeutic** (0.75–2.0 µg/ml) and **toxic** (>2.0 µg/ml) concentrations is narrow.

b. **Clinical utility.** Mexiletine can be used alone or in combination with a class Ia drug for treatment of ventricular arrhythmias. When it is used in combination with quinidine, a synergistic interaction may allow a lower dose of each agent to be used. It is not effective for the treatment of supraventricular arrhythmias.

  c. **Toxicity and precautions.** Side effects of long-term oral therapy are dose dependent. The frequency and severity of adverse effects are markedly increased with plasma concentrations above 2.0 μg/ml.

  (1) Central nervous system toxicity includes fine tremor, dizziness, and blurred vision. Higher levels of mexiletine may result in dysarthria, diplopia, nystagmus, and an impaired level of consciousness.

  (2) Nausea or vomiting is common. Symptoms may be reduced by administering mexiletine with food.

  (3) A depressant effect on sinus node function may be observed in patients with sick sinus syndrome. Mexiletine should be used with caution in patients who have conduction system disease. It has minimal myocardial depressant effects; however, it should be used cautiously in patients with advanced heart failure. Hypotension may occur with higher doses.

  d. **Drug interactions.** Cumulative toxicity may be observed with concomitant use of mexiletine and lidocaine. Rifampin and phenytoin reduce plasma levels of mexiletine by enhancing hepatic metabolism. Mexiletine can increase theophylline plasma levels.

  e. **Preparations and dosage.** Mexiletine is available as 150-, 200-, and 250-mg capsules. A loading dose of 400 mg can be administered when rapid control of ventricular arrhythmias is essential. The usual maintenance dosage is 200 mg PO q8h. Some patients may require up to 1200 mg/day, but toxicity is dose dependent. Patients may have fewer side effects if mexiletine is taken with food. A minimum of 2–3 days between dosage adjustments is recommended.

3. **Tocainide**

  a. **Pharmacokinetics.** Approximately 95% of tocainide is absorbed, with peak plasma concentrations occurring within 2 hours. Absorption is complete but delayed if tocainide is given with meals. Approximately 40% of an administered dose is eliminated in the urine, and much of the remainder undergoes hepatic metabolism. Renal clearance is reduced by alkalinization of the urine. The half-life ranges from 10–14 hours and appears to be prolonged in patients with acute myocardial infarction. **Therapeutic serum levels** are 4–10 μg/ml. Increased toxicity is observed with levels exceeding 10 μg/ml.

  b. **Clinical utility.** Tocainide can be used alone or in combination with class Ia drugs for treatment of ventricular arrhythmias. It is not recommended for supraventricular arrhythmias.

  c. **Toxicity and precautions**

  (1) Neurologic symptoms such as dizziness, tremor, paresthesias, and confusion are the most commonly reported adverse reactions.

  (2) Nausea or vomiting is relatively common. Symptoms may be reduced by administering tocainide with food.

  (3) A lupus-like illness is a rare complication.

  (4) Tocainide has little effect on sinus node automaticity or intracardiac conduction, but it should be used with caution in patients with sinus node dysfunction. Although hemodynamic effects are minor, tocainide should be used cautiously in patients with advanced heart failure.

  (5) Pulmonary fibrosis, interstitial pneumonitis, and fibrosing alveolitis have been reported in 0.1% of patients.

  (6) Agranulocytosis, leukopenia, hypoplastic anemia, and thrombocytopenia have been reported in 0.18% of patients. Complete blood counts should be monitored during long-term therapy.

  d. **Drug interactions.** The electrophysiologic effects of tocainide are additive with other antiarrhythmic agents, particularly lidocaine.

  e. **Preparations and dosage.** Tocainide is available as 400- and 600-mg tablets. The usual daily dose of tocainide is 1200–1800 mg given orally in divided doses q8–12h. Patients may have fewer side effects if tocainide is taken with food.

4. **Phenytoin (intravenous)**
   a. **Pharmacokinetics.** The onset of action after IV administration is prompt. Phenytoin is hydroxylated in the liver and then excreted in the urine. Approximately 90% of the drug is protein bound. The serum half-life is 22–25 hours in adults, but cardiac tissue levels decline more slowly. **Therapeutic serum levels** are 10–20 μg/ml, and levels exceeding 20 μg/ml are associated with toxicity.
   b. **Clinical utility.** Phenytoin is used primarily in the treatment of digitalis-induced ventricular and supraventricular arrhythmias. Since phenytoin slows atrial conduction and increases AV conduction, the ventricular response to paroxysmal atrial tachycardia with block may transiently increase before conversion to sinus rhythm. It is of little benefit as a primary agent in the treatment of arrhythmias not due to digoxin.
   c. **Acute toxicity**
      (1) Hypotension, sinus bradycardia, and respiratory depression may occur with rapid IV administration. These effects may be mediated by the IV vehicle (alcohol propylene glycol) and can be minimized by slow administration (maximum 50 mg/min).
      (2) Nystagmus, nausea, vertigo, ataxia, and cerebellar dysfunction are signs of toxicity.
      (3) Thrombophlebitis may occur as a result of the acidity of the parenteral drug.
   d. **Intravenous preparations and dosage.** The loading dose is 250 mg diluted in normal saline (crystallization occurs in dextrose-containing solutions) and given slowly over 10 minutes. Subsequent doses of 100 mg can be given q5min as needed to a total of 1000 mg. Digitalis-induced arrhythmias frequently respond to the initial 250-mg dose and rarely require large amounts of the drug. Frequent monitoring of the ECG and blood pressure and examination for signs of nystagmus are required. A continuous infusion should not be used.

C. **Class Ic agents. Encainide, flecainide, and propafenone** (see Table 7-3) profoundly depress the maximum rate of rise of phase 0 of the action potential and markedly slow conduction. Accordingly, these agents have pronounced effects on conduction in the His-Purkinje system and ventricular myocardium. They also slow conduction in the AV node. Automaticity is decreased in the sinus node, Purkinje fibers, and ventricular tissue. Propafenone exerts modest beta antagonism. The ECG characteristically shows a widening of the QRS and lengthening of the QT_c intervals, which is attributable to QRS prolongation.

1. **Toxicity and precautions.** Several adverse effects are shared by these agents; however, the occurrence of these effects with one agent does not reliably predict a response to the other.
   a. Flecainide, encainide, and propafenone have **marked effects on cardiac conduction** and should be used with caution in patients with AV conduction delay. A 20% increase in the PR and QRS intervals is commonly observed and is not cause for concern. Patients who have an increase of more than 50% in the PR and QRS intervals should be closely monitored. The dose should be reduced or the drug discontinued if the PR interval exceeds 0.3 seconds, the QRS duration exceeds 0.2 seconds, or bifascicular block, second-degree AV block, or third-degree AV block occurs.
   b. **Pacing thresholds** of the atria and ventricles may increase by as much as 200%. These agents should be used cautiously in pacemaker-dependent patients, and chronic use may require adjustment in pacemaker parameters.
   c. **Exacerbation of ventricular arrhythmias** has been reported in 5–10% of patients. This risk may be higher in patients with underlying heart disease or malignant ventricular arrhythmias. Flecainide serum levels

above 1.0 μg/ml appear to be associated with a higher risk of sustained ventricular arrhythmias that may be refractory to conventional resuscitative measures.

d. Sinus node dysfunction may be exacerbated by these agents, particularly propafenone. They should be used with caution in patients with sick sinus syndrome.

e. Other common side effects include blurred vision, dizziness, nausea, and headache. Propafenone can cause bronchospasm.

2. Clinical utility

a. Ventricular arrhythmias. Class Ic drugs prevent induction of sustained VT in approximately 30% of patients with a prior history of VT. The risk of serious proarrhythmic effects in patients with sustained VT or VF mandates close observation during initiation of therapy. These drugs are not recommended for suppression of ventricular ectopy.

b. Supraventricular tachycardia. Flecainide, but not encainide nor propafenone, has been approved for treatment of supraventricular tachycardia in patients with normal ventricular function. Results indicate that the efficacy of these drugs for atrial fibrillation and atrial flutter is comparable to that of class Ia agents. Class Ic drugs prolong the refractory properties of accessory pathways and are useful in treating patients with WPW syndrome.

3. Encainide (withdrawn from commercial sale in December 1991)

a. Pharmacokinetics. Absorption of encainide is rapid and complete. It undergoes extensive hepatic metabolism to metabolites that are more active than encainide and contribute to the observed electrophysiologic effects. The elimination half-life of encainide is 1–2 hours in extensive metabolizers and 6–11 hours in slow metabolizers. The half-lives of the active metabolites are much longer (3–12 hours). A subset of patients (8%) lack the ability to extensively metabolize encainide levels. Since encainide and its metabolites are excreted primarily by the kidney, patients with renal failure require dosage adjustment. Patients with liver disease generally need no major dose adjustment.

b. Drug interactions. Cimetidine is an inhibitor of the P450 hepatic enzyme system, which extensively metabolizes encainide. Concurrent use of cimetidine increases plasma levels of encainide and its metabolites by 30–40%. Encainide does not alter digoxin levels and can be safely administered with anticoagulants.

c. Hemodynamic effects. The negative inotropic effects of encainide are less than those of flecainide, but encainide should be used cautiously in patients with congestive heart failure.

d. Preparations and dosage. Encainide is formulated in 25-, 35-, and 50-mg capsules. The initial dosage is 25 mg tid. The dosage can be increased cautiously to 35 mg tid after 3–5 days. If the arrhythmia is not controlled, after an additional 3–5 days the dosage can be increased to 50 mg tid. An occasional patient may require a dosage of 50 mg qid, but doses beyond 200 mg daily are not recommended. In patients with severe renal impairment, the initial dose is 25 mg daily.

4. Flecainide

a. Pharmacokinetics. Absorption is complete and is not affected by food. Peak plasma levels are observed in about 3 hours. The mean plasma elimination half-life in patients is 20 hours (range, 12–27). Approximately two thirds of flecainide undergoes hepatic metabolism to inactive metabolites, and one third is excreted unchanged in the urine.

b. Drug interactions. Modest increases in plasma digoxin levels will occur when flecainide is administered. Plasma levels of both flecainide and propranolol are increased when these agents are used concurrently. Amiodarone increases flecainide levels, requiring a one-third reduction in dosage of flecainide.

c. Hemodynamic effects. Flecainide has significant negative inotropic effects and should be avoided in patients with depressed ventricular function.

d. Preparations and dosage. Flecainide is available in 100-mg scored tablets. It requires 5–7 days to reach a steady-state plasma level. The initial dosage is 100 mg PO bid. The dosage can be increased cautiously by an increment of 50 mg bid every fourth day until clinical efficacy is obtained or a total dose of 400 mg per day (200 mg bid) is reached. Doses exceeding 400 mg per day should be avoided. In patients with heart failure or renal failure, dosage adjustment should be made at intervals greater than 4 days and should be guided by plasma levels. Therapeutic serum levels range from 0.4–0.9 μg/ml. Some patients may require q8h dosage intervals.

5. Propafenone. Propafenone is structurally related to both other Ic agents and to some beta antagonists. At therapeutic levels it has moderate beta-adrenergic antagonism and can cause an increase in airway reactivity in patients with asthma. Heart rate and contractility can be depressed (see sec. **II**). The effects on the ECG are similar to those of other Ic agents (increased PR, QRS, and QT).

a. Pharmacokinetics. Propafenone is well absorbed following oral administration, and is 85–95% protein bound. Metabolism occurs in the liver and, as with encainide, depends on the P450 cytochrome. The dose for patients with hepatic insufficiency is 20–30% of the usual dose. In the 93% of the population who are normal metabolizers, the half-life is 2–10 hours. The 7% of patients who are slow metabolizers have a drug half-life of 12–32 hours. Caution is advised in renal insufficiency because the parent drug and the metabolites are eliminated in the urine. Plasma levels rise nonlinearly with the dose, so disproportionately large increases in serum concentration can result when the dose is increased.

b. Drug interactions. Cimetidine inhibits the P450 system and may inhibit propafenone metabolism. Plasma digoxin and warfarin concentrations and effects are increased by propafenone. Metoprolol and propranolol clearances are reduced, and the doses should be decreased if used with propafenone.

c. Hemodynamic effects. Both the drug and its metabolites have negative inotropic effects. In patients with preexisting ventricular dysfunction, heart failure may develop. Bradycardias can occur due to the beta-antagonist and Ic effects on the sinus node.

d. Preparations and dosage. Propafenone is available in 150- and 300-mg tablets. The starting dosage is 150 mg tid, which can be increased at 3- to 4-day intervals to 225 mg tid, and then 300 mg tid. The starting dose should be low and increased cautiously in patients with hepatic or renal insufficiency. The relationship between serum level and effect is poor. Neurologic side effects are more common with levels over 0.9 mg/ml.

II. Class II agents: Beta antagonists (Table 7-4). The principal effects of these agents result from competitive beta-antagonist actions. Beta-adrenergic stimulation causes a marked increase in automaticity in isolated Purkinje and sinus node tissues and can induce abnormal automatic rhythms due to depolarizations. Beta stimulation enhances AV node conduction and shortens refractoriness. As a result, beta-blockade is **effective in decreasing automaticity and abolishing reentrant arrhythmias involving the AV node.** In ventricular tissue, beta antagonists have little direct effect on action potential characteristics of ventricular muscle but significantly shorten action potential duration and the refractory period of Purkinje fibers, resulting in a more homogeneous recovery throughout the ventricular conduction system. In concentrations that exceed therapeutic use, propranolol has direct membrane depressant properties. Finally, beta antagonists can favorably influence arrhythmias by their effects on myocardial oxygen supply–demand relations. The beta-antagonist effects also account for their cardiac toxicity. The negative inotropic and chronotropic effects of sympathetic blockade may exacerbate sinus bradycardia, inhibit AV node conduction, and cause myocardial depression.

Table 7-4. Dosages of class II, III, and IV antiarrhythmic agents and adenosine

Drug	Half-life		Route of metabolism	Oral dose	IV dose
	Normal	ESRD			
II					
Propranolol	3–6h	1–6h	Hepatic	20–60 mg q6h	1–3mg diluted in normal saline; max dose 0.15 mg/kg
Esmolol	9 min	—	RBC esterase	—	500 μg/kg over 1 min loading infusion; 50–200 μg/kg/min maintenance infusion
III					
Bretylium	4–17h	36h	Renal 80%; hepatic 20%	—	VF: 5–10 mg/kg bolus; VT: 5–10 mg/kg diluted 1:4 over 8 min; then 1–2 mg/min infusion
Amiodarone	18–40d	—	Unknown (not renal)	800–1600 mg qd for 7–14d; then maintenance dose, 200–600 mg qd	5 mg/kg IV over 2–3 min; then 10 mg/kg/d; use central IV line
IV					
Verapamil	4–12h	—	Hepatic 96%; renal 4%	40–80 mg q6h	5–10 mg IV over 2–3 min; can repeat q30min prn
Other					
Adenosine	Seconds	—	Endothelial uptake and metabolism	—	6–12 mg rapid IV bolus through antecubital vein

Key: ESRD = end-stage renal disease.
Note: Dosage reductions are often indicated in the presence of renal or hepatic dysfunction.

A. Toxicity and precautions

1. Because of their **negative inotropic** properties, beta antagonists should not be used in patients with severe heart failure or shock unless the condition is secondary to a tachyarrhythmia. The myocardial depressant effects can be treated with inotropic agents such as dopamine and dobutamine.

2. Blood pressure should be closely monitored during intravenous infusions of either propranolol or esmolol because **hypotension** is commonly induced.

3. **Negative chronotropic effects** slow the heart rate and exacerbate conduction disturbances of the AV node.

4. **Cardiac arrhythmias** or **angina** may be precipitated by the abrupt withdrawal of beta antagonists. Whenever possible, after chronic administration, the drug should be tapered over several days.

5. Beta-antagonist properties may inhibit recovery from and mask the symptoms of acute hypoglycemia.

6. Propranolol should not be used in patients with asthma, chronic obstructive pulmonary disease, or allergic rhinitis. Esmolol is less likely to cause bronchospasm in patients with asthma because it is more cardioselective, but caution is still advised.

7. Other side effects include nausea, vomiting, lightheadedness, depression, rash, fever, paresthesias, impotence, and visual disturbances.

B. Clinical utility

1. **Atrial fibrillation and atrial flutter.** Beta antagonists reduce the ventricular response and may be effective when digitalis has failed. They also enhance the responsiveness to vagal stimulation.

2. Beta antagonists may terminate and prevent **automatic and reentrant SVTs,** particularly SVTs that utilize the AV node as part or all of the reentrant circuit.

3. **Ventricular arrhythmias** are less responsive to beta antagonists than to class I drugs except those that are clearly catecholamine related.

4. **Digitalis-induced arrhythmias,** in the absence of high-degree AV block, may respond to beta antagonists. However, this indication applies only after potassium and phenytoin have been tried.

5. Sinus tachycardia rarely requires specific treatment and frequently is needed to maintain cardiac output. When treatment is indicated, propranolol or esmolol is effective.

C. Propranolol

1. **Pharmacokinetics.** Following oral administration, propranolol is rapidly and completely absorbed. More than 90% of circulating propranolol is bound to plasma protein. Hepatic extraction is high (50–80%), so that little free compound is available to the circulation after a single oral dose. Variations in hepatic metabolism and blood flow may cause marked variations in serum levels for a given dose. The serum half-life of small oral doses of propranolol is 2–3 hours; however, with larger doses and long-term administration, the half-life ranges from 3–6 hours. The serum half-life is not prolonged markedly in patients with diminished renal function. Propranolol may decrease its own elimination rate by decreasing cardiac output and hepatic blood flow. Following IV administration, beta-blockade occurs almost immediately. An IV dose of 1 mg is approximately equal to 10 mg administered orally.

2. **Drug interactions.** Propranolol may accentuate the negative chronotropic effects of digoxin and the negative inotropic effects of other antiarrhythmic agents.

3. **Preparations and dosage**

   a. **Oral.** Propranolol is available in 10-, 20-, 40-, 60-, 80-, and 90-mg tablets. The dosage may vary considerably, but 20–80 mg PO q6h is usually adequate for antiarrhythmic efficacy. Sustained-release preparations of 60, 80, 120, and 160 mg are available.

   b. **Intravenous.** When needed emergently, propranolol should be given in 1-mg aliquots diluted in normal saline; 1–3 mg is generally sufficient. The maximum acute dose is 0.15 mg/kg.

D. Esmolol

1. **Pharmacokinetics.** Esmolol is a beta$_1$ selective adrenergic antagonist that undergoes hydrolysis by a red blood cell esterase to an inactive acid metabolite and methanol. The acid metabolite undergoes renal excretion, and methanol levels during 24-hour infusions remain within endogenous levels. The distribution half-life of esmolol is 2 minutes, and the elimination half-life is about 9 minutes. After termination of infusion, recovery from beta-blockade is observed within 10–20 minutes. The dose of esmolol is not altered by renal or hepatic disease; however, because the metabolite is excreted in the urine, esmolol should be used with caution in patients with impaired renal function.

2. **Drug interactions.** Esmolol does not significantly affect plasma digoxin or warfarin levels.

3. **Preparations and dosage.** Esmolol is supplied in 10-ml ampules containing 2.5 g each. This concentrated solution must be diluted and should not be administered with sodium bicarbonate or other drugs. Two ampules (5 g) should be added to 500 ml glucose, saline, or lactated Ringer's solution. A loading dose of 0.5 mg/kg is given over 1 minute, followed by a 4-minute maintenance infusion of 50 μg/kg/minute. If an adequate response is not observed, the same loading dose is repeated and the maintenance infusion is increased to 100 μg/kg/minute. The dose is titrated by repeating the loading dose and increasing the maintenance infusion by increments of 50 μg/kg/minute every 4 minutes to a maximum of 200 μg/kg/minute. As the desired response is approached, the loading dose can be omitted and the maintenance dose increment reduced. Blood pressure, heart rate, and respiratory function must be closely monitored. For less urgent situations, esmolol infusion can be initiated at 50 μg/kg/minute without a loading dose. Infusion rate can be increased by 50 μg/kg/minute increments at 30- to 40-minute intervals.

III. Class III agents. Amiodarone and bretylium (see Table 7-4) are powerful drugs that markedly prolong action potential duration and repolarization to a greater extent than they depress conduction velocity. As a consequence, refractoriness is prolonged and the ability of the membrane to undergo spontaneous diastolic depolarization is delayed. These drugs appear to suppress arrhythmias mediated by reentry as well as those due to disturbances in automaticity.

A. Amiodarone. Amiodarone is a benzofuran derivative with a chemical structure similar to that of thyroxine (T$_4$). Amiodarone prolongs action potential duration, repolarization, and refractoriness in atrial and ventricular tissue. It slows the sinus node rate and recovery time and prolongs AV node conduction. Amiodarone blocks the peripheral conversion of T$_4$ to triiodothyronine (T$_3$). It is a noncompetitive alpha and beta antagonist and inhibits release of neurotransmitter from presynaptic adrenergic neurons. Systemic vascular resistance and mean arterial blood pressure are reduced without a significant change in left ventricular function; however, hemodynamic deterioration has been reported in patients with severe underlying left ventricular failure.

1. **Pharmacokinetics.** Approximately 50% of an oral dose is absorbed and a peak plasma concentration occurs 3–8 hours after ingestion. Amiodarone undergoes a complex distribution and equilibrium. It is highly lipophilic and is detected in many organs and tissues. A loading period of 10 days or longer is required. The slow uptake and release from reservoir tissues contribute to its long half-life. It has a biphasic elimination pattern suggesting discordant rates of release from different tissue compartments. The main route of elimination is via hepatic excretion into the bile. The kinetics in patients with hepatic insufficiency require further study. Renal elimination of amiodarone and its metabolite desethylamiodarone is negligible. The terminal half-life of amiodarone is in the range of 40–55 days in most patients. There is substantial overlap between therapeutic (1.5–3.0 μg/ml) and toxic serum levels. Measurements of serum concentrations of amiodarone are of only limited value in monitoring a maintenance dose but are helpful in documenting compliance and absorption.

2. **Clinical utility.** Amiodarone is a potent antiarrhythmic agent with significant toxicity (*J. Am. Coll. Cardiol.* 13:442, 1989). It has been approved for use in patients with documented sustained ventricular arrhythmias. It should be reserved for patients with arrhythmias that are refractory to more conventional agents or patients in whom conventional agents produce intolerable side effects.

   a. **Supraventricular arrhythmias.** Amiodarone has been reported to prevent recurrences of atrial fibrillation and atrial flutter and can result in chemical conversion of atrial fibrillation to sinus rhythm. It effectively slows the ventricular response in patients having chronic atrial fibrillation, but the onset of this effect is slow in comparison to conventional agents.

   b. **Sustained VT or VF.** Amiodarone prevents the recurrence of sustained spontaneous VT or VF (not associated with acute myocardial infarction) in up to 60% of patients. A therapeutic latency of 5–15 days exists before beneficial antiarrhythmic effects are observed, and full suppression of arrhythmias may not be obtained for a month or more after initiating therapy.

3. **Toxicity and precautions**

   a. **Corneal microdeposits,** detectable on slit-lamp examination, develop in virtually all patients. Their occurrence is dose dependent and is reversible with discontinuation of the drug. These deposits rarely interfere with vision, although a small number of patients may notice halos around lights at night.

   b. **Photosensitivity** is a common adverse reaction, and in some patients a violaceous facial discoloration develops.

   c. **Hypothyroidism** and **hyperthyroidism** have been reported with an incidence of approximately 3%. Thyroid function should be monitored routinely. Amiodarone blocks peripheral conversion of T_4 to T_3; thus, most euthyroid patients treated with amiodarone demonstrate mild elevations of T_4 and a decrease in T_3 levels. The diagnosis of **hyperthyroidism** may be obscured by elevation of T_4 observed routinely during chronic amiodarone therapy but is confirmed by high free T_3 levels or failure of thyroid-stimulating hormone (TSH) to respond to administration of thyrotropin-releasing hormone. **Hypothyroidism** is diagnosed by the clinical features, low T_3 and T_4 levels, and a markedly increased TSH level.

   d. **Pulmonary fibrosis** has been reported with an incidence of 5–15% (*Circulation* 82:51, 1990). It may occur early or late in the course of therapy at a wide range of doses. Patients characteristically have dry cough and dyspnea associated with pulmonary infiltrates and rales. The process appears to be reversible if detected early. Serial chest x-rays should be obtained every 3–6 months to detect interstitial changes. Changes in pulmonary function tests, especially a decrease in diffusing capacity, and abnormal radioisotope uptake revealed on gallium lung scans are of value in the diagnosis of amiodarone pulmonary toxicity.

   e. **Cardiovascular.** Asymptomatic sinus bradycardia and prolonged AV node conduction are frequently observed; however, in rare instances a permanent pacemaker may be required to treat severe bradycardia or high-grade AV block (more often in patients with preexisting conduction abnormalities). Exacerbation of ventricular arrhythmias has been reported but occurs less commonly than with class I agents. The ECG effects of amiodarone are a lengthened PR interval, QRS duration, and QT interval. Torsades de pointes is a rare complication of amiodarone therapy.

   f. **Miscellaneous.** Nausea, anorexia, and constipation may occur.

   g. **A transient rise in hepatic transaminases** is commonly observed early in the course of therapy but is usually asymptomatic. If the increase exceeds three times normal or doubles in a patient with an elevated baseline, amiodarone should be discontinued or the dose reduced. Tremor, ataxia, and peripheral neuropathy have been reported.

   h. Drug interactions. Amiodarone has been reported to markedly potentiate the effects of **warfarin** and to increase **flecainide** and **digoxin** levels. Maintenance doses of digoxin should be routinely reduced by one half when amiodarone is started.
   4. Preparations and dosage. Amiodarone is available as a 200-mg scored tablet. The initial loading schedules are empiric and vary between 800 and 1600 mg PO qd for 1–2 weeks. The usual maintenance dose is 200–600 mg qd (5–10 mg/kg).

B. Bretylium tosylate. Bretylium has direct electrophysiologic effects as well as important interactions with the autonomic nervous system. Automaticity transiently increases after drug exposure because of the initial release of norepinephrine from adrenergic nerve terminals. Bretylium markedly prolongs action potential duration and refractoriness in Purkinje fibers and ventricular muscle. Efficacy in terminating reentrant arrhythmias is probably related to marked alterations in refractoriness or stabilization of sympathetic tone.

The **toxicity** of this agent is primarily due to its interaction with the autonomic nervous system. Bretylium accumulates in peripheral adrenergic nerve terminals, resulting in an initial release of norepinephrine, producing a sympathomimetic effect. Subsequently, bretylium inhibits the release of norepinephrine by producing adrenergic neuronal blockade and may cause hypotension.

   1. Pharmacokinetics. The onset of action is prompt with IV administration, **although maximum efficacy may require 15–20 minutes.** The serum half-life varies from 4–17 hours. Myocardial binding is avid, and serum levels may not reflect pharmacologic efficacy. After 24 hours, 70–80% of bretylium is excreted unchanged in the urine.
   2. Clinical utility
      a. Refractory ventricular arrhythmias, including VT and VF, constitute the primary indication for the use of this drug. It may be effective in cardiac arrest, even if VF has been present for long periods and is refractory to conventional maneuvers including lidocaine and defibrillation.
      b. Ventricular arrhythmias associated with digitalis intoxication may respond to bretylium, but conventional agents (potassium, phenytoin) should be tried first.
   3. Toxicity and precautions
      a. Supine and orthostatic **hypotension.**
      b. Initial elaboration of catecholamines may exacerbate arrhythmias (including those caused by toxicity to digitalis) and may cause a transient mild increase in blood pressure.
      c. Other side effects include nausea, vomiting, parotid pain and swelling, lightheadedness, rash, emotional lability, and renal dysfunction.
   4. Drug interactions
      a. Bretylium's effectiveness may be reduced when used with other antiarrhythmic drugs.
      b. Bretylium may heighten the response to infused catecholamines.
      c. The hypotensive effects of diuretics or vasodilator drugs may be augmented during bretylium administration.
   5. Preparations and dosage
      a. Ventricular fibrillation. A 5-mg/kg undiluted bolus is given rapidly IV, and defibrillation is attempted again after 1–2 minutes. If VF recurs or persists, a second bolus of 10 mg/kg can be given and repeated at intervals of 15 minutes to a maximum dose of 30 mg/kg.
      b. Ventricular tachycardia. Rapid injections of bretylium may cause hypotension, nausea, and vomiting. For patients with refractory or recurrent VT who do not require immediate cardioversion, 5–10 mg/kg bretylium should be injected over 10 minutes, followed by an infusion of 2 mg/min. A solution containing 500 mg bretylium in 50 ml D_5W provides a concentration of 10 mg/ml.

IV. Class IV agents. Verapamil (see Table 7-4) selectively **blocks the slow inward current** carried primarily by calcium ions. The slow inward current is responsible for normal depolarization of sinus and AV nodal cells but may be pathologically induced in diseased atrial or ventricular muscle and thereby plays an important role in mediating ischemic and digitalis-induced arrhythmias. In tissues dependent on slow-channel activity, verapamil induces a concentration-dependent depression in phase 4 depolarization, resting membrane potential, and a prolongation in refractoriness, resulting in depressed automaticity and slowed conduction. It has no significant effect on the action potential parameters of fast-response fibers normally located in atrial and ventricular muscle and the His-Purkinje system.

Clinically, the **major action** of verapamil is to slow conduction in the AV node. This effect is the principal mechanism by which the ventricular response in atrial fibrillation and flutter is controlled, and SVTs utilizing the AV node as all or part of their reentrant circuit are abolished. Verapamil has little net effect on normal sinus rate, but it may depress sinus node function in patients with sick sinus syndrome.

At therapeutic levels, verapamil has mild **negative inotropic effects** that result from impairment of excitation–contraction coupling. In most patients, including those with organic heart disease, this effect is partially nullified by a reduction in afterload mediated through verapamil's direct dilating action on vascular smooth muscle. The hypotensive effect is generally mild and transient.

A. **Pharmacokinetics.** Following IV administration, the **onset of action is within 1–2 minutes,** with a peak effect occurring in 10–15 minutes. Depression of AV node conduction is detectable up to 6 hours after drug administration. In contrast, hemodynamic effects occur between 3 and 5 minutes after bolus injection but usually are dissipated by 10–20 minutes. More than 90% of an orally administered dose is absorbed, but it undergoes rapid first-pass metabolism by the liver. Ninety percent of the drug is protein bound. Peak plasma concentrations are reached 1–2 hours after an oral dose. The half-life is 4–12 hours in normal patients but is prolonged with hepatic dysfunction.

B. **Clinical utility**
   1. Intravenous formulations are useful for rapid conversion to sinus rhythm of paroxysmal reentrant SVTs that incorporate the AV node as part or all of the reentrant circuit. These include AV nodal SVT and SVTs utilizing either manifest or concealed accessory pathways.
   2. **Temporary control** of rapid ventricular rates in atrial flutter or atrial fibrillation can be rapidly achieved in most patients.
   3. Verapamil is used for chronic prophylactic therapy of SVT, but it is not as effective for chronic prophylaxis as it is for the acute termination of SVT. It is contraindicated for patients with a manifest accessory pathway (WPW syndrome) who are at risk of atrial fibrillation or atrial flutter.

C. **Toxicity and precautions**
   1. Bradycardia, high-degree AV block, and asystole have been reported. **Verapamil should not be administered** to patients with preexisting second- or third-degree AV block or to patients with sinus node dysfunction unless a temporary or permanent pacemaker is operative.
   2. In patients with the **WPW syndrome** and atrial fibrillation, verapamil may augment the ventricular response rate by enhancing anterograde conduction over the accessory pathway.
   3. Transient ventricular ectopy may be seen following verapamil-induced termination of reentrant SVTs. The cause of these arrhythmias is unknown, but they are generally self-limited.
   4. Toxic levels may be reached quickly in patients with hepatic dysfunction who receive multiple doses.
   5. Marked **hypotension** may occur after IV administration. Therapy with IV fluids and pressor agents is generally effective. Verapamil should be used cautiously in patients with mild to moderate heart failure and in the elderly and is **contraindicated** in the presence of severe heart failure or hypotension.

D. **Drug interactions**
   1. Verapamil's **negative inotropic and chronotropic effects are additive** with

those of other antiarrhythmic agents, and combination therapy should be used with caution in patients with heart failure or preexisting conduction system disease.

2. **Serious adverse effects** have been reported with concomitant use of verapamil and IV beta antagonists in patients with impaired ventricular function or impaired AV nodal conduction.

3. Verapamil can be used with digoxin. However, since both drugs impair AV conduction, patients should be monitored for AV block or profound bradycardia.

E. **Preparations and dosage**

1. **Oral.** Verapamil is available in 40-, 80-, and 120-mg tablets. The usual initial dosage is 80 mg q6–8h. The total daily dose ranges from 240–480 mg; however, lower doses are required for patients with liver disease. Sustained-release tablets (160, 240 mg) permit a dosing interval of once daily.

2. **Intravenous.** Verapamil is supplied in 20-ml vials, each containing 5 mg of drug. An initial dose of 5–10 mg (0.075–0.15 mg/kg) should be administered as a slow IV bolus over 2–3 minutes. This dose can be repeated after 15–30 minutes if the initial response is unsatisfactory. If required, a continuous infusion of verapamil can be initiated after the initial 10-mg injection. A rapid loading infusion (in isotonic saline) of 0.375 mg/minute for 30 minutes is followed by a maintenance infusion of 0.125 mg/minute. The heart rhythm and vital signs should be closely monitored.

V. **Adenosine** is an endogenous nucleoside with significant electrophysiologic effects that include inhibition of sinus node automaticity, depression of AV node conduction, and prolongation of AV nodal refractoriness. Adenosine is indicated for the treatment of reentrant SVT that can be terminated by blocking AV node conduction. The efficacies (90–95%) of adenosine and verapamil are comparable for termination of AV nodal reentry and orthodromic SVT (WPW syndrome) (*Ann. Intern. Med.* 113:104, 1990). Adenosine is not effective in converting atrial flutter, atrial fibrillation, or VT to sinus rhythm. Although adenosine is a potent vasodilator, the recommended doses have no systemic hemodynamic effects.

A. **Pharmacokinetics.** Following an IV bolus adenosine is rapidly taken up by erythrocytes and endothelial cells and converted to the electrophysiologically inactive metabolites inosine and adenosine monophosphate. The half-life of adenosine, which is approximately 10 seconds, is not affected by hepatic or renal failure.

B. **Toxicity and precautions**

1. Adenosine is contraindicated in patients with sick sinus syndrome and second- or third-degree AV block.

2. A continuous infusion of adenosine should not be used for control of supraventricular arrhythmias.

3. Facial flushing (18%), dyspnea (12%), and chest pressure (7%) are common but brief effects with therapeutic doses.

C. **Drug interactions**

1. The effects of adenosine are antagonized by **methylxanthines** such as caffeine or theophylline. Accordingly, adenosine may be ineffective or larger doses may be required in patients who have taken methylxanthines.

2. The effects of adenosine are potentiated by **dipyridamole,** which blocks cellular uptake of adenosine and thereby delays its metabolism. Carbamazepine also potentiates the effects of adenosine.

D. **Preparation and dosage.** Adenosine is supplied in vials containing 6 mg/2 ml. The recommended initial dose is 6 mg given IV as a rapid bolus via an antecubital vein (efficacy 62%). If SVT is not terminated within 1–2 minutes, 12 mg should be given (efficacy 91%) and can be repeated if necessary. A lower initial dose (1–3 mg) should be used if the drug is injected through a central venous line.

VI. **Assessment of drug efficacy**

A. **Continuous ECG monitoring** in a coronary care unit (CCU) or telemetry unit is advisable for patients with incessant arrhythmias. Alternatively, Holter monitoring can be used for patients whose conditions are more stable. Because of large variability in arrhythmia frequency, an 80–90% reduction in VPDs and elimination of nonsustained VT are needed to be considered an efficacious response to drug therapy. This approach is useful for individuals with a high frequency of spontaneous ventricular arrhythmias; however, approximately 20–30% of patients with sustained ventricular arrhythmias have a low frequency of ventricular ectopy. In such patients drug efficacy cannot be adequately assessed by continuous monitoring. Conversely, complex ventricular ectopy may persist in subjects who are successfully treated with antiarrhythmic agents. The response to treatment of ventricular ectopy may not predict the response to programmed stimulation. Controlled studies are in progress to compare the predictive value of noninvasive testing to results of programmed electrical stimulation for the assessment of drug efficacy.

B. Exercise testing is useful in assessing arrhythmias that are triggered by exertion or changes in sympathetic tone. As a rule, however, exercise testing is less sensitive than a 24-hour ECG recording for detecting atrial or ventricular arrhythmias.

C. Programmed electrical stimulation (See Recognition and Management, sec. **VII**).

Cardioversion

The most common cardioverter–defibrillator is the capacitor–discharge unit, which delivers an external electrical impulse and can be synchronized to the QRS to avoid discharge during the vulnerable period of the ventricle. The amount of energy delivered to the heart depends on many factors, but cardioversion should be accomplished at the lowest possible energy level to reduce the incidence of complications and the degree of discomfort. The incidence of major complications with cardioversion is small. Successful reversion to sinus rhythm occurs in more than 90% of patients with recent-onset atrial flutter and fibrillation, reentrant SVTs, and VT. Successful cardioversion does not obviate the need to administer antiarrhythmic drugs.

I. Indications. Immediate cardioversion is mandatory if the arrhythmia causes angina, hypotension, or heart failure.

A. Atrial fibrillation is one of the most common indications for cardioversion; generally, a minimum of 100 joules is required. Elective DC cardioversion is the preferred technique for converting atrial fibrillation to sinus rhythm. Patients are unlikely to maintain sinus rhythm if atrial fibrillation is of longstanding duration or the echocardiographically determined left atrial dimension exceeds 4.5 cm. Cardioversion is more likely to be complicated by systemic emboli in patients with atrial fibrillation of more than 3 days' duration.

B. Atrial flutter is one of the easiest rhythms to convert to sinus rhythm. Cardioversion frequently requires less than 50 joules, but atrial flutter is often converted to atrial fibrillation by low energy discharges (5–10 joules).

C. Reentrant SVTs. Cardioversion of reentrant SVTs due to dual AV nodal pathways or accessory pathways generally requires 25–100 joules.

D. Ventricular tachycardia. Synchronized cardioversion may be accomplished with as little as 20–50 joules. However, the patient without blood pressure or pulse should be given 200 joules; if there is no immediate response, 360 joules should be delivered. Brief paroxysmal episodes of VT should not be treated with cardioversion.

E. Ventricular fibrillation (see Chap. 8)

II. Contraindications. Cardioversion is relatively contraindicated in the following circumstances.

A. Digitalis toxicity. Therapeutic levels of digoxin are not contraindications to cardioversion; however, if there is a question of high serum levels of digoxin, cardioversion should begin at low energy levels utilizing prophylactic lidocaine therapy. The energy delivered should be progressively increased until reversion occurs or evidence of increased ventricular irritability appears. **Elective cardioversion should not be performed in the presence of potentially toxic levels of digoxin.** Cardioversion may be required on an emergent basis to terminate sustained ventricular arrhythmias due to digoxin toxicity. Concomitant medical therapy (see Antiarrhythmic Agents) is required to prevent recurrent arrhythmias.

B. **Repetitive, short-lived tachycardias**
C. **Multifocal atrial tachycardia** or other automatic arrhythmias.
D. Hemodynamically stable atrial fibrillation associated with rheumatic heart disease in the immediate preoperative or postoperative period. If hemodynamic compromise is present, cardioversion may be of short-term benefit. Elective cardioversion should not be done immediately preoperatively or postoperatively, since recurrence is common.
E. Patients with supraventricular arrhythmias and **hyperthyroidism** should be euthyroid before elective cardioversion.
F. **Recurrent supraventricular arrhythmias** previously converted to sinus rhythm should not be treated by repeated cardioversion. However, if the patient has not had adequate maintenance antiarrhythmic therapy, a second cardioversion can be considered. Frequently, rapid atrial pacing is a better approach for recurrent reentrant SVT or atrial flutter, since it allows for multiple conversions over a short period while different antiarrhythmic regimens are evaluated. Rapid atrial pacing is not effective in atrial fibrillation or automatic SVTs.
G. Supraventricular tachyarrhythmias with **complete AV block**
H. Cardioversion should be done cautiously in (1) elderly patients with coronary artery disease and disease of the conduction system, (2) patients with atrial fibrillation and a slow ventricular response in the absence of digitalis or verapamil, and (3) those with evidence of sick sinus syndrome. In such patients either a transcutaneous pacemaker should be available or a temporary pacemaker should be placed before cardioversion.

III. **Technique of cardioversion**
A. The procedure is explained to the patient to decrease anxiety and written informed consent is obtained.
B. In patients treated with digoxin, serum levels are recommended before cardioversion to exclude potential toxicity.
C. The patient should take nothing by mouth for 6–8 hours before elective cardioversion.
D. **Anticoagulants** should be administered for up to 3 weeks before the procedure (see Recognition and Management, sec. **II.F.3**).
E. In patients with atrial fibrillation or flutter, quinidine or procainamide should be started 24–48 hours before the procedure.
F. A reliable IV line should be established.
G. The ECG should be continuously monitored.
H. Oxygen and the equipment needed for intubation and manual ventilation should be available.
I. The paddles should be generously coated with electrode paste or defibrillation pads applied and positioned with the anterior paddle to the right of the sternum at the level of the third or fourth intercostal space, and the second paddle just outside the cardiac apex or posteriorly at the left infrascapular region. Paddles should be at least 6 cm from permanent pacemaker generators.
J. **Amnesia** should be induced with midazolam (1 mg/ml, 1–2 mg IV q2min to a maximum of 5 mg) or methohexital (25–75 mg IV) until the patient is drowsy. The blood pressure and respirations should be carefully monitored. If possible, an anesthetist should be present for optimal airway management.
K. **The synchronization artifact should be checked on the defibrillator monitor.** Firm pressure (20 lb) should be applied to the paddles. Direct contact with the patient or the bed should be avoided. After a stable baseline is obtained, the unit is discharged. As a result of synchronization, the discharge may be delayed a short time; do not remove the anterior paddle prematurely. Initial synchronized energy settings for stable patients are **25 joules for atrial flutter, 50 joules for**

SVT and stable VT, and 100 joules for atrial fibrillation. Sequential increases to 100, 200, 300, and 360 joules may be necessary. **A 200-joule unsynchronized discharge should be delivered for unstable atrial fibrillation and VT.** If normal sinus rhythm is achieved only transiently, a higher energy setting is of no value. If ventricular arrhythmias develop before cardioversion, a 50- to 100-mg bolus of lidocaine should be administered if the procedure is to be continued. If brady-cardia is noted, atropine, 0.6–1.0 mg IV, is generally helpful. An initial **unsynchronized discharge of 200–300 joules is recommended for VF.**

IV. **Adverse effects.** Muscle soreness, with a concomitant rise in lactic dehydrogenase (LDH), SGOT, and creatine kinase (CK), and irritation of the skin at the paddle site, are common. Elevation of MB-CK is related to the total amount of energy delivered to the patient and generally does not occur until a cumulative discharge greater than 425 joules has been given. **Arrhythmias** may occur because of the release of catecholamines, acetylcholine, and potassium, or the interaction of these substances with cardioactive drugs. Sinus pauses, as well as atrial, junctional, or ventricular ectopic beats, may occur transiently after restoration of sinus rhythm, especially in patients with longstanding atrial fibrillation and a slow ventricular response. Reports of serious arrhythmias, such as VT, VF, or cardiac standstill, are unusual. These complications are more likely in patients with digitalis intoxication or when the defibrillator is not synchronized properly. Pulmonary edema and systemic or pulmonary embolism are rare complications.

Cardiac Pacing

Technical advances in pacing technology over the past decade have greatly improved the performance of cardiac pacemakers. Recent designs maintain atrio-ventricular synchrony and adapt the rate of pacing to optimize the physiologic response to exertion. When cardiac pacemakers are used appropriately, they enhance the quality of life in patients with symptomatic bradyarrhythmias. Before the decision is made to implant a pacemaker, however, the indications, appropriate mode of pacing, and arrangements for follow-up study should be carefully consid-ered.

I. **Pacing modalities**

An alphabetical code has been devised to identify the various pacing modalities available for the treatment of bradyarrhythmias, which comprise the major indica-tions for cardiac pacing. The first initial defines the chamber paced (**V**entricle, **A**trial, **D**ouble), the second identifies the sensing chamber, and the third indicates the response to a sensed event (**I**nhibited, **T**riggered, and **D**ouble). The letter D in the response position indicates that atrial sensing will inhibit the atrial stimulus and trigger a ventricular response after an appointed interval, and ventricular sensing will inhibit both ventricular and atrial outputs. The VVI, DVI, and DDD modes are most commonly employed. VVI units pace and sense in the ventricle; a sensed event inhibits the ventricular stimulus. DVI units pace both chambers. Atrial sensing does not occur, but an event sensed in the ventricle inhibits both the atrial and ventricular stimuli. DDD units pace and sense in both chambers and respond in the manner previously described. In addition, rate-adaptive pacemakers sense motion or physiologic changes (temperature, respiratory minute volume, QT interval, ventricular impedance) associated with exercise and adjust the pacing rate to increase cardiac output. These are indicated by the letter **R** (rate adaptive) in the pacemaker code.

The optimal hemodynamic response to cardiac pacing is achieved when atrioven-tricular synchrony and rate responsiveness to exercise are preserved. In normal subjects a reduction in cardiac output on the order of 20% may be observed with loss of atrial synchrony, but this effect may be more pronounced in patients with noncompliant ventricles and high diastolic filling pressures. In most patients, however, an increase in cardiac output with exertion primarily depends on heart rate. Dual-chamber pacemakers with atrial sensing (DDD) provide both atrioven-tricular synchrony and rate responsiveness in patients with normal sinus node function. Dual-chamber pacing also prevents the development of pacemaker syndrome (see sec. **IV.J**), which has been reported in 5–10% of patients with VVI pacemakers. However, dual-chamber pacemakers are not appropriate for patients with chronic atrial fibrillation or atrial flutter. A VVI unit with or without rate adaptation should be considered for the patient whose cardiac output is not significantly changed by loss of atrioventricular synchrony.

II. Bradyarrhythmias

  A. Indications for temporary pacing (the external transcutaneous pacemaker will often provide support until the temporary transvenous pacemaker can be inserted).

  1. Symptomatic second- or third-degree heart block due to transient drug intoxication or electrolyte imbalance.

  2. Complete heart block, Mobitz II, or bifascicular block in the setting of acute myocardial infarction (*Circulation* 58:689, 1978). It is our preference to insert a temporary pacemaker when new right or left bundle branch block occurs in acute myocardial infarction. A temporary pacemaker is indicated for treatment of Mobitz I AV block if the arrhythmia causes hemodynamic compromise or angina.

  3. Symptomatic sinus bradycardia, atrial fibrillation with a slow ventricular response, or other bradycardic manifestations of conduction system disease may necessitate temporary pacing until a permanent pacemaker can be inserted.

  B. Indications for permanent pacing. The decision to implant a permanent pacemaker is predicated on the natural history of cardiac rhythm disorders and the general medical condition of the patient. Several indications for permanent pacing have been established (*Circulation* 70:331A, 1984); however, in many conditions there is a divergence of opinion. Asymptomatic patients with chronic bundle branch block do not require a permanent pacemaker because the progression to complete heart block is only 1% per year. Patients with chronic bundle branch block and symptoms suggesting transient atrioventricular block pose a difficult problem if a bradyarrhythmia has not been documented, because syncope is often due to causes other than complete heart block. Extended periods of monitoring, an exercise test, or an electrophysiologic study may determine the etiology of symptoms. Implantation of a permanent pacemaker is rarely warranted in the absence of a **documented symptomatic** bradyarrhythmia. There is general consensus regarding the following indications:

  1. Congenital complete heart block associated with symptoms, bradycardia, or failure to demonstrate an appropriate increase in rate with exercise.

  2. Symptomatic second- or third-degree AV node block.

  3. Second- or third-degree intra-His or infra-His block.

  4. Bifascicular block that progresses to complete heart block in the setting of acute myocardial infarction, whether or not there is resolution of complete heart block during the evolution of the infarction.

  5. Symptomatic sinus bradycardia.

III. Pacemaker follow-up. The patient should take his or her pulse daily for a full minute and report variations greater than 3–5 beats/min when the pacemaker is operational. The ECG should be repeated if symptoms occur and at selected intervals to determine the discharge rate of the pacemaker and the presence of competitive rhythms. The amplitude of the stimulus artifact may vary with digital ECG recorders. Transtelephonic monitoring can be utilized to supplement other observations. Pacemaker function should be checked via telephone transmission once a month as the projected end of battery life approaches. Particular attention should be given to potential changes in the stimulation threshold when patients are treated with antiarrhythmic agents. Antibiotic prophylaxis should be employed for dental and operative procedures that carry a risk of bacteremia.

IV. Complications

  A. Battery depletion is a common cause of pacemaker failure.

  B. Electrode fracture tends to occur at the point where the lead enters the venous system or at the point at which fixation sutures are applied and may be evident on the chest x-ray.

C. Electrode dislodgment may occur, particularly early after placement, but can be detected by changes in both the pacing and sensing thresholds and by the chest radiograph.

D. Infection may occur in the pacemaker site or pacemaker pocket, frequently necessitating removal of the pacemaker. However, **bacteremia alone is not an indication for pacemaker removal.**

E. Perforation of the myocardium can occur, causing loss of sensing or capture or a change in the ECG of the paced beat from the usual left bundle branch block morphology to a right bundle branch block morphology.

F. Myopotential sensing, which may occur with unipolar pacemakers, inhibits the output of the pacemaker and may cause syncope. Occasionally, unipolar pacemakers stimulate muscle near the pulse generator, causing twitching that is synchronized to pacing.

G. Pacemakers may irritate the ventricular cavities, resulting in mechanically induced ventricular ectopy.

H. Acceleration of the pacemaker rate is seen rarely (except in rate-responsive pacemakers).

I. Pacemaker-mediated tachycardia may occur in the DDD mode. It can be terminated immediately by applying a magnet or programming to a different mode (DVI, VVI). Adjustment of other pacing parameters generally allows the DDD mode to be resumed.

J. Pacemaker syndrome may result from the loss of atrioventricular synchrony during ventricular pacing and is usually associated with retrograde atrial conduction. Symptoms of dizziness and syncope predominate. In the patient with noncompliant ventricles and a high diastolic filling pressure, the loss of atrial synchrony may lead to profound hypotension and pulmonary congestion (*Ann. Intern. Med.* 103:420, 1985).

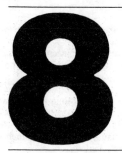

Basic and Advanced Cardiac Life Support

John R. Onufer

Cardiopulmonary resuscitation (CPR) was developed to rescue patients with acute circulatory or respiratory failure, or both. The time from the arrest to initiation of basic life support (BLS) and advanced cardiac life support (ACLS) and the time to the restoration of a rhythm associated with adequate organ perfusion are critical for a successful outcome. The use and potential benefit of this therapeutic modality should be anticipated, especially in the hospitalized patient, and should be discussed with the patient, family, and ancillary staff (*N. Engl. J. Med.* 318:25, 1988). The decision to perform CPR is a dynamic one. The potential benefit of BLS and ACLS must be evaluated before and during the active resuscitative process. The following sequences were developed by the American Heart Association (AHA) to standardize treatment and are useful guides for the treatment of the majority of patients (*J.A.M.A.* 255:2905, 1986). They do not preclude other measures that may be indicated on the basis of specific characteristics of each patient.

Basic Life Support

The ABCs of basic life support, **A**irway, **B**reathing, and **C**irculation, are essential to successful resuscitative efforts. Attempts at restoring circulation will be futile if adequate respiratory function is not achieved. When one encounters an unconscious patient, the following procedures are recommended.

  I. **Determine responsiveness** by gently shaking the patient. **Do not shake the head or neck unless trauma to this area has been excluded.**
 II. **Call for help** if there is no response.
III. **Position the patient** on a firm, flat surface.
 IV. **Open the mouth,** leaving dentures in place as they facilitate a good mouth-to-mouth seal.
  V. **Open the airway.** Unless head or neck trauma is suspected, place the palm of one hand on the patient's forehead and apply firm pressure to tilt the head backward. At the same time, place the index and middle fingers of the other hand under the chin and displace the mandible anteriorly. This will raise the tongue away from the posterior pharynx (head-tilt/chin-lift maneuver) (*J.A.C.E.P.* 5:588, 1976). The mouth can be kept open by retracting the lower lip with the tongue. The upper and lower teeth should be nearly in apposition. If a neck injury is suspected, the neck tilt should be avoided and the modified jaw thrust should be used. This is performed by grasping the angles of the mandible with the fingers of both hands and moving the mandible anteriorly.
 VI. **Assess for the presence of respiration** with the airway open. The rescuer should place his or her ear above the patient's mouth to listen and feel for airflow while observing for movement of the patient's chest. Maintenance of an open airway may be all that is necessary for spontaneous respirations to resume and continue.
VII. **If spontaneous respiration is not present,** gently pinch the nose closed with the index finger and thumb of the hand that is on the forehead. Make a tight seal over the patient's mouth and ventilate twice with slow, full breaths (1–1.5 seconds each).

A 2-second pause should be interspersed between breaths. Rapid and high-pressure breaths will result in gastric distention. Health care professionals should be proficient in the use of the pocket mask to help prevent the transmission of infection during BLS. Proper technique involves holding the mask in place with the thenar aspects of both thumbs while applying upward pressure with the middle and ring fingers of the hands at the angle of the mandible while executing the head-tilt maneuver. Because it is difficult to maintain a leakproof seal, a bag–valve device with a mask should be used only by well-trained and experienced personnel. **Indicators** of adequate ventilation are the rise and fall of the chest and detection of escaping air during exhalation. If several rescuers are present, one should displace the cricoid cartilage toward the cervical vertebrae to prevent regurgitation (the Sellick maneuver) (*Lancet* 2:404, 1961). Improper chin or head position is the most common cause of difficulty with ventilation. If the patient cannot be ventilated, the head should be repositioned and ventilation attempted again. If ventilation is still unsuccessful, obstructed airway maneuvers should be used (see sec. **XI**).

VIII. **Palpate the carotid pulse** for at least 5 seconds. If a carotid pulse is present, rescue breathing should be continued at a rate of 12 slow breaths per minute.

IX. **Deliver chest compressions** in the absence of a carotid pulse. If in bed, a wide board should be placed under the patient. Chest compressions are performed by placing the heel of one hand on the back of the other; the fingers can be extended or interlocked. The hands are then positioned 1 in. above (cephalad to) the xiphoid process, with the shoulders of the rescuer directly above the hands and the elbows in a locked position. With the heel of the hand, the sternum is compressed 1.5–2.0 in., thrusting straight down toward the spine. Fingers should remain off the chest. Compressions should be smooth and regular, with an equal amount of time allowed for compression and release. Pressure must be completely released from the chest after each compression, but the heel of the hand should remain in contact with the chest. The recommended compression rate is 80–100 per minute. The rescuer responsible for airway management should assess the adequacy of compressions by periodically palpating for the carotid pulse. During one-rescuer BLS, 15 chest compressions should be performed before ventilating twice, as described previously. For two-rescuer BLS, the compression-ventilation ratio is 5:1, with a 1–1.5 second pause for ventilation after every 5 compressions. Once the patient is intubated, ventilations can be given at a rate of 12–15 per minute, without pausing for compressions.

X. **Basic life support should be stopped for 5 seconds at the end of the first minute and every 2–3 minutes thereafter to determine whether the patient has resumed spontaneous breathing or circulation.** If a spontaneous pulse has returned, ventilation should be continued as needed. Basic life support should otherwise not be stopped for more than 5 seconds except to intubate or defibrillate. Not more than 30 seconds should be allotted for intubation.

XI. **If an unconscious patient cannot be ventilated** after two attempts at positioning the head and chin, abdominal thrusts should be performed. Careful technique should be used, because improper hand position may damage internal organs. The rescuer should straddle the patient's thighs and place the heel of one hand against the patient's abdomen slightly above the navel and well below the tip of the xiphoid. The second hand should be placed directly on top of the first. The rescuer should then press posteriorly and cephalad with 6–10 quick upward thrusts. This maneuver should be followed by sweeping debris from the mouth with a finger and reattempting ventilation. When removing debris from the mouth, the tongue and lower jaw are grasped as a unit with the thumb and fingers of one hand and lifted anteriorly and caudad. The index finger of the opposite hand is placed down along the inside of the cheek deeply into the throat to the base of the tongue. A hooking action is then used to dislodge a foreign body and move it into the mouth where it can be grasped and removed. Gloves should be used. If attempts are unsuccessful in relieving the obstruction, the aforementioned sequence should be repeated. Cricothyrotomy and transtracheal ventilation should be necessary only rarely (see Chap. 26).

Advanced Cardiac Life Support

I. **General considerations.** Without well-performed BLS, advanced cardiac life support (ACLS) is futile. The exact clinical circumstances in which an arrest occurs may mandate changes in resuscitative management. Proper leadership of resuscitative efforts is essential. Supervision is the responsibility of the team leader, who must ensure that (1) **BLS** is performed adequately, (2) **early defibrillation** is employed expediently when appropriate, (3) **adequate intravenous** access is accomplished and maintained, (4) **intubation** occurs as early as possible without excessive (>30 sec) interruption of BLS, (5) **necessary equipment** is accessible at the arrest site, and (6) **pharmacologic treatment** is initiated in the proper sequence and at the proper dose. The team leader also has the responsibility of deciding when resuscitative efforts should be terminated.

II. **Primary therapies**

A. **Electrical defibrillation** is the most effective therapy for terminating ventricular fibrillation. External CPR is merely a temporizing measure as this results in low perfusion pressures and reduced blood flow to vital organs.

Thus, the monitor/defibrillator should be applied to assess the cardiac rhythm as soon as it is available; if pulseless ventricular tachycardia (VT) or ventricular fibrillation (VF) is present, defibrillation should be performed immediately. Ventricular fibrillation may appear as a "flat line" (asystole) with rhythm recordings from a single placement of the monitor/defibrillator paddles. Therefore, if asystole is initially recorded, the monitoring paddles should be placed at 90 degrees to the first recording sites on the chest. Subsequently, ECG monitoring leads can be placed so that reliance on the paddles for rhythm analysis is reduced. Blind defibrillation (defibrillation in the absence of a rhythm diagnosis) is rarely necessary because of the availability of monitoring capabilities on most modern defibrillators but is recommended when monitoring is unavailable.

Proper technique is essential to the success of defibrillation. One paddle should be placed along the upper right sternal border below the clavicle and the other lateral to the nipple centered in the midaxillary line. Conductive gel or pads should be used, with firm paddle pressure (about 25 lb) applied to reduce transthoracic resistance; excessive gel should be avoided. **Individuals using the paddles must ensure that no one is touching the bed or the patient during defibrillation.** (See Figs. 8-1, 8-2, and 8-5 for defibrillator settings.)

Patients with an automatic implantable cardioverter/defibrillator (AICD) or a pacemaker can be externally defibrillated without damage to the device provided a defibrillation paddle is not placed over the device. Higher energy levels (>200 joules) and anterior-posterior paddle positions may be necessary for defibrillation in patients with an AICD because of the insulating effects of the AICD epicardial patch electrodes.

B. **Airway management and oxygen therapy** are essential parts of any resuscitative effort. One hundred percent oxygen should be administered and endotracheal intubation accomplished by a qualified individual as soon as possible. Endotracheal tube (ETT) position must be immediately assessed after placement. Equal bilateral breath sounds during ventilation should be present to

---

Fig. 8-1. Ventricular fibrillation and pulseless ventricular tachycardia.▶ Some patients may require care not specified herein. This algorithm should not be construed as prohibiting such flexibility. Flow of algorithm presumes that VF is continuing. (VT = ventricular tachycardia; VF = ventricular fibrillation.) (From Part III. Adult advanced cardiac life support. *J.A.M.A.* 255:2933, 1986. Copyright 1986, American Medical Association.)

Ventricular fibrillation and sustained ventricular tachycardia

Witnessed arrest
▼
Check pulse—if no pulse
▼
Precordial thump
▼
Check pulse—if no pulse

Unwitnessed arrest
▼
Check pulse—if no pulse

CPR until a defibrillator is available
▼
Check monitor for rhythm—if VF or VT[a]
▼
Defibrillate, 200 joules[b]
▼
Defibrillate, 200-300 joules[b]
▼
Defibrillate with up to 360 joules[b]
▼
CPR if no pulse
▼
Establish IV access
▼
Epinephrine, 1:10,000, 0.5-1.0 mg IV push[c]
▼
Intubate if possible[d]
▼
Defibrillate with up to 360 joules[b]
▼
Lidocaine, 1 mg/kg IV push
▼
Defibrillate with up to 360 joules[b]
▼
Bretylium, 5 mg/kg IV push[e]
▼
(Consider bicarbonate)[f]
▼
Defibrillate with up to 360 joules[b]
▼
Bretylium, 10 mg/kg IV push[e]
▼
Defibrillate with up to 360 joules[b]
▼
Repeat lidocaine or bretylium
▼
Defibrillate with up to 360 joules[b]

[a] Pulseless VT should be treated identically to VF.

[b] Check pulse and rhythm after each shock. If VF recurs after transiently converting (rather than persists without ever converting), use whatever energy level has previously been successful for defibrillation.

[c] Epinephrine should be repeated every five minutes.

[d] Intubation is preferable. If it can be accomplished simultaneously with other techniques, then the earlier the better. However, defibrillation and epinephrine are more important initially if the patient can be ventilated without intubation.

[e] Some may prefer repeated doses of lidocaine (0.5-mg boluses q8min to a total dose of 3 mg/kg).

[f] Value of sodium bicarbonate is questionable during cardiac arrest, and it is not recommended for routine cardiac arrest sequence. Consideration of its use in a dose of 1 mEq/kg is appropriate at this point. Half of the original dose may be repeated q10min if it is used.

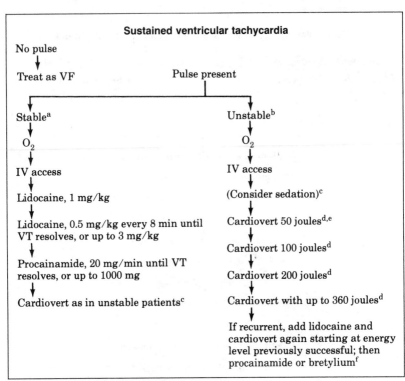

Fig. 8-2. Sustained ventricular tachycardia. Some patients may require care not specified herein. This algorithm should not be construed as prohibiting such flexibility. Flow of algorithm presumes VT is continuing. (VT = ventricular tachycardia; VF = ventricular fibrillation.) (From Part III. Adult advanced cardiac life support. *J.A.M.A.* 255:2933, 1986. Copyright 1986, American Medical Association.)

[a] If a patient becomes unstable at any time, move to "Unstable" arm of algorithm.
[b] Unstable indicates symptoms (e.g., chest pain or dyspnea), hypotension (systolic BP <90 mm Hg), congestive heart failure, ischemia, or infarction.
[c] Sedation should be considered for all patients, including those defined as "unstable," except those who are hemodynamically unstable (e.g., hypotension, in pulmonary edema, or unconscious).
[d] If hypotension, pulmonary edema, or unconsciousness is present, unsynchronized cardioversion should be done to avoid delay associated with synchronization.
[e] In the absence of hypotension, pulmonary edema, or unconsciousness, a precordial thump may be given before cardioversion.
[f] Once VT has resolved, begin IV infusion of antiarrhythmic agent that has aided resolution of VT. If hypotension, pulmonary edema, or unconsciousness is present, use lidocaine if cardioversion alone is unsuccessful, followed by bretylium. In all other patients, recommended order of therapy is lidocaine, procainamide, and then bretylium.

ensure that a mainstem bronchus has not been intubated. Auscultating over the stomach is also necessary to determine accidental esophageal intubation. A disposable colorimetric end-tidal carbon dioxide detector can be easily placed between the ET and ventilatory device to assist in the determination of esophageal intubation (*Anesth. Analg.* 70:191, 1990). Basic life support should not be interrupted for more than 30 seconds for intubation. Ventilation with a well-fitting pocket mask and protection of the airway by suctioning is preferable to making repeated unsuccessful attempts at intubation. Because of difficulty in maintaining a leakproof seal, a bag-valve device with a mask should only be used by experienced personnel. The use of an esophageal obturator airway should never be necessary in hospitalized patients. If airway obstruction is present and cannot be relieved by abdominal thrusts, transtracheal catheter ventilation or cricothyrotomy is indicated.

C. Route of drug administration. An internal jugular or subclavian central venous line should be used for drug administration **if in place before the arrest.** If central access is not available, an antecubital vein should be cannulated so that BLS is not interrupted. The distal wrist, hand, and saphenous veins provide poor access to the central circulation, and the femoral venous route is not adequate unless a long catheter is used that reaches above the diaphragm. When an antecubital vein is used, rapid entry of drugs into the central circulation can be facilitated by using a long IV catheter, elevating the extremity, and flushing with large volumes (50 ml) of solution. If there is a delay in gaining venous access, isotonic agents such as atropine, lidocaine, epinephrine, naloxone, isoproterenol, and bretylium may be diluted in 10 ml saline and injected into the endotracheal tube and distributed into the bronchi by several forceful lung inflations. The dosage for drugs used in this manner should be in the upper range of those recommended for each agent. If circulation is not rapidly restored after initial drug administration via a peripheral IV line, a subclavian or internal jugular IV line should be placed with minimal interruption of BLS. Intracardiac injections are not recommended. Intraosseous access has been used effectively in pediatric resuscitation. This has also been reported to be feasible in adult resuscitation efforts for drug administration (*J. Emerg. Med.* 7:587, 1989). Low flow rates preclude volume resuscitation in the adult with this technique.

D. Assessment of CPR effectiveness. Carotid pulse, femoral pulse, pupillary signs, and arterial blood gases have not correlated with successful resuscitation and may be misleading. Continuous end-tidal carbon dioxide concentration measured during the resuscitative process appears to correlate better with cardiac output, myocardial perfusion pressure, and resuscitation success (*J.A.M.A.* 262:1347, 1989). This measurement, however, is not yet widely available, and its role in prehospital resuscitation is not yet defined.

E. Antiarrhythmic agents (see Chap. 7)

III. Adjunctive therapies

A. Cough. When an arrest or impending arrest is recognized before loss of consciousness, self-induced forceful coughing can generate sufficient blood flow to the brain to maintain consciousness until definitive treatment can be initiated (*Circulation* 74 (Suppl. IV):42, 1986).

B. A solitary precordial "thump" can be accomplished quickly and may convert VT, VF, asystole, marked bradycardia, or complete atrioventricular (AV) block to a more stable rhythm (*Br. Med. J.* 291:627, 1985). A precordial thump should be used only for witnessed arrests in patients without a pulse if a defibrillator is not immediately available. In patients who have a pulse, a defibrillator must be available before a precordial thump is administered as it may induce VF.

C. Epinephrine (0.5–1.0 mg IV or by ETT q5min) is a pharmacologic adjunct used to increase coronary and systemic blood flow during CPR. Its use is predicated on its alpha- rather than beta-adrenergic properties, and it is presently the catecholamine of choice for resuscitative efforts (*Anesthesiology* 71:133, 1989). Ongoing trials are testing strategies employing higher doses of epinephrine.

D. Atropine sulfate (0.5 mg IV or by ETT q5min to a maximum total dose of 2 mg) is the treatment of choice for symptomatic bradycardia (i.e., a heart rate inappropriate for the hemodynamic state). There is anecdotal evidence that atropine 1 mg, administered twice, may be effective for the treatment of asystole (*Ann. Emerg. Med.* 13:815, 1984).

E. Internal cardiac compression and defibrillation should be considered in cardiac arrest patients in the following situations: (1) penetrating chest trauma, (2) anatomic deformity of the chest or severe emphysema that precludes adequate chest compressions, (3) severe hypothermia, (4) ruptured aortic aneurysm or pericardial tamponade unresponsive to pericardiocentesis, (5) during or shortly after procedures requiring open thoracotomy (e.g., coronary artery bypass graft [CABG]), and (6) when VF is refractory to standard techniques. In general, this procedure is successful only if implemented early during the arrest sequence by experienced personnel rather than as a last resort. When electrodes are directly applied to the heart, defibrillation energies starting at 5 joules are recommended with no more than 50 joules used per discharge.

F. Intravenous fluids for volume expansion are not recommended in the patient with routine cardiac arrest unless there is an indication of volume depletion. Excessive volume expansion may diminish blood flow to the cerebral and coronary circulations (*Circulation* 69:181, 1984).

G. Sodium bicarbonate is not recommended for routine use early during the resuscitative effort. In most patients with cardiac arrest, acidosis is uncommon if BLS is performed correctly; if present, it is usually due to inadequate ventilation, and treatment should be directed at increasing minute ventilation (*Am. J. Emerg. Med.* 3:498, 1985). Therefore, bicarbonate administration is rarely required to treat acidosis. Sodium bicarbonate may produce a paradoxical exacerbation of intracellular acidosis that may inhibit cardiac function. Its use during the resuscitation period should be predicated on a clearly defined diagnosis such as hyperkalemia or previously existing metabolic acidosis. If indicated, the initial dosage is 1.0 mEq/kg given IV followed by 0.5 mEq/kg every 10 minutes. **Bicarbonate should not be administered through the same site as calcium or catecholamine preparations,** as it precipitates the former and may inactivate the latter.

H. Calcium has not been shown to improve survival in patients with cardiac arrest (*Ann. Emerg. Med.* 13:820, 1984). Like bicarbonate, its use should be limited to situations in which definite indications exist (e.g., hyperkalemia, hypocalcemia, or calcium antagonist toxicity). Potential detrimental effects (e.g., exacerbation of postresuscitation cerebral or myocardial ischemia) cause further reservation in the routine use of calcium. When indicated, **10% calcium chloride** is the preferred preparation and is given as an IV bolus of 2–4 mg/kg; **caution should be used in patients taking digitalis,** because its toxic effects may be potentiated by calcium.

I. External cardiac pacing. Improved survival for patients with hemodynamically significant bradycardia has been observed with external cardiac pacing (*Ann. Emerg. Med.* 17:1221, 1988). This therapy has no impact on the successful treatment of asystole or electromechanical dissociation. When instituted early, external pacing is associated with increased resuscitation rates. Pacing effectiveness should be monitored with the palpation of femoral, radial, or brachial pulses since electrical capture can be obscured by the pacing artifact. Transthoracic or transvenous pacing can be considered if external pacing is not available. In the postresuscitation period, transvenous pacing is more stable and can be placed more safely than during active resuscitation.

J. Automated external defibrillators (AED) are now being employed in the prehospital setting, allowing a shortened time between collapse and defibrillation and increased range of personnel who can use a defibrillator. The AED is attached only to the pulseless, unconscious patient through two adhesive pads that function as both recording and active electrodes. The device is designed to analyze the rhythm and, if VF or VT above a defined threshold rate is detected, the defibrillator capacitors are automatically charged and a defibrillatory

---

Asystole

If rhythm is unclear and possibly ventricular fibrillation, defibrillate as for VF.
If asystole is present[a]

↓

Continue CPR

↓

Establish IV access

↓

Epinephrine, 1:10,000, 0.5-1.0 mg IV push[b]

↓

Intubate when possible[c]

↓

Atropine, 1.0 mg IV push (repeated in 5 min)

↓

(Consider bicarbonate)[d]

↓

Consider pacing

Fig. 8-3. Asystole. Some patients may require care not specified herein. This algorithm should not be construed to prohibit such flexibility. (VF = ventricular fibrillation.) (From Part III. Adult advanced cardiac life support. *J.A.M.A.* 255:2933, 1986. Copyright 1986, American Medical Association.)

[a] Asystole should be confirmed in two leads.
[b] Epinephrine should be repeated every five minutes.
[c] Intubation is preferable. If it can be accomplished simultaneously with other techniques, then the earlier the better. However, CPR and epinephrine are more important initially if the patient can be ventilated without intubation (endotracheal epinephrine can be used).
[d] Value of sodium bicarbonate is questionable during cardiac arrest and is not recommended for routine cardiac arrest sequence. Consideration of its use in a dose of 1 mEq/kg is appropriate at this point. Half the original dose may be repeated q10min if it is used.

impulse is delivered. Semiautomatic external defibrillators are also in use that require the ACLS provider to initiate the system analysis and approve the delivery of the defibrillatory shock after being "advised" by the device. The accuracy and effectiveness of the AED have been tested and are excellent (*Circulation* 73:701, 1986).

K. Emergency cardiopulmonary bypass may be lifesaving in certain cases of circulatory arrest, such as massive pulmonary embolism or acute coronary occlusion when coronary anatomy is known and an operating room is immediately available.

Specific Arrest Sequences

The following sequences are useful in treating a broad range of patients with arrhythmias but should be modified as the clinical situation warrants (*J.A.M.A.* 255:2905, 1986). Figures 8-1 through 8-6 outline the algorithms recommended by the AHA. The success of treatment depends in large part on adequate BLS. Basic life support should not be stopped for more than 5 seconds except to defibrillate or intubate, when a maximum of 30 seconds is acceptable.

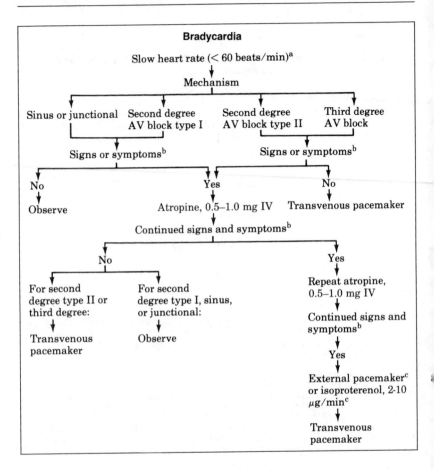

Bradycardia

Slow heart rate (< 60 beats/min)[a]

↓

Mechanism

Sinus or junctional | Second degree AV block type I | Second degree AV block type II | Third degree AV block

Signs or symptoms[b]

Signs or symptoms[b]

No → Observe

Yes → Atropine, 0.5–1.0 mg IV

No → Transvenous pacemaker

Continued signs and symptoms[b]

No:
For second degree type II or third degree: → Transvenous pacemaker
For second degree type I, sinus, or junctional: → Observe

Yes:
Repeat atropine, 0.5–1.0 mg IV
↓
Continued signs and symptoms[b]
↓
Yes
↓
External pacemaker[c] or isoproterenol, 2-10 µg/min[c]
↓
Transvenous pacemaker

Fig. 8-4. Bradycardia. Some patients may require care not specified herein. This algorithm should not be construed to prohibit such flexibility. (AV = atrioventricular.) (From Part III. Adult advanced cardiac life support. *J.A.M.A.* 255:2933, 1986. Copyright 1986, American Medical Association.)

[a] A solitary chest thump or cough may stimulate cardiac electrical activity and result in improved cardiac output and may be used at this point.
[b] Hypotension (systolic BP <90 mm Hg), premature ventricular contractions, altered mental status or symptoms (e.g., chest pain or dyspnea), ischemia, or infarction.
[c] Temporizing therapy.

    I. Ventricular fibrillation is often the result of ischemic heart disease. Definitive treatment with immediate defibrillation should be carried out whenever possible, with the correction of underlying etiologic abnormalities (e.g., hypokalemia, myocardial infarction, hypoxia) undertaken shortly thereafter. A solitary precordial thump can be used if the onset of VF is witnessed and a defibrillator is not immediately available (see Fig. 8-1).

    A. The patient's pulse and rhythm should be assessed after each defibrillation attempt.

    B. Epinephrine should be repeated every 5 minutes until a pulse is established.

    C. Continue to attempt defibrillation with 360 joules after each subsequent dose of antiarrhythmic medication.

Paroxysmal supraventricular tachycardia

Unstable	Stable
↓	↓
Synchronous cardioversion 75-100 joules	Vagal maneuvers
↓	↓
Synchronous cardioversion 200 joules	Verapamil, 5 mg IV[a]
↓	↓
Synchronous cardioversion 360 joules	Verapamil, 10 mg IV (in 15-20 min)
↓	↓
Correct underlying abnormalities	Cardioversion, digoxin, beta-blockers, pacing as indicated (see text)[b]
↓	
Pharmacologic therapy + cardioversion[b]	

[a] Adenosine (6–12 mg IV, to be repeated twice q2min if no response) may be administered instead of verapamil.

[b] If cardioversion occurs but PSVT recurs, repetitive electrical cardioversion is not indicated until further pharmacologic intervention has been undertaken. Sedation should be used as time permits.

Fig. 8-5. Paroxysmal supraventricular tachycardia (PSVT). Some patients may require care not specified herein. This algorithm should not be construed as prohibiting such flexibility. Flow of algorithm presumes PSVT is continuing. (Adapted from Part III. Adult advanced cardiac life support. *J.A.M.A.* 255:2933, 1986.)

   D. If VF is refractory to the treatments outlined in Fig. 8-1, procainamide or internal cardiac defibrillation should be considered.
   E. If VF recurs during the arrest sequence rather than persists, defibrillation should be reinitiated at previously successful energy levels.
II. Ventricular tachycardia in the absence of a pulse is treated as VF (see Fig. 8-1). Intravenous administration of amiodarone can be used for refractory ventricular tachycardia or ventricular fibrillation after the above sequences have been exhausted (*Ann. Intern. Med.* 110:839, 1989).
III. Sustained VT in the presence of pulse is managed according to the condition of the patient (see Fig. 8-2). A solitary precordial thump can be used before cardioversion; however, a defibrillator must be available, since this maneuver may cause the rhythm to degenerate into VF.
   A. Hemodynamically unstable patients (e.g., loss of consciousness, hypotension, or pulmonary edema) require immediate attempts at **unsynchronized** cardioversion with 50 joules. Sedation is generally not indicated in these patients.
   B. Hemodynamically stable patients who are symptomatic (e.g., chest pain, dyspnea, or myocardial infarction) are treated as previously outlined for the unstable patient, except that **synchronized** cardioversion is used and procainamide is given before bretylium. Sedation should be considered.
   C. Stable patients who are asymptomatic should be treated with antiarrhythmic therapy. If unsuccessful, synchronized cardioversion as described for symptomatic patients is indicated. The patient should be sedated. If the patient's condition deteriorates, immediate therapeutic adjustments must be made. Note: **Wide complex tachycardias of uncertain etiology (i.e., VT versus supraventricular tachycardia with aberrancy) should be treated as VT.** Verapamil is contraindicated.
IV. Asystole is usually associated with severe underlying cardiac disease and often occurs in the hospitalized patient (see Fig. 8-3). The likelihood of successful

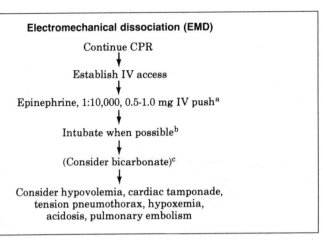

Electromechanical dissociation (EMD)

Continue CPR

↓

Establish IV access

↓

Epinephrine, 1:10,000, 0.5-1.0 mg IV push[a]

↓

Intubate when possible[b]

↓

(Consider bicarbonate)[c]

↓

Consider hypovolemia, cardiac tamponade,
tension pneumothorax, hypoxemia,
acidosis, pulmonary embolism

Fig. 8-6. Electromechanical dissociation. Some patients may require care not specified herein. This algorithm should not be construed to prohibit such flexibility. (From Part III. Adult advanced cardiac life support. *J.A.M.A.* 255:2933, 1986. Copyright 1986, American Medical Association.)

[a] Epinephrine should be repeated every five minutes.
[b] Intubation is preferable. If it can be accomplished simultaneously with other techniques, then the earlier the better. However, epinephrine is more important initially if the patient can be ventilated without intubation.
[c] Value of sodium bicarbonate is questionable during cardiac arrest and is not recommended for routine cardiac arrest sequence. Consideration of its use in a dose of 1 mEq/kg is appropriate at this point. Half of original dose may be repeated q10min if it is used.

resuscitation is poor. Asystole should be confirmed in two leads, as it can be difficult to distinguish fine VF from asystole. If the diagnosis is unclear, the presence of fine VF should be assumed. Metabolic abnormalities, including hyperkalemia or severe preexisting acidosis, may contribute to the genesis of asystole and may respond to bicarbonate therapy.

V. Bradycardic arrest is managed according to the patient's hemodynamic stability and the exact type of arrhythmia. Efforts should focus on those activities that increase the heart rate, or attempts should be made to pace the heart (see Fig. 8-4). The development of effective external pacing devices has made this an option in many situations.

   A. Sinus bradycardia, junctional rhythm, or type I second-degree AV block should be observed in the asymptomatic patient.

   B. Type II second-degree and complete AV block are unstable rhythms and may progress to asystole or ventricular fibrillation. A pacemaker is required even in the absence of symptoms. Atropine, isoproterenol, or external pacing can be used in the symptomatic patient until a transvenous pacemaker can be placed.

VI. Supraventricular tachycardia with a narrow complex QRS may result from a variety of mechanisms. Management depends on accurate characterization of the arrhythmia and the hemodynamic stability of the patient. **Unstable patients** with angina, congestive heart failure, or hypotension require immediate **synchronized cardioversion** starting with 100 joules (see Fig. 8-5). **Stable patients** can initially be treated with vagal maneuvers (i.e., carotid sinus massage) followed by verapamil (5 mg IV over 5 min) or propranolol (1–3 mg IV q5min, not to exceed a total dose of 0.1 mg/kg). Adenosine (6–12 mg rapid IV push to be repeated twice q2min if no response), although not in the AHA algorithm, may also be effective. Intravenous procainamide or cardioversion may be necessary if the above therapies are unsuccessful.

VII. Electromechanical dissociation (EMD) is almost uniformly fatal unless an underlying etiology can be identified and treated (see Fig. 8-6). Potentially reversible underlying etiologies should be considered, including the following:

   A. Hypovolemia, especially due to hemorrhage. Once the diagnosis is established, aggressive volume repletion should be instituted. When trauma is present, military antishock (MAST) trousers should be used if appropriate.

   B. Massive pulmonary embolism. Rarely, the embolus may break up during prolonged resuscitative efforts.

   C. Tension pneumothorax, especially in patients with underlying lung disease or chest trauma or those receiving mechanical ventilation. If tension pneumothorax (e.g., tracheal deviation) is suspected, a large-bore (14 gauge) angiocatheter should be inserted into the pleural space in the second intercostal space in the midclavicular line over the superior aspect of the rib. The needle should be removed and the catheter left open to air. A chest tube should then be placed later by experienced personnel.

   D. Pericardial tamponade, especially in patients with a recent myocardial infarction or uremia with EMD. If tamponade is suspected, blind pericardiocentesis is warranted; definitive therapy with pericardiotomy or catheter drainage should follow shortly thereafter.

   E. Obstruction to cardiac inflow or outflow by an intracardiac thrombus, myxoma, or malfunctioning prosthetic valve requires immediate surgical therapy.

Postresuscitation Management

Management of successfully resuscitated patients depends on their underlying disease process and continued maintenance of electrical and hemodynamic stability. All patients should be transferred to an intensive care unit with cardiac monitoring capabilities. Meticulous evaluation and management of **electrolytes, volume status, and previously initiated therapies** (e.g., antiarrhythmics or pacing) are essential to successful long-term survival. Diagnosis and management of specific disorders are described in their specific chapters. Therapeutic issues unique to the arrest and the immediate postarrest period are as follows:

   I. Dopamine is an excellent vasopressor, with alpha-, beta-, and dopaminergic effects. As hypotension is common following resuscitation from cardiac arrest, dopamine is often useful in the postresuscitative phase (with spontaneous circulation). Several minutes of observation before vasopressor administration is suggested, as hypotension will often abate without therapy.

   II. Isoproterenol is a pure beta-adrenergic agonist that stimulates vascular $beta_2$ and cardiac $beta_1$ receptors. The use of isoproterenol should be limited to temporary control of hemodynamically significant bradycardia that is refractory to atropine; it is not indicated in the treatment of electromechanical dissociation.

   III. Intra-aortic balloon counterpulsation pump (IABP) is of no benefit in the absence of spontaneous circulation and thus should not be used as primary therapy in the cardiac arrest patient. If an IABP is in place at the time of arrest, it should be set to an asynchronous mode.

   IV. Thrombolytic therapy. Sudden cardiac death may be the presenting manifestation of acute coronary ischemia in 20% of out-of-hospital arrests. Although cardiac resuscitation can be traumatic if not properly performed, patients who have received uncomplicated CPR of up to 10 minutes' duration have been treated with tissue plasminogen activator (TPA) without complication (*J.A.C.C.* 12:24A, 1988).

   V. Barbiturates have no role in averting irreversible anoxia of ischemic brain damage due to cardiopulmonary arrests.

   VI. Electrophysiologic evaluation is often warranted in the survivor of sudden death not associated with an acute myocardial infarction (*N. Engl. J. Med.* 318:19, 1988).

   VII. The discontinuation of CPR is the responsibility of the physician. No workable guidelines for terminating resuscitative efforts are available. The outcome of resuscitative efforts is very much influenced by pre–CPR conditions (*Resuscitation*

17:S11, 1989). Although the duration of the resuscitative effort is correlated with successful outcome, this is not absolute. Neither the presence nor absence of any neurologic sign short of regaining consciousness provides a reliable end point for resuscitative efforts. Therefore, the decision to terminate resuscitative efforts should be individualized and based on the lack of cardiovascular responsiveness to acceptable resuscitative techniques (*J.A.M.A.* 244:511, 1980).

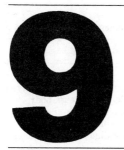

Acute Respiratory Failure

James D. Kaplan

General Considerations

The major function of the respiratory system is to ensure an adequate exchange of oxygen (O_2) and carbon dioxide (CO_2). Normally, this system transfers enough oxygen to saturate circulating hemoglobin and eliminates adequate carbon dioxide to maintain a normal arterial pH. **Respiratory failure** results when either of these two end points of gas exchange cannot be met (Table 9-1). Failure of the lungs' gas-exchanging function usually causes hypoxemia, with either normocapnia or hypocapnia. Failure of the ventilatory apparatus results in hypoventilation, which causes hypercapnia and, to a lesser extent, hypoxemia.

I. **Diagnosis.** The detection of acute respiratory failure (ARF) may require a high index of suspicion. Any symptoms or signs of respiratory impairment should prompt an analysis of **arterial blood gases** (ABGs). A hemoglobin saturation (SaO_2) less than 90%, which usually corresponds to an arterial oxygen tension (PaO_2) less than 60 mm Hg, seriously compromises tissue oxygenation. An acute rise in arterial carbon dioxide tension ($PaCO_2$) to greater than 45–50 mm Hg implies seriously impaired alveolar ventilation. When $PaCO_2$ is elevated for prolonged periods, renal bicarbonate buffer production tends to normalize arterial pH. Therefore, arterial pH is a valuable index of ventilatory function, but absolute $PaCO_2$ values are not independently important. Respiratory failure can be defined as (1) a PaO_2 less than 60 mm Hg on room air or (2) a pH less than 7.35 with a $PaCO_2$ greater than 50 mm Hg.

II. **Pathophysiologic mechanisms.** Respiratory failure includes both oxygenation and ventilation failure. Although the two may occur together, it is useful to separate them to understand their pathophysiology and management.

A. **Oxygenation failure.** A decreased PaO_2 can be caused by (1) mismatch between ventilation and perfusion, (2) right-to-left intrapulmonary shunting of blood, (3) low inspired or mixed venous oxygen tension, (4) diffusion impairment at the alveolar capillary membrane, and (5) alveolar hypoventilation. In ARF, ventilation-perfusion mismatch, right-to-left intrapulmonary shunting, and a low mixed venous oxygen tension are the most common mechanisms of hypoxemia. Diffusion impairment and hypoventilation probably do not contribute significantly in most cases of ARF. The simplified **alveolar gas equation** estimates the alveolar oxygen tension (PaO_2):

$$P_AO_2 = (P_B - PH_2O)(F_IO_2) - \frac{(PaCO_2)}{R}$$

where P_B is the barometric pressure (760 mm Hg at sea level), PH_2O is the partial pressure of water vapor (47 mm Hg), and F_IO_2 is the fractional concentration of oxygen in inspired gas. R, the respiratory exchange ratio of carbon dioxide excretion to total oxygen uptake by the lungs, is 0.8 when metabolizing a normal diet under nonstressed conditions. However, hemodialysis (particularly with an acetate bath), starvation, excessive caloric administration (especially with excess carbohydrates), or sepsis may alter R. Although R can be measured by expired gas collection, the accuracy and clinical utility of this measurement remain controversial. The **alveolar-arterial oxygen tension difference,** $P_{(A-a)}O_2$, is the difference between calculated P_AO_2 and measured

Table 9-1. Components of the respiratory system and common causes of malfunction

Components	Selected causes of malfunction
Lungs	
Airways	Laryngospasm, asthma, chronic obstructive pulmonary disease (COPD), foreign body
Parenchyma	Adult respiratory distress syndrome (ARDS), pneumonia, fibrosis, emphysema
Vasculature	Pulmonary emboli, cardiac and noncardiogenic pulmonary edema
Pump	
Central nervous system	Drug overdose, cerebrovascular accident, hypothyroidism, spinal cord injury
Peripheral nervous system and respiratory muscles	Guillain-Barré syndrome, myasthenia gravis, tetanus, inspiratory muscle fatigue
Thoracic cage and abdomen	Trauma, kyphoscoliosis, thoracic or upper abdominal surgery

PaO_2; it is normally less than 10–15 mm Hg. When alveolar hypoventilation, a low inspired oxygen tension, or a decrease in R is solely responsible for a decreased PaO_2, the $P(A\text{-}a)O_2$ remains normal. In contrast, impaired diffusion, ventilation-perfusion mismatching, or intrapulmonary shunting will increase the $P(A\text{-}a)O_2$.

1. **Ventilation-perfusion ($\dot{V}_A/\dot{Q}$) mismatch** is minimal in the normal lung, such that the average $\dot{V}_A/\dot{Q}$ is near 1. In ARF, airway or parenchymal disease disrupts this balance of ventilation and perfusion, increasing the proportion of lung units with low $\dot{V}_A/\dot{Q}$ ratios.

2. **Intrapulmonary shunt** from right to left exists when blood flows to completely unventilated lung units ($\dot{V}_A/\dot{Q} = 0$). During pulmonary edema (cardiogenic or noncardiogenic), alveolar flooding and collapse create large regions of intrapulmonary shunt. Hypoxemia during these conditions is refractory to increases in FiO_2 and often requires the use of positive airway pressure to reverse atelectasis and achieve adequate oxygenation.

3. **Low mixed venous oxygen tension.** Normally, the lungs fully oxygenate pulmonary arterial blood, and mixed venous oxygen tension does not affect arterial oxygen tension. However, a decreased mixed venous oxygen tension may significantly lower the PaO_2 when either intrapulmonary shunting or $\dot{V}_A/\dot{Q}$ mismatching is present. The causes of a low mixed venous oxygen tension are discussed in sec. II.C.

B. **Ventilation failure** is present when the $PaCO_2$ is elevated and the pH is less than 7.35.

1. Ventilation failure can occur when minute ventilation is inappropriately decreased or when it fails to increase in compensation for an increase in carbon dioxide production or dead space.

   a. **Increased carbon dioxide production not matched by a rise in alveolar ventilation** may arise from a variety of causes, including fever, sepsis, seizures, and excessive carbohydrate loads during parenteral alimentation.

   b. **An increase in dead space**, or in the proportion of dead space ventilated with each breath ($\dot{V}_D/\dot{V}_T$), occurs when (1) areas of the lung are ventilated but not perfused or (2) decreases in regional perfusion exceed decreases in ventilation.

   c. **Decreased total minute ventilation** may result from central nervous system depression, neuromuscular disease, or respiratory muscle fatigue.

2. **Respiratory muscle fatigue** or weakness occurs when the inspiratory muscles, particularly the diaphragm, are unable to generate the pressure necessary to maintain adequate ventilation. Early signs of inspiratory muscle fatigue often

precede a significant decrease in alveolar ventilation and a resulting increase in $PaCO_2$. An initial stage of rapid, shallow breathing, followed by uncoordinated inspiratory muscle activity characterized by respiratory alternans (alternating rib cage and abdominal breathing) and paradoxical abdominal motion (inward movement of the abdominal wall during inspiration), can indicate impending respiratory acidosis and respiratory arrest.

C. **Oxygen delivery to the tissues** depends on (1) an intact respiratory system to provide oxygen for hemoglobin saturation, (2) the concentration of hemoglobin (Hb), (3) the cardiac output and regional microvasculature, and (4) an oxyhemoglobin unloading mechanism. Oxygen delivery is the product of cardiac output and arterial oxygen content (CaO_2). CaO_2 is the sum of hemoglobin-bound and dissolved oxygen:

$$CaO_2 \text{ (ml/dl)} = 1.36 \times Hb \text{ (g/dl)} \times (SaO_2) + 0.003 \times PaO_2 \text{ (mm Hg)}$$

where SaO_2 is the oxyhemoglobin saturation. **Oxygen delivery may be improved by increasing SaO_2, Hb, or cardiac output;** however, correction of a low Hb most efficiently increases CaO_2. The relationship of SaO_2 to PaO_2 is such that little is gained in oxygen content by striving for a PaO_2 higher than 60 mm Hg. However, below a PaO_2 of 60 mm Hg, small changes in PaO_2 result in large changes in SaO_2 and in oxygen content. **Oxygen consumption** is determined by metabolic requirements and cannot be readily manipulated, although it **can be minimized by treating fever and reducing physical activity, including the work of breathing.** One parameter for assessing the balance between oxygen supply and demand is the **mixed venous tension** ($P\bar{v}O_2$) or **saturation** ($S\bar{v}O_2$). These can be measured with a pulmonary artery catheter by direct blood sampling from the proximal pulmonary artery or by continuous reflection spectrophotometry. Normal values of $P\bar{v}O_2$ range from 35–40 mm Hg, and correspond to $S\bar{v}O_2$ values from 0.65–0.75. When $S\bar{v}O_2$ falls below 0.60 acutely, tissue hypoxia and lactic acidosis are likely. Factors that may contribute to a low $S\bar{v}O_2$ in ARF include anemia, hypoxemia, inadequate cardiac output, and increased oxygen consumption. Factors that may elevate measured $S\bar{v}O_2$ despite tissue hypoxia include peripheral arteriovenous shunting, the blood flow maldistribution commonly seen in sepsis, a hyperdynamic circulation, or cellular poisoning such as with cyanide toxicity.

III. **Principles of therapy.** The underlying process that precipitated ARF should dictate specific therapy. However, some supportive measures apply to most situations.

A. **Improving oxygenation.** The goal of oxygen therapy is to relieve critical hypoxemia. Although clinical criteria are important, serial ABGs are crucial in planning and evaluating treatment.

1. **Methods of oxygen administration**

a. **Without intubation,** patients can receive supplemental oxygen in several ways (Table 9–2). Nasal prongs and nonreservoir masks deliver oxygen at a predetermined flow rate; the remaining inspired gas is entrained room air. Patients with high minute ventilations entrain more room air, diluting the oxygen source and lowering the FiO_2. Thus, the initial flow rate setting is empiric and is titrated to achieve a PaO_2 of at least 55–60 mm Hg.

b. **Intubation** provides more reliable oxygen concentrations to patients with marginal gas exchange because the endotracheal tube cuff seal provides a predictable FiO_2. In addition, the increased airway pressure provided by mechanical ventilation (especially with positive end-expiratory pressure) opens terminal airways and decreases shunt.

2. **Hazards.** Oxygen is a treatment that should be administered in a dose that provides maximal benefits with minimal risk.

a. **Adequate humidification** with bubble-jet or aerosol humidifiers is necessary to prevent drying of respiratory secretions.

b. **Atelectasis.** High concentrations of oxygen eliminate the nitrogen normally present in alveoli, causing instability of terminal respiratory units and atelectasis.

Table 9-2. Oxygen delivery systems

Type	FiO_2 capability	Comments
Nasal cannula		
Standard	True FiO_2 uncertain and highly dependent on inspiratory flow rate	Flow rates should be limited to <5 liters/minute
Reservoir type	True FiO_2 uncertain and highly dependent on inspiratory flow rate	Several fold less flow required than with standard cannula
Transtracheal cannula	FiO_2 less dependent on inspiratory flow rate	Usual flow rates of 0.25–3.0 liters/minute
Ventimask	Available at 24, 28, 31, 35, 40, and 50%	Less comfortable, but provides a relatively controlled FiO_2 Poorly humidified gas at maximum FiO_2
High humidity mask	Variable from 28 to nearly 100%	Levels >60% may require additional oxygen bleed-in Flow rates should be 2–3 times minute ventilation Excellent humidification
Reservoir mask		
Nonrebreathing	Not specified, but about 90% if well fitted	Reservoir fills during expiration and provides an additional source of gas during inspiration to decrease entrainment of room air
Partial rebreathing	Not specified, but about 60–80%	
Face tent	Variable; same as high humidity mask	Mixing with room air makes actual O_2 concentration inspired unpredictable
T tube	Variable; same as high humidity mask	For spontaneous breathing through endotracheal or tracheostomy tube Flow rates should be 2–3 times minute ventilation

    c. Oxygen toxicity produces worsening oxygen transfer accompanied by diffuse pulmonary infiltrates (*Chest* 88:900, 1985). Because the concentration of inspired oxygen, the duration of exposure, and the presence of concomitant lung injury can modify the severity of oxygen toxicity, it is difficult to define the exact level of FiO_2 that can be considered toxic. In intubated patients, exposure to greater than 60% oxygen for longer than 48 hours poses a significant risk. In nonintubated patients breathing oxygen by face mask, the risk is less clear. Although many masks have a nominal FiO_2 of greater than 60%, entrainment of some room air is common; therefore, the actual intratracheal FiO_2 is unknown but is often lower than specified.

B. Improving ventilation in patients with hypercapnia that is unresponsive to standard treatment requires assisted mechanical ventilation. **Intermittent pos-**

itive pressure breathing (IPPB), delivered by mouthpiece or face mask, is a temporizing measure that may improve alveolar ventilation and increase functional residual capacity (FRC). A 15- to 20-minute treatment can be given every 1–4 hours using a 10–12 ml/kg tidal volume with a pressure limit of 30–40 cm H_2O. Patients must maintain effective carbon dioxide elimination and perform the work of breathing between each IPPB treatment. IPPB is most useful in chronic neuromuscular diseases and thoracic cage deformities. The tight-fitting face mask for continuous positive airway pressure (CPAP) is poorly tolerated for long periods (>24–48 hours) or at CPAP levels greater than 7–10 cm H_2O.

C. Airway care. A patent, secretion-free airway is crucial to patient care during respiratory failure. Humidifying inspired gases prevents drying of the airway. Methods for mobilizing and clearing secretions include deep breathing and coughing, suctioning, and chest physical therapy (percussion or vibration and postural drainage). Chest physical therapy given more frequently than q4–6h may cause chest soreness and interfere with effective coughing. Suctioning via a fiberoptic bronchoscope is no more effective than conservative measures in most cases. Bronchoscopic suctioning is most useful in removing mucus plugs in large airways and identifying unsuspected obstructive lesions, including foreign bodies.

1. Response to oxygen administration depends on the underlying pathophysiology. Three patterns are common.

a. Hypoxemia caused by mild to moderate $\dot{V}_A/\dot{Q}$ mismatching is usually reversible with supplemental oxygen. This pattern is typical of pneumonia, pulmonary embolism, and asthma.

b. Hypoxemia caused by severe $\dot{V}_A/\dot{Q}$ mismatching and intrapulmonary shunting is more refractory to supplemental oxygen. Potentially toxic concentrations of oxygen are often necessary. This pattern is typical of severe pulmonary edema and adult respiratory distress syndrome (ARDS). Positive end-expiratory pressure (PEEP) may help reverse atelectasis and achieve adequate oxygenation with a nontoxic FiO_2 in this setting (see Mechanical Ventilation, sec. **IV.C.**).

c. Hypoxemia caused by mild to moderate $\dot{V}_A/\dot{Q}$ mismatching associated with ventilation failure is commonly seen in exacerbations of chronic obstructive pulmonary disease (COPD). Supplemental oxygen in nontoxic concentrations will often reverse the hypoxemia; however, a rise in $PaCo_2$ and a worsening respiratory acidosis may result. Nonetheless, adequate oxygenation (as judged by a PaO_2 of at least 55–60 mm Hg) must be achieved. Treatment of underlying processes and administration of oxygen in low concentrations may accomplish this goal without catastrophic rises in $PaCO_2$. **If hypercapnia and respiratory acidosis progress to an unacceptable degree, intubation and mechanical ventilation are indicated.** Discontinuation of oxygen therapy to avoid progressive hypercapnia may result in even more severe hypoxemia and is not an acceptable alternative.

Endotracheal Intubation and Tracheostomy

The most common medical indication for intubation is initiation of mechanical ventilation for ARF. Other reasons include airway protection, prevention of aspiration, airway hygiene, and relief of upper airway obstruction.

I. Endotracheal intubation performed by skilled personnel has minimal complications. Table 9–3 outlines a protocol for intubation. Techniques include (1) blind nasotracheal, (2) direct laryngoscopic, and (3) flexible fiberoptic intubation. When time permits, any of these methods can be used; the flexible fiberoptic approach may be helpful if difficulty is anticipated. For emergency intubation, the direct laryngoscopic approach for **orotracheal** placement is preferred and allows the use of large

Table 9-3. Protocol for intubation and initiation of mechanical ventilation

1.	Prepare endotracheal tube, laryngoscope, and suction apparatus.
2.	Clear the airway. Place an oral or nasopharyngeal airway.
3.	Ventilate with a resuscitation bag and mask attached to high-flow oxygen.
4.	Intubate by nasal or oral route. If not successful after 30 seconds, stop and resume ventilation with bag and mask, then repeat attempt.
5.	Inflate the cuff and ventilate with the resuscitation bag.
6.	Auscultate over chest and stomach for proper tube placement; order a chest x-ray for confirmation.
7.	Secure the airway with tape and suction using sterile technique.
8.	Order initial ventilator settings: FIO_2: 0.9–1.0 Tidal volume: 10–15 ml/kg Mode/rate: IMV or A/C at 8–14 breaths/minute
9.	Ensure proper function of alarms, humidifier, and pressure limit.
10.	Remain at the bedside and watch the patient being ventilated. Adjust rate, tidal volume, and mode to meet respiratory demands.
11.	Check ABGs after 10–20 minutes; make additional ventilator adjustments accordingly.

endotracheal tubes. **Nasotracheal** tube placement is acceptable for short intubation periods and can be performed with the patient in the upright position. The smaller tube size necessitated by the nasal approach may make weaning more difficult. After 5–7 days of nasotracheal intubation, the risk of middle ear and sinus infection is considerable, and changing to an orotracheal tube should be strongly considered.

II. **Endotracheal tubes** are classified by size according to their internal lumen diameter (for example, a No. 8 tube has an 8-mm lumen). Since the resistance to airflow is proportional to the fourth power of tube radius, a No. 8 or larger tube is preferable to reduce airway resistance and work of breathing in ARF. A large tube also permits easier suctioning and allows passage of a bronchoscope when indicated.

III. **Tracheostomy** is indicated when prolonged mechanical ventilation or airway care is necessary. With modern low-pressure cuffs, there is no clear time limit for endotracheal intubation. A tracheostomy should be considered after 2 weeks of intubation but can be performed earlier when a prolonged intubation is anticipated or can be postponed safely for up to 4 weeks if weaning from mechanical ventilation is imminent. The sizing nomenclature of both cuffed and uncuffed tracheostomy tubes is not well standardized, but the internal diameter is usually specified. Various types of cuffed tubes are available, differing primarily in (1) the type of cuff (balloon versus foam), (2) the mechanism for regulating cuff inflation pressure, and (3) the presence or absence of fenestra above the cuff. Foam cuffs do not require cuff pressure monitoring, but they may not seal well with PEEP and may require more frequent tube changes. Cuff pressure should be monitored as described in sec. IV; some balloon-cuffed tubes have a mechanism to prevent overinflation. Fenestrated tubes are designed mainly for the patient who does not need continuous mechanical ventilation; with the cuff down and the fenestra open, there is little obstruction by the tube, and air can be directed through the larynx for talking. Metal, uncuffed tracheostomy tubes can keep a stoma patent in spontaneously breathing patients until it is no longer needed.

IV. **Cuff care** is important with both endotracheal and tracheostomy tubes. High-volume, low-pressure cuffs seal the airway with minimal pressure against the tracheal wall, thereby avoiding tracheal ischemia. Cuff pressure should be monitored q8h with a manometer and maintained below capillary filling pressure (i.e., <25 mm Hg). Periodic cuff deflation, formerly thought necessary to reduce tracheal trauma, is no longer recommended.

V. **Problems and complications**

A. **Improper tube placement.** Intubation of the esophagus or right main-stem bronchus may cause inadequate ventilation, hypoxemia, or barotrauma. Suspected esophageal intubation can be rapidly confirmed noninvasively by a very low end-tidal carbon dioxide tension ($P_{ET}CO_2$) or failure to improve SaO_2. With full extension or flexion of the neck, an endotracheal tube may move up or down 2 cm, respectively; therefore, tube stabilization approximately 2 cm above the carina is important. The tube may also migrate during routine manipulations such as retaping. Therefore, tube position should be checked carefully on all chest x-rays.

B. Endotracheal tube dislodgment or cuff leak should be suspected when there is a sudden decrease in expired volume associated with a fall in airway pressure. A new endotracheal tube should be inserted following the guidelines in Table 9–3. Using a laryngoscope to visualize the damaged tube in the glottic opening may facilitate a rapid change with less risk of losing airway control.

C. Tracheostomy tube dislodgment and cuff leaks are potentially more complicated than endotracheal tube failure. A new tracheostomy site takes at least 72 hours to mature. During this period, blind attempts at tracheostomy tube reinsertion can lead to malposition of the new tube in the pretracheal space, or elsewhere outside the trachea, with catastrophic results. Therefore, tracheostomy tube dislodgement during this early period should be managed in consultation with the responsible surgical service. If the airway cannot be identified readily, a tracheostomy hook may be used to retract the tissues to locate the stoma. A catheter (red rubber or other type) inserted through a damaged tube into the trachea can guide tube replacement. Coughing during this maneuver can be suppressed by instilling 5–10 ml of 2% aqueous lidocaine into the trachea. **However, if a new tracheostomy tube cannot be reinserted safely and confidently, routine orotracheal intubation should be performed** (unless the upper airway is obstructed). After 72 hours, a tracheostomy site has usually matured and the well-formed track from the skin to the trachea makes such measures unnecessary.

D. Cuff overinflation frequently produces late development of tracheal stricture or tracheomalacia. Excessive inflation may also cause the cuff to herniate over the end of the endotracheal tube and obstruct the airway. Careful adherence to inflation guidelines may prevent these complications (see sec. **IV**).

E. Tracheoesophageal fistula, a rare but serious complication, requires immediate attention. Mediastinal malignancies, mediastinal irradiation, and the use of large-bore nasogastric tubes in intubated patients predispose to this complication.

F. Erosion into the innominate artery with hemorrhage is a rare, catastrophic event associated with a low-lying tracheostomy (fifth tracheal ring or below) and poor airway stabilization.

Mechanical Ventilation

Mechanical ventilation can improve both alveolar ventilation and oxygenation and can reduce the work of breathing while other therapies are instituted to treat underlying disease processes.

I. Indications. The decision to begin mechanical ventilation must take into account the reversibility of the process that caused ARF as well as the patient's overall condition. Mechanical ventilation may be required when (1) gas exchange is severely impaired, (2) the onset of ARF is rapid, (3) the response to treatment is inadequate, or (4) respiratory work becomes overwhelming in the face of other organ system failure. Table 9–4 presents some guidelines for common situations, but clinical judgment should ultimately determine whether a patient requires intubation.

II. Intubation and initiation of mechanical ventilation should be carried out as outlined in Table 9–3 and under Endotracheal Intubation and Tracheostomy (*J. Intensive Care Med.* 3:6, 1988).

Table 9-4. Guidelines for elective intubation and mechanical ventilation for acute respiratory failure

Process	Usual indication(s)	Useful parameters	Comment
Acute respiratory failure without underlying respiratory disease			
Neuromuscular illness (e.g., Guillain-Barré syndrome, myasthenia gravis)	Imminent failure of respiratory pump	Inspiratory pressure <25 cm H_2O; vital capacity <15 ml/kg; respiratory rate >30–40/min	Onset of abnormalities in gas exchange is often sudden and follows signs of weakness
Central airway obstruction	Presence of inspiratory stridor		Emergency tracheostomy may be necessary
Lung parenchymal or airway disease (e.g., ARDS, pulmonary edema, pneumonia, asthma)	Progressive refractory hypoxemia Progressive respiratory acidosis Excessive work of breathing	PaO_2 <60 mm Hg, with FiO_2 >0.6 $PaCO_2$ >50 mm Hg; pH <7.3 Respiratory rate >30–40 min	Hypercapnia is often a late manifestation
Stupor or coma (e.g., drug overdose)	Airway protection	Poor gag reflex, ineffective cough	Onset of apnea may be abrupt
Circulatory failure (e.g., myocardial infarction, cardiogenic shock)	Inadequate gas exchange; increased O_2 consumption	As above in lung parenchymal disease	Decreased workload for the severely failing or ischemic heart can be critical
Acute-on-chronic respiratory failure (e.g., acute exacerbations of COPD or chronic neuromuscular disease)	Impaired mental status; refractory hypoxemia; progressive respiratory acidosis	PaO_2 <35–45 mm Hg despite controlled O_2 therapy; pH <7.2–7.25; respiratory rate >30–40 min	Implies hypoxia or CO_2 narcosis; O_2 therapy resulting in progressive respiratory acidosis is an indication for mechanical ventilation

III. Modes of mechanical ventilation
A. Common modes
1. **In the assist/control (A/C)** mode, every inspiratory effort by the patient triggers a ventilator-delivered breath at the selected tidal volume. Controlled ventilator-initiated breaths are automatically delivered when the spontaneous rate falls below a selected backup rate. Because all breaths are delivered by the ventilator, the work of breathing is minimized in this mode, although the diaphragm continues to perform some work (*Am. Rev. Respir. Dis.* 134:902, 1986). Respiratory alkalosis may develop in patients with tachypnea. Complete ventilatory support for patients with no spontaneous respirations may be provided by setting an appropriate rate.
2. During **intermittent mandatory ventilation (IMV)**, the patient can breathe at a spontaneous rate and tidal volume without triggering the ventilator, while the ventilator adds mechanical breaths at a preset rate and tidal volume. Potential advantages of IMV include (1) less respiratory alkalosis, (2) fewer adverse cardiovascular effects of mechanical ventilation due to lower intrathoracic pressures, (3) less requirement for sedation or paralysis, (4) maintenance of respiratory muscle function, and (5) facilitation of weaning. Little scientific support exists for these advantages, however. Potential disadvantages of IMV include (1) a lack of response to increased ventilatory demand, (2) increased work of breathing, (3) potential respiratory muscle fatigue, and (4) inappropriately prolonged weaning. The source of gas for spontaneous breathing during IMV may be provided by two different means. Older ventilators usually supply a continuous flow of gas. Many newer ventilators use a demand valve that opens a reservoir of fresh gas when activated by a spontaneous breath. The latter arrangement may require more respiratory work. Low levels of pressure support ventilation (4–8 cm H_2O pressure) can augment spontaneous inspiratory efforts and reduce the work imposed by these demand valves (see sec. **III.B.1**).

B. Less frequently employed modes
1. **Pressure-controlled ventilation** allows the patient to determine tidal volume, inspiratory time, and flow rate, while the airway pressure is set by the physician. Small amounts of inspiratory pressure support can overcome ventilator circuit and endotracheal tube inspiratory resistance; however, patients should be monitored closely for progressively increasing tidal volumes with resultant air trapping and barotrauma (see secs. **VII.G** and **VII.H**). This mode has been used primarily during weaning (see sec. **VIII.A.2(c)**) alone or combined with IMV and PEEP.
2. **Independent lung ventilation (ILV)** uses two independent ventilators and a double-lumen endotracheal tube. When used during severe unilateral lung disease, ILV can minimize barotrauma to the normal lung, in contrast to conventional ventilation, which would deliver most of the minute ventilation and positive airway pressure to the normal lung. With ILV, rate, tidal volume, FiO_2, and PEEP can be set separately for each lung and the ventilators do not need synchronization. Neuromuscular paralysis and sedation are often required.
3. **Inverse ratio ventilation (IRV)** uses an inspiratory to expiratory (I:E) ratio greater than the standard 1:2 (e.g., 1:1 to 4:1) to stabilize terminal respiratory units and improve gas diffusion. The goal is to decrease peak airway pressure while maintaining adequate alveolar ventilation and improved oxygenation. IRV should be reserved for patients with diffuse lung disease and oxygenation failure despite high levels of PEEP. It is available only with selected ventilators. Tidal volume, respiratory rate, FiO_2, PEEP, and I:E ratio are adjusted based on frequent ABGs. Neuromuscular paralysis and sedation are required. The major untoward effect of this mode is hypotension from decreased cardiac output due to increased intrathoracic pressure; therefore, some patients may require invasive hemodynamic monitoring. No controlled studies have yet documented decreased barotrauma, morbidity, or mortality.
4. **High-frequency ventilation (HFV)** uses rates substantially faster

(60–3000/min) than conventional ventilation with small tidal volumes (2–4 ml/kg). Because of the associated mechanical difficulties in ventilator management and lack of proven efficacy, HFV cannot yet be recommended for the adult intensive care unit patient except for carefully selected individuals with mechanically unstable airway trauma or bronchopleural fistulas with refractory hypoxemia.

IV. Ventilator management

A. FiO_2. Hypoxemia is more dangerous than brief exposure to high FiO_2; therefore, the initial ventilation FiO_2 setting should be 0.9–1.0. Noninvasive pulse oximetry or ABGs can then guide FiO_2 adjustments to maintain PaO_2 greater than 60 mm Hg with an FiO_2 <0.60 (see Cardiopulmonary Monitoring, sec. **III.A**).

B. Rate and tidal volume. The minute ventilation ($\dot{V}E$) provided by the ventilator is the product of its rate and tidal volume. An appropriate initial $\dot{V}E$ of 100 ml/kg may be accomplished at 8–14 breaths/min with a tidal volume of 10–15 ml/kg. Minute ventilation should be regulated to achieve a normal pH, but not necessarily a normal $PaCO_2$. For example, in patients with COPD and chronic hypercapnia, the minute ventilation should allow a $PaCO_2$ near the previous baseline. When possible, the tidal volume should be adjusted to keep peak airway pressures below 40–50 cm H_2O. For a given respiratory system compliance, smaller tidal volumes will cause lower peak airway pressures. When greater alveolar ventilation is the goal, an increase in tidal volume is more efficient than an increase in rate unless peak airway pressure guidelines are exceeded.

C. Positive end-expiratory pressure may improve oxygenation by increasing $\dot{V}A/\dot{Q}$ in terminal respiratory units that collapse at low airway pressures. Adding PEEP will usually allow the FiO_2 to be lowered, thus decreasing the oxygen toxicity risk. It is added in 3- to 5-cm H_2O increments until oxygenation is adequate with an FiO_2 less than 0.6. Although PEEP improves overall lung compliance, competing deleterious effects on oxygen delivery to the tissues may occur from reduced cardiac output. The net effect on oxygen delivery can be difficult to predict. Therefore, cardiac output and $P\bar{v}O_2$ or $S\bar{v}O_2$ monitoring are usually necessary with high levels of PEEP. Increases in peak and mean airway pressures usually accompany increases in PEEP, and thus the incidence of barotrauma can increase. When levels >15 cm H_2O are used, equipment necessary to manage a pneumothorax should be readily available (see sec. **VII.H**).

V. Sedation and neuromuscular paralysis

A. Sedation is often necessary in mechanically ventilated patients to control anxiety, allow rest and sleep, and synchronize breathing with the ventilator. A suitable agent should be chosen from the benzodiazepines, barbiturates, or opioids and the dose titrated to achieve the desired effect with minimal hemodynamic and respiratory depression. One of these agents in combination with IV or IM haloperidol is usually very effective (see Chap. 1).

B. Neuromuscular paralysis is occasionally necessary to control ventilation when sedation alone has been inadequate. Succinylcholine will provide a very brief period of paralysis lasting 6–8 minutes when given in a dose of 1 mg/kg IV. Pancuronium and vecuronium are long-acting agents for prolonged paralysis. An initial dose is 0.08 mg/kg IV, followed by maintenance doses of 0.01–0.04 mg/kg IV as needed. Routine dosing of a sedative capable of inducing unawareness (e.g., diazepam) should be provided before paralysis and while paralysis is present. **Careful monitoring of the paralyzed patient is critical because ventilator disconnection is rapidly fatal.**

VI. Nutrition is important during mechanical ventilation, but its role in improving
patient outcome remains ill-defined. Providing nutrition is prudent in patients who require mechanical ventilation for more than a few days. Enteral alimentation through an enteric feeding tube is preferable when possible, but parenteral alimentation is often necessary (see Chap. 2). If a pulmonary artery catheter is in place, energy expenditure (EE) can be calculated from oxygen consumption derived from the cardiovascular Fick equation:

$$EE \text{ (kcal/day)} = Q \text{ (liters/min)} \times Hb \text{ (g/dl)} \times (SaO_2 - S\bar{v}O_2) \times 95$$

where Q is cardiac output (*Chest* 91:562, 1987). Most nonsurgical patients on mechanical ventilation require less than 2000 kcal/day. Lipids should provide 40–60% of the total nonprotein calories supplied to most ventilated patients if tolerated, since the increased oxygen consumption and carbon dioxide production associated with carbohydrate-predominant diets can compromise ventilatory status.

VII. Problems and complications

A. Airway problems (see Endotracheal Intubation and Tracheostomy, sec. **V**)

B. Respiratory distress may develop suddenly and may be due to a change in the patient's status or to a ventilator malfunction. The first priority is to ensure adequate ventilation and oxygenation while beginning an evaluation.

1. Briefly note ventilator alarms, airway pressures, and tidal volume.

2. Disconnect the patient and manually ventilate with an anesthesia bag using 100% oxygen.

3. If manual ventilation is difficult, check airway patency and suction through the endotracheal tube or tracheostomy.

4. Check vital signs and perform a rapid physical examination with attention to cardiopulmonary aspects. Note other parameters, including ECG and hemodynamics.

5. Treat appropriately any specific problem identified; institute supportive therapy while collecting more information (e.g., ABGs, chest x-ray).

6. Return the patient to the ventilator only after checking its function. Following such an event, escalate the degree of ventilator support (i.e., higher rate if using IMV, higher F_1O_2) until the patient's condition stabilizes and until other information has been obtained and evaluated.

C. High airway pressure. Either an increase in airway resistance or a decrease in respiratory compliance can cause high airway pressure. An abrupt airway pressure increase may be due to (1) endotracheal tube malposition (in a main-stem bronchus), (2) blockage of the tube or major airway with secretions, (3) bronchospasm, (4) pneumothorax, or (5) a new or worsening pulmonary process.

D. Loss of tidal volume. A difference between the tidal volume setting and the delivered tidal volume implies a leak in the ventilator or inspiratory line. A difference between the delivered tidal volume and the expired tidal volume implies an airway leak, which may be caused by a poor seal between the cuff and the airway or malposition of the cuff in the subglottic area.

E. Asynchronous breathing ("fighting the ventilator") occurs when the patient's breathing coordinates poorly with the ventilator. This may indicate unmet respiratory demands. A careful adjustment of mode, rate, tidal volume, and inspiratory flow may alleviate the problem. If these adjustments are not successful, sedation should be attempted. Neuromuscular paralysis should be reserved for those cases in which effective ventilation cannot be achieved with other measures (see sec. **V.B**).

F. Hemodynamic effects of positive pressure ventilation include decreased venous return. This may decrease cardiac output and blood pressure, especially in the setting of intravascular volume depletion. Volume expansion with isotonic saline, plasma expanders (e.g., albumin solutions, dextran, or hetastarch), or blood (if transfusion is indicated) may increase venous return and restore blood pressure. Brief use of vasopressor drugs may be required while volume expansion is undertaken.

G. End-expiratory lung volume, the balance of lung elastic recoil and chest wall elastance, can exceed the predicted functional residual capacity (FRC) when (1) airflow resistance increases and causes dynamic airway collapse during expiration, or when (2) alveolar pressure cannot reach equilibrium with downstream airway pressure in the time available for expiration. This occult pressure at end expiration, called auto-PEEP, is common (1) during severe bronchospasm, (2) when secretions partially obstruct airways, or (3) when ventilator rate or tidal volume is excessive for respiratory system resistance and compliance. Graphic tracings suggest auto-PEEP when airflow persists during end expiration. Auto-PEEP is estimated in the paralyzed patient by monitoring continuous pressure and flow tracings or in the spontaneously breathing patient by brief expiratory port occlusion just before inspiration, placing the ventilator manometer in continuity with airway pressure. Auto-PEEP can be a hidden source of increased work of breathing and can contribute to barotrauma and impaired venous return.

H. **Barotrauma.** Subcutaneous emphysema, pneumomediastinum, and pneumothorax (PTX) are associated with high peak airway pressures and PEEP. **Subcutaneous emphysema** and **pneumomediastinum** seldom threaten the patient's well-being and require no specific therapy. In some cases, their occurrence may indicate the need for a reduction in PEEP or peak airway pressure. **Pneumothorax,** on the other hand, is potentially life threatening and should be considered when airway pressure rises, breath sounds are diminished unilaterally, or blood pressure falls abruptly. The degree of respiratory impairment caused by a PTX in the mechanically ventilated patient depends on the extent of lung collapse and the degree of underlying lung disease. During a tension PTX, air continues to fill the hemithorax through the ruptured pleura, displacing the heart and ipsilateral diaphragm, and compressing the venae cavae as they enter the chest. This may cause profound respiratory and hemodynamic impairment. In most cases, acute tension PTX should be quickly treated by inserting a needle or small catheter into the pleural space at the xiphoid level in the midaxillary line. Anterior placement is much less safe and is usually not necessary. Chest tube insertion should follow. A large nontension PTX also usually requires chest tube evacuation. A small PTX (<15%) may resolve over several days without a chest tube and may not cause significant respiratory impairment.

I. **Positive fluid balance and hyponatremia** often develop in mechanically ventilated patients from several factors including applied PEEP, humidification of inspired gases, and circulating hormone release.

J. **Cardiac arrhythmias,** particularly multifocal atrial tachycardia, are common in respiratory failure and should be treated as outlined in Chap. 7.

K. **Aspiration** commonly occurs despite use of a cuffed endotracheal tube, especially in patients receiving enteral nutrition. Demonstrating glucose in tracheal secretions with glucose oxidase reagent strips or observing blue tracheal secretions after the enteral administration of methylene blue confirms aspiration.

L. **Upper gastrointestinal bleeding** may develop secondary to gastritis or ulceration (*J. Intensive Care Med.* 3:109, 1988). Frequent antacid titration, keeping the gastric pH greater than 5, significantly decreases the incidence of bleeding. Parenteral H_2 antagonists achieve the same goal and avoid increasing gastric volume. Sucralfate has also been used for prophylaxis. The relative efficacy of each of these therapies is not yet established.

M. **Deep venous thrombosis** due to immobilization and venous stasis may be avoided by prophylactic use of subcutaneous heparin, 5000 units SQ q8–12h, or sequential compression stockings.

N. **Nosocomial infections** may be reduced by strict adherence to sterile technique during intratracheal suctioning, avoidance of cross-contamination (especially by careful hand washings), and frequent changes of ventilator tubing and equipment.

O. **Acid-base complications** are common in the critically ill patient (see also Chap. 3).
   1. **Non–anion gap metabolic acidosis** may make weaning difficult, since minute ventilation must increase to normalize pH.
   2. **Metabolic alkalosis** may compromise weaning by blunting ventilatory drive to maintain a normal pH. In patients with chronic ventilatory insufficiency (such as those with emphysema), correction of metabolic alkalosis is inappropriate and may cause an unsustainable minute ventilation requirement (see sec. **IV.B**).
   3. **Respiratory alkalosis** may develop rapidly during mechanical ventilation, particularly in tachypneic patients in the A/C mode. When severe, it can lead

Table 9-5. Guidelines for assessing withdrawal of mechanical ventilation

1. An awake and alert mental state.
2. PaO_2 >60 mm Hg with an FiO_2 <0.5.
3. PEEP <5 cm H_2O.
4. $PaCO_2$ acceptable, with pH in the normal range.
5. Vital capacity >10–15 ml/kg.
6. Minute ventilation <10 liters/min; respiratory rate <25/min.
7. Maximum voluntary ventilation double that of minute ventilation.
8. Peak inspiratory pressure more negative than -25 cm H_2O.
9. Spontaneous ventilation via T tube (with or without CPAP) for 1–4 hours with acceptable blood gases and without marked increases in respiratory rate, heart rate, or change in general status.

to arrhythmias, CNS disturbances (including seizures), and a decrease in cardiac output. Changing the ventilator settings (see sec. **IV**) or the mode of ventilation (sec. **III**) usually corrects this alkalosis. However, some patients (such as those with interstitial disease or bronchospasm) are driven to high respiratory rates by local pulmonary stimuli. In these cases, an attempt to normalize pH by drastically reducing ventilatory support will result in profound fatigue. In such patients, sedation or paralysis is indicated during the acute phase of respiratory compromise.

   P. Oxygen toxicity (see General Considerations, sec. **III.A.2**)
VIII. Weaning and extubation
   A. Weaning is the gradual withdrawal of mechanical ventilatory support (*J. Intensive Care Med.* 3:109, 1988). Successful weaning depends on the condition of the patient and the status of the cardiovascular and respiratory systems. In patients who have had brief periods of mechanical ventilation, the manner in which support is discontinued is often not critical. In patients with marginal respiratory function, chronic underlying lung disease, or incompletely resolved respiratory impairment, the weaning method may be crucial to a favorable outcome. Decreasing mechanical ventilation too early during an illness may induce a state of chronic respiratory muscle fatigue. In addition, concerns that long periods of respiratory muscle disuse may induce atrophy and cause ventilator dependence are generally unwarranted. Recent evidence suggests that respiratory muscles work continuously, even during ventilatory support. Therefore, it is prudent to begin weaning the patient from ventilatory support as soon as the overall condition permits. Table 9–5 presents some guidelines for assessing the withdrawal of mechanical ventilation; however, some patients, especially those with COPD, can be weaned despite failure to meet these criteria. Common problems that prolong the weaning process include (1) incompletely treated pulmonary infection, (2) bronchospasm, (3) excessive airway secretions, (4) depressed cardiac output, (5) respiratory muscle weakness, and (6) small endotracheal tubes.
      1. When oxygenation failure is the major clinical problem, weaning involves the gradual decrease of positive airway pressure (primarily PEEP) and FiO_2 until the patient can sustain a PaO_2 greater than 60 mm Hg on an FiO_2 less than 0.50 and PEEP less than 5 cm H_2O. Until this point, the ventilator mode, rate, and tidal volume should be adjusted in tandem, carefully following ABGs and the patient's respiratory effort. After the PEEP requirement for oxygenation is less than 5 cm H_2O (with an FiO_2 less than 0.50), weaning can usually be rapid. Extubation can be considered after a trial of 30–60 minutes of unassisted ventilation.
      2. When ventilation failure is the primary clinical problem, the focus must be on tidal volume and rate. Several weaning methods are available.
         a. The intermittent mandatory ventilation technique allows a change from mechanical ventilation to spontaneous breathing by gradually decreasing the ventilator rate. However, the weaning process may be prolonged if

Table 9-6. Extubation procedure

1.	Begin early in the day.
2.	Educate the patient about the procedure.
3.	Elevate head and trunk 20–90 degrees.
4.	Check the clinical baseline (vital signs and ABGs).
5.	Have a high-humidity, oxygen-enriched gas source with a higher than current F_1O_2 available at bedside.
6.	Have equipment available in case reintubation becomes necessary.
7.	Carefully suction the airway and the oropharynx above the cuff.
8.	Deflate the cuff completely, extubate, and administer high-humidity oxygen.
9.	Encourage vigorous coughing; suction as necessary.
10.	Check vital signs and ABGs; watch for evidence of laryngospasm (e.g., listen with a stethoscope for inspiratory stridor).
11.	Reintubate for progressive hypoxemia, hypercapnia, acidosis, or laryngospasm not responsive to therapy.

ventilator changes are not made often enough. Prolonged periods at low rates (<6/min) may promote a state of respiratory muscle fatigue because of the work of breathing through a high-resistance ventilator circuit. Pressure support ventilation may alleviate this but can prolong the weaning process if not rapidly titrated.

b. The T-tube technique intersperses periods of unassisted spontaneous breathing through a T-tube (or other continuous flow circuit) with periods of ventilator support. Short daytime periods (5–15 minutes 2–6 times/day) are used initially and then are progressively increased in duration or frequency. Small amounts (3–5 cm H_2O) of CPAP during these periods may prevent airway closure and microatelectasis. Small amounts of pressure support ventilation (4–8 cm H_2O) decrease inspiratory resistance imposed by the ventilator circuit and endotracheal tube. Extubation may be appropriate when the patient tolerates 30–90 minutes on the T tube. More prolonged periods of T-tube breathing may be fatiguing, especially if the endotracheal tube is small.

c. Pressure support ventilation (PSV) (see sec. **III.B.1**) may be preferred when respiratory muscle weakness appears to be compromising weaning. It is available only on selected newer ventilators. PSV may reduce the work of breathing through a tracheal tube and ventilator circuit, although this concept has not been clearly established (*Chest* 89:677, 1986). In this mode, the patient initiates each breath with a small amount of negative pressure. The respiratory rate, tidal volume, inspiratory time, and flow rate are governed by the patient rather than being set at the ventilator. The physician sets the amount of positive pressure (usually 15–25 cm H_2O) necessary to increase the spontaneous tidal volume to 7–15 ml/kg. As lung mechanics improve, the amount of pressure support is gradually decreased until the patient requires little support to maintain a satisfactory minute ventilation. Only 5–8 cm H_2O of pressure support is needed to overcome the resistance of the endotracheal tube and ventilator circuit. Removal of these low levels of PSV is not usually necessary before extubation. However, in the patient with very high compliance (e.g., from emphysema), surprisingly low levels of PSV may provide considerable mechanical support.

B. Extubation can be performed when weaning is completed and airway control is no longer necessary. Table 9–6 outlines the extubation procedure.

C. Common causes of extubation failure

    1. Inadequate clearance of tracheobronchial secretions will increase airway resistance and worsen $\dot{V}_A/\dot{Q}$ mismatch; the consequences are an increased work of breathing and a deterioration in gas exchange. Causes include (1) excessive secretions, usually from inadequately treated pulmonary infections, and (2) insufficient pulmonary toilet, which may be the result of a weakened cough, impaired mucociliary clearance, or ineffective suctioning. Therapy should include appropriate antibiotic treatment as well as other techniques of airway care (see General Considerations, sec. **III.C**).

2. **Upper airway obstruction.** Glottic and subglottic edema may cause inspiratory stridor within 24 hours of extubation. If clinical status permits, treatment with 2.5% racemic epinephrine (0.5 ml in 3 ml normal saline) via nebulization and inhalation should be tried. If successful, this treatment can be repeated as needed every 20–30 minutes for an additional 1–2 doses. If the clinical response is not rapid, reintubation may be necessary. Extubation should not be attempted again for 48–72 hours to allow time for improvement in edema. Steroids are of no immediate benefit but are occasionally given to diminish inflammation, which may hinder subsequent extubation attempts. Recurrent or severe upper airway obstruction or subglottic stenosis may require a tracheostomy.

3. **Inspiratory muscle fatigue** (see General Considerations, sec. **II.B.2**) has many causes and may contribute to otherwise unexplained extubation failures. Causes include (1) increased work of breathing due to persistent underlying lung disease that has been inadequately treated or is unresolved, (2) decreased cardiac output, (3) poor nutritional status, (4) hypoxemia, (5) inspiratory muscle deconditioning during mechanical ventilation, (6) inappropriate weaning methods, and (7) metabolic disturbances (especially severe hypophosphatemia, hypokalemia, or hypomagnesemia).

4. **New untoward events** in the postextubation period may require reintubation if respiratory function remains compromised.

Cardiopulmonary Monitoring

Cardiopulmonary monitoring is widely used for ARF management. These data must be accurately collected and thoughtfully interpreted to be valuable in clinical decision making.

I. **Pulmonary artery catheterization** with a balloon-flotation catheter allows measurement of (1) right atrial, right ventricular, pulmonary artery, and pulmonary artery occlusive pressures; (2) thermodilution cardiac output; and (3) mixed venous oxygen tension and saturation. It can be helpful (1) in separating cardiogenic from noncardiogenic pulmonary edema, (2) in evaluating volume or cardiovascular status when empiric therapy is unsafe or has failed, and (3) in guiding therapy with PEEP, fluids, and cardiovascular drugs. Confirming a catheter tip position in a lung zone where both pulmonary artery pressure and pulmonary venous pressure exceed alveolar pressure is necessary to avoid measuring alveolar pressure instead of intravascular pressure. If the catheter tip is at or below the gravitational level of the left atrium, it is usually in such a zone. **Complications** of pulmonary artery catheterization include inadvertent arterial puncture, pneumothorax, venous thrombosis or phlebitis, infection, air embolism, cardiac arrhythmias and bundle branch block, pulmonary infarction, and pulmonary artery rupture. The conversion of intravascular pressures into digital and graphic displays is complex. Equipment malfunction or operator error may result in a spurious measurement. Any data that do not correlate with clinical circumstances should be repeated after system recalibration.

A. **Pulmonary artery occlusive pressure** (PAOP) measurements often guide fluid therapy during ARF (*Am. Rev. Respir. Dis.* 128:319, 1983). **The trend in PAOP measurements** is often more valuable than any single determination; reproducibility should be within 10%. If the PAOP is less than 10 mm Hg, volume expansion can be undertaken to treat hypotension. If the PAOP is greater than 20–25 mm Hg and hypotension is not a problem, a diuretic can generally be given for pulmonary edema. If PAOP is between 10 and 20 mm Hg, a therapeutic trial of volume infusion, diuresis, or a positive inotropic or vasoactive agent can be initiated and the response assessed by the changes in PAOP and cardiac output. The following paragraphs outline several factors that often complicate interpretation of PAOP tracings.

1. **Transmural pressure,** the difference between intravascular and extravascular pressure, is the true determinant of hemodynamic behavior. The PAOP is an intravascular, not a transmural, pressure. During quiet, spontaneous breathing, pleural pressure is only slightly below atmospheric pressure and changes little during the respiratory cycle; hence, there is no significant discrepancy between the PAOP and the true transmural pressure. In contrast, during mechanical ventilation with PEEP, pleural pressure is significantly above atmospheric pressure and varies throughout the respiratory cycle. When pleural pressure is positive, the PAOP measured relative to atmospheric pressure may rise, whereas transmural pressure actually falls. For example, a patient with a PAOP of 12 mm Hg may have a measured PAOP of 18 after 10 mm Hg PEEP has been added to the ventilator circuit. This patient's transmural pressure would actually be 8 mm Hg (18 mm Hg − 10 mm Hg) if all the pleural pressure were transmitted to the pericardial space. Differences between the measured PAOP and the true transmural pressure are rarely significant when PEEP is less than 10 cm H_2O. However, above this PEEP level, the difference is unpredictable. Discontinuing PEEP to make pressure measurements is potentially detrimental and rarely useful. The beneficial effects of PEEP are lost rapidly and restored slowly, such that serious hypoxemia may result. It is therefore preferable to obtain the measurements on PEEP and correlate them with trends in other data (for example, $S\bar{v}O_2$ and cardiac output).

2. **Respiratory variation may make reliable PAOP measurement difficult.** Pressure measurements should be made at end exhalation directly from a graphic tracing. Digital readings alone can seriously overestimate or underestimate the actual value. Occasionally, respiratory variation renders pressure tracings uninterpretable. If this fails in the sedated or unconscious mechanically ventilated patient, neuromuscular paralysis with succinylcholine, 40–60 mg IV (see Mechanical Ventilation, sec. **V.B**), allows a brief period of respiratory control for high-quality pressure tracings. During paralysis, the ventilator rate should ensure adequate minute ventilation.

3. **Although the PAOP measures left atrial diastolic pressure, it is clinically used to estimate ventricular preload.** Because the true determinant of ventricular preload is end-diastolic volume, PAOP measurements **can be misleading.** During ARF, ventricular compliance, the relationship between end-diastolic volume and end-diastolic pressure, may be below normal and may change with alterations in PEEP, the severity of the underlying process, or other factors. Therefore, PAOP values must often be correlated with stroke volume measurements to be properly interpreted.

B. **Pulmonary artery diastolic (PAD)** pressure is occasionally used to estimate PAOP when a catheter cannot be advanced into a wedge position. A close correlation exists between these parameters when pulmonary vascular resistance and heart rate are normal; however, tachycardia and pulmonary hypertension commonly disrupt this correlation in ARF so that PAD may overestimate PAOP.

C. **Thermodilution cardiac output** measurement is accurate over the range of most normal values. It is most prone to error at very low cardiac outputs and is not valid in the presence of an intracardic shunt or tricuspid regurgitation. Thermodilution cardiac output values vary with the phase of respiration; mechanical ventilation and PEEP exaggerate these variations. Measurement at end exhalation is ideal but impractical during mechanical ventilation; hence, three consecutive random determinations are averaged.

D. **Mixed venous oxygen saturation** can be useful for assessing the overall adequacy of tissue oxygenation in the absence of sepsis or significant arteriovenous shunting (see General Considerations, sec. **II.C**). The goal is to maintain $P\bar{v}O_2$ greater than 35 mm Hg or $S\bar{v}O_2$ greater than 0.65. Aspirating blood from the distal port of the pulmonary artery catheter in the unwedged position provides a mixed venous sample. Rapid blood withdrawal, severe mitral insufficiency, or left-to-right intracardiac shunting may result in an unreliable sample. Pulmonary artery catheters that continuously monitor mixed venous oxygen saturation reduce the need for frequent mixed venous blood samplings and may be useful in adjusting vasoactive drug therapy.

II. **Systemic artery catheterization** via the radial, brachial, or femoral artery allows continuous monitoring of systemic blood pressure. Indications include hypotensive states, where cuff pressures are difficult to obtain, and hemodynamic instability during vasodilator or vasopressor therapy. Indwelling arterial cannula complications include arterial laceration, bleeding, thrombosis, infection, and distal ischemia.

III. **Gas exchange** can be monitored by ABGs or noninvasive methods.

   A. **Pulse oximetry** provides a quantitative assessment of arterial oxygen saturation and, in most circumstances, closely correlates with oxygen saturation obtained by ABGs. It is less reliable during severe peripheral hypoperfusion, during carbon monoxide poisoning, when skin pigmentation is extremely dark, or when saturation is below 70%.

   B. **Mass spectrometry and capnography** allow rapid analysis of carbon dioxide concentrations in expired gas. The $P_{ET}CO_2$ value is close to the value for $PaCO_2$ in patients with normal lungs, but not in patients with acute or chronic lung diseases. Nevertheless, after an initial correlation to $PaCO_2$, the trend in $P_{ET}CO_2$ values can often guide ventilator management. A rise in $P_{ET}CO_2$ reflects a rise in $PaCO_2$, which can indicate a decrease in alveolar ventilation or an increase in carbon dioxide production, as is seen with overfeeding, sepsis, fever, exercise, or acute increases in cardiac output. A fall in $P_{ET}CO_2$ indicates either an increase in alveolar ventilation or an increase in dead space, as is seen with massive pulmonary thromboembolism or air embolism, endotracheal tube obstruction, ventilator circuit leak, or a sudden drop in cardiac output. Significant changes in $P_{ET}CO_2$ should alert the physician to obtain ABGs and recheck $PaCO_2$.

IV. **Measurements of mechanical properties of the respiratory system**

   A. **Respiratory rate, tidal volume, vital capacity, minute ventilation, maximal voluntary ventilation, and maximum negative inspiratory pressure** can all be measured at the bedside with a Wright spirometer and pressure manometer. These measurements are most useful in assessing the need for continued mechanical ventilation (see Mechanical Ventilation, sec. **VIII**). The minute ventilation required to maintain a given $PaCO_2$ reflects ventilatory demands and is a major determinant of respiratory work. The maximum negative inspiratory pressure is a measure of respiratory muscle strength, and the maximum voluntary minute ventilation is a gauge of respiratory muscle endurance.

   B. **Peak airway pressure** changes of 10 cm H_2O or greater during mechanical ventilation at unchanged tidal volume and PEEP settings usually represent a change in lung, thoracic cage, or abdominal compliance or airway resistance. Lung compliance is the change in lung volume for a given change in transpulmonary pressure. Although measurements of both static and dynamic compliance can be made, they are not routine.

V. **Extravascular lung water** measurement is possible with a double-indicator (thermal–indocyanine green dye) dilution technique, using commercially available equipment (*Crit. Care Clin.* 2:511, 1986). The clinical utility of this information in the management of pulmonary edema has not been firmly established.

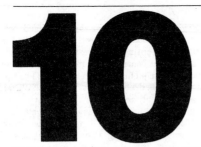

Pulmonary Diseases

J. Randall Hansbrough and
Steven D. Shapiro

Asthma

Asthma is a clinical syndrome characterized by increased responsiveness of the tracheobronchial tree to a variety of stimuli that result in variable airway obstruction. Reduced airflow is caused by bronchial smooth muscle contraction (bronchospasm), edema of the bronchial mucosa, inflammatory infiltration of the bronchial mucosa or submucosa, and plugging of small airways with secretions. Other causes of airway obstruction that may mimic asthma include pulmonary edema, exacerbation of chronic obstructive pulmonary disease (COPD), bronchiectasis, and airway obstruction by tumor or foreign body.

I. **Diagnosis**
  A. **Clinical presentation.** Patients typically have a history of wheezing, cough, breathlessness, and chest tightness. Severity ranges from intermittent mild symptoms requiring no therapy to continuous, disabling respiratory symptoms despite intensive therapy.
  B. **Pulmonary function tests** are often normal during remission. During an acute attack, and occasionally when symptoms are absent, there is a reduction in the forced expiratory volume in one second (FEV_1) and often a proportionally smaller reduction in the forced vital capacity (FVC), producing a decreased FEV_1/FVC ratio (<0.75). Hyperinflation, with increased residual volume (RV) and functional residual capacity (FRC), may be observed. Bronchial provocation testing (methacholine challenge) is occasionally useful in the evaluation of atypical presentations.

II. **Assessment of severity of an asthma attack** is critical for proper management of the patient.
  A. **History.** Patients with a prolonged history of asthma can often compare the present attack to prior attacks. Previous or current use of corticosteroids, frequent hospitalizations, previous need for mechanical ventilation, or recent emergency room visits may be indicative of a more severe or unresponsive attack that requires hospitalization.
  B. **Physical examination.** A severe attack is suggested by respiratory distress at rest, difficulty speaking in sentences, diaphoresis, or use of accessory muscles. A respiratory rate greater than 30 breaths/minute, pulse greater than 120 beats/minute, and pulsus paradoxus greater than 18 mm Hg indicate a dangerously severe episode (*N. Engl. J. Med.* 305:783, 1981). The intensity of wheezing is an unreliable indicator. Subcutaneous emphysema suggests an associated pneumothorax or pneumomediastinum.
  C. **Laboratory studies**
    1. **Spirometry.** Objective measurements of airflow are essential in evaluating and treating an attack. Hospitalization is recommended if the initial FEV_1 is less than 30% of the predicted value or does not increase to at least 40% of the predicted value after 1 hour of vigorous therapy (*Am. J. Med.* 72:416, 1982). When spirometry is not readily available, peak expiratory flow rates can be easily obtained with a Wright peak flowmeter. Generally, hospitalization is recommended if peak flow is less than 60 liters/minute initially or does not improve to greater than 50% predicted after 1 hour of treatment.

2. **Arterial blood gases.** Mismatching of ventilation and perfusion ($\dot{V}/\dot{Q}$ mismatch) (see Chap. 9) due to airway obstruction results in an increased alveolar-arterial oxygen tension difference [$P(A\text{-}a)O_2$], which correlates roughly with the severity of the attack. An arterial oxygen tension (PaO_2) less than 60 mm Hg may be a sign of a severe attack or a complicating condition. Almost all asthmatic patients experiencing a mild to moderately severe episode will hyperventilate and have an arterial carbon dioxide tension ($PaCO_2$) of less than 35 mm Hg. With a severe or prolonged attack, the $PaCO_2$ may rise as a result of a combination of severe airway obstruction, areas of high $\dot{V}/\dot{Q}$ ratio causing increased dead space ventilation, and respiratory muscle fatigue. A "normal" or increased $PaCO_2$ may be a sign of impending respiratory failure. Patients who are in respiratory distress and have a sustained $PaCO_2$ greater than 40 mm Hg, accompanied by other signs of severe asthma, should be managed in an intensive care unit with careful and frequent evaluation for the need for intubation and mechanical ventilation.

3. **Chest radiography** is indicated in all but mild attacks. The radiograph may suggest or confirm a diagnosis of pneumonia, exclude complications such as pneumothorax or pneumomediastinum, and reveal evidence of other conditions that mimic asthma.

III. **Therapy of acute asthma attacks.** The immediate goals of therapy are to ensure adequate gas exchange while reducing airway obstruction.

A. **Oxygen.** Adequate supplemental oxygen should be given; low flow rates (2–3 liters/min by nasal cannula) are usually sufficient.

B. **Intubation and mechanical ventilation** are not usually required but are mandatory in patients with severe respiratory distress, mental status changes, obvious exhaustion, or progressively increasing $PaCO_2$ (see sec. **II.C.2**). Intubation of patients with asthma may be difficult; anxiolytic agents may be indicated, but only in preparation for intubation by experienced personnel or after mechanical ventilation is initiated. Mechanical ventilation may require very high inspiratory pressures; neuromuscular blockade, in addition to sedatives, may be helpful in achieving adequate ventilation (see Chap. 9). Occasionally, mechanically controlled hypoventilation must be implemented to avoid or minimize the complications of extremely high airway pressures (*Am. Rev. Respir. Dis.* 129:385, 1984; *Am. J. Med.* 89:42, 1990).

C. **Beta-adrenergic agonists** are the most effective bronchodilators in asthma and should be instituted immediately on presentation. Beta$_2$ selective agonists produce fewer cardiac side effects than nonselective agents, but minor side effects, including tremor, nervousness, and tachycardia, may occur. Beta$_2$-adrenergic agonists can be given in aerosolized, parenteral, and oral forms. Aerosolized preparations are the preferred mode of delivery. Parenteral administration (SQ) is unnecessary if adequate inhaled medications can be administered quickly and effectively. Oral administration has no role in the treatment of acute asthma.

1. **Metered-dose inhaler** (MDI) is the optimal means of delivery in both acute and chronic settings. For most patients, bronchodilator administration by MDI with a spacer device or reservoir is as effective as delivery by nebulizer (*Chest* 98:822, 1987). Albuterol, terbutaline, and metaproterenol MDIs have both beta$_2$ selectivity and long duration of action. The optimal dose and frequency of administration in the acute setting have not been determined. In comparison with maintenance therapy, however, the frequent administration of large doses may be beneficial in seriously ill patients (*N. Engl. J. Med.* 315:870, 1986). Two to four initial puffs can be followed by 1–2 puffs q10–20min until improvement is obtained or significant toxicity, such as unacceptable tremor, tachycardia, or cardiac arrhythmia, is noted. Thereafter, 2 puffs q4h can be given until the patient's condition becomes stable. Patient instruction and supervised administration are essential initially to ensure that effective delivery is achieved.

2. **Administration by nebulizer.** Albuterol and metaproterenol are available as

solutions for nebulization. Albuterol (2.5 mg/ml) or metaproterenol (50 mg/ml), 0.25–0.5 ml in 3 ml of normal saline, can be inhaled from an updraft nebulizer over 5–15 minutes. A minimum of 4 hours between treatments is generally recommended. Treatment can be intensified initially (see MDIs, above).

3. **Parenteral administration** is unnecessary if adequate inhaled medications can be administered quickly and effectively. In the rare situations in which parenteral therapy is necessary, epinephrine (0.3 ml 1:1000 SQ q15–20min for up to three doses) can be used. Patients should have electrocardiographic monitoring; ischemic heart disease is a relative contraindication to its use.

D. **Corticosteroids.** Systemic corticosteroids reduce airway obstruction by reducing inflammation. There are no clinically significant effects for the first 4–6 hours of therapy. In all but mild attacks, steroids should be administered if substantial improvement does not occur within the first hour of intensive bronchodilator therapy. Methylprednisolone, 0.5–1.0 mg/kg IV q6h, is recommended. Larger dosages (e.g., 125 mg IV q6h) may result in more rapid improvement but have not been shown to improve outcome (*Arch. Intern. Med.* 143:1324, 1983).

E. **Theophylline,** a xanthine derivative and adenosine receptor antagonist, is a weak bronchodilator that may also prevent muscle fatigue and consequent respiratory failure. Although data suggest that no further benefit is derived from the acute addition of theophylline to an adequate beta-agonist regimen (*Chest* 98:44, 1990), it may be of benefit in chronic management (see sec. **IV.E**) and is frequently used in acute management of asthma.

1. **Route of administration.** Theophylline is generally administered intravenously in acute asthma to quickly attain and sustain therapeutic plasma levels. Oral administration may also be reasonable even in the acute setting.

2. **Dosage.** Theophylline must be converted to a water-soluble salt form (aminophylline) for IV use. Aminophylline contains 80% theophylline by weight. The loading dose of aminophylline is 6 mg/kg ideal body weight, infused IV over 20 minutes. The loading dose should be reduced or omitted if the patient has recently taken theophylline. A maintenance dose is given by constant IV infusion at a rate of 0.5–0.6 mg/kg/hr. Lower infusion rates (0.2–0.4 mg/kg/hr) should be used in patients with heart failure or liver dysfunction and in the elderly. Medications such as cimetidine and erythromycin (see Appendix B) decrease theophylline clearance and may require reduction of infusion rates. Adolescents, smokers, and patients taking phenytoin metabolize theophylline more rapidly and may require higher infusion rates (0.7–0.9 mg/kg/hr).

3. **Serum theophylline** concentrations must be monitored. The dosage is usually adjusted to maintain serum levels of 10–20 mg/liter. Levels greater than 12 mg/liter may be more effective in some individuals but are also more frequently associated with nausea, vomiting, diarrhea, and atrial arrhythmias. More serious toxicities, particularly seizures and ventricular arrhythmias, usually do not occur when serum levels are below 30–40 mg/liter. They can occur at lower levels, however, and may occur without any preceding signs of toxicity.

F. **Hydration** is indicated only to correct dehydration, which may be significant due to the diuretic effect of theophylline and the increased insensible losses that result from increased ventilation. There is no evidence that vigorous hydration decreases mucus viscosity.

G. **Chest physiotherapy** (see Chronic Obstructive Pulmonary Disease) has not been definitively evaluated in asthma and may aggravate bronchospasm (*Chest* 88:436, 1985).

IV. **Maintenance therapy.** All patients with asthma, except those with mild and infrequent episodes of bronchospasm, should be continuously treated with appropriate medications, even when asymptomatic between acute attacks. Recent trends in asthma maintenance therapy have placed greater emphasis on the use of inhaled cromolyn and inhaled corticosteroids along with inhaled beta agonists as first-line drugs. Theophylline is more often used as a second- or third-line agent in combination therapy or in special situations (i.e., evening doses for the control of nocturnal symptoms) (*N. Engl. J. Med.* 321:1517, 1989).

A. Known precipitating factors should be avoided if possible. Stimuli that may provoke bronchospasm include allergens, cold weather, exercise, chemical irritants, viral infections, and medications such as aspirin, nonsteroidal anti-inflammatory drugs (NSAIDs), beta-adrenergic antagonists, and cholinergic drugs (including eye drops).

B. Inhaled beta-adrenergic agonists. Following proper patient instruction, MDIs (with spacer devices or reservoirs when appropriate) should be used regularly in patients with significant asthma. The usual regimen is albuterol, terbutaline, or metaproterenol, 2 puffs q4–6h. Oral sympathomimetic agents are rarely a necessary or helpful addition to inhaled bronchodilators.

C. Inhaled corticosteroids. Beclomethasone, triamcinolone, or flunisolide, delivered by MDI, may prevent frequent attacks and reduce or eliminate the need for systemic steroids. The usual dose is 2 puffs qid (bid for flunisolide) 5–10 minutes after administration of inhaled bronchodilators, followed by rinsing of the oropharynx and gargling (with water) to reduce the risk of oral candidiasis. Larger doses of inhaled steroids (up to 4 times the starting dose) may be required to adequately control some patients. Inhaled corticosteroids have no significant systemic side effects.

D. Cromolyn sodium (2 puffs qid by MDI) is effective in the maintenance therapy of asthma, particularly when exercise is a precipitating factor (*Am. Rev. Respir. Dis.* 139:694, 1989). Since only a subgroup of adult patients will respond to cromolyn, a trial of 4–6 weeks of cromolyn therapy is required to assess the effectiveness in an individual patient.

E. Theophylline preparations can be added to the patient's regimen if inhaled agents fail to control asthma. Usually, 200–400 mg PO bid of a long-acting preparation will achieve therapeutic, nontoxic levels, but serum drug concentrations should be measured (see sec. **III.E**). Following improvement from an acute attack treated with IV aminophylline, oral theophylline therapy can be initiated by administering an amount of theophylline equal to 80% of the total daily aminophylline dose (in milligrams). The total calculated dose is then divided by 2–3 and administered equally q12h or q8h, respectively, using sustained-release dosage forms. Blood levels should be monitored.

F. Anticholinergic agents (see Chronic Obstructive Pulmonary Disease). Ipratropium bromide by MDI, 2 puffs qid, may be useful in cases of refractory asthma or when there are intolerable side effects from other agents.

G. Oral corticosteroids. During treatment of an acute attack, prednisone, 40–60 mg PO qd, can be substituted for parenteral therapy when airflow improves and the patient is comfortable. Steroids should be gradually tapered, and inhaled corticosteroids can be substituted for oral corticosteroids (see sec. **IV.C**). Long-term systemic corticosteroids should be used only in **rare** instances when frequent, severe attacks persist despite maximal therapy. The lowest effective dose should be used and alternate-day therapy is preferred when effective.

H. Methotrexate. Studies have suggested that low-dose methotrexate may be useful in the management of steroid-dependent asthma by stabilizing the disease and allowing reduction in corticosteroid dosages (*Ann. Intern. Med.* 112:577, 1990; *Lancet* 336:137, 1990). Methotrexate should be administered only to those asthmatics who are not well controlled on moderate doses of corticosteroids or to patients who experience unacceptable side effects from chronic corticosteroid use. All other therapeutic modalities should be attempted before methotrexate is used, and such therapy should be directed by a medical specialist who has experience with the management of refractory asthma. Consideration should also be given to preexisting hematopoietic disorders, hepatic or renal dysfunction, insulin-dependent diabetes mellitus, and morbid obesity or alcohol use, all of which may increase the toxicity of methotrexate. Sulfa-containing drugs, weak organic acids (including salicylates, penicillins), and blockers of renal tubular secretion (probenecid) may potentiate drug toxicity. Potential side effects include: (1) elevated hepatic transaminases with the risk of permanent liver damage; (2) gastrointestinal symptoms including anorexia, vomiting, and diarrhea; (3) dermatitis; (4) stomatitis; (5) bone marrow suppression; (6) **teratogenesis;** (7) alopecia; and (8) an acute drug-induced pneumonitis.

Chronic Obstructive Pulmonary Disease

Chronic obstructive pulmonary disease is a clinical syndrome of chronic dyspnea with expiratory airflow obstruction due to chronic bronchitis and emphysema. **Chronic bronchitis** is a clinical syndrome of chronic productive cough with no other identifiable cause. Although diagnosed clinically, pulmonary **emphysema** is a pathologic diagnosis, characterized by enlarged air spaces distal to the terminal bronchioles with associated destruction of alveolar septae. Chronic bronchitis and emphysema coexist in most patients. Expiratory airflow obstruction occurs predominantly because of loss of supporting structures for small airways and, to a lesser extent, loss of lung elastic recoil. Airflow obstruction may be worsened by bronchospasm, airway thickening, and mucus plugging of small airways.

I. **Diagnosis and evaluation**
   A. **History and physical examination.** Patients typically have a chronic productive cough for many years, followed by slowly progressive breathlessness with decreasing amounts of exertion. COPD is unusual in the absence of a significant history of cigarette smoking. Alpha$_1$-antitrypsin deficiency should be considered in nonsmokers or young patients (age < 50 years) with emphysema. On examination, tachypnea, pursed-lip breathing, and use of accessory muscles of respiration are commonly observed. The chest may be hyperresonant to percussion, breath sounds may be decreased, and adventitious sounds (wheezes, midinspiratory crackles, and large airway sounds) may be present. Clubbing of the digits is not commonly associated with COPD and suggests the presence of another disease. Signs of cor pulmonale may be present in severe or long-standing disease.
   B. **Chest radiographs** often show low, flattened diaphragms. In severe emphysema, the lung fields may be hyperlucent, with diminished vascular markings and bullae. Disease is often most prominent in the upper lung zones except in alpha$_1$-antitrypsin deficiency, which may show a basilar predominance. Chest radiographs are of value during an acute exacerbation to exclude complications such as pneumonia and pneumothorax.
   C. **Pulmonary function testing.** The FEV_1 and all other measurements of expiratory airflow are reduced. Total lung capacity (TLC), FRC, and RV may be increased. The diffusion capacity of carbon monoxide (DL_{CO}) is reduced in the presence of emphysema.
   D. **Arterial blood gases**
      1. **Stable COPD.** Gas exchange abnormalities vary with the type and severity of $\dot{V}/\dot{Q}$ abnormalities. Perfusion of poorly ventilated areas of the lungs (i.e., areas with low $\dot{V}/\dot{Q}$) results in an increased $P(A\text{-}a)O_2$ and hypoxemia. Ventilation of poorly perfused areas (i.e., high $\dot{V}/\dot{Q}$) results in increased dead space, requiring a higher minute ventilation to maintain a normal $PaCO_2$. A subpopulation of patients with severe airway obstruction will have chronically increased arterial $PaCO_2$, but metabolic compensation (increased serum bicarbonate) will maintain the arterial pH near normal.
      2. **Acute ventilatory failure.** During an acute exacerbation of COPD, worsening airway obstruction, increased dead space ventilation, and respiratory muscle fatigue may lead to rapid rises in $PaCO_2$ with subsequent acute respiratory acidosis (see Chap. 9).
   E. **Serum alpha$_1$-antitrypsin levels.** Alpha$_1$-antitrypsin deficiency can be identified by the absence of the alpha-globulin peak on the densitometric tracing of a serum protein electrophoresis (the reported alpha-globulin level is not helpful). Quantitative determination of alpha$_1$-antitrypsin or alpha$_1$-antitrypsin phenotyping can be performed when appropriate (see sec. **I.A**).

II. **Management of acute exacerbations.** A variety of insults may provoke broncho-spasm or an increase in mucus secretion and plugging. The resulting increase in airway obstruction may cause worsening dyspnea, fatigue, and, sometimes, respi-ratory failure. Upper respiratory infections are the most common identifiable cause of acute exacerbations. In addition, pneumonia (especially with *Streptococcus pneumoniae* and *Haemophilus influenzae*), pulmonary emboli, pulmonary edema, and pneumothorax may all worsen gas exchange and increase breathlessness in patients with COPD. These and other causes of dyspnea should be considered in patients with apparent acute exacerbations of COPD.

A. **Maintenance of adequate gas exchange**

1. **Oxygen** should be administered to achieve and maintain a PaO_2 of 55–60 mm Hg (88–90% oxyhemoglobin saturation). The effectiveness of supplemen-tal oxygen should be evaluated by serial arterial blood gas determinations. Low-flow oxygen (1–3 liters/min by nasal cannula or 24–35% oxygen by Venturi mask) is almost always adequate. Higher levels of supplemental oxygen are rarely necessary and may result in elevation of $PaCO_2$, with consequent depression of mental status, hypoventilation, and further impair-ment of gas exchange. Nevertheless, adequate oxygenation must be main-tained, even in the face of increasing hypercapnia (see Chap. 9). Requirement for high concentrations of supplemental oxygen suggests a complicating condition.

2. **Mechanical ventilation** should be considered in patients with acute ventila-tory failure (see Chap. 9).

B. **Inhaled beta$_2$-adrenergic agonists.** As in asthma, inhaled medications are best given by MDI (with a spacer device or reservoir if appropriate) with careful patient instruction. Inhaled beta$_2$-adrenergic agonists such as metaproterenol, terbutaline, or albuterol, 2–4 puffs initially, followed by 2 puffs q4h, are currently first-line therapy for acute exacerbations of COPD.

C. **Anticholinergic agents** (see sec. **III.C.1**). Ipratropium bromide may decrease obstruction to airflow in COPD, but published experience with anticholinergic agents in the treatment of acute exacerbations is limited.

D. **Corticosteroids.** Methylprednisolone, 0.5 mg/kg IV q6h for 3 days, is used in acute exacerbations of COPD. This therapy is based on data that demonstrate significant improvements in airflow in some patients. Oral prednisone, 40–60 mg PO qd, is usually started after a few days. Steroids should be tapered as tolerated, following the same guidelines as in asthma (see Asthma, sec. **IV.G.**).

E. **Theophylline** administration should be considered in patients who respond poorly to inhaled bronchodilators. As in asthma, however, the benefit of adding theophylline to an adequate inhaled bronchodilator regimen in acute exacerba-tions of COPD is unclear (*Ann. Intern. Med.* 107:305, 1987). Dosage and administration are similar to those for asthma (see Asthma, sec. **III.E.**)

F. **Antimicrobial therapy.** Appropriate IV antimicrobials should be used for pneu-monia (see Chaps. 12 and 13). For routine exacerbations of COPD, in the absence of pneumonia, a 7- to 10-day course of oral antimicrobial therapy (e.g., amoxicillin, 250 mg PO tid, or trimethoprim-sulfamethoxazole, 160 mg/800 mg [1 double-strength tablet] PO bid) may be beneficial in some patients (*Ann. Intern. Med.* 106:196, 1987).

G. **Chest physiotherapy** is useful to improve clearance of secretions in patients with copious respiratory secretions (>50 ml/day). Patients without excessive secretions have not been shown to benefit from such therapy.

III. **Long-term management** is aimed at (1) providing symptomatic relief, (2) decreas-ing the frequency and severity of acute exacerbations, and (3) treating hypoxemia and its complications.

A. **Smoking cessation.** The primary determinant of smoking cessation is patient motivation. Nevertheless, interventions should include (1) repetitive counseling on the preventable health risks of smoking and advice to stop smoking, (2) encouraging patients to make further attempts to stop smoking even if they have failed previously, and (3) providing smoking cessation materials to patients. Nicotine-containing chewing gum (2 mg chewed slowly over 20–30 minutes, repeated up to 60 mg/day) may reduce nicotine withdrawal symptoms and promote abstinence in some patients. It is most effective when used short term in conjunction with formal smoking cessation programs or close medical follow-up.

B. Education. Patients must be made aware of the deleterious effects of continued smoking so that abstinence can be maintained. Patients should learn the correct use of medicines and the proper techniques of administration. Patients and families should learn to recognize early symptoms of acute exacerbations, including subtle but common manifestations such as hypersomnolence and agitation.

C. Bronchodilators. The optimal bronchodilator regimen for long-term management of COPD has not been established. **Inhaled anticholinergic** agents and inhaled beta-adrenergic agonists may be beneficial in stable COPD. Studies of the relative efficacy of these agents alone or in combination have had conflicting results.

   1. Anticholinergic agents. Ipratropium bromide is a nonabsorbable anticholinergic agent that reduces vagal tone and is the drug of choice for many patients with stable COPD. The drug is available as an MDI and is generally given in a dosage of 2 puffs q4–6h, although higher doses can be used. Ipratropium is generally well tolerated; minor side effects include cough and dry mouth.

   2. Beta-adrenergic agonists, such as albuterol, terbutaline, or metaproterenol, are typically administered in dosages of 2 puffs q4–6h.

   3. Oral theophylline preparations can be administered in dosages similar to those used for maintenance therapy of asthma (see Asthma, sec. **IV.E.**).

D. Corticosteroids. In patients with disabling airway obstruction despite optimal bronchodilator therapy, a 2-week trial of methylprednisolone 32 mg PO qd or prednisone 40 mg PO qd will identify a small subpopulation with steroid responsiveness (*Ann. Intern. Med.* 96:17, 1982). Steroid therapy should be continued *only if* pulmonary function test (PFT) values improve significantly (e.g., 15% improvement in FEV_1 or 20% improvement in FVC) on repeat testing in 3 weeks. The lowest effective dose should be used and alternate-day therapy is preferred. Inhaled steroids should be substituted for systemic steroids when possible. However, only a minority of responders will maintain an objective response with inhaled corticosteroids alone (*Am. J. Med.* 78:655, 1985).

E. Oxygen therapy has been shown to improve survival and quality of life in patients with COPD and chronic hypoxemia. Results are best with continuous oxygen administration (*Ann. Intern. Med.* 93:391, 1980). PaO_2 should be maintained at approximately 60 mm Hg. Increased oxygen delivery may be required with exercise and sleep. Criteria for long-term oxygen therapy include (1) PaO_2 consistently less than 55 mm Hg or oxyhemoglobin saturation less than 88% by pulse oximetry despite optimal medical therapy; or (2) PaO_2 of 55–59 mm Hg with evidence of cor pulmonale or secondary polycythemia (hematocrit >55%). In addition, oxygen therapy during exercise may improve endurance in patients with exertional hypoxemia. Nocturnal oxygen therapy may reduce arrhythmias and retard the development of cor pulmonale in patients with documented sleep-induced hypoxemia.

F. A general rehabilitation program, including exercise training and proper nutrition, may help improve the patient's exercise tolerance and sense of well-being, even without a measurable improvement in pulmonary function tests.

G. Influenza and pneumococcal vaccines are recommended for patients with COPD (see Appendix E and Table E-1).

H. Sedatives and tranquilizers should be avoided because they suppress respiratory drive and cough. In addition, the nervousness and irritability for which they may be prescribed can be early signs of a COPD exacerbation.

I. Alpha₁-proteinase inhibitor administration may be appropriate in patients with documented alpha₁-antitrypsin deficiency and emphysema, but treatment with this agent is expensive and its long-term efficacy has not been established.

Table 10-1. Frequency of symptoms and signs in pulmonary embolism

Symptom	%	Sign	%
Chest pain		Tachypnea ($\geq$20/min)	85
Pleuritic	74	Tachycardia ($\geq$100/min)	58
Nonpleuritic	14	Accentuated P_2	57
Dyspnea	84	Rales	56
Apprehension	63	Fever ($\geq$38.5°C)	50
Cough	50	Phlebitis	32
Hemoptysis	28	Cyanosis	19
Syncope	13	Pleural rub	18

Source: Adapted from W. R. Bell and T. L. Simon. Current status of pulmonary thromboembolic disease: Pathophysiology, diagnosis, prevention, and treatment. *Am. Heart J.* 103:239, 1982.

Pulmonary Embolism

Pulmonary thromboembolism is an important cause of morbidity and mortality, especially among hospitalized patients. The majority of clinically significant pulmonary emboli arise from deep venous thromboses (DVTs) in the iliofemoral system; many of the remainder arise in the pelvic venous plexus as postsurgical or gynecologic complications. Predisposing factors for thromboembolic disease include venous disease of the lower extremities, carcinoma, heart failure (HF), recent pelvic or lower abdominal surgery, prolonged immobilization, pregnancy, and administration of estrogens. The clinical manifestations of acute pulmonary embolism may be nonspecific and vary widely, ranging from subtle signs and symptoms to hypotension and sudden death. The most common symptoms are dyspnea, pleuritic chest pain, apprehension, and cough; frequent physical findings include tachypnea, tachycardia, accentuation of the pulmonic component of the second heart sound, and inspiratory crackles (*Am. Heart J.* 103:239, 1982) (Table 10-1). Pleuritic chest pain and hemoptysis suggest pulmonary infarction.

I. **Diagnosis** of pulmonary embolism is based on clinical suspicion, ancillary laboratory data, and the results of specific diagnostic studies.

   A. **A general diagnostic evaluation** should include arterial blood gases, which may demonstrate an increased $P(\text{A-a})O_2$ (see Chap. 9). Arterial hypoxemia with a PaO_2 below 80 mm Hg occurs in the majority of patients without underlying cardiopulmonary disease (*Chest* 81:495, 1982) and is usually accompanied by hypocapnia. The ECG most often demonstrates sinus tachycardia and may show signs of right heart strain; rhythm disturbances such as atrial fibrillation or flutter occur less frequently. Chest radiographs are generally unremarkable or demonstrate subsegmental atelectasis. Pleural effusion occurs in 30–50% of cases but is often small. Although uncommon, pleural-based infiltrates may be present, especially in the lower lobes. Areas of hyperlucency in the lung fields may result from oligemia.

   B. **Specific diagnostic studies** are necessary in patients suspected of having pulmonary emboli. The patient's clinical status and previously obtained data determine which tests to order and the sequence in which they should be performed.

      1. **Ventilation-perfusion ($\dot{V}/\dot{Q}$) lung scans** should be performed in all clinically stable patients with suspected pulmonary emboli. Perfusion defects that are greater than or equal to one pulmonary segment and are unmatched by ventilation defects indicate a high probability of pulmonary embolism. A normal lung scan excludes the diagnosis of pulmonary embolism in almost all cases. Low, intermediate, or indeterminate probability may also be designated based on the relative size of perfusion and ventilation defects and radiographic abnormalities. Further evaluation is usually indicated in patients with nondiagnostic $\dot{V}/\dot{Q}$ scans and in patients with low probability

studies when the clinical suspicion for pulmonary embolism is high (*Ann. Intern. Med.* 98:891, 1983; *J.A.M.A.* 263:2753, 1990).

2. **Evaluation for deep vein thrombosis** provides a less invasive means than pulmonary angiography for supporting a diagnosis of thromboembolic disease in patients in whom a V̇/Q̇ scan is nondiagnostic. Impedance plethysmography and Doppler ultrasonography are the most sensitive noninvasive techniques for the diagnosis of DVT in the thigh. Venous duplex scanning, which provides ultrasonic venous imaging with Doppler blood flow imaging, may have greater accuracy than either technique. ^{125}I-fibrinogen scans are better for detecting calf vein thromboses, although these rarely embolize unless they extend proximal to the knee. These noninvasive tests can be used individually or in combination, depending on availability and expertise in interpretation. Venography may be needed to make a definitive diagnosis.

3. **Pulmonary angiography** should be performed whenever clinical data and noninvasive tests are equivocal or contradictory. When reasonable clinical suspicion of pulmonary emboli exists, the risks of untreated pulmonary embolism or of complications from unnecessary anticoagulation outweigh the morbidity and mortality of pulmonary angiography (*Am. J. Med.* 70:17, 1981). In addition, pulmonary angiography is appropriate in patients with a high probability of pulmonary embolism by V̇/Q̇ scan, if the risks of anticoagulation are high or if vena caval interruption or thrombolytic therapy is being considered. Pulmonary angiography may be the appropriate initial diagnostic test in patients who are hemodynamically unstable and in whom the clinical suspicion of pulmonary embolism is high.

II. Treatment

A. **Supportive care** may be needed for patients with massive pulmonary emboli or preexisting cardiopulmonary disease. Supplemental oxygen should be given to correct hypoxemia. Hypotension and reduced cardiac output that do not rapidly respond to IV saline should be treated with vasopressors and can be considered an indication for thrombolytic therapy or surgical intervention (see sec. **II.C**).

B. **Prophylaxis against further emboli** is sufficient to yield clinical improvement in most cases.

1. **Anticoagulation** (see Chap. 17) should be started with IV heparin for the first 7–10 days. Adjusted-dose SQ heparin is also acceptable. Oral warfarin therapy should be initiated several days before discontinuation of heparin. Warfarin is then continued alone for approximately 3 months, or indefinitely if risk factors are still present or thromboembolism is recurrent.

2. **Inferior vena caval interruption** is required in selected patients to prevent further emboli. Accepted indications include patients at high risk of a fatal pulmonary embolus if there is recurrence early in therapy, a major bleeding complication from anticoagulation, the presence of a contraindication to anticoagulants (see Chap. 17), and cases when emboli recur despite adequate anticoagulation. Before a vena caval device is inserted, the diagnosis of pulmonary embolism should be confirmed by pulmonary angiography and followed by a venocavogram to exclude venous anomalies, assess the level of thrombus formation, and allow optimal placement of the device. Vena caval interruption is then usually achieved with a transvenous filter. Laparotomy with ligation of the vena cava is reserved for septic emboli arising from below the diaphragm or for rare cases in which filter placement is not possible (e.g., with altered venous anatomy).

C. **Specific therapy**

1. **Systemic thrombolytic therapy** with streptokinase, urokinase, or tissue plasminogen activator hastens the resolution of thrombi and may be more effective than heparin alone in reducing mortality in patients with hypotension secondary to massive or submassive pulmonary emboli (*Chest* 89:426, 1986). Other indications are controversial. Details of administration and contraindications are provided elsewhere (see Chap. 5).

2. **Pulmonary embolectomy** should be considered only in the rare patient with angiographically proven pulmonary emboli (1) who remains in shock despite

thrombolytic therapy and supportive care, or (2) in whom thrombolytic therapy would be appropriate but is contraindicated.

Adult Respiratory Distress Syndrome

The adult respiratory distress syndrome (ARDS) is acute lung injury due to a wide variety of insults. The predominant medical risk factor for ARDS is sepsis, particularly from an abdominal source (*Am. Rev. Respir. Dis.* 132:485, 1985). Other predisposing conditions include major trauma, aspiration of gastric contents, and drug overdose (including heroin, methadone, and barbiturates). The common end result is disruption of pulmonary endothelial and epithelial barriers. Vascular permeability to large molecular weight proteins is increased, resulting in noncardiogenic pulmonary edema.

I. **Diagnosis** requires exclusion of other causes of pulmonary edema. Patients with ARDS are in respiratory distress with severe hypoxemia despite a high fractional concentration of inspired oxygen (FiO_2). Chest radiographs demonstrate diffuse infiltrates without cardiomegaly or pulmonary vascular redistribution. Significant pleural effusions are unusual in ARDS unless there is a complicating illness.

II. **Therapy** centers on maintaining adequate tissue oxygen delivery while minimizing the risk of oxygen toxicity from prolonged exposure to high concentrations of supplemental oxygen (i.e. $FiO_2 > 0.5$) (see Chap. 9). Additional goals of therapy include identification and treatment of the underlying disorder and prevention of complications. Empiric antimicrobial therapy is often appropriate until infection can be excluded.

A. **Oxygenation.** Mechanical ventilation with positive end-expiratory pressure (PEEP) usually allows maintenance of an adequate PaO_2 with an acceptably low FiO_2 (see Chap. 9). Because of the possibility of adverse hemodynamic consequences with high levels of PEEP (i.e., >10 cm H_2O), invasive hemodynamic monitoring may be indicated (see sec. **II.B**). Patients must also be monitored carefully for other complications of mechanical ventilation, especially barotrauma (see Chap. 9).

B. **Invasive monitoring** with a pulmonary artery catheter may be useful for (1) ensuring adequate cardiac output and mixed venous oxygen content when using high levels of PEEP, and (2) obtaining the lowest pulmonary artery occlusive pressure (PAOP) or lung water compatible with an adequate cardiac output.

C. **Intravascular volume.** Pulmonary edema may be minimized by maintaining the lowest intravascular volume compatible with adequate tissue perfusion. Blood hemoglobin should be kept greater than 10 mg/dl to optimize oxygen delivery.

D. **Complications.** Despite supportive measures, mortality remains high (60% overall and 90% when associated with sepsis). If the patient survives the acute phase, secondary pulmonary infection is the most frequent cause of death (*Am. Rev. Respir. Dis.* 134:12, 1986). Superimposed pneumonia is difficult to diagnose in patients with diffuse pulmonary infiltrates. Therefore, if clinical and radiographic changes consistent with pneumonia develop, aggressive antimicrobial therapy is indicated.

Pneumonia, Pulmonary Aspiration, and Lung Abscess

I. **Pneumonia**

A. **Pneumonia in the immunocompetent host.** Diagnosis and treatment of community-acquired and nosocomial pneumonia in the normal host is discussed in Chap. 13.

B. **Pulmonary infiltrates in the immunocompromised host.** Immunocompromised patients include those with severe defects in lymphocyte or granulocyte number or function. Host defenses are significantly impaired in patients with AIDS (see sec. I.C and Chap. 13), with hematologic malignancy, and in those undergoing immunosuppressive therapy for malignancy or organ transplantation.

1. **Causes of pulmonary infiltrates** in this population are diverse, but the differential diagnosis may be narrowed by noting the specific host immune defect and the rate of onset and radiographic appearance of the pulmonary process (*Mayo Clin. Proc.* 60:610, 1985). Noninfectious etiologies include spread of malignancy, cytotoxic drug reactions, radiation pneumonitis, pulmonary hemorrhage, pulmonary edema, and pulmonary embolus. Infectious etiologies, however, account for the majority of infiltrates and have a mortality approaching 50%. During the first month following **organ transplantation,** bacterial infections predominate; over the next several months, when immunosuppression is greatest, opportunistic infections are common and are due to organisms such as *Nocardia* spp, fungi (e.g., *Aspergillus* spp), viruses (especially cytomegalovirus [CMV]), and *Pneumocystis carinii.* Patients with **severe neutropenia** (absolute granulocyte count <500/μl) are also at markedly increased risk for infection with these organisms and are particularly susceptible to infection with *Pseudomonas aeruginosa* and *Aspergillus* spp. Specific pulmonary problems related to **AIDS** are discussed in sec. I.C.

2. **Diagnostic evaluation.** Empiric antimicrobial therapy is usually initiated after a rapid clinical evaluation is performed and cultures are obtained. In patients without rapid clinical improvement (e.g., within 1–3 days), invasive procedures are generally pursued because of the large differential diagnosis, the necessity for effective antimicrobial therapy, and the potential toxicity of unnecessary therapy.

   a. **Fiberoptic bronchoscopy (FOB)** with bronchoalveolar lavage (BAL) and transbronchial lung biopsies has a 90% sensitivity for identifying an infectious source when present, especially in the presence of diffuse pulmonary involvement (*Am. Rev. Respir. Dis.* 131:880, 1985). Bacteria, atypical mycobacteria, and fungi recovered from washings may reflect upper airway colonization, and confirmation with special stains of biopsy specimens is helpful in identifying true pathogens. FOB is less sensitive in diagnosing noninfectious causes of pulmonary infiltrates. Transbronchial biopsy is relatively contraindicated in the presence of bleeding diathesis, severe hypoxemia, and mechanical ventilation.

   b. **Open lung biopsy** requires a thoracotomy but allows for better control of bleeding and air leaks. Diagnostic yield, particularly for noninfectious etiologies, is higher than with FOB. This procedure is generally reserved for patients who are rapidly deteriorating, have contraindications to transbronchial biopsy, or have had nondiagnostic FOB and are not improving clinically.

3. **Treatment of pneumonia in immunocompromised patients.** Therapy includes supportive measures, supplemental oxygen, antibiotics, and mechanical ventilation if respiratory failure develops. Empiric broad-spectrum antimicrobial therapy should include coverage for *P. aeruginosa* and *Staphylococcus aureus* (see Chap. 13). Amphotericin is often added if the patient fails to respond to initial antimicrobial therapy, especially if there is evidence of superficial fungal colonization or infection; however, a tissue diagnosis of invasive fungal infection should be pursued (*Am. J. Med.* 72:101, 1982). Therapy should be adjusted if a specific etiologic diagnosis is obtained. The greatest impact on ultimate outcome is the response to therapy or resolution of the underlying disorder that initially produced the patient's immunodeficiency.

C. **Pulmonary infiltrates in patients with AIDS.** Almost 50% of AIDS patients initially present with pulmonary disease, most commonly on the basis of an opportunistic pulmonary infection (*Am. Rev. Respir. Dis.* 135:504, 1987). The most common pulmonary infection in this population is *P. carinii* pneumonia

(PCP), although prophylactic therapy (see Chap. 13) has been effective in reducing the incidence of this diagnosis.

1. **Clinical manifestations of PCP** often include the acute or insidious onset of nonproductive cough and dyspnea. The lung examination may be normal, or scattered crackles may be present. The chest radiograph often demonstrates diffuse interstitial or alveolar infiltrates. Occasionally, focal infiltrates are seen or the radiograph appears normal. In patients who have been receiving prophylactic aerosolized pentamidine, PCP may occur as upper lobe infiltrates. Gas exchange abnormalities are usually present.

2. **Differential diagnosis**
   a. **Opportunistic infections** account for most of the pulmonary complications of AIDS. The majority of pulmonary infiltrates are due to PCP (*J. Infect. Dis.* 157:1115, 1988). Other common opportunistic infections occurring alone, or more often in addition to PCP, include those due to *Mycobacterium avium-intracellulare* (MAI) and CMV. *Cryptococcus neoformans, Histoplasma capsulatum, Toxoplasma gondii, Coccidioides immitis, Blastomyces dermatitidis,* and herpes simplex virus pneumonia also occur but are less common.
   b. **Nonopportunistic pathogenic organisms** associated with human immunodeficiency virus (HIV) infection include pyogenic bacteria (especially *Strep. pneumoniae* and *H. influenzae*) and *Mycobacterium tuberculosis.* Tuberculosis often presents with atypical, noncavitary infiltrates and mediastinal and hilar adenopathy in this patient population.
   c. **Neoplasms.** Kaposi's sarcoma is common and may involve the lung. Pulmonary involvement of non-Hodgkin's lymphomas also complicates AIDS.
   d. **Lymphocytic and idiopathic interstitial pneumonitis** may be seen on biopsy, but the implications of these diagnoses are unclear.

3. **Diagnostic evaluation** of patients with pulmonary symptoms who have or are at high risk for AIDS should be undertaken if (1) an infiltrate is seen on chest radiograph or (2) gas exchange abnormalities are present (i.e., increased $P(A-a)O_2$ at rest or with exercise, or a decreased DL_{CO}). Intravenous drug abuse alone may produce similar abnormalities as a result of both infectious etiologies and the reactions to intravenous contaminants and particles from injected materials. Gallium scanning has been used as a sensitive but nonspecific test for pulmonary infections, especially in the presence of a normal chest x-ray. It is not clear that gallium scans provide benefit over assessment of DL_{CO} or exercise-induced gas exchange abnormalities (*Am. Rev. Respir. Dis.* 139:1324, 1989). Evaluation should be directed toward identifying treatable infections.
   a. **Sputum** samples can be used to detect *P. carinii* by the **cytologic identification of organisms** or by the use of *P. carinii* antigen detection assays; the reliability of these methods depends on expertise in collection and interpretation of these specimens. **Stains and cultures** of sputum for mycobacteria, fungi, and bacteria should also be performed. **Cytology** is occasionally diagnostic.
   b. **Fiberoptic bronchoscopy** with BAL and transbronchial biopsy have a 90% sensitivity for diagnosing infectious processes in patients with AIDS and have a higher yield for PCP. Kaposi's sarcoma appears as characteristic, slightly raised cherry-red lesions in the bronchi, which establishes a presumptive diagnosis by fiberoptic bronchoscopy.
   c. **Open lung biopsy** may be necessary to establish noninfectious diagnoses. However, there is currently little benefit from making noninfectious diagnoses in patients with AIDS. Therefore, this procedure is generally reserved for patients unable to safely undergo transbronchial biopsy and in whom BAL is nondiagnostic.

4. **Therapy.** Empiric therapy for PCP is recommended only while awaiting completion of FOB and interpretation of the results, because of the high frequency of adverse drug reactions in this population. Corticosteroid therapy appears to have benefit in patients with moderately severe PCP (defined by

PaO$_2$ <70 mm Hg on room air). Specific treatment should be instituted for documented *P. carinii,* fungal, bacterial, and *M. tuberculosis* infections (see Chap. 13). MAI appears to be resistant to therapy, although the clinical significance of this infection is unclear. Neoplasms causing symptomatic airway obstruction or hemoptysis may be controlled with radiotherapy.

II. **Pulmonary aspiration syndromes** occur most often in patients with decreased level of consciousness, esophageal disorders that predispose patients to reflux, or impaired mucociliary clearance.

    A. Aspiration of gastric contents may have a variety of consequences.

        1. Aspiration pneumonitis is a chemical injury that occurs within hours, presenting with fever, increased P(A-a)O$_2$, and pulmonary infiltrates. If aspiration is massive, ARDS may develop.

        2. Aspiration pneumonia occurs most commonly 2–5 days after the initial event and is often polymicrobial. It may be difficult to discriminate between bacterial pneumonia and chemical pneumonitis. Prophylactic antibiotics do not appear to prevent pneumonia but should be initiated if pneumonitis persists or the patient's clinical status is deteriorating. Penicillin G or clindamycin is usually effective, but broader coverage should be considered in hospitalized patients because they are more likely to be colonized with gram-negative bacilli and *Staph. aureus* (see Chap. 13).

        3. Aspiration of foreign bodies may obstruct the airway and cause atelectasis or lobar collapse. The possible presence of aspirated food particles must always be considered in patients with known aspiration of gastric contents and focal infiltrates. Early bronchoscopy is frequently indicated, especially if the patient has signs of parenchymal volume loss, segmental or lobar collapse, or atelectasis.

    B. Aspiration of oropharyngeal flora predisposes the patient to anaerobic pneumonias and lung abscess (see sec. **III**).

III. **Lung abscess** most often follows aspiration of oropharyngeal contents containing large numbers of anaerobes. Extensive gingival and dental disease facilitate the growth of anaerobic organisms and thus predispose to such infections. The onset of illness may be insidious with constitutional symptoms, fever, and weight loss. Foul-smelling sputum suggests infection with anaerobic bacteria.

    A. Evaluation. Other causes of cavitary lung disease should be considered, including tuberculosis, fungal disease, acute necrotizing pneumonia (e.g., gram-negative bacilli and *Staph. aureus*), carcinoma, vasculitis, septic embolism, and pulmonary embolism with infarction. Sputum should be cultured for mycobacteria and fungi, and skin testing with an intermediate-strength purified protein derivative (PPD) should be performed. Bronchoscopy is indicated if an obstructing tumor or foreign body is suspected.

    B. Therapy. Postural drainage of the involved segment is mandatory. Antibiotic treatment with aqueous penicillin G, 1.5–2.0 million units IV q4h, is satisfactory, although treatment with clindamycin may hasten the resolution of anaerobic lung abscesses (*Ann. Intern. Med.* 98:486, 1983). Therapy can be switched to oral penicillin VK, 500 mg PO q6h, once there is a definite clinical response, and should be continued until the cavity closes. Even with adequate treatment, fever may persist for up to 3 weeks, the cavity may be present for 10–12 weeks, and an infiltrate may be evident for 18–20 weeks. Surgical resection or percutaneous drainage of a lung abscess is only rarely required for a nonresolving abscess with persistent symptoms in spite of prolonged antibiotic therapy, the development of a bronchopleural fistula or empyema, or persistent hemoptysis.

Interstitial Lung Disease

The interstitial lung diseases are a heterogeneous group of disorders. Pathologically, these diseases are characterized by inflammation and exudate in the alveolar spaces and by diffuse microatelectasis, as well as by cellular and connective tissue changes in the interstitial spaces. These changes may result in progressive, irreversible

Table 10-2. Common causes of interstitial lung disease

Known etiologies
　Pulmonary edema
　Infections
　Drugs
　　Cytotoxic agents (e.g., bleomycin)
　　Allergic or other mechanisms (e.g., gold)
　Radiation exposure
　Occupational and environmental inhalants
　　Dusts (organic, inorganic); gases; fumes
　Neoplasms
　　Lymphangitic spread of carcinoma
　　Alveolar-cell carcinoma; lymphoma
Unknown etiologies
　Sarcoidosis and other granulomatous disorders
　Idiopathic pulmonary fibrosis
　Fibrosis associated with collagen vascular diseases

pulmonary fibrosis. The differential diagnosis of interstitial lung disease is extensive (Table 10-2).

I. **Clinical manifestations**
　A. **General.** Patients typically present with breathlessness and a nonproductive cough. The physical examination, chest radiograph, PFTs, and arterial blood gas (ABG) abnormalities vary depending on the underlying etiology.
　B. Clinical manifestations of **idiopathic pulmonary fibrosis (IPF).** IPF is the most common interstitial lung disease. Physical examination reveals bibasilar end-inspiratory crackles; clubbing of the digits may occasionally be present. Chest radiographs usually demonstrate diffuse bilateral reticular infiltrates; rarely, patients have normal chest radiographs. Early gas exchange abnormalities include a decrease in the DL_{CO} and oxygen desaturation during exercise. Arterial blood gases may show variable degrees of hypoxemia at rest and a chronic respiratory alkalosis; with more severe disease, $PaCO_2$ may rise and acidosis may occur. PFTs demonstrate a restrictive abnormality with decreased lung volumes (especially TLC), but usually no evidence of airflow obstruction ($FEV_1/FVC > 0.75$).

II. **Initial evaluation** should include a careful history focusing on possible reversible causes of lung injury. Particular attention should be given to exposure to dusts, fumes, and drugs with known pulmonary toxicity. In addition, the duration of illness should be estimated by noting the rate of progression of symptoms, and especially by reviewing previous chest radiographs. This information may be useful in limiting the differential diagnosis as well as in planning subsequent diagnostic tests. Although the etiology may be identified from a careful history, diagnosis often requires microscopic examination of lung tissue. Histologic diagnosis is advisable unless the injury is due to a known etiology or the patient's condition is improving. A pathologic diagnosis should be obtained before initiation of steroid or immunosuppressive therapy. The method of lung biopsy utilized depends on the suspected diagnosis.
　A. **FOB with transbronchial lung biopsy** provides small samples but should be the initial procedure if the leading diagnostic possibilities are infection, cancer, sarcoidosis, or other conditions with specific, well-defined, widespread histologic abnormalities. **BAL** may provide evidence for CMV, PCP, and rare conditions such as alveolar proteinosis (lipoproteinaceous material), eosinophilic granuloma (X-bodies), and idiopathic hemosiderosis (iron-laden macrophages). BAL does not aid in the diagnosis of idiopathic pulmonary fibrosis, although the cell count and differential of the BAL fluid may have limited prognostic value.
　B. **Open lung biopsy** requires thoracotomy but provides an opportunity to study a relatively large amount of tissue for diagnosis. This is the procedure of choice

when transbronchial lung biopsy is nondiagnostic or contraindicated (see Pneumonia, Pulmonary Aspiration, and Lung Abscess) or when IPF or another syndrome with a variable and patchy histologic appearance is likely. A large biopsy sample also allows a more accurate assessment of the relative degree of active inflammation versus fibrosis.

C. **Monitoring of disease activity.** Serial evaluation of the severity of breathlessness, radiographic changes, and physiologic derangements as judged by PFTs and arterial blood gases is used to assess the rate of progression of disease and to facilitate decisions concerning the initiation, continuation, and termination of therapy. [67]Gallium scans and BAL are procedures of uncertain utility in following the course of disease. Data regarding their usefulness in predicting the degree of inflammatory activity are conflicting, and these tests are not recommended for routine follow-up study of patients with IPF.

III. **Therapy**

A. **General therapy.** Potentially injurious occupational, environmental, and drug exposures should be discontinued if possible. Appropriate therapy should be directed toward management of heart failure, infection, or other identified treatable etiologies for interstitial lung disease.

B. **Supplemental oxygen.** PaO_2 or oxygen saturation should be evaluated both at rest and during exercise. Supplemental oxygen, with appropriate increases during exercise, should be prescribed when appropriate.

C. **Treatment of specific interstitial lung diseases**

1. **Sarcoidosis** is a granulomatous disease of unknown etiology with protean clinical manifestations and an unpredictable natural course. Up to two thirds of patients who initially present with sarcoidosis will have resolution or improvement in symptoms or radiographic abnormalities over the following several years, with chronic disease developing in only a minority of patients. Because of the waxing and waning nature of the illness and the lack of controlled studies, it has been difficult to prove that steroids actually improve outcome. Steroids are, however, indicated for ophthalmologic disease or for significant impairment of pulmonary, cardiac, neurologic, renal, or endocrine function (i.e., hypercalcemia). In an asymptomatic patient with parenchymal infiltrates and a mild to moderate restrictive defect, decisions regarding initiation of therapy should be individualized. If steroids are withheld, the patient must be closely followed. Deterioration of vital capacity, gas exchange, or diffusing capacity is an indication for initiation of steroid therapy. Prednisone, 30–40 mg qd, is an effective starting dose. If studies obtained 4–8 weeks later show no response, steroids should be discontinued gradually. If a clinical response is obtained, prednisone should be tapered to the lowest dose that maintains the clinical response (usually >15 mg qod) and maintained for approximately 1 year before one attempts to discontinue therapy completely. Serial evaluation should be performed every 2 months initially, gradually lengthening the intervals to about 4–5 months; patients should be carefully followed for at least 2 years after steroids have been stopped. Immunosuppressive agents and inhaled corticosteroids have not been definitively shown to be beneficial in sarcoidosis lung disease. However, chloroquine, hydroxychloroquine, and methotrexate have all been used successfully in the management of severe mucocutaneous sarcoidosis.

2. **IPF** has a highly variable but progressive course, with a median survival of less than 5 years from presentation. Relatively good prognostic factors include young age, recent onset of symptoms, less severe breathlessness and infiltrates at presentation, predominantly cellular histology (as opposed to fibrosis), and initial responsiveness to steroids (*Thorax* 35:171, 1980). Longitudinal evaluation of clinical, radiographic, and physiologic data has been shown to predict cellular and fibrotic pathology and, more important, to determine clinical impairment in patients with IPF (*Am. Rev. Respir. Dis.* 133:97, 1986).

   a. **Steroids** (prednisone, 40–60 mg PO qd) should be initiated early in the course of the illness. Patients should be monitored as in sarcoidosis (see sec. **III.C.1**) and therapy discontinued or tapered to the lowest dose after

3–6 months if there has been a response. Fifty percent of treated patients have a subjective improvement, whereas 25% demonstrate objective improvement (*Thorax* 38:349, 1983).

    b. Cyclophosphamide, 100–120 mg PO qd (adjusted to maintain a white blood cell count >3000/μl), alone or in combination with low-dose steroids, may result in improvement in some cases that are unresponsive to steroids alone.

    c. Organ transplantation. Unilateral lung transplantation for IPF appears promising in patients with end-stage disease who are young and free of infection. Patients who are receiving even small dosages of maintenance steroids preoperatively may be at increased risk for infection or poor healing of the bronchial anastomosis following transplantation.

3. Radiation pneumonitis is a subacute inflammatory pneumonitis that occurs in response to radiation exposure to the lung, most commonly in the form of radiotherapy for malignant diseases. Symptoms are nonspecific—usually cough, dyspnea, and low-grade fevers. Radiographically, the presence of an infiltrate corresponding to the region of radiation exposure is characteristic. The incidence, severity, and time of onset of symptoms depend on several factors, the most important of which are the total radiation dose, the fractionation schedule, and the volume of lung irradiated. In general the onset of symptoms occurs 6–12 weeks after completion of radiotherapy; however, the onset can range from 1–6 months. Management of radiation pneumonitis involves first excluding other causes for pulmonary infiltrates, especially infections, recurrent tumors, and lymphangitic carcinomatosis. Mild symptoms can be managed with cough suppressants, antipyretics, and rest. Patients with more severe symptoms and a deterioration in gas exchange should be treated with corticosteroids. Prednisone is started at 60–100 mg/day, is continued until symptoms and gas exchange improve (usually 3–5 days), and then is tapered to 20–40 mg/day. After 4 weeks of treatment, attempts should be made to gradually taper the patient completely off prednisone. Only half of patients with radiation pneumonitis will respond to corticosteroid therapy.

Pulmonary Hypertension

Pulmonary hypertension may result from a variety of underlying diseases, including pulmonary venous hypertension (e.g., mitral stenosis), chronic hypoxemia (e.g., COPD), left-to-right shunts (e.g., atrial septal defects), or vascular diseases of the lungs (e.g., thromboembolic disease). Primary pulmonary hypertension (PPH) is an uncommon disease of unknown etiology characterized by dyspnea, fatigue, and occasionally syncope. It is a diagnosis of exclusion. It occurs most often in young women and usually results in death within several years of diagnosis. Evaluation of the patient should include chest radiography, PFTs, echocardiography, $\dot{V}/\dot{Q}$ scanning, and pulmonary artery catheterization. Pulmonary angiography and open lung biopsy may be appropriate in some patients. Treatment should include therapy for the underlying disease in cases of secondary pulmonary hypertension.

I. Supplemental oxygen is beneficial in patients who are hypoxic.

II. Vasodilator therapy is effective in some patients with PPH but is infrequently helpful in secondary pulmonary hypertension. No single agent has been proven routinely effective, and long-term responses are infrequent. Because of the high risk of an adverse hemodynamic response (e.g., hypotension, arterial oxygen desaturation, worsening pulmonary hypertension), **therapy with these agents should only be initiated with the aid of invasive hemodynamic monitoring.** A vasodilator should not be used unless a beneficial effect (e.g., a decrease in pulmonary vascular resistance relative to systemic vascular resistance) can be demonstrated for that drug (*Ann. Intern. Med.* 103:258, 1985).

III. Anticoagulants should be used for thromboembolic pulmonary disease, but their role in PPH is controversial. Some evidence suggests that chronic microvascular thrombosis in the abnormal pulmonary vascular bed is involved in the pathophysiology of this disease, at least in a subset of patients with PPH (*Circulation* 82:841, 1990; *Circulation* 70:580, 1984). Because of this evidence, many centers advocate anticoagulation in patients with PPH.

IV. **Lung transplantation or heart-lung transplantation** may be appropriate in selected patients.

Hemoptysis

Hemoptysis is a nonspecific sign associated with many pulmonary diseases, including infection (e.g., bronchitis, lung abscess, tuberculosis, pneumonia), neoplasm (e.g., carcinoma, bronchial adenoma), cardiovascular disease (e.g., mitral stenosis, pulmonary embolus, pulmonary vascular malformations), and autoimmune disorders (e.g., Wegener's granulomatosis, Goodpasture's syndrome). Often, the specific etiology of hemoptysis is never determined.

I. **Diagnosis**

A. **History and physical examination.** The source of bleeding should be confirmed to be the respiratory tract and not the gastrointestinal tract or nasopharynx (see Chap. 14). An attempt should be made to estimate the amount of bleeding, although quantification is often difficult. The remainder of the clinical evaluation should focus on obtaining clues to the cause of hemoptysis.

B. **Laboratory studies** include a chest radiograph, sputum cytology, appropriate sputum stains and cultures, arterial blood gases, tests of hemostasis, and urinalysis to detect red cells or red cell casts that may be associated with Wegener's granulomatosis or Goodpasture's syndrome.

C. **Bronchoscopy** is indicated in patients with hemoptysis who have a risk factor for carcinoma, even if hemoptysis is minor and the radiograph normal. Risk factors include (1) age greater than 40 years, (2) significant smoking history, (3) hemoptysis of greater than 1-week duration, and (4) unexplained abnormality on chest radiograph (*Chest* 87:142, 1985). If bleeding is brisk, rigid bronchoscopy is required.

II. **Therapy** is tailored to the severity of the episode and the findings at bronchoscopy.

A. **Minor hemoptysis.** Therapy for minor bleeding or blood-streaked sputum should be directed at the underlying etiology.

B. **Massive hemoptysis** is defined as greater than 600 ml over 48 hours or quantities sufficient to impair gas exchange. The primary goals of therapy are to provide cardiopulmonary support and control bleeding while preventing asphyxiation, the major cause of mortality in patients with massive hemoptysis.

1. **Supportive care.** While awaiting surgical consultation, clinically stable patients should be positioned with the bleeding side in a dependent position to reduce aspiration of blood into the contralateral lung. Sedatives aid patient cooperation, but excessive sedation may suppress airway protection and mask signs of respiratory decompensation. Bed rest and mild cough suppression are helpful.

2. **Definitive therapy.** Prompt surgical resection of the bleeding site is the therapy of choice. Rigid bronchoscopy should be performed first to localize the the site of bleeding if possible and to isolate and ventilate the uninvolved lung. Contraindications to surgical resection include inoperable lung cancer and previous pulmonary function studies precluding pulmonary resection (e.g., a predicted postoperative FEV_1 of less than 800 ml). Potential therapeutic maneuvers in inoperable patients include tamponade of the bleeding bronchial segment with a balloon catheter, endobronchial cold saline or fibrinogen-thrombin solution lavage, intravenous vasopressin, and embolization of the bronchial artery supply to the bleeding segment. The use of angiography with selective bronchial artery embolization has gained increased acceptance in conditions of massive or submassive hemoptysis, especially in chronic lung diseases for which preservation of functional lung parenchyma is a consideration.

Pleural Effusion

Fluid normally travels from parietal pleura (systemic circulation) through the pleural space to the visceral pleura (pulmonary circulation) without accumulation of fluid in the pleural space. This movement of fluid through the pleural space is governed by hydrostatic and colloid-osmotic pressure differences between the systemic and pulmonary circulation. Transudative pleural effusions are formed when the normal hydrostatic or oncotic pressures are perturbed (e.g., increased mean capillary pressure in parietal pleural [right heart failure] or visceral pleural [left heart failure]; or decreased oncotic pressures in cirrhosis or nephrotic syndrome). Exudative pleural effusions occur when there is damage or disruption of the normal pleural membranes or vasculature leading to increased capillary permeability or decreased lymphatic drainage (e.g., tumor involvement of the pleural space, infection, inflammatory conditions, or trauma).

I. **Diagnosis.** Most pleural effusions require further evaluation unless their origin is clear (e.g., heart failure) and they are responding well to therapy.

   A. **Thoracentesis** can be safely performed, in the absence of disorders of hemostasis (see Chap. 18), on effusions demonstrating a thickness of greater than 10 mm on lateral decubitus films. Loculated effusions can be localized with ultrasonography or computed tomography. Proper technique will minimize the risk of pneumothorax and other complications.

      1. **Gross appearance.** Frank pus is diagnostic of an empyema (see sec. **II.B**), but confusion with chylous effusions can occur. Bloody effusions may be caused by trauma, tumor, or pulmonary infarction; however, introduction of as little as 1 ml blood into 500 ml fluid during a thoracentesis will impart a blood-tinged appearance to the effusion.

      2. **Lactic dehydrogenase (LDH) and protein concentrations** are useful for distinguishing transudative from exudative pleural effusions. Pleural fluid is considered exudative if (1) the ratio of pleural fluid protein to serum protein is greater than 0.5, (2) the ratio of pleural fluid LDH to serum LDH is greater than 0.6, or (3) pleural fluid LDH is greater than 200 IU/liter. Pleural effusions lacking all these characteristics are considered transudates. Most transudates are caused by HF, hepatic cirrhosis, or nephrotic syndrome and generally require no further investigation of the pleural space. Exudates have a large differential diagnosis, including infections, malignancy, collagen vascular diseases, drug reactions, and pulmonary infarction.

      3. **Other laboratory tests** are useful primarily for further evaluation of an exudate.

         a. **Cytology** is positive in approximately 60% of malignant effusions (*Mayo Clin. Proc.* 60:158, 1985). At least 100 ml fluid should be submitted to maximize diagnostic yield.

         b. **Stains and cultures** should be performed for aerobic and anaerobic bacteria, mycobacteria, and fungi.

         c. **Cell count and differential** are of limited value. The red blood cell count may be misleading (see sec. **I.A.1**). A predominance of lymphocytes (>50% of nucleated cells) should raise suspicion for lymphoma and tuberculosis but may be present in any chronic inflammatory exudate.

         d. **Amylase** in the effusion in a concentration that exceeds that of serum suggests pancreatitis or esophageal rupture.

         e. **Triglyceride** levels greater than 110 mg/dl indicate chylous effusions, which are caused by thoracic duct rupture from trauma, surgery, or malignancy (usually lymphoma).

         f. **Glucose** may be less than 60 mg/dl in parapneumonic effusions, rheumatoid arthritis, and tuberculosis.

         g. **pH** may be less than 7.30 in parapneumonic effusions, malignancy, tuberculosis, collagen vascular disease, esophageal rupture, or systemic acidosis.

   B. **Closed pleural biopsy** should be performed when the cause of an exudative pleural effusion cannot be determined by thoracentesis. For tuberculous effusions, pleural fluid cultures alone are positive in only 20–25% of cases; however, the combination of fluid studies and pleural biopsy (demonstrating granulomas or organisms) is 90% sensitive in establishing tuberculosis as the etiology of the effusion (*Arch. Intern. Med.* 144:325, 1984). For malignant effusions, pleural biopsies add a small but significant diagnostic yield to fluid cytology alone.

   C. Other diagnostic procedures. In patients in whom the results of two pleural biopsies and pleural fluid cytologies are nondiagnostic, up to 25% will ultimately be found to have malignancy. If malignancy is suspected, biopsy of other abnormal sites (e.g., a mediastinal or lung mass) may provide a tissue diagnosis. Open pleural biopsy improves the diagnostic yield for pleural metastases and mesothelioma. Evaluation for pulmonary emboli should always be considered for undiagnosed pleural effusions.

II. Treatment

   A. Symptomatic pleural effusions may require removal of large amounts of pleural fluid. The rapid removal of more than 1 liter of pleural fluid may rarely result in ipsilateral pulmonary edema, especially when reexpansion of the lung is accomplished with suction.

   B. Parapneumonic effusions are pleural effusions associated with bacterial pneumonia. Thoracentesis is required both as a reliable means of identifying a pathogen and as a guide to further management of the pleural space.

   1. Complicated parapneumonic effusions include those composed of gross pus and those with a positive Gram's stain or bacterial culture, a glucose less than 40 mg/dl, a pH less than 7.0, or a pH of 7.0–7.2 with LDH greater than 1000 IU/liter. The presence of any of these characteristics predicts the need for chest tube drainage of the pleural space (*Am. J. Med.* 69:507, 1980). Chronic empyemas may not drain completely with closed chest tubes; in these cases, thoracotomy with decortication is the most effective intervention. However, this procedure is generally reserved for young, otherwise healthy patients or those in whom more conservative measures such as open drainage fail. Instillation of streptokinase into the pleural cavity may occasionally promote chest tube drainage. There is no established role for repeated therapeutic thoracenteses in the treatment of complicated parapneumonic effusions.

   2. Uncomplicated parapneumonic effusions lack the aforementioned characteristics and should resolve with antimicrobial therapy for the underlying pneumonia. If the volume of fluid does not progressively decrease, the pleural fluid should be reevaluated.

   C. Malignant pleural effusions arise from tumor involvement of the pleura or mediastinum. Patients with malignancy are also at increased risk for pleural effusions from postobstructive pneumonia, pulmonary emboli, chylothorax, and drug or radiation reactions. If pleural tissue or cytology is positive for malignancy, or if other causes of effusion are reasonably excluded in a patient with malignancy, several therapeutic options exist.

   1. Therapeutic thoracentesis may improve patient comfort and relieve dyspnea. The subjective response to drainage and the rate of fluid reaccumulation should be monitored. Repeated thoracenteses are reasonable if there is symptomatic relief and if fluid reaccumulation is slow.

   2. Complete drainage via chest tube followed by sclerosis is an effective therapy for recurrent effusions. This treatment is recommended in patients whose symptoms are relieved with initial drainage but who have rapid reaccumulation of fluid. Doxycycline, 500 mg in 50 ml normal saline (NS), or minocycline, 300 mg in 50 ml NS, can be instilled in the pleural space. If, after 48 hours, the chest tube drainage remains high (>100 ml/day), a second dose of the sclerosing agent can be administered. The relative efficacy of these two agents as well as the value of a second sclerosis attempt are being evaluated. Bleomycin may also be an effective sclerosing agent, but it is generally more expensive. The use of lidocaine in the sclerosing agent solution (3 mg/kg to a maximum of 150 mg) helps decrease the discomfort associated with the procedure.

3. **Pleurectomy or pleural abrasion** requires thoracotomy and should be reserved for patients with a good prognosis when sclerosis has been ineffective.

4. **Chemotherapy and mediastinal radiation therapy** may control effusions in responsive tumors such as lymphoma or small-cell bronchogenic carcinoma but are seldom useful in metastatic carcinoma (see Chap. 19).

5. **Observation** alone may be appropriate in asymptomatic patients, particularly when they are in poor general condition and have other significant complications of malignancy.

Lung Transplantation

The results of lung transplantation have steadily improved over the last several years to the point where it is a viable option for patients with end-stage lung disease (*Clin. Chest Med.* 11:347, 1990). Patients with idiopathic pulmonary fibrosis, chronic obstructive lung disease, cystic fibrosis, and primary pulmonary hypertension have had successful transplants. Single lung transplantation (SLT), double lung transplantation (DLT), and heart-lung transplantation (HLT) are the currently used procedures. In general, selection criteria include the following: (1) a limited life expectancy based on the severity of the lung disease, (2) the absence of underlying systemic disease, (3) no mitigating psychosocial problems, and (4) a good emotional support structure. The age of the patient is also a consideration, with 45 to 60 years being the upper limits in most cases. Prior major thoracic surgery or pleurodesis also is a consideration in some cases due to the expected pleural adhesions that might complicate operative procedures. Systemic steroids have an adverse effect on the healing of bronchial anastomosis in SLT and DLT and should be reduced or discontinued if possible. Early referral of a prospective transplant candidate is suggested.

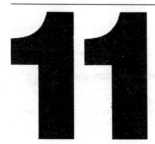

Renal Diseases

Steven B. Miller

Evaluation of the Patient with Renal Disease

The patient with renal disease may present with a variety of signs and symptoms. A careful history and physical examination will often lead to the correct diagnosis. Initial evaluation should emphasize identifying reversible causes of renal dysfunction.

I. **Initial studies** should include a **urinalysis** of a freshly voided specimen to look for proteinuria, hematuria, and pyuria, and to assess urine pH. Dirty brown sediment with epithelial cells and granular casts is seen with ischemic damage of the tubules. White blood cell casts are seen in pyelonephritis and red blood cell casts in glomerulonephritis. **Serum chemistries** should include electrolytes, creatinine (Cr), BUN, calcium, magnesium, phosphate, uric acid, and protein. If the serum Cr is stable, the **glomerular filtration rate** (GFR) can be estimated by using the following empiric formula for creatinine clearance (Cl_{Cr}):

$$Cl_{Cr} \ (ml/min) = \frac{(140 - age) \times weight \ (kg)}{72 \times serum \ Cr \ (mg/dl)} \times (0.85 \ for \ women)$$

This equation provides only a rough estimate of GFR and should not be used in place of a 24-hour urine collection for Cl_{Cr}. Weight should reflect ideal body weight.

II. **Supplementary studies** can be useful to further assess renal function and may aid in identifying specific disorders.

A. Twenty-four–hour urine studies include measurement of **urine volume, Cr, and protein.** GFR can be estimated by measurement of the Cl_{Cr}, which is calculated as follows:

$$Cl_{Cr} \ (ml/min) = \frac{urine \ Cr \ (mg/dl) \times volume \ (ml)}{plasma \ Cr \ (mg/dl) \times time \ (min)}$$

This value is useful in predicting remaining renal function, timing placement of dialysis access, and adjustment of drug dosage in renal insufficiency. When GFR is markedly reduced, measurement of Cl_{Cr} may actually overestimate true GFR. If the 24-hour Cr is less than 15–20 mg/kg lean body weight, the collection may be incomplete, leading to an underestimate of GFR. Twenty-four–hour protein studies are necessary for diagnosis of the nephrotic syndrome and are useful for following the response of certain glomerular diseases to treatment. Measurements of **24-hour urinary calcium, phosphate, oxalate, and uric acid** are indicated in the evaluation of some patients with renal stones.

B. **Supplementary blood tests.** Erythrocyte sedimentation rate, antinuclear and antiglomerular basement membrane antibody studies, antineutrophil cytoplasmic antibodies, angiotensin-converting enzyme and complement levels, cryoglobulin studies, hepatitis B serology, and antistreptococcal antibody titers are often useful for laboratory evaluation of glomerular disease. Serum protein electrophoresis should also be performed in selected patients with proteinuria to exclude multiple myeloma.

C. **Renal ultrasonography** noninvasively assesses kidney size and evaluates the collecting system. Small kidneys generally reflect chronic renal disease, although kidney size may not be diminished in some common chronic processes such as diabetes, amyloidosis, and multiple myeloma. Ultrasound is also used in the evaluation of acute renal failure, as the presence of hydronephrosis suggests an obstructive nephropathy.

D. Radionuclide scanning uses an isotope of hippuran to define effective renal plasma flow and a technetium-labeled isotope to estimate GFR. The renal scan also allows an assessment of the relative contribution of each kidney to overall renal function. This provides important information if unilateral nephrectomy is being considered. Renal scanning is useful when disruption of renal blood flow is suspected; the absence of perfusion of either kidney on scan should prompt further investigation of the renal vasculature. In addition, radionuclide studies can be used to follow renal function and rejection in transplanted kidneys.

E. Renal biopsy is an invasive procedure that may be indicated in patients with proteinuria (or nephrotic syndrome), hematuria, or casts suggestive of glomerular disease. Biopsy may also be useful in guiding the therapy of some glomerular diseases (e.g., associated with systemic lupus erythematosus) and often provides prognostic information. Finally, biopsy may be useful in patients with renal failure and kidneys of normal size when other studies fail to reveal a diagnosis. Prior to biopsy, the presence of two kidneys should be established, sterility of the urine ensured, and hypertension and abnormalities of hemostasis corrected. Packed red blood cells should be available for transfusion. The patient should not take drugs that interfere with platelet function (e.g., aspirin) before or immediately following the biopsy. Patients on dialysis who require a biopsy should have their dialysis sessions planned to avoid heparinization immediately after the biopsy.

Acute Renal Failure

Although there are many causes of acute renal failure (ARF) (Table 11-1), the syndrome uniformly presents with a sudden decline in the ability of the kidney to maintain homeostasis, resulting in failure to clear metabolic wastes, as well as electrolyte, acid-base, and volume disturbances. Renal failure may be oliguric (urine output <500 ml/day) or nonoliguric. The approach to patients with ARF is simplified by classifying it as prerenal, intrinsic, or postrenal obstructive. Table 11-2 includes laboratory tests that are helpful in differentiating *oliguric* prerenal azotemia (early, reversible injury) from *oliguric*, intrinsic ARF. Serum and urine should be obtained simultaneously before a fluid challenge or diuretic use is initiated. A fresh urine sample is essential, as urine retained in the bladder may not reflect current renal function. Temporary bladder catheterization is recommended to exclude lower urinary tract obstruction. It should be removed promptly unless obstruction is present.

I. Prerenal azotemia is a functional disorder that results from a decrease in effective arterial blood volume. Early correction of this decreased renal perfusion, with volume expansion, blood pressure support, or treatment of heart failure, may result in reversal of renal insufficiency; prolonged hypoperfusion may cause permanent renal damage. In prerenal states, the kidney attempts to reabsorb filtered sodium and the FE_{Na} is usually less than 1%. Intrinsic renal failure with damaged tubules results in sodium loss and an FE_{Na} greater than 1%. This calculation may not be diagnostic in patients who are elderly, who have received diuretics, or who have preexisting renal disease, acute glomerulonephritis (GN), vasculitis, radiocontrast-induced renal failure, or cirrhosis.

A. Hemodynamic monitoring is sometimes needed to assess intravascular volume, especially in patients with poor cardiac function. There is danger of excessive volume expansion in oliguric patients and a risk of inadequate volume replacement in prerenal patients. Invasive monitoring with a central venous pressure (CVP) or Swan-Ganz catheter is indicated if an accurate assessment of intravascular volume cannot be obtained by physical examination and an initial volume challenge.

Table 11-1. Causes of acute renal failure

  I. Prerenal (ischemic)
      A. Volume contraction
      B. Hypotension
      C. Heart failure (severe)
      D. Liver failure (?)

 II. Intrinsic renal failure
      A. Acute tubular necrosis (prolonged ischemia; nephrotoxic agents
          such as heavy metals, aminoglycosides, radiographic contrast
          media)
      B. Arteriolar injury
          1. Accelerated hypertension
          2. Vasculitis
          3. Microangiopathic (thrombotic thrombocytopenic purpura,
              hemolytic-uremic syndrome)
      C. Glomerulonephritis
      D. Acute interstitial nephritis (drug induced)
      E. Intrarenal deposition or sludging (uric acid, myeloma)

III. Postrenal
      A. Ureteral obstruction (clot, calculus, tumor, sloughed papillae,
          external compression)
      B. Bladder outlet obstruction (neurogenic bladder, prostatic hypertro-
          phy, carcinoma, calculus, clot, urethral stricture)

Table 11-2. Laboratory examination in oliguric ARF

Diagnosis	U/P Cr	U_{Na}	$FE_{Na}(\%)$	U osmolality
Prerenal azotemia	>40	<20	<1	>500
Oliguric ARF	<20	>40	>1	<350

Key: U = urine; P = plasma; FE_{Na} = fractional excretion of sodium = 100 × (U/P sodium)/(U/P creatinine).

B. Fluid challenge may be appropriate in oliguric patients who are not volume overloaded. The quantity of fluid to be given must be determined on an individual basis, but typically 500–1000 ml normal saline is infused over 30–60 minutes. Frequent cardiopulmonary examination is necessary. Such a volume challenge may result in increased urine flow in prerenal azotemia, but some cases of intrinsic renal failure may also respond with increased urine output; therefore, the response to volume challenge must be interpreted with caution. If there is no response, volume infusion can be followed by 100–400 mg IV furosemide in an effort to promote urine flow. Occasionally, the addition of metolazone, 5–10 mg PO, will facilitate initiation of diuresis induced by volume repletion and furosemide. If successful, the lowest effective dose of furosemide can be continued in the volume-repleted patient, with careful monitoring to avoid volume depletion. Diuretic administration may convert oliguric ARF to nonoliguric ARF, which simplifies management and may improve prognosis. It should be noted, however, that large doses of furosemide given intravenously for prolonged periods may cause hearing loss, particularly when renal function is impaired.
II. Obstructive nephropathy. Acute renal failure may be secondary to upper or lower urinary tract obstruction. Early diagnosis and relief of obstruction are essential to prevent permanent renal damage. Lower tract obstruction can be assessed (and relieved) by temporary bladder catheterization, while renal ultrasonography will aid in the diagnosis of upper tract obstruction. Urine flow often increases dramat-

ically after relief of obstruction. This postobstructive diuresis is often physiologic and reflects excretion of fluid, urea, and sodium accumulated during the period of obstruction; however, inappropriate loss of volume and electrolytes may occur after relief of severe acute bilateral obstruction. If the **postobstructive diuresis** appears excessive, replacement of fluid and electrolytes should be guided by daily weights, urine output, orthostatic blood pressure changes, and serum and urine electrolyte concentrations. The appropriate initial replacement fluid in such cases is usually 0.45% saline.

III. **Intrinsic renal failure** results from a variety of injuries to the renal blood vessels, glomeruli, tubules, or interstitium (see Table 11-1). These insults may be toxic, immunologic, or idiopathic; they may be iatrogenic and may develop as part of a systemic disorder or as a primary renal disease. Specific syndromes that are preventable or treatable are discussed in the following paragraphs.

A. **Radiocontrast nephropathy** occurs with increased frequency in patients with long-standing diabetes mellitus or preexisting renal insufficiency. Volume depletion, multiple myeloma, heart failure (HF), and age greater than 65 years may also be risk factors. The ARF of contrast nephropathy tends to be oliguric and the serum creatinine peaks in the first 72 hours. Patients often recover renal function over 7–14 days. Preventive measures may decrease the incidence of ARF. Patients at risk who require contrast studies should be well hydrated, preferably for 24 hours prior to the study. Patients with normal cardiac function can receive mannitol, 25 g in 100 ml of 0.45% saline IV over 30 minutes, 1 hour before the study, followed by 25 g mannitol in 500 ml of 0.45% saline IV at 150–200 ml/hour during and for 2 hours after the procedure. Subsequently, urinary volume loss should be replaced by infusion of 0.45% saline for 24 hours. Serum electrolytes should be monitored.

B. **Aminoglycoside nephrotoxicity** may cause ARF that is often nonoliguric and results from direct toxicity to the proximal tubules. Predisposing factors include prolonged exposure to these drugs, advanced age, volume depletion, liver disease, and preexisting renal disease. Patients in whom ARF develops from aminoglycoside therapy have usually received the medication for at least 5 days. The risk of aminoglycoside nephrotoxicity may be minimized by frequent monitoring of drug levels with appropriate dosage adjustments to keep levels in the therapeutic range.

C. **Pigment-induced renal injury** occurs during **hemolysis** or **rhabdomyolysis.** With rhabdomyolysis, early aggressive hydration to replace the fluid that is lost into necrotic muscle may be beneficial. Diuresis to decrease tubular pigment reabsorption may be promoted by mannitol, 25 g IV. If sufficient urine flow can be established, IV infusion of bicarbonate, 2–3 ampules in 1 liter of 5% dextrose in water (D/W) to maintain urine pH greater than 6.5 may also be useful by preventing dissociation of myoglobin and hemoglobin into potentially toxic compounds.

D. **Acute uric acid nephropathy** may result from cell lysis with consequent hyperuricemia during the course of cytotoxic therapy of hematologic malignancies. Renal failure results from intratubular precipitation of uric acid. Prevention involves decreasing uric acid production prior to cytotoxic therapy with allopurinol, 600 mg PO initially, followed by 100–300 mg/day. In addition, forced alkaline diuresis to maintain a urine pH of 6.5–7.0 will help prevent uric acid precipitation. This may be accomplished with acetazolamide, 250 mg PO qid, or infusion of sodium bicarbonate, 2–3 ampules in 1 liter of 5% D/W. If tumor lysis results in hyperphosphatemia, alkalinization should be avoided because of the increased risk of calcium phosphate precipitation.

E. **Allergic interstitial nephritis** secondary to drugs is often unrecognized and may result in classic signs that include fever, rash, and renal dysfunction. When present, eosinophilia, elevated serum immunoglobulin E (IgE), and eosinophiluria suggest the diagnosis. A high index of suspicion for interstitial nephritis must be maintained in patients taking drugs such as the penicillins, sulfonamides, and nonsteroidal anti-inflammatory drugs (NSAIDs). In most cases, renal insufficiency will resolve with discontinuation of the offending agent. In severe or prolonged cases, however, a 1-week course of prednisone, 60 mg PO qd, may hasten recovery (*Ann. Intern. Med.* 93:735, 1980).

F. **Glomerular disease** of a rapidly progressive nature can result in ARF. Histologically, glomeruli demonstrate extensive crescent formation on biopsy, but this morphologic end point is shared by a variety of antecedent events (see The Glomerulonephropathies).

IV. **Management of ARF** can often be accomplished with conservative measures alone. Dialysis may be required depending on the severity of renal impairment, the resulting complications, and the presence of other diseases.

A. **Conservative medical management** of ARF is facilitated by weighing the patient daily, accurately recording fluid intake and output, and frequently (at least 3 times/week) measuring serum electrolytes, BUN, Cr, calcium, and phosphate.

1. **Fluid management** requires accurate clinical judgment of intravascular volume. Volume depletion may contribute to ARF by decreasing renal perfusion and must be corrected, occasionally with the aid of invasive hemodynamic monitoring (see sec. **I.A**). Once any volume deficit has been corrected, fluid and sodium balance must be carefully regulated to avoid volume overload. Fluid replacement should be equal to insensible loss (about 500 ml/day in afebrile patients) plus urinary and other drainage losses. Daily salt intake should be restricted to 2–4 g NaCl. The larger urine output and diuretic responsiveness in nonoliguric ARF allow more liberal administration of fluids (and nutrients), facilitating the general care of the patient. Because patients with nonoliguric ARF may lose significant amounts of fluid and electrolytes in the urine, careful attention to volume status and serum electrolyte levels is necessary to avoid electrolyte and water depletion. Hyponatremia in patients with ARF is usually secondary to volume expansion, whereas hypernatremia is most often caused by overly aggressive diuresis with inadequate intake of free water.

2. **Dietary modification. Protein** intake should be limited to approximately 0.5 g/kg/day to decrease nitrogenous waste production. Total caloric intake should be 35–50 kcal/kg/day to avoid catabolism. Patients who are highly catabolic (e.g., postsurgical and burn patients) or malnourished require higher protein intake and should be considered for early institution of dialysis (see sec. **IV.B**). Restricting intake of salt to 2–4 g/day NaCl will facilitate volume management. **Potassium** intake should be restricted to 40 mEq/day and **phosphorus** to 800 mg/day. Ingestion of **magnesium**-containing compounds should be avoided.

3. **Blood pressure. Hypotension** should be promptly evaluated and corrected with volume expansion or vasopressors, depending on the patient's intravascular volume status. **Hypertension** should be managed aggressively. Volume overload is frequently a contributing factor. Antihypertensive medications that do not decrease renal blood flow (e.g., clonidine, prazosin) or vasodilators are preferred. Hypertensive crises can be managed with IV sodium nitroprusside (see Chap. 4), but thiocyanate, a toxic metabolite of nitroprusside, is excreted by the kidneys and may accumulate in renal failure. Thiocyanate levels should therefore be closely monitored during therapy with this agent. Intravenous labetalol is an effective alternative and avoids the problem of thiocyanate toxicity (*N. Engl. J. Med.* 323:1177, 1990).

4. **Phosphate and calcium.** Phosphate levels may remain elevated despite dietary restriction. Aluminum hydroxide–containing antacids such as Basaljel or Amphojel, 15–30 ml PO tid with meals, are used to decrease intestinal absorption of phosphate. Concomitant with elevated phosphate, serum calcium is often low but usually does not require specific treatment. The calcium-phosphate product should be kept less than 60 to avoid metastatic calcification.

5. **Uric acid.** Mild elevations of uric acid levels are frequent in ARF but do not have any clearly deleterious effect on the kidneys. In some types of ARF (e.g.,

associated with rhabdomyolysis), however, uric acid may be quite elevated (>20 mg/dl) and should be treated with allopurinol, 100 mg PO qd.

6. **Hyperkalemia** is common and, if mild (<6 mEq/liter), can be treated with dietary restriction and potassium-binding resins. More marked hyperkalemia, or hyperkalemia accompanied by ECG or neuromuscular abnormalities, requires immediate medical therapy (see Chap. 3). Hyperkalemia refractory to medical therapy is an indication for dialysis.

7. **Metabolic acidosis.** Mild acidosis (serum bicarbonate level ≥ 16 mEq/liter) does not require therapy. More marked acidosis should be corrected with sodium bicarbonate, 325–650 mg PO tid. Severe uncompensated acidosis (serum pH <7.2) requires prompt medical therapy with parenteral sodium bicarbonate (see Chap. 3). Caution must be exercised with sodium bicarbonate therapy, however, since the additional sodium may exacerbate volume overload. In addition, excessive alkali use may decrease the ionized calcium concentration and cause tetany. Correctable causes of metabolic acidosis should be sought and treated. Acidosis unresponsive to medical therapy is an indication for dialysis.

8. **Drug dosages** of agents excreted by the kidney must be adjusted for the level of renal function (see Appendix D).

9. **Infection** is common and accounts for a significant proportion of deaths associated with ARF. Antimicrobial therapy is dictated by the infectious process; potentially nephrotoxic agents should not be withheld if needed. Most antimicrobial dosages need to be adjusted for the degree of renal failure.

10. **Gastrointestinal bleeding** may occur in ARF, reflecting both mucosal changes and altered platelet function secondary to uremia. Major bleeding sources should be excluded (see Chap. 14 for management).

11. **Anemia** is common and usually caused by decreased red cell production and increased blood loss. The hematocrit often falls below 30%. Transfusion is appropriate for patients with active bleeding or symptoms referable to anemia (see Chap. 18).

B. **Dialysis** for ARF is indicated when **severe hyperkalemia, acidosis,** or **volume overload** cannot be controlled by conservative measures. Additional indications include **uremic pericarditis, encephalopathy,** or **nutritional requirements** that would precipitate volume overload or uremia. A patient may not need dialysis early in the course of ARF but should be evaluated daily to assess the need for such intervention. Technical aspects of dialysis are considered under Renal Replacement Therapies.

1. **Uremic signs and symptoms** become prominent as BUN and Cr rise. Morbidity and mortality may be reduced if the BUN is maintained below 100 mg/dl, and dialysis is often started empirically as the BUN approaches this level. **Neurologic manifestations** (e.g., lethargy, seizures, myoclonus, asterixis, and peripheral polyneuropathies) may develop with uremia and are an indication for dialysis. **Uremic pericarditis** is often manifested only as a pericardial friction rub and should be treated with dialysis; heparin use during dialysis should be minimized in these patients (see Renal Replacement Therapies, sec **I.C**). Patients with pericarditis who do not respond to dialysis, or in whom signs of pericardial tamponade develop, require pericardial drainage.

2. **Nutritional considerations.** Patients with ARF are often highly catabolic or need dietary supplementation to promote wound healing. Dialysis is indicated in patients who need aggressive nutritional therapy (e.g., hyperalimentation) that cannot be provided within the limitations imposed by the volume and dietary restrictions of conservative management.

V. **Management of the recovery phase of ARF** is best accomplished by careful monitoring of serum electrolytes, volume status, and urinary fluid and electrolyte loss. As with obstructive nephropathy, a diuretic phase may occur during recovery and is often physiologic. Management is similar to that for postobstructive diuresis (see sec. **II**). Renal function may continue to improve for several weeks to months after the patient enters the recovery phase.

The Glomerulonephropathies

Glomerular disease may be **primary** or **secondary** to a systemic process and may present in a variety of ways. **Acute glomerulonephritis** (GN) is often characterized by hematuria, red blood cell casts, and proteinuria, along with hypertension, edema, and deteriorating renal function. Other glomerulopathies may present primarily with significant proteinuria, an unremarkable urine sediment, and a relatively preserved GFR. Renal biopsy often provides useful diagnostic, therapeutic, and prognostic information in glomerular disease. Treatment usually involves the use of corticosteroids. In the following sections, cytotoxic therapy is recommended for certain types of GN in consultation with a nephrologist. Initial dosages of these agents are suggested, but these may require adjustment to keep the WBC count above 3000–3500/μl. White blood cell counts should be checked weekly while cytotoxic agents are administered to decrease the potential for excessive immunosuppression and infectious complications.

I. **Minimal change disease** (MCD) presents with nephrotic syndrome (see The Nephrotic Syndrome). The pathologic diagnosis is confirmed by normal light microscopy, negative immunofluorescence, and foot process fusion on electron microscopy. About 80% of adults with MCD respond to prednisone, 1 mg/kg/day PO, with a decrease in proteinuria to less than 3 g/day, or a remission of the nephrotic syndrome. Patients who respond should have steroids tapered over 3 months and discontinued. Failure to respond may reflect an error in diagnosis; MCD is most commonly confused with early focal segmental glomerulosclerosis. Urinary protein should be carefully monitored during steroid taper. If relapse is documented, reinstitution of prednisone is often effective. Treatment with cytotoxic agents may be indicated in patients who relapse frequently or who do not respond to or cannot be tapered off high dosages of steroids. Cyclophosphamide, 2 mg/kg/day PO for 8 weeks, or chlorambucil, 0.2 mg/kg/day PO for 8–12 weeks, are typical regimens. Progression to chronic renal failure is unusual. Certain neoplastic disorders such as Hodgkin's disease and non-Hodgkin's lymphoma have been associated with the development of MCD and should be considered in the appropriate setting.

II. **Focal segmental glomerulosclerosis** is an idiopathic glomerular disorder usually characterized by hypertension, renal insufficiency, and nephrotic syndrome. Histologic findings include foot process fusion and segmental sclerosis of glomeruli. The disease slowly progresses to chronic renal failure within 5 to 10 years of diagnosis. No therapy has been proved to be of benefit in the treatment of this disorder, but a trial of prednisone, 60 mg PO qd, for at least 1 month may be appropriate in an effort to reduce proteinuria and slow progression to chronic renal failure (*Medicine* 65:304, 1986). Cyclosporine may provide some therapeutic benefit but is experimental at this time.

III. **Membranous glomerulonephropathy** characteristically presents with the nephrotic syndrome, although some patients have non-nephrotic proteinuria. The GFR is usually normal or near normal, and the urinary sediment is often unremarkable. Biopsy demonstrates thickening of the glomerular capillary wall secondary to subepithelial deposits of IgG and C3. Membranous nephropathy may be a primary renal disease or may be associated with systemic diseases (e.g., malignancies, systemic lupus erythematosus) or drug ingestions (e.g., penicillamine, gold). The natural history of the disease includes spontaneous remissions and exacerbations, making evaluation of potential therapy difficult. About 20% of patients will progress to end-stage renal disease, whereas the remainder will have variable degrees of remission. The optimal therapy of membranous glomerulonephropathy has not been established. Treatment options include high-dose alternate-day steroids (*N. Engl. J. Med.* 320:210, 1989) and the combination of a cytotoxic agent (e.g., chlorambucil) and steroids (*N. Engl. J. Med.* 320:8, 1989). **Renal vein thrombosis** with the potential for systemic thromboembolism may complicate this disease. A sudden decrease in GFR should prompt evaluation for renal vein thrombosis with Doppler ultrasonography or MRI; in some cases, venography may be required.

IV. **Membranoproliferative glomerulonephritis** (MPGN) has a variety of clinical presentations, including acute GN, nephrotic syndrome (see The Nephrotic Syndrome), and asymptomatic hematuria and proteinuria. The diagnosis should be suspected if these clinical findings are associated with low complement levels. Histologic findings include mesangial proliferation and alterations of the glomerular basement membrane (GBM) with subendothelial (type I) or intramembranous (type II) deposits. MPGN progresses slowly to renal failure. No therapy, including the use of dipyridamole and aspirin, has been shown to improve disease-free survival, despite a trend toward better outcome in some studies (*Am. J. Kidney Dis.* 15:445, 1989).

V. **Idiopathic rapidly progressive glomerulonephritis** (RPGN) presents with an acute deterioration in renal function, proteinuria (sometimes nephrotic range), and an active urinary sediment with hematuria and red cell casts. Oliguria may be present. Many patients note a preceding viral-like illness. As many as 75% of patients with idiopathic RPGN may respond to high-dose pulse steroid therapy—for example, methylprednisolone, 30 mg/kg (up to 3 g) IV qod for 3 doses, followed by prednisone, 2 mg/kg PO qod for 2 months, with a subsequent taper over 4 months (*Am. J. Nephrol.* 2:57, 1982). In patients with extrarenal disease suggestive of vasculitis or a renal biopsy demonstrating necrotizing glomerulonephritis, the addition of cyclophosphamide, 2 mg/kg PO qd, may be beneficial.

VI. **Anti-GBM antibody disease** may present with lung and renal involvement (Goodpasture's syndrome) or with renal disease alone. Diagnosis is based on either the presence of anti-GBM antibodies in the serum or the linear deposition of antibody along the basement membrane on renal biopsy. Anti-GBM disease is often rapidly progressive, requiring urgent diagnosis and treatment. Therapy may not be effective if the patient is already oliguric or receiving dialysis, or has a Cr greater than 6.5 mg/dl. The accepted therapeutic strategy in this disease is clearance of anti-GBM antibodies from the serum with concomitant suppression of formation of new antibodies. Daily total volume plasmapheresis for approximately 2 weeks, in combination with cyclophosphamide, 2 mg/kg PO qd for 8 weeks, and prednisone, 60 mg PO qd tapered over 8 weeks, may be effective. Progress is monitored by frequent clinical evaluation and measurement of anti-GBM antibody titers. Immune suppression should be continued until the anti-GBM antibody is undetectable. Relapse is common and tends to occur within the first several months.

VII. **Systemic lupus erythematosus** (SLE) may involve the kidney and can present as slowly progressive azotemia with urinary abnormalities, as nephrotic syndrome, or as rapidly progressive renal insufficiency. A wide variety of histologic changes may be seen on renal biopsy, including mesangial, membranous, focal or diffuse proliferative, and crescentic GN. Renal biopsy is useful in SLE for evaluating disease activity and assessing irreversible changes such as glomerular sclerosis, tubular atrophy, and interstitial fibrosis. A predominance of irreversible changes with little acute inflammation portends a poor response to therapy and should modify the aggressiveness of immunosuppressive treatment. Steroids are the mainstay of treatment. Patients with severe renal disease are initially treated with methylprednisolone, 500 mg IV q12h for 3 days, followed by oral prednisone, 0.5–1.0 mg/kg PO qd. Prednisone should then be tapered over 6–8 weeks to the lowest dosage that controls disease activity, preferably using an alternate-day regimen. The addition of cytotoxic agents to maintenance steroid therapy may result in better preservation of renal function and may decrease the progression of renal scarring (*N. Engl. J. Med.* 311:491, 1984; *N. Engl. J. Med.* 314:614, 1986). The use of plasmapheresis remains controversial.

VIII. **Systemic vasculitides** (see Chap. 24) often present with clinical features of acute GN that may be rapidly progressive. Wegener's granulomatosis usually responds to a combination of (1) cyclophosphamide, 2 mg/kg/day PO continued for at least 1 year beyond induction of remission with subsequent taper, plus (2) prednisone, 1 mg/kg PO qd for 4 weeks followed by slow taper and conversion to alternate-day therapy over the next 6–9 months (*Ann. Intern. Med.* 98:16, 1983). The combination of prednisone and cyclophosphamide may also be effective in other forms of necrotizing GN, such as microscopic polyarteritis nodosa.

IX. Infection-related glomerulonephritis may occur in association with a variety of infectious processes, including bacterial endocarditis, visceral abscesses, and infected shunts. Treatment of the underlying infection (e.g., antimicrobials, drainage) may result in improvement or resolution of renal disease. **Poststreptococcal glomerulonephritis** may follow group A beta-hemolytic streptococcal infection of the upper respiratory tract or skin. There is no specific therapy, and treatment consists of supportive measures. Some groups have reported a human immunodeficiency virus (HIV)-associated GN that is similar to focal segmental glomerulosclerosis and is usually seen in patients who abuse IV drugs (*Am. J. Nephrol.* 9:441, 1989).

The Nephrotic Syndrome

The nephrotic syndrome is a glomerulonephropathy that is characterized by proteinuria (>3.5 g/day), hypoalbuminemia, hyperlipidemia, and edema. It may appear as a manifestation of primary glomerular disease or may be associated with systemic diseases such as diabetes mellitus, amyloidosis, multiple myeloma, SLE, or many other disorders. Therapy includes treatment of the underlying disease and symptomatic management.

I. Edema should be controlled with bed rest, salt restriction (2–3 g/day), and judicious use of diuretics. Despite massive edema, these patients are subject to intravascular volume depletion, and diuretic therapy may lead to severe volume contraction with decreased renal perfusion. Nevertheless, diuretic therapy is appropriate for controlling edema that is causing respiratory compromise, skin breakdown, or difficulty in ambulation. Furosemide alone or in combination with metolazone is often effective; the dosage must be individualized. Occasionally, parenteral furosemide is necessary, with or without prior infusion of albumin to mobilize fluid into the vascular space.

II. Hyperlipidemia due to the nephrotic syndrome is difficult to treat, and its role in cardiovascular morbidity in nephrotic patients is controversial (*Nephron* 27:53, 1981). Dietary restriction of cholesterol and saturated fat seems prudent. Lovastatin is effective in improving the lipoprotein profile in patients with the nephrotic syndrome, but the efficacy and long-term benefit of treatment with lipid-lowering drugs have not been established (*Am. J. Kidney Dis.* 15:8, 1990).

III. Thromboembolic complications. The nephrotic syndrome produces a hypercoagulable state, and the clinician should maintain a high index of suspicion for thromboemboli. Renal vein thrombosis is common. If embolization occurs, anticoagulation with heparin followed by long-term warfarin therapy is indicated (see Chap. 17).

IV. Dietary protein restriction, 0.6–0.7 g/kg, may be appropriate for nephrotic patients with renal insufficiency (see Chronic Renal Failure, sec. **II.A.1**), but an amount of protein equal to that lost in the urine should be added to the calculated protein restriction to give the total daily protein intake.

Chronic Renal Failure

Chronic renal failure (CRF) may result from many different renal insults. Because of the compensatory ability of remaining nephrons, declining renal function is often asymptomatic until the very late stages of the process. When CRF progresses to end-stage renal disease (ESRD), renal replacement therapy may be required. The decline in GFR may be followed by recording the reciprocal of serum Cr versus time. The resulting plot is usually linear, unless there is a superimposed renal insult, and is useful in end-stage planning and predicting the time when dialysis is needed (usually when GFR is less than 10 ml/min). Conservative medical treatment of CRF and attention to factors that are known to cause an acute decline in renal function may postpone the need for dialysis in these patients.

Table 11-3. Causes of a rapid deterioration of renal function in chronic renal failure

---

I. Decrease in effective arterial blood volume
   A. Volume depletion
   B. Worsening congestive heart failure

II. Alterations in blood pressure
   A. Hypertension
   B. Hypotension, including that induced by antihypertensive medication

III. Infection

IV. Urinary tract obstruction

V. Nephrotoxic agents

VI. Renal vein thrombosis

I. **Acute deterioration in CRF** (Table 11-3). A sudden decline in GFR that is more rapid than expected should prompt a search for a superimposed, reversible process.

   A. **Volume depletion** resulting in decreased renal perfusion is a common cause of deterioration of renal function in CRF. Ideally, patients with CRF should be well hydrated as suggested by the presence of trace pedal edema.

   B. **Depression of cardiac output** may impair renal perfusion, thereby worsening CRF. Treatment that increases cardiac output may therefore improve renal function through enhanced renal blood flow. Afterload reduction may be particularly useful in these patients (see Chap. 6).

   C. **Drugs** may exacerbate CRF through direct toxicity to renal structures (e.g., aminoglycosides) or decreased renal perfusion (e.g., NSAIDs). Careful attention to drug dosing in patients with decreased GFR and avoidance of the unnecessary use of nephrotoxic agents is appropriate.

II. **Conservative management of CRF** includes measures intended to prevent and correct the metabolic derangements of renal failure and to preserve remaining renal function.

   A. **Dietary modification** is important as a method for controlling metabolic abnormalities and possibly for slowing progression of renal failure.

      1. **Protein restriction** will reduce accumulation of nitrogenous waste products. In addition, a low-protein diet may slow the progression of renal failure. Intake should be reduced to 0.6–0.7 g/kg/day of high biologic value protein when GFR falls below 30 ml/min. Adequate caloric intake (35–50 kcal/kg/day) must be provided to avoid endogenous protein catabolism, and patients should be followed carefully for evidence of malnutrition.

      2. **Potassium** should be restricted to 40 mEq/day when GFR falls below 20 ml/min.

      3. **Phosphate and calcium.** Renal failure results in phosphate retention with elevation of serum phosphate and a reciprocal fall in serum calcium. In addition, decreased generation of 1,25-dihydroxyvitamin D and skeletal resistance to the action of parathyroid hormone (PTH) further exacerbate hyperphosphatemia and hypocalcemia. These alterations result in elevation of PTH and secondary hyperparathyroidism, which, left unchecked, contributes to the renal osteodystrophy seen in CRF (see sec. III). Elevated phosphate may also play a role in the progression of renal failure. Dietary phosphorus should be restricted to 800–1000 mg/day when GFR is less than 50 ml/min. As GFR falls further, phosphate restriction becomes less effective and the addition of phosphate binders that prevent gastrointestinal phosphate absorption is indicated. These include aluminum hydroxide antacids, such as Amphojel or Basaljel, 15–30 ml or 1–3 capsules PO with meals, and calcium carbonate, 1–2 g PO with meals. The disadvantage of aluminum-containing phosphate binders is accumulation of aluminum in patients with CRF. Elevated tissue aluminum levels can cause osteomalacia and have been

implicated as a cause of encephalopathy in patients with CRF. Although calcium carbonate avoids these problems, large doses may be required to control phosphate levels and may result in hypercalcemia with the potential for extraskeletal calcification. Calcium carbonate should not be used until serum phosphate is less than 7 mg/dl, and a calcium–phosphate product less than 60 should be maintained to avoid the possibility of metastatic calcification. Vitamin D metabolites may be required in the treatment of hypocalcemia (see Chap. 23).

4. **Sodium and fluid restriction** must be determined on an individual basis, taking the patient's cardiovascular status into consideration. For most patients, a no-added salt diet (8 g NaCl/day) is palatable and adequate. If necessary, 24-hour urinary sodium loss can be determined to aid in sodium intake planning. Once a patient has reached an acceptable volume status, fluid intake should equal daily urine output plus an additional 500 ml for insensible loss. Fluid restriction is appropriate in patients with dilutional hyponatremia or excessive weight gain. The presence of heart failure or refractory hypertension requires greater restriction of salt and water.

5. **Magnesium** is excreted by the kidney and accumulates in CRF. Extradietary intake of magnesium (e.g., some antacids and cathartics) should be avoided.

B. **Hypertension** may accelerate the rate of decline of renal function in patients with CRF and should be treated aggressively (see Acute Renal Failure, sec. **IV.A.3,** and Chap. 4). Diuretic use must be carefully monitored to avoid volume depletion. Loop diuretics (e.g., furosemide) remain efficacious when GFR is less than 25 ml/min.

C. **Acidosis** is treated with oral sodium bicarbonate, 300–600 mg PO tid, when serum bicarbonate falls below 16 mEq/liter. The additional sodium load from such therapy, however, may require further dietary sodium restriction or administration of a diuretic.

D. **Anemia** is responsible for many of the symptoms of chronic renal failure and can be corrected with the use of recombinant human erythropoietin both in dialysis and predialysis patients. One should consider initiating treatment in patients with symptoms or earlier in patients with known cardiovascular disease. Starting dosage is 50 U/kg SQ 3 times a week (*Am. J. Kidney Dis.* 10:128, 1990) (see Chap. 18). Hypertension may complicate therapy and should be aggressively treated.

III. **Renal osteodystrophy** (*Kidney Int.* 38:193, 1990) refers to the skeletal disorders seen in chronic renal failure. The major histologic categories are (1) **secondary hyperparathyroidism** (high-turnover bone disease, osteitis fibrosa), due to hyperphosphatemia, hypocalcemia, deficient production of calcitriol [1,25(OH)$_2$D], and skeletal resistance to PTH; (2) **low-turnover bone disease** (osteomalacia and aplastic bone disease), most often due to aluminum (Al) retention from Al-containing phosphate binders and dialysate; and (3) **mixed renal osteodystrophy,** with features of both.

A. **Clinical manifestations** include bone pain, fractures, skeletal deformity, proximal muscle weakness, pruritus, and extraskeletal calcification. Serum phosphorus is elevated and serum calcium is usually low. Hypercalcemia may develop in Al-related bone disease, marked parathyroid hyperplasia, or during treatment with calcium and calcitriol. Serum PTH, measured by immunoassays for intact hormone, is markedly elevated in osteitis fibrosa, and much less elevated in low-turnover bone disease. X-ray findings of osteitis fibrosa include subperiosteal resorption and patchy osteosclerosis; pseudofractures may be seen in osteomalacia.

B. **Diagnosis.** Certain clinical features suggest a particular histologic category. Pruritus or periarticular calcification points to hyperparathyroidism as the dominant lesion, while spontaneous fractures, relatively low serum PTH levels, or hypercalcemia suggest Al-related bone disease. Serum Al levels do not reflect tissue Al content; definitive diagnosis of Al-related bone disease requires bone biopsy.

C. **Management.** Therapy should be started early in the course of progressive renal failure. Goals include (1) maintenance of normal serum calcium and phosphorus levels, (2) suppression of secondary hyperparathyroidism, (3) prevention of extraskeletal calcification, (4) reversal of histologic abnormalities of bone, and (5) prevention and therapy of Al toxicity.

1. **Correction of hyperphosphatemia** (see Chap. 23). Dietary phosphate should be restricted to 0.6–0.9 g/day. Calcium carbonate is the phosphate binder of choice. Calcium citrate and other citrate preparations (e.g., Shohl's solution) should not be used because they promote intestinal Al absorption. The goal is to maintain predialysis serum phosphorus levels between 4.5 and 6.0 mg/dl. Use of Al-containing phosphate binders should be kept to a minimum.

2. **Calcitriol,** or 1,25(OH)$_2$D (see Chap. 23) is often required to suppress hyperparathyroidism despite control of hyperphosphatemia. The usual dose is 0.25–1.0 μg PO qd, which is adjusted to maintain serum calcium between 10.5 and 11.0 mg/dl. Serum calcium should be measured twice a week and the dose can be adjusted at 2- to 4-week intervals. The major side effect is hypercalcemia, which is especially likely if Al-related bone disease is present. If low doses of oral calcitriol cause hypercalcemia, substitution of IV calcitriol, 1.0–2.5 μg 3 times a week, may suppress hyperparathyroidism more effectively, with less hypercalcemia (*N. Engl. J. Med.* 321:274, 1989).

3. **Parathyroidectomy** may be required to control severe hyperparathyroidism (*Am. J. Med.* 84:23, 1988). A bone biopsy must be done to confirm the presence of osteitis fibrosa and exclude Al-related bone disease. Indications include (1) persistent severe hypercalcemia (after other causes of hypercalcemia are excluded), (2) pruritus unresponsive to dialysis or medical therapy, (3) progressive extraskeletal calcification, (4) severe skeletal pain or fractures, and (5) calciphylaxis (ischemic necrosis of skin or soft tissue associated with vascular calcification). The risk of Al toxicity is increased after parathyroidectomy and, thus, only calcium carbonate should be used as a phosphate binder.

4. **Management of Al toxicity.** Asymptomatic patients with evidence of Al-related bone disease should avoid Al-containing phosphate binders. In symptomatic patients with biopsy-proven Al-related bone disease, deferoxamine (Desferal), 1–3 g infused IV over 2 hours weekly, increases removal of Al by dialysis, and improves symptoms over a period of 6–12 months. Side effects include nausea, vomiting, hypotension, cataracts, and other visual abnormalities, and predisposition to bacteremia and mucormycosis.

Renal Replacement Therapies

As CRF progresses and metabolic abnormalities can no longer be controlled with conservative management, signs and symptoms of uremia develop, and the patient requires renal replacement therapy. The indications for dialysis in CRF are similar to those for ARF (see Acute Renal Failure, sec. **IV.B**). The patient with end-stage renal disease now has a variety of therapeutic options.

I. **Hemodialysis** (HD) works by diffusion of small molecular weight solutes across a semipermeable membrane. Fluid removal occurs via ultrafiltration (see sec. **III.A**). To perform HD, access to the vasculature for blood outflow and return is needed. Temporary access can be achieved via subclavian or femoral venous catheters. Permanent vascular access requires creation of a primary arteriovenous (AV) anastomosis or a synthetic (e.g., polytetrafluorethylene) AV graft. Since these grafts must heal before use, they should be placed when Cl$_{Cr}$ is 10–15 ml/minute. The frequency and duration of dialysis and the type of artificial kidney used are based on the patient's metabolic, nutritional, and volume status. When HD is instituted, dietary protein should be increased to 1.0–1.2 g/kg/day. Fluid intake should also be adjusted to permit a weight gain of about 2 kg between dialysis sessions. Antihypertensive medication may no longer be needed and often needs to be withheld on dialysis days. Complications of HD are discussed in the following paragraphs.

A. Active bleeding and coagulopathies may be exacerbated by the systemic anticoagulation needed in HD. The heparin dosage used for hemodialysis should be minimized in these patients or a switch to peritoneal dialysis considered. When uremic patients require therapy for active bleeding, the use of IV diamino-8-D-arginine-vasopressin (DDAVP; 0.3 µg/kg in 50 ml saline every 4–8 hours), IV estrogen (0.6 mg/kg/day for 5 days), or intranasal DDAVP (3.0 µg/kg every 4–6 hours) may shorten bleeding time (see Chap. 14).

B. Dialysis disequilibrium is a syndrome that may occur during the first few treatments of profoundly uremic patients and is attributed to CNS edema from rapid osmolar shifts. Symptoms include nausea, emesis, and headache, with occasional progression to confusion and seizures. This complication may be prevented or ameliorated by using low blood flows and shortened treatment duration during initial dialysis sessions.

C. Pericarditis may occur in patients undergoing dialysis and appears to be different than uremic pericarditis. Treatment involves intensification of dialysis to 6–7 times a week. If this therapy fails or if there is evidence of tamponade, pericardiectomy is indicated. Anticoagulation during HD must be minimized or discontinued until pericarditis resolves.

D. Hypotension during dialysis may be the result of many contributing factors, including volume depletion, low dialysate sodium content, use of antihypertensive medications before dialysis, allergic reactions to the dialyzer, intolerance to acetate-containing dialysate, left ventricular dysfunction, and autonomic insufficiency. Acute treatment includes infusion of normal saline, reduction of dialyzer blood flow, and reduction of the ultrafiltration rate. Other causes of hypotension such as myocardial infarction (MI), cardiac tamponade, sepsis, and bleeding should be excluded. In patients exhibiting acetate intolerance, a switch to bicarbonate-based dialysate is often beneficial.

E. Vascular access complications

  1. Vascular access infections may produce local or systemic signs but are often "silent." Prompt therapy with IV antibiotics should be started after blood cultures are obtained. Careful examination and ultrasound of the access site may reveal a local abscess, which should be cultured and drained. Initial therapy must include coverage for staphylococci and should be continued for at least 4 weeks. Removal of an infected access is often necessary.

  2. Vascular access thrombosis. A clotted access can be recanalized by balloon catheter embolectomy. The access can usually be used immediately after declotting.

F. Dialysis dementia is a progressive dementing syndrome secondary to CNS accumulation of aluminum. Hesitant, nonfluent speech is frequently the presenting sign. Awareness of the potential toxicity of aluminum has led to monitoring of blood and dialysate levels and to careful use of aluminum-containing phosphate binders. Chelation therapy with deferoxamine may improve or stop progression of dialysis dementia in some patients.

II. Peritoneal dialysis (PD) uses the peritoneum as a dialysis membrane. It can be performed acutely for ARF by bedside placement of a temporary peritoneal catheter, or on a chronic basis after surgical placement of a catheter. Solutes are removed by diffusion into the dialysate. Fluid removal is controlled by the addition of dextrose to the dialysate to create an osmotic gradient. Dextrose concentrations are usually 1.5–4.25 g/dl. Higher dextrose concentrations and more frequent exchanges increase the rate of fluid removal. A typical dialysis exchange is performed by infusion of 2 liters of fluid into the peritoneal cavity, followed by an equilibration period and dialysate drainage. In acute PD, exchanges can be performed as often as every hour. **Continuous ambulatory peritoneal dialysis** (CAPD) usually involves 4–5 exchanges/day performed by the patient. A modification of CAPD uses an automatic cycler to perform exchanges during sleep (continuous cyclic peritoneal dialysis, or CCPD). Peritoneal dialysis should be avoided in patients with recent abdominal surgery or a history of multiple surgeries with adhesions. Strict sterile technique is

Table 11-4. Intraperitoneal antibiotics in peritoneal dialysis

Antibiotic	Loading dose	Maintenance dose (mg/liter)
Cefazolin	500 mg/liter IP	125
Cephalothin	500 mg/liter IP	125
Vancomycin	1 g IV	25
Gentamicin	2 mg/kg IV	6–8
Tobramycin	2 mg/kg IV	6–8
Ampicillin	500 mg/liter IP	50

mandatory when performing exchanges. Compared with HD, PD is less efficient and less useful in highly catabolic patients. Because PD does not require systemic anticoagulation and produces less stress on the cardiovascular system, it may offer advantages over HD in certain situations. In addition, PD causes fewer abrupt changes in blood pressure and electrolytes, and allows patients greater independence than HD. Complications of PD are as follows.

A. Infections are the most significant problem in PD and include peritonitis, infection of the catheter tunnel, and infection of the catheter exit site. Peritonitis is usually secondary to a break in sterile technique during fluid exchanges. Most episodes of peritonitis are mild and can be treated on an outpatient basis, with the patient initiating therapy; however, patients should save infected dialysate for culture. Initial treatment is accomplished with two rapid exchanges, followed by exchanges q1–2h until abdominal pain stops. Antimicrobials and heparin (500 units/liter) should be added to the dialysate after the first two exchanges. Fluid balance must be closely monitored and dialysate concentration adjusted to avoid dehydration or volume overload. Treatment is continued with routine exchanges for 10 days. Antimicrobial therapy should include coverage for skin organisms, especially staphylococci. Intraperitoneal cephalosporins, or a combination of gentamicin and vancomycin, are appropriate choices (Table 11-4). Hospitalization is indicated in patients with frank sepsis, resistant or recurrent infections, or suspicion of organ perforation or abscess formation. Tunnel or exit site infections also involve skin organisms, are frequently difficult to treat, and may require catheter removal and temporary HD until the infection resolves.

B. Hyperglycemia may occur from absorption of glucose in PD fluid. If necessary, regular insulin can be added directly to the dialysate (e.g., 2 units to 2 liters of 1.5% dextrose, 6 units to 2 liters of 4.25% dextrose). In diabetic patients, intraperitoneal insulin is effective in controlling blood sugar. Conversion from SQ insulin to intraperitoneal insulin is best accomplished in the hospital, where proper glucose monitoring can be ensured. Initially, the patient's usual total daily subcutaneous insulin dose is divided by the number of exchanges he or she will receive and is given as regular insulin in each CAPD exchange. Additional insulin to cover glucose in the PD fluid (see above) should be included. Insulin must be added using sterile technique to avoid contamination and peritonitis.

C. Since **protein loss** in PD can be excessive, dietary protein intake should be increased to 1.2–1.4 g/kg/day.

III. Ultrafiltration and hemofiltration remove large volumes of fluid with minimal removal of metabolic wastes. These filtration techniques are useful for removing fluid in patients with renal insufficiency and volume overload who do not need concomitant dialysis.

A. Ultrafiltration is performed with standard hemodialysis cartridges and equipment. A blood pump perfuses the cartridges with the patient's blood, but no dialysate is used. By manipulation of the transmembrane pressure gradient, an ultrafiltrate of plasma is formed and removed. Because large volumes of fluid are removed in a short period of time, the patient may experience hypotension. Ultrafiltration can be performed alone or in combination with hemodialysis.

B. Continuous arteriovenous hemofiltration (CAVH) or hemodialysis (CAVHD) uses a highly permeable membrane to filter blood from a femoral or extremity artery. Blood is returned to the patient through a femoral or extremity vein. The driving force for filtration is the patient's blood pressure; no blood pump is needed. CAVH is better tolerated than ultrafiltration in hemodynamically unstable patients because fluid removal is slow and continuous. Another advantage of this technique is the simplicity of the equipment. However, the patient must be continuously heparinized and is virtually bed bound. In addition, fluid balance must be closely monitored to avoid massive volume depletion. Fluid removal rates can be adjusted frequently to compensate for fluid input. This procedure should be carried out only in an intensive care setting.

IV. **Renal transplantation** has enjoyed considerable success as a result of improved donor–recipient selection, immunosuppressive drug regimens, and methods of treating allograft rejection. One-year graft survival rates are as high as 87% for cadaver allografts and 98% for living-related donor grafts (*Mayo Clin. Proc.* 61:523, 1986). Transplantation represents the only therapeutic option that may allow patients with ESRD to return to their premorbid lifestyles. Selected medical aspects of transplant therapy are presented in the following paragraphs.

   A. **Pretransplant evaluation** of the recipient includes assessment of cardiovascular status and any structural abnormalities of the urinary tract, correction of potential sources of infection (e.g., dental hygiene problems), HLA typing, and evaluation for preformed antibodies against potential donor antigens. The latter, along with blood group compatibility testing, should prevent hyperacute rejection in most cases.

   B. **Immunosuppression** after transplantation is essential for prevention of allograft rejection. A variety of immunosuppressive regimens have been used, and the choice of immune suppression varies with the type of transplant (i.e., cadaver versus living-related donor). The most frequently used regimens employ a combination of prednisone and either cyclosporine (CsA) or azathioprine, but some regimens use all three agents. The advent of CsA has improved cadaver allograft survival rates by 10–20% and has reduced rejection episodes. Its major toxicity is acute and chronic renal failure. A rising creatinine in a patient receiving CsA may thus indicate rejection or CsA nephrotoxicity. Acute nephrotoxicity often responds to a decrease in dosage or discontinuation of CsA. CsA may rarely produce a hemolytic-uremic–like syndrome, which results in significant allograft loss. Chronic CsA nephrotoxicity produces irreversible interstitial fibrosis. Other adverse effects of CsA include hypertension, hyperkalemia, predisposition to lymphoproliferative malignancy, tremor, seizure, and hepatotoxicity. CsA levels can be measured and the incidence of toxic side effects is increased when trough levels are elevated. CsA is metabolized by the liver. Concomitant drug use may affect CsA metabolism; erythromycin and ketoconazole increase, and phenytoin decreases, CsA blood levels. Such drug interactions should be sought and appropriate dosage adjustments made in patients taking CsA.

   C. **Allograft rejection** may be acute or chronic and is suggested by rising creatinine, allograft tenderness, and decreasing urine output. Other causes of renal impairment such as volume depletion, obstruction, problems of vascular supply, drug nephrotoxicity, and recurrent or de novo renal disease should be excluded. Evaluation of suspected rejection generally requires allograft biopsy. Therapy of rejection is best carried out by an experienced transplant team.

      1. **Acute cellular rejection** typically produces a lymphocytic interstitial infiltrate with destruction of epithelial cells and is often amenable to treatment. Currently used modalities for treatment of acute rejection include high-dose IV methylprednisolone, anti-lymphocyte globulin, and anti–T-lymphocyte monoclonal antibody (OKT3) administration.

      2. **Chronic rejection** is characterized by interstitial fibrosis, tubular atrophy, and arterial intimal proliferation and generally progresses to allograft failure over months to years. There is no specific treatment for chronic rejection; general measures for conservative management of chronic renal insufficiency should be instituted.

D. Infections are a major cause of morbidity and mortality in the transplant patient and must be sought when fever is present (see Chap. 13).

Nephrolithiasis

I. **Clinical manifestations** of nephrolithiasis include hematuria, predisposition to urinary tract infection, and pain (usually flank) with passage of the stone. Renal stones may also be an incidental finding on radiographic studies. Oliguria and ARF may occur when both collecting systems are blocked by stones.

II. **Diagnostic evaluation** of an acute episode of flank pain and hematuria should include a plain abdominal roentgenogram, as the majority of renal stones are radiopaque. Exceptions include cystine stones, which may be of intermediate opacity, and uric acid stones, which are radiolucent. Intravenous pyelography should be performed acutely if renal colic is severe and obstruction is suspected. IVP is also useful in evaluating the anatomy of the kidneys and collecting systems. Urine should be examined for pH and crystals, and cultured. Other initial studies include serum electrolytes, creatinine, calcium, uric acid, and phosphorus. All passed stones should be saved for analysis. After resolution of the acute episode, further diagnostic evaluation can be guided by stone composition. The extent of the metabolic evaluation that should be undertaken for the patient with a single calcium stone has not been established, but recurrent calcium nephrolithiasis warrants complete investigation. Patients with non-calcium stones should undergo complete evaluation after the first episode. Further studies may include PTH levels (if hypercalcemia is present) and 24-hour urine studies for measurement of calcium, phosphate, urate, oxalate, citrate, creatinine, sodium, urea nitrogen, and cystine. Yearly follow-up examination of the patient with nephrolithiasis includes abdominal roentgenograms to check for new stone formation or growth of existing stones, and repeat metabolic studies to assess the effects of specific therapies.

III. **Treatment.** Acute management of patients with stones includes analgesia and hydration. If the stone is obstructing outflow or is accompanied by infection, removal is indicated. After passage of a stone, treatment is directed at prevention of recurrent stone formation. In most patients, the foundation of general therapy is maintenance of high urine output (>2.5 liters/day) through oral hydration and avoidance of dietary excesses. Specific treatments are discussed in the following paragraphs.

A. **Calcium stones** account for about 80% of all stones and are composed of calcium oxalate and phosphate. Hypercalciuria is usually present and may be idiopathic or secondary to an identifiable disease. Calcium stones may also precipitate around a uric acid nidus in patients with hyperuricosuria, even in the absence of hypercalciuria (see sec. **III.B**). Other conditions associated with calcium stone formation include hyperoxaluria (commonly seen in patients with inflammatory bowel disorders), distal renal tubular acidosis, medullary sponge kidney, and sarcoidosis.

1. **Hypercalciuria** (calcium excretion >4 mg/kg/day with a normal calcium intake [800–1000 mg/day]) may be due to increased gastrointestinal absorption of calcium, impaired renal tubular calcium reabsorption, or excessive skeletal resorption as in primary hyperparathyroidism. Hypercalciuria can be treated conservatively by limiting calcium intake to 500 mg/day and protein to 1 g/kg/day and by maintaining a high fluid intake. Excess sodium intake (i.e., >10 g salt/day) should be avoided, and restriction of salt intake to less than 6 g/day may be beneficial (*Kidney Int.* 34:544, 1988). If dietary measures alone are not effective, addition of a thiazide diuretic (hydrochlorothiazide, 25–50 mg PO bid) to increase calcium reabsorption is often useful. Careful follow-up is important in these patients to ensure that therapy has decreased calcium excretion and has not caused adverse alterations in serum electrolyte concentrations.

2. **Hyperparathyroidism** resulting in renal stone formation should be treated with parathyroidectomy.

3. **Hyperoxaluria** (urinary oxalate excretion >0.7 mg/kg/day) requires dietary oxalate restriction.

4. **Hypocitraturia.** Urine citrate (an inhibitor of calcium oxalate precipitation) is frequently low in patients with calcium stones. Therapy with potassium citrate, 20 mEq PO tid, is often effective.

B. **Uric acid stone** formation is favored by conditions of uric acid overproduction (urine uric acid excretion >11 mg/kg/day), low urinary volume, and persistently acid urine pH. Conservative therapy involves maintenance of urine volume greater than 2 liters/day through oral hydration, and alkalinization of urine to pH 6.5–7.0 with an oral alkali preparation (e.g., Shohl's solution, 20 ml PO bid-tid). Patients should be instructed in the home measurement of urine pH so that the oral alkali dose can be appropriately titrated. If these measures fail, administration of allopurinol, 300 mg PO qd, is indicated. Probenecid and other uricosuric drugs should be avoided as they may increase the risk of uric acid or calcium oxalate stone formation.

C. **Cystine stones** arise from an inborn error in amino acid transport with consequent cystinuria. Cystine crystals are hexagonal on microscopic examination of the urine. Treatment includes maintenance of urine volume of greater than 3 liters/day and alkalinization of urine to a pH greater than 7.5 with Shohl's solution, 30 ml PO qid. D-penicillamine, 1–2 g/day PO, can be used in refractory cases, but this therapy is often complicated by side effects such as nephrotoxicity, allergic reactions, and hematologic abnormalities (see Chap. 24).

D. **Struvite stones** (staghorn calculi) occur under conditions of high urinary pH, reflecting infection with urea-splitting organisms (e.g., *Proteus mirabilis*). For antimicrobial therapy to be effective, the infected stone material must be removed.

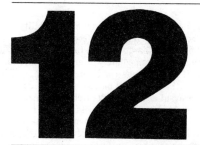

Antimicrobials

Victoria J. Fraser and
William Claiborne Dunagan

Principles of Antimicrobial Therapy

Use of antimicrobial agents. The decision to institute antimicrobial chemotherapy should be made carefully. Antimicrobials have potentially serious adverse effects and are often expensive. In addition, the widespread use of antibiotics leads to the development of resistant organisms, a problem that might be ameliorated by more appropriate use. When antimicrobial therapy is indicated, a number of factors must be considered in selecting an appropriate regimen.

I. **Choice of initial antimicrobial therapy.** The infecting organism is usually unknown when therapy is begun; consequently, initial empiric therapy should be directed against the most likely pathogens. Therapy can then be altered in accordance with the patient's course and laboratory results.

   A. **Gram's stain.** During the initial evaluation, all potentially infected material should be examined with a Gram's stain. A careful examination often permits a rapid presumptive etiologic diagnosis and may be essential for interpretation of subsequent culture results.

   B. **Local susceptibility** patterns must be considered in selecting empiric therapy because patterns vary widely among communities and hospitals.

   C. **Cultures** are necessary for precise diagnosis and for susceptibility testing. Specimens obtained for culture should be delivered promptly to the laboratory, as delays may allow fastidious organisms to die and contaminating flora to overgrow. Whenever organisms with special growth requirements are suspected, the microbiology laboratory should be consulted to ensure appropriate transport and processing. If anaerobes are suspected, specimens must be kept free of air and cultured as soon as possible.

   D. **Antimicrobial susceptibility testing.** Susceptibility testing permits a rational selection of antimicrobial agents. Disk–diffusion susceptibility testing is usually sufficient. In serious infections, such as infective endocarditis, quantification of the drug concentrations that inhibit and kill the pathogen may be useful. The lowest drug concentration that prevents the growth of a defined inoculum of the isolated pathogen is the **minimal inhibitory concentration (MIC)**; the lowest concentration that kills 99.9% of an inoculum is the **minimal bactericidal concentration (MBC).** For bactericidal drugs, the MIC and MBC are usually similar. The antimicrobial activity of a treated patient's serum can be estimated by measuring **serum bactericidal titers.** Intravascular infections are usually controlled when the peak serum bactericidal titer is 1:8 or greater (*N. Engl. J. Med.* 312:968, 1985).

   E. **An acute-phase serum specimen** is often valuable when uncertainty exists in diagnosis. Serum should be collected and frozen until a convalescent sample is obtained. Demonstration of a high serologic titer or of changing titers against an infectious agent may be diagnostic, particularly in atypical pneumonias, systemic mycoses such as histoplasmosis and coccidioidomycosis, infectious vasculitides, viral illnesses, and parasitic diseases.

II. **Status of the host.** The clinical status of the patient determines the speed with which therapy must be instituted, as well as the route of administration and type of therapy. Patients should be quickly evaluated for hemodynamic stability, rapidly progressive or life-threatening infections, and immune defects.

A. **Timing of the initiation of antimicrobial therapy.** When the clinical situation is acute, empiric therapy is usually begun immediately after appropriate cultures have been obtained. However, if the patient's condition is stable, a delay of several days may permit specific therapy based on the results of culture and susceptibility testing and may prevent adverse effects from the use of unnecessary drugs. **Urgent therapy** is indicated in febrile patients who are neutropenic, asplenic, or otherwise immunosuppressed. Sepsis, meningitis, and rapidly progressive anaerobic or necrotizing infections should always be treated with antimicrobial therapy as quickly as possible.

B. **Route of administration.** Patients with serious infection should be given antimicrobial agents intravenously. In less urgent circumstances, intramuscular or oral therapy is usually sufficient. Oral therapy is acceptable when it can be tolerated by the patient and when it produces adequate drug concentrations at the site of infection.

C. **Type of therapy.** Bactericidal therapy is indicated for patients with immunologic compromise or life-threatening infection. It is also preferred for infections characterized by impaired regional host defenses, such as endocarditis, meningitis, and osteomyelitis. Other infections can be treated effectively with either bactericidal or bacteriostatic drugs (*Infect. Dis. Clin. North Am.* 3:389, 1989).

D. **Underlying renal or hepatic disease.** Renal and hepatic metabolism and excretion are the major pathways of antimicrobial elimination. Antimicrobials such as the aminoglycosides are excreted by the kidney and require dosage reductions in patients with renal insufficiency (see Appendix D). Likewise, hepatically excreted or metabolized drugs may require dosage reduction in patients with significant liver disease. Drugs excreted primarily by the kidney may be particularly useful in patients with liver disease. Measurement of serum drug levels is especially helpful in the treatment of patients with hepatic or renal failure.

E. **Pregnancy and the puerperium.** Although no antimicrobial is known to be completely safe in pregnancy, the penicillins and cephalosporins are used most often. Tetracycline and quinolones are specifically contraindicated, and the sulfonamides and aminoglycosides should not be used if alternative agents are available. Dosages of most antimicrobials should be increased to compensate for an increased maternal volume of distribution in pregnancy. In addition, most antibiotics administered in therapeutic dosages will appear in breast milk and should be used with caution in patients who are breast-feeding.

III. **Drug interactions.** The possibility of incompatibilities in solution or of in vivo drug interactions should be considered each time a new drug is prescribed (see Appendix B).

IV. **Antimicrobial combinations.** The use of multiple antimicrobials is justified in seriously ill patients when (1) the identity of an infecting organism is not apparent, (2) the suspected pathogen has a variable antimicrobial susceptibility, or (3) failure to initiate effective antimicrobial therapy will significantly increase morbidity or mortality. Antimicrobial combinations are specifically indicated (1) to produce synergism (e.g., in enterococcal endocarditis or gram-negative sepsis in neutropenic patients), (2) to treat infections probably caused by multiple pathogens (e.g., peritonitis following a ruptured viscus), and (3) to prevent the emergence of antimicrobial resistance (e.g., tuberculosis, *Pseudomonas* infections). The indiscriminate use of antimicrobial combinations should be avoided because of the potential for increased toxicity, pharmacologic antagonism, and the development of resistant organisms.

V. **Duration of therapy.** Treatment of acute, uncomplicated infections should be continued until the patient has been afebrile and clinically well for a minimum of 72 hours. Infections at certain sites (e.g., endocarditis, septic arthritis, osteomyelitis) require long-term therapy, and periodic cultures may be useful in these cases to assess the response to treatment.

Antimicrobials

I. **Beta-lactam antibiotics** include the penicillins, cephalosporins, cephamycins, oxa-beta-lactams, carbapenems, and monobactams. These highly effective antimicrobials bind to specific binding proteins on the bacterial cell membrane and interfere with cell wall synthesis. Resistance to beta-lactams may be intrinsic (e.g., due to an altered target site) or enzymatic (i.e., mediated by drug-inactivating enzymes [beta-lactamases]).

A. **Penicillins (PCNs)** remain among the most effective and least toxic antimicrobials available and are often the drug of choice for treatment of susceptible pathogens. Most PCNs are rapidly excreted by the kidney; therefore, dosages must be reduced in renal insufficiency. **Probenecid** (500 mg PO q6h) interferes with tubular secretion of PCNs and can be used to increase their serum half-life. **Hypersensitivity** is the most common side effect of the PCNs and may produce fever, eosinophilia, serum sickness, or anaphylaxis (*Ann. Intern. Med.* 107:204, 1987). Metabolites of the PCNs form covalent bonds with serum and tissue proteins and are highly immunogenic. Penicillins have a common immunogenicity; thus, persons known to be allergic to one PCN preparation should not be given another PCN if an acceptable alternative is available. In questionable cases or when there is no alternative to the use of a PCN, **skin testing** can be performed. A negative reaction makes anaphylaxis unlikely if the PCN is given immediately but does not preclude other allergic reactions or the possibility of anaphylaxis if the patient is rechallenged with PCN at a later date. **Desensitization** is rarely required and should be performed only in a closely monitored setting (*J. Allergy Clin. Immunol.* 69:275, 1982). Coombs'-positive hemolytic anemia, leukopenia, and thrombocytopenia are rare. Seizures may occur with very high dosages of PCN, particularly in patients with renal failure. Interstitial nephritis is an unusual side effect, most commonly seen with ampicillin and the penicillinase-resistant PCNs (see Chap. 11).

1. **Penicillin G (benzyl penicillin)** is hydrolyzed by gastric acid and in general is ineffective when taken orally. Penicillin G is active against most gram-positive and gram-negative aerobic cocci that do not produce beta-lactamase and against many anaerobes, including anaerobic cocci and *Clostridium* spp. Dosages vary depending on the disease being treated.

a. **Aqueous penicillin G (IM or IV)** is usually supplied as the potassium salt (1.7 mEq K^+/million units), although sodium salts are available and may be useful for patients with hyperkalemia or renal failure.

b. **Procaine penicillin G** is a relatively insoluble salt that yields sustained serum levels when given intramuscularly. It is useful for treatment of gonorrhea and streptococcal infections, particularly when compliance with oral therapy may be a problem. Procaine hypersensitivity is a contraindication to its use.

c. **Benzathine penicillin G (IM)** is another insoluble salt that produces low sustained serum levels of PCN G for 1–3 weeks. Its use is limited to prophylaxis of rheumatic fever and treatment of syphilis. Cerebrospinal fluid (CSF) penetration is unreliable.

2. **Penicillin V** (250–500 mg PO q6h) is relatively resistant to hydrolysis by gastric acid and can be given PO. In general, food diminishes its absorption. Penicillin V is the oral drug of choice for infections caused by gram-positive cocci that do not produce beta-lactamase (e.g., group A streptococci).

3. **Penicillinase-resistant semisynthetic penicillins (PRSP)** are indicated for the treatment of infections caused by penicillinase-producing staphylococci. They are less active than PCN G and PCN V against non–beta-lactamase–producing gram-positive cocci. Staphylococci that are resistant to one of the PRSPs are also resistant to other PRSPs and to the cephalosporins as well. Notable toxicities of these agents include interstitial nephritis, elevations of serum transaminases, cholestatic jaundice, and neutropenia.

a. **Oxacillin** (1–2 g IV q4–6h) and **nafcillin** (1–2 g IV q4–6h) are the preferred agents for parenteral therapy. Nafcillin is excreted by the liver and may be preferable when treating patients with renal dysfunction.

   b. Dicloxacillin (250–500 mg PO q6h) is similar to oxacillin and is the preferred agent for oral use, because its absorption is better than that of cloxacillin or oxacillin. It should be given on an empty stomach.

   c. Methicillin may be associated with a higher incidence of interstitial nephritis than the other semisynthetic PCNs. Therefore, many physicians prefer to avoid its use.

4. Extended-spectrum PCNs are also semisynthetic derivatives and provide coverage against many gram-negative bacilli. They are usually not recommended for treatment of infection caused by streptococci because PCN G and PCN V are more active against these organisms in vitro and are less expensive.

   a. Ampicillin (500 mg PO q6h for mild infections, 1.0–2.0 g IV q4–6h for moderate to severe infections) is active against many of the Enterobacteriaceae and against *Haemophilus influenzae* and *Neisseria* spp. However, ampicillin is hydrolyzed by beta-lactamase and is therefore inactive against most strains of *Staphylococcus, Pseudomonas, Enterobacter, Klebsiella,* and 20–30% of *H. influenzae.*

   b. Amoxicillin (250–500 mg PO q8h) is an analog of ampicillin with a nearly identical antibacterial spectrum. Amoxicillin is associated with less diarrhea than ampicillin but is also less effective in the treatment of shigellosis.

5. Carboxy and ureido PCNs are extended-spectrum agents indicated primarily for treatment of infection due to *Pseudomonas aeruginosa* and other gram-negative bacilli. They are effective against a larger number of gram-negative organisms than ampicillin and are active against many strains of *Bacteroides fragilis.* All these drugs are susceptible to staphylococcal beta-lactamase and should not be used to treat infections caused by *Staphylococcus aureus.* In treating serious infections due to susceptible gram-negative organisms such as *P. aeruginosa, Enterobacter* spp, and *Serratia,* these agents should probably be **combined with an aminoglycoside** to take advantage of potential synergy and to prevent emergence of resistance. CNS penetration of these agents is modest (10% of serum levels), and they are not recommended for the treatment of gram-negative bacillary meningitis. **Adverse effects** of these agents are similar to those of other PCNs. In addition, phlebitis, hypokalemia, and prolongation of bleeding time may occur (*Ann. Intern. Med.* 105:924, 1986).

   a. Carboxy PCNs include **carbenicillin** (5 g IV q4h) and **ticarcillin** (3 g IV q4–6h). These agents are not active against enterococci and most *Klebsiella* spp. Carbenicillin and ticarcillin contain 4.7 and 5.2 mEq sodium/g, respectively, which must be considered when used in patients susceptible to volume overload.

   b. Ureido PCNs include **azlocillin, mezlocillin,** and **piperacillin** (3 g IV q4h or 4 g IV q6h). The ureido PCNs have activity against *Enterococcus* spp approaching that of ampicillin. In addition, mezlocillin and piperacillin are active in vitro against most strains of *Klebsiella.* The ureido PCNs may inhibit *P. aeruginosa* strains that are resistant to the carboxy PCNs. Individual ureido PCNs offer no clear therapeutic advantage over carboxy PCNs when treating infections due to susceptible organisms.

   c. Indanyl carbenicillin (1–2 tablets PO q6h), an oral preparation of carbenicillin, is effective for urinary tract infections (UTI) caused by *Pseudomonas* spp and some other ampicillin-resistant organisms. Because it produces low serum levels, it should not be used for the treatment of systemic infections.

6. Amdinocillin (mecillinam) has a high degree of activity in vitro against many gram-negative bacilli, but is inactive against gram-positive cocci, *Pseudomonas* spp, and anaerobes. Amdinocillin, alone or in combination, appears to offer no advantage over other antimicrobial regimens.

B. Cephalosporins, cephamycins, and **oxa-beta-lactams.** These agents can be classified by generations, the members of which share similar antibacterial activity and pharmacokinetics. **None of these agents are indicated for treatment of enterococcal infections.** Higher generations of cephalosporins tend to have increased activity against gram-negative bacilli, usually at the expense of gram-positive activity. The increased use of these broad-spectrum second- and third-generation agents has been accompanied by the development of bacteria with clinically significant drug resistance (*J. Infect. Dis.* 151:399, 1985). Cross-resistance for other beta-lactam agents also occurs. Resistance is particularly common with *Enterobacter, Pseudomonas, Acinetobacter, Serratia,* and indole-positive *Proteus* spp. In situations in which these bacteria are potential pathogens, combination therapy with an aminoglycoside is recommended. These drugs may produce **hypersensitivity** reactions, and some PCN-allergic patients are also allergic to the cephalosporins. Other **adverse reactions** include phlebitis (with IV administration), sterile abscesses (when given IM), and diarrhea. In addition, cephalosporins that contain an N–methylthiotetrazole (MTT) side chain (cefamandole, cefoperazone, cefotetan, and moxalactam) may produce a coagulopathy by interfering with the synthesis of vitamin K–dependent clotting factors. This effect is reversed by administration of vitamin K. Ingestion of ethanol may also induce a disulfiram-like reaction in patients receiving agents with the MTT side chain. Most cephalosporins are renally excreted, and dosages should be reduced in renal failure.

1. **First-generation cephalosporins** have activity against most gram-positive cocci, including beta-lactamase–producing strains, and against the gram-negative bacilli that cause most community-acquired infections, including *Escherichia coli* and *Klebsiella* spp. However, *B. fragilis, P. aeruginosa,* and *Enterobacter* spp are typically resistant, as are methicillin-resistant staphylococci. None of these agents cross the meninges in concentrations sufficient for the treatment of meningitis.

   a. **Cephalothin, cephapirin,** and **cephradine** (all 1–2 g IV q4–6h) have similar pharmacokinetics and toxicity. Oral cephradine is equivalent to cephalexin (see sec. **I.B.1.c**).

   b. **Cefazolin** (1–2 g IV or IM q8h) produces higher and more sustained serum levels and is less painful when given intramuscularly than the other first-generation cephalosporins.

   c. **Cephalexin** (250–500 mg PO q6h) and **cefadroxil** (1–2 g/day PO in 1 or 2 doses) are used primarily in the treatment of UTI and are not optimal for systemic infections at standard doses because achievable serum levels are low. Large doses of cephalexin, combined with probenecid, have been used for the oral therapy of osteomyelitis and other systemic infections after an initial response to 2–4 weeks of parenteral therapy.

2. **Second-generation cephalosporins** offer expanded coverage against gram-negative bacilli compared to first-generation agents. There are sufficient differences among their antibacterial spectra to require individual susceptibility testing of clinical isolates. Their major role is in the treatment of infections due to cephalothin-resistant gram-negative bacilli. **Aside from cefuroxime, none of the second-generation agents has reliable CSF penetration and they should not be used to treat meningitis.**

   a. **Cefamandole** (1–2 g IM or IV q4–6h) and **cefonicid** (1–2 g IM or IV qd) are active in vitro against most Enterobacteriaceae and *H. influenzae.* They are not active against *P. aeruginosa, B. fragilis,* or *Serratia marcescens.* Cefamandole may produce MTT side chain–associated toxicity (see sec. **I.B**). **Ceforanide** is similar to cefamandole but is less active in vitro against *Staph. aureus* and *H. influenzae;* it has no advantage over other agents in this class.

   b. **Cefuroxime** (0.75–2.0 g IV q8h) has a spectrum of activity similar to that of cefamandole but is more resistant to beta-lactamases, including those produced by *H. influenzae.* Cefuroxime enters the CSF in sufficient concentration to be useful in the treatment of meningitis due to susceptible organisms, although data suggest that third-generation cephalosporins may be more effective (*J. Pediatr.* 114:1049, 1989).

c. **Cefuroxime axetil** (250 mg PO q12h) can be used to treat otitis media, UTI, and some respiratory infections, but equally effective and less expensive drugs are often available.

d. **Cefoxitin** (1–2 g IM or IV q4–8h), **cefotetan** (1–3 g IM or IV q12h), and **cefmetazole** (2 g IV or IM q6–12h) are cephamycins that are particularly resistant to beta-lactamase and are active against *B. fragilis, S. marcescens,* and beta-lactamase–producing *Neisseria gonorrhoeae.* Cefotetan and cefmetazole also possess the MTT side chain (see sec. **I.B**). Despite minor differences in in vitro activity, there is no clear therapeutic advantage among any of these agents for treatment of infections due to susceptible bacteria and choices can be made based on local cost considerations.

e. **Cefaclor** (250–500 mg PO q8h) has a spectrum of activity similar to that of cephalexin but with enhanced activity against *H. influenzae,* including beta-lactamase–producing strains. Serum sickness has been reported, usually in children during the second course of therapy.

3. **Third-generation cephalosporins** are more active in vitro against gram-negative bacilli and less active against gram-positive cocci, especially *Staph. aureus,* than the first- and second-generation agents. Most agents are not effective for infections due to *Pseudomonas* spp, and none are effective for enterococcal infections, even if used in combination with an aminoglycoside. **The third-generation cephalosporins are the drugs of choice for gram-negative bacillary meningitis.** They are also useful for treatment of other gram-negative bacillary infections, but widespread use may lead to the emergence of resistant flora and superinfection with enterococci and other resistant bacteria. These agents are not indicated for routine surgical prophylaxis.

a. **Cefotaxime** (1–2 g IV q4–8h), **ceftizoxime** (1–2 g IV q6–8h), **ceftriaxone** (1–2 g IV q12–24h), and **moxalactam** have similar spectra of activity. The dosages of cefotaxime and ceftizoxime should be reduced in renal insufficiency. The dosage of ceftriaxone, which has both renal and hepatic excretion, needs to be reduced only in patients with combined renal and hepatic dysfunction. Ceftriaxone is useful for the treatment of gonorrhea due to penicillinase-producing *N. gonorrhoeae.* Its long half-life may also facilitate long-term parenteral therapy. Moxalactam has been associated with frequent bleeding complications, and its use is not recommended.

b. **Ceftazidime** (1–2 g IV q8h) is the most active of the cephalosporins against *P. aeruginosa.* Its activity against other gram-negative rods is equivalent to that of cefotaxime, but it is less active than other third-generation agents against gram-positive cocci.

c. **Cefoperazone** (1–2 g IV q8–12h) is less active than other third-generation agents against most gram-negative pathogens. It does not penetrate the CSF well and is not recommended for the treatment of meningitis. Because of its hepatic excretion, dosage reduction may be necessary in severe liver disease. Cefoperazone also possesses the MTT side chain (see sec. **I.B**).

d. **Cefixime** (400 mg PO/day in 1 or 2 doses) is the first oral third-generation cephalosporin. Its activity is similar to that of other third-generation agents against streptococci, *Neisseria* spp, *H. influenzae,* and *Branhamella catarrhalis;* however, it has poor activity against staphylococci and anaerobes and *Pseudomonas, Enterobacter,* and *Acinetobacter* spp. **The dosage should be reduced in patients with renal dysfunction.**

C. **Aztreonam** (0.5–1.0 g IV q8–12h for mild infections and 1–2 g IV q6–8h for moderate to serious infections) is a monobactam, with activity exclusively against aerobic gram-negative bacilli, including most strains of *P. aeruginosa* and *Serratia.* It is inactive against gram-positive cocci and anaerobes. **Aztreonam may be useful in patients allergic to PCN, as there is no apparent cross-reactivity in these patients** (*Rev. Infect. Dis.* 7 [suppl 4]:S613, 1985). Otherwise, it has no clear advantage over other broad-spectrum beta-lactam agents. Its role as a substitute for an aminoglycoside in combination regimens is not yet defined, but **it should not be used in place of aminoglycosides when synergistic therapy is desired** (e.g., treatment of enterococcal infections). Resistance may occur, sometimes with cross-resistance to third-generation cephalosporins.

D. Imipenem (0.5–1.0 g IV q6–8h), a carbapenem antibiotic, given in a fixed combination with cilastatin (an inhibitor of imipenem metabolism) has potent broad-spectrum activity against many bacteria, including anaerobes, most gram-positive cocci (except *Enterococcus faecium* and methicillin-resistant staphylococci), and gram-negative bacilli (excluding *Xanthomonas maltophilia* and some *Pseudomonas cepacia*). As with other beta-lactam antibiotics, resistance has emerged during imipenem therapy, particularly among strains of *P. aeruginosa*. Whether concurrent use of an aminoglycoside will prevent the emergence of resistance has not yet been determined. The dosage should be decreased in patients with renal dysfunction.

   1. Indications. Imipenem is useful for the treatment of infections due to multiply resistant organisms, including *Enterobacter* and *Acinetobacter* spp, and is also useful as empiric single-drug therapy for mixed aerobic/anaerobic infections when the potential toxicity of alternative antimicrobial combinations is unacceptable.

   2. Adverse reactions. Toxicity is similar to that of the PCNs, and there may be immunologic cross-reactivity in some PCN-allergic patients. Seizures occur more frequently than with the PCNs, especially in patients with predisposing factors or renal insufficiency.

E. Inhibitors of beta-lactamase. Clavulanic acid and sulbactam are beta-lactam molecules that have minimal intrinsic antibacterial activity but are potent inhibitors of many beta-lactamases, including some of those produced by *Staph. aureus, H. influenzae, E. coli,* and *Klebsiella pneumoniae.* The enzymes produced by *P. aeruginosa* and *Serratia* and *Enterobacter* spp are resistant to these agents, and methicillin-resistant staphylococci are not susceptible to antimicrobials containing clavulanic acid or sulbactam. Cerebrospinal fluid penetration of clavulanic acid and sulbactam is unreliable, and they should not be used to treat meningitis.

   1. Amoxicillin with clavulanic acid (250–500 mg PO q8h) is useful in the treatment of UTI, otitis media, sinusitis, and bite wounds. There is an increased incidence of gastrointestinal side effects compared with amoxicillin alone.

   2. Ticarcillin with clavulanic acid (3.1 g IV q4–6h) may be useful for therapy of selected polymicrobial infections such as infected diabetic foot ulcers.

   3. Ampicillin with sulbactam (1.5–3.0 g IV or IM q6h) may be useful for therapy of uncomplicated or community-acquired intra-abdominal or pelvic infections or polymicrobial upper and lower respiratory infections.

II. Macrolide and azalide antimicrobials are bacteriostatic agents with a large volume of distribution producing high tissue concentrations but **unreliable CSF penetration.** These drugs are excreted primarily by the liver, with about 20% renal excretion. Reduced dosages should be used with severe hepatic dysfunction. Macrolide and azalide antimicrobials can **increase plasma levels of theophylline, carbamazepine, cyclosporine, digoxin, and warfarin** as well as other drugs, so special attention to drug interactions is necessary. Gastric irritation and diarrhea are common side effects with erythromycin; however, azithromycin and clarithromycin produce fewer GI symptoms.

A. Erythromycin (250–500 mg PO q6h or 0.5–1.0 g IV q6h) is used most frequently as an alternative to PCNs for PCN-allergic patients with infection caused by streptococci or staphylococci. Erythromycin is the drug of choice for infections due to *Legionella* or *Mycoplasma* spp and can be used in the treatment of chlamydial infections, chancroid, and *helicobacter* (campylobacter) enteritis. Phlebitis is common with IV administration. Reversible ototoxicity is a rare complication. The erythromycin estolate formulation is hepatotoxic and should not be used in adults.

B. Clindamycin (150–450 mg PO q6h or 600–900 mg IV q8h) has a gram-positive spectrum similar to that of erythromycin and is also active against most anaerobes, including *B. fragilis;* however, resistance among *Bacteroides* spp is increasing. Except for anaerobic infections, it is rarely the drug of choice. Clindamycin is well absorbed orally. Its most common side effects are rashes and diarrhea. **Pseudomembranous colitis** occurs in a significant number of patients (see Chap. 13).

C. Clarithromycin (250–500 mg PO q12h) is a semisynthetic macrolide antibiotic with a spectrum similar to erythromycin but that also covers *Haemophilus influenzae* and *Moraxella (Branhamella) catarrhalis*. It can be used for mild to moderate upper and lower respiratory tract infections and skin or soft tissue infections. Clarithromycin also has in vitro activity against mycobacteria and may be useful in treatment regimens for MAI and other nontuberculous mycobacterial infections. Clarithromycin is contraindicated in pregnancy, and the dosage should be reduced for severe renal insufficiency.

D. Azithromycin (250–500 mg PO qd) is an azalide antimicrobial chemically related to erythromycin, but with a broader spectrum, longer half-life, and greater tissue penetration. Azithromycin has an extended spectrum similar to clarithromycin but also has activity against genitourinary pathogens including *Chlamydia trachomatis*. Azithromycin can be used for respiratory tract infections, skin and soft tissue infections, and cervicitis or urethritis due to chlamydia. Azithromycin should not be given concurrently with ergot alkaloids due to the risk of precipitating ergotism.

III. Vancomycin (1 g IV q12h) is a bactericidal agent active only against gram-positive organisms.

A. Indications include treatment of infections due to methicillin-resistant staphylococci and of infections due to susceptible organism in patients allergic to both PCNs and cephalosporins. Vancomycin in combination with an aminoglycoside is also effective for the treatment of enterococcal endocarditis. Vancomycin is particularly well suited for use in dialysis patients, since 1 g IV provides adequate blood levels for up to 7–10 days. Oral vancomycin (250–500 mg PO q6h for 10 days) is not well absorbed and is therefore useful in the treatment of *Clostridium difficile* diarrhea (see Chap. 13).

B. Administration. Vancomycin should be given intravenously at a maximum rate of 1 g/hour to avoid the "red-man" syndrome. Vancomycin is excreted by the kidney; its dosage must be adjusted in the presence of renal insufficiency. Serum levels should be monitored routinely to ensure adequate therapy and to minimize toxicity.

C. Adverse effects. Rapid administration of vancomycin often results in a histamine-mediated reaction characterized by tingling and flushing of the face, neck, and upper torso **(the red-man syndrome)**, sometimes with hypotension. Deafness, skin rash, phlebitis, chills, and, rarely, reversible neutropenia have also been described. **Ototoxicity** has rarely been observed with serum levels less than 50 μg/ml, 60 minutes after IV infusion. Significant nephrotoxicity is not clearly associated with current preparations, but there may be synergistic toxicity when vancomycin is given concurrently with an aminoglycoside (*Antimicrob. Agents Chemother.* 23:138, 1983).

IV. Tetracyclines are bacteriostatic agents with a broad spectrum of activity, including *Rickettsia, Chlamydia, Nocardia,* and *Actinomyces* spp. However, resistance is widespread, especially among *Staph. aureus* and gram-negative bacilli.

A. Indications include treatment of nongonococcal urethritis, rickettsial disease, exacerbations of chronic bronchitis, early Lyme disease, and acne. They are alternatives for the PCN-allergic patient with syphilis or *Pasteurella multocida* infection.

B. Pharmacokinetics. The tetracyclines are well absorbed when taken on an empty stomach. However, their absorption is decreased if they are taken with milk, antacids, calcium, or iron. Tetracyclines are distributed throughout the extracellular fluid (ECF). **Cerebrospinal fluid penetration is unreliable.**

C. Preparations and dosages. Tetracycline hydrochloride (250–500 mg PO q6h) is excreted primarily by the kidney. **Doxycycline** (100 mg PO bid) is well absorbed orally and has a prolonged serum half-life (17–20 hours). Because it is excreted by the liver, doxycycline is preferred in patients with renal insufficiency. Doxycycline, 100 mg IV bid, is also available.

D. Adverse effects include oral or vaginal candidiasis with prolonged use, gastrointestinal upset, photosensitivity (especially with doxycycline), and elevation of BUN. Tetracyclines should not be administered to pregnant women or to children younger than 10 years of age because of adverse effects on developing teeth and bones. Intravenous dosages should not exceed 2 g/day because of the risk of fatty degeneration of the liver.

V. Chloramphenicol (500–750 mg PO q6h or 1.0–1.5 g IV q6h) is a bacteriostatic agent active against a wide variety of gram-negative and gram-positive organisms, including anaerobes.

A. Indications include the treatment of infections due to ampicillin-resistant *H. influenzae, Salmonella* (especially typhoid fever), *Rickettsia,* and anaerobes including *B. fragilis.* Because of its toxicity, use of chloramphenicol should be restricted to seriously ill patients in whom its potential toxicity can be justified.

B. Pharmacokinetics. Chloramphenicol can be given orally or intravenously; intramuscular administration results in unreliable absorption. It penetrates into all body tissues, including the CSF (where concentrations 30–50% of serum levels are attained), the eye, and the fetal circulation. Chloramphenicol is metabolized in the liver; dosage adjustment must be made in the presence of liver disease.

C. Adverse effects. Hematopoietic toxicity, including reversible bone-marrow suppression and irreversible aplasia, may occur. Aplastic anemia is a late idiosyncratic reaction to the drug and is usually fatal. It has a frequency (1:25,000) similar to the risk of fatal anaphylaxis with penicillin. Reversible leukopenia, thrombocytopenia, and suppression of erythropoiesis are dose related and can usually be avoided by maintaining peak serum levels less than 25 μg/ml. Other adverse effects include hemolysis (in glucose-6-phosphate dehydrogenase [G-6-PD]-deficient patients), allergic reactions, and peripheral neuritis.

VI. Aminoglycoside antibiotics are bactericidal for numerous gram-positive and gram-negative organisms and mycobacteria. They are not active in an oxygen-poor environment or at a low pH and are therefore ineffective against anaerobes and unsuitable for the treatment of abscesses. Resistance to aminoglycosides is plasmid mediated; therefore, organisms that are resistant to one aminoglycoside may be susceptible to another. Consequently, susceptibility testing should be used when selecting an aminoglycoside for therapeutic use. Resistance to streptomycin is widespread among the Enterobacteriaceae and neither streptomycin nor kanamycin has reliable activity against *Pseudomonas* spp.

A. Pharmacokinetics. Aminoglycosides are distributed throughout the extracellular space, excluding the CSF, and are rapidly excreted by normally functioning kidneys. Parenteral administration is necessary to produce therapeutic levels because of poor gastrointestinal absorption, although significant amounts of the aminoglycosides may be absorbed if the mucosa of the gastrointestinal tract is inflamed or disrupted. Factors that increase the volume of distribution (e.g., pregnancy, burns, peritonitis, retroperitoneal infections) increase the amount of aminoglycoside necessary to achieve an effective peak serum level. Critically ill or young patients with an increased cardiac output and glomerular filtration rate require more frequent doses. In contrast, renal failure prolongs the half-life of aminoglycosides and necessitates a decrease in dose or a lengthening of the dosing interval. Measurement of serum drug levels is invaluable in most chronically or critically ill patients to prevent drug accumulation and in young patients may help prevent subtherapeutic regimens.

B. Indications. Aminoglycosides are useful (usually in combination with a beta-lactam antibiotic) for the treatment of serious infections caused by susceptible gram-negative bacilli, especially *Pseudomonas* spp and other resistant organisms. They have proven particularly effective in bacteremia in immunocompromised hosts. Aminoglycosides are also useful for therapy of streptococcal (especially enterococcal) endocarditis when used with PCN or ampicillin. The **limited indications for streptomycin** include bubonic plague, tularemia, brucellosis, serious enterococcal infections, and tuberculosis. **Parenteral aminoglycosides are not effective for meningitis** because they do not cross the blood-brain barrier. These agents are not used for most gram-positive infections because the PCNs and cephalosporins are less toxic. Aminoglycosides alone are not recommended for treatment of methicillin-resistant staphylococcal infections despite in vitro susceptibility.

C. **Dosage.** Aminoglycosides can be given intravenously or intramuscularly. The **loading dose** for gentamicin, tobramycin, and netilmicin is 1.5–2.0 mg/kg and for amikacin and kanamycin is 5.0–7.5 mg/kg. The **maintenance dosage** is 3–5 mg/kg/day in 3 doses for gentamicin and tobramycin, 4–6 mg/kg/day in 3 doses for netilmicin, and 15 mg/kg/day in 2–3 divided doses for amikacin and kanamycin. **Maintenance dosages must be reduced in patients with renal insufficiency and in the elderly** (see Appendix D).

D. **Adverse effects.** Nephrotoxicity and ototoxicity are the major adverse effects of the aminoglycosides. Nephrotoxicity is usually reversible, but **acute renal failure** with azotemia may occur. **Ototoxicity** may be cochlear or vestibular and is more likely to occur with prolonged use (more than 14 days) and with concurrent use of other ototoxic drugs, especially loop diuretics. If possible, serial audiometry should be conducted on patients treated for extended periods. Netilmicin may be less ototoxic and streptomycin more ototoxic than the other aminoglycosides. **Neuromuscular blockade** is a rare complication of aminoglycoside use. The risks of toxicity appear to be dose related. In monitoring for toxicity, appropriate trough levels should be less than 2 µg/ml for gentamicin and tobramycin, and less than 10 µg/ml for amikacin.

VII. **Sulfonamides** are bacteriostatic agents that interfere with folic acid synthesis.

A. **Indications** for the sulfonamides are few because many organisms are resistant to them. However, they are useful in the treatment of uncomplicated UTI, nocardiosis, and chancroid, and in the topical therapy of burns and ocular infections.

B. **Pharmacokinetics.** Gastrointestinal absorption is rapid and **therapeutic CSF levels are achieved.** Only oral preparations are currently available in the United States. Sulfonamides are excreted by the kidney, and their dosages should be reduced in renal failure.

C. **Selected preparations and dosages. Sulfisoxazole** (1 g PO q6h) is used in the treatment of UTI. **Sulfadiazine** (1.0–1.5 g PO q6h) is often used for nocardiosis and in combination with pyrimethamine for toxoplasmosis. **Sulfamethoxazole** (2 g load, then 1 g PO q12h) has a longer half-life but is more likely to produce crystalluria.

D. **Adverse effects** occur in 5–10% of treated patients. **Hypersensitivity** reactions are common and include a variety of skin rashes, vasculitis, and drug fever. Erythema multiforme and the Stevens-Johnson syndrome may occur. The sulfonamides can induce hemolytic anemia in patients with G-6-PD deficiency. The sulfonamides are contraindicated in the latter stage of pregnancy because of the risk of neonatal kernicterus.

VIII. **Trimethoprim** (100 mg PO bid) has a slow bactericidal effect against many gram-negative bacteria but not *P. aeruginosa*. It can be used alone for therapy of UTI. **Side effects** include megaloblastic anemia, bone-marrow suppression, and skin rashes.

IX. **Trimethoprim/sulfamethoxazole (cotrimoxazole) (TMP/SMZ)** is a fixed-dose combination of trimethoprim and sulfamethoxazole in a ratio of 1:5. The antibacterial spectrum of TMP/SMZ includes most gram-positive and gram-negative pathogens except *P. aeruginosa* and enterococci. Both agents are excreted by the kidney, and the dosage should be decreased in patients with renal dysfunction.

A. **Indications. TMP/SMZ** is useful in the treatment of UTI, prostatitis, acute and chronic bronchitis, acute otitis media, sinusitis, gonorrhea, chancroid, nocardiosis, shigellosis, and salmonellosis. It is the agent of choice in the treatment of

Pneumocystis carinii infection. TMP/SMZ can also be used to treat serious infections caused by susceptible gram-negative bacilli resistant to other antimicrobials (e.g., meningitis, osteomyelitis).

B. Administration (1 double-strength tablet PO bid for mild to moderate infections; 8/40–20/100 mg/kg/day PO or IV in 2–4 doses for serious infections). Monitoring sulfa or trimethoprim levels is useful when using high doses, particularly in patients with renal insufficiency (see Appendix D).

C. Adverse effects. This combination shares all the potential toxicities of its component drugs (see sec. **VII.D.** and sec. **VIII**) and should not be administered to patients with a history of sensitivity to sulfonamides. Megaloblastic anemia, leukopenia, or thrombocytopenia may occur as a result of folate deficiency. Bone-marrow suppression may occur, especially at high dosages. Patients with **AIDS seem particularly susceptible to drug toxicity from TMP/SMZ.** The large fluid volumes required for parenteral TMP/SMZ may complicate the care of patients with renal or cardiac disease.

X. Quinolones (quinolone carboxylic acids) are generally well tolerated. Among adverse reactions, gastrointestinal symptoms such as nausea, vomiting, diarrhea, and abdominal pain are most frequent. Rashes and CNS side effects (e.g., drowsiness, headache, insomnia, restlessness, dizziness, subjective visual disturbances, and, rarely, seizures) are less common. These drugs should be avoided in pregnant women and children. The fluoroquinolones may interfere with hepatic metabolism of theophylline and caffeine and may increase theophylline levels in some patients. Aluminum- and magnesium-containing antacids interfere with absorption of the quinolones.

A. Nalidixic acid (1 g PO q6h) is the prototype of this family. Its spectrum of activity includes most gram-negative bacilli except *P. aeruginosa*. Poor absorption and a high frequency of mutational resistance have limited its utility in the treatment of UTI.

B. Fluoroquinolones. Norfloxacin, ciprofloxacin, and ofloxacin are effective against most gram-negative bacilli, including *P. aeruginosa,* and many gram-positive cocci, including *Staph. aureus.* They have variable activity against streptococci, especially *Enterococcus* spp, and are inactive against anaerobic bacteria and most nonaeruginosa strains of *Pseudomonas.* These agents are highly active against *N. gonorrhoeae* and *Haemophilus ducreyi,* but none are effective against syphilis. Ciprofloxacin and ofloxacin also have activity against *Mycobacterium tuberculosis* and atypical mycobacteria. **The dosage of all of these drugs should be reduced in renal failure.** None of these agents should be used in children, or in pregnant or lactating women.

  1. Norfloxacin (400 mg PO q12h) is useful in the treatment of UTI, gonorrhea (including PCN-resistant *N. gonorrhoeae*), and bacterial enteric infections. Serum levels are relatively low; therefore, norfloxacin is not recommended for systemic or serious local infections.

  2. Ofloxacin (200–400 mg PO q12h) achieves significant serum concentrations. It can be used in the treatment of acute uncomplicated urethral or cervical gonorrhea. It may also be effective in nongonococcal urethritis or cervicitis due to *Chlamydia trachomatis,* but data are limited. Ofloxacin may also be useful in the treatment of UTIs, prostatitis, or respiratory infections.

  3. Ciprofloxacin (250–750 mg PO q12h and 200–400 mg IV q12h) also achieves significant serum concentrations after oral administration and has excellent penetration into a variety of tissues. In addition to the above indications, ciprofloxacin may be useful in the treatment of osteomyelitis, pneumonia, skin infections due to susceptible organisms, and treatment of infectious diarrhea (*Campylobacter,* toxigenic *E. coli,* and *Shigella*).

XI. Metronidazole is a nitroimidazole active against most gram-negative anaerobic bacteria, including *B. fragilis,* and many *Clostridium* spp. Many anaerobic streptococci are resistant to this agent. Metronidazole is also active against several protozoan parasites, *Trichomonas vaginalis, Giardia lamblia, Entamoeba histolytica,* and *Dracunculus medinensis.*

A. Indications. Metronidazole is useful in the treatment of anaerobic bacterial infections, including abdominal and pelvic infections, brain abscess, and osteomyelitis, and in the rare patient with *B. fragilis* endocarditis. Oral metronidazole is effective for the treatment of pseudomembranous colitis. Metronidazole must be combined with other antimicrobials when treating mixed aerobic and anaerobic infections.

B. Administration (500 mg IV q6–8h; a 1-g loading dose can be used for serious infections, 250–500 mg PO q8h for less severe infections). The gastrointestinal absorption of metronidazole is excellent. Its distribution is widespread, including the CSF, where therapeutic levels are obtained. Metronidazole is metabolized in the liver before excretion by the kidney, and the dosage should be reduced in patients with severe hepatic dysfunction.

C. Adverse effects include nausea, dry mouth, alterations in taste, disulfiram-like effects with alcohol, and uncommon neurologic reactions. Because of potential teratogenicity, it should not be used in pregnant women.

XII. Pentamidine isethionate (4 mg/kg/day IV or IM) is an aromatic diamidine indicated for therapy of *P. carinii* pneumonia (PCP). Its mechanism of action is poorly understood. Painful sterile abscesses at IM injection sites are common, making IV administration preferable. For IV use, the drug should be infused over 2 hours to minimize the risk of hypotension. **Adverse reactions** are common and include hypotension, renal failure, hypoglycemia and hyperglycemia due to pancreatic islet cell destruction, cardiac arrhythmias, leukopenia, and thrombocytopenia. Fatal pancreatitis has been reported. **Aerosolized pentamidine** (300 mg/once a month) is useful as prophylactic suppressive therapy against PCP; however, extrapulmonary *Pneumocystis* infections have been reported in patients receiving aerosolized pentamidine. The metabolism of pentamidine is not well understood, but the dosage should be reduced in patients with renal dysfunction.

Antimycobacterial Agents

I. Primary drugs

A. Isoniazid (INH) (300 mg PO qd) is bactericidal for *Mycobacterium tuberculosis*, *M. kansasii*, and *M. bovis*.

1. Administration. Isoniazid is well absorbed orally and is widely distributed throughout the body, including the CSF. It can be given in supervised short-course protocols as 15 mg/kg PO (maximum dose, 900 mg) twice a week. Larger dosages (10 mg/kg/day) can be used in more severe disease but are associated with increased toxicity.

2. Adverse effects

a. Hepatotoxicity. Asymptomatic elevation of serum transaminases may occur during the first few months of therapy in up to 20% of patients receiving INH but usually resolves as drug therapy continues. **Hepatitis** is an idiosyncratic toxicity. The incidence of INH-induced hepatitis increases with age (i.e., from 0.3% for patients 20–34 years old to approximately 2.3% for patients 50 years of age or older) (*Am. Rev. Respir. Dis.* 117:991, 1978). Daily alcohol consumption and alcoholic liver disease increase the risk of INH-induced hepatitis; however, a prior history of nonalcoholic liver disease may not. Isoniazid-induced hepatitis usually resolves after discontinuation of the drug.

b. Peripheral neuropathy is a dose-related complication of INH therapy probably due to enhanced excretion of pyridoxine. Poorly nourished patients and those predisposed to neuropathy by diabetes, uremia, or alcoholism are at particular risk and should receive **pyridoxine**, 50 mg PO qd. Patients receiving large dosages of INH, pregnant women, and those with seizure disorders should also receive pyridoxine. Other nervous system toxicities are not clearly related to pyridoxine deficiency but have been reported to respond to supplementation.

B. Rifampin (600 mg PO qd) is bactericidal for gram-positive cocci, many gram-negative bacilli, and most species of *Mycobacterium*, including intracellular and extracellular organisms. Absorption and distribution, including CNS penetration, are excellent. Rifampin undergoes enterohepatic circulation and is progressively metabolized by the liver. Rifampin induces hepatic microsomal enzymes and may alter the metabolism of many drugs. Patients should be warned about the orange-red discoloration of secretions (e.g., tears, urine, and sweat) that occurs with rifampin; it is harmless but will permanently discolor soft contact lenses. **Toxicities** include rash, mild gastrointestinal disturbances, hepatitis that may be potentiated by other types of liver disease, and CNS side effects. A rare influenza-like syndrome associated with a variety of hematologic and renal abnormalities has been reported.

II. **Secondary drugs** are used in the treatment of complicated or resistant tuberculosis and for infections with atypical mycobacteria. Selection of these agents may be aided by in vitro susceptibility studies.

  A. **Pyrazinamide (PZA)** (15–30 mg/kg/day PO; maximum, 2.0 g/day) is bactericidal for intracellular mycobacteria. A dosage of 50–70 mg/kg PO twice a week can be used in supervised settings. The drug is excreted by the kidneys. The major side effect is hepatotoxicity.

  B. **Ethambutol** (15 mg/kg/day PO) is a bacteriostatic agent. For more serious disease an initial dosage of 25 mg/kg/day can be used. The drug is excreted primarily by the kidneys, and the dosage should be reduced in patients with renal failure. The only significant dose-related toxicity is **optic neuritis,** which occurs in fewer than 1% of patients treated with 15 mg/kg/day but is seen more frequently at higher dosages. The earliest manifestations may include decreased color perception, visual field deficits, or reduced visual acuity. Routine eye examinations should be included in the care of these patients, because the ophthalmic complications are often reversible with early drug withdrawal.

  C. **Streptomycin** (0.5–1.0 mg/kg/day IM) is an aminoglycoside that is bactericidal for extracellular mycobacteria. A dosage of 25–30 mg/kg IM twice a week can also be used in supervised settings. It is not presently available in the U.S.

III. **Tertiary agents** have the lowest therapeutic ratio for the treatment of mycobacterial disease and should not be used without subspecialty consultation and susceptibility testing.

  A. **Ethionamide** (0.5–1.0 g/day PO in 3 doses) is widely distributed, including the CSF. Adverse effects include gastric irritation, hepatotoxicity, and ganglionic blockade.

  B. **Cycloserine** (0.5–1.0 g/day PO in 2–3 divided doses) is widely distributed with good CSF penetration. Side effects include behavioral disturbances, as well as seizures, somnolence, and muscle twitching.

  C. **Other aminoglycosides.** Although experience is limited, **amikacin** may be preferable as a second-line aminoglycoside for the treatment of tuberculous disease, including *Mycobacterium avium* complex, as drug assays for monitoring levels are more readily available. Kanamycin can also be used.

  D. **Clofazimine** (200–300 mg PO qd) has been used in the treatment of leprosy and *M. avium* complex infections. Toxicities include gastrointestinal intolerance and red-brown to blue discoloration of the skin.

Antiviral Agents

Viruses are obligate intracellular parasites that utilize host-specific biosynthetic mechanisms for replication. Current antiviral agents suppress viral replication; viral containment or elimination requires an intact host immune response.

I. **Amantadine** blocks an early step in replication of the influenza A virus. It has no effect against infections caused by influenza B or C.

  A. **Indications.** Uncomplicated influenza A infection usually resolves within 3–7 days, and most patients do not need prophylaxis or treatment with amantadine. However, this drug should be used for patients at high risk of complications from influenza (e.g., immunocompromised patients, the elderly, patients with pulmonary or cardiac disease) when they have influenza. During an epidemic, prophylactic amantadine should be strongly considered for patients or staff members of nursing homes or hospitals, where epidemic spread of influenza can be devastating.

B. Administration. Amantadine (100 mg PO bid) is excreted by the kidneys, and its use should be restricted to patients with adequate renal function. **Prophylaxis** should begin when influenza A is documented in the community. Amantadine can be started concurrently with vaccination for influenza A and discontinued 14 days later when protective antibodies have developed. Treatment of nonimmune individuals should begin as soon as possible after exposure or within 48 hours of the onset of symptoms and can be discontinued after 7–10 days, or 48 hours after symptoms disappear. Vaccination remains the most effective method of controlling influenza.

C. Adverse effects are uncommon and are primarily neurologic. They include confusion, slurring of speech, blurred vision, and sleep disturbance. Amantadine is teratogenic and should not be given to pregnant women.

II. Nucleoside analogs

A. Acyclovir (acycloguanosine) is most active against herpes simplex virus (HSV) types 1 and 2 and varicella–zoster virus (VZV). It has no effect on the latency of the herpes viruses. High doses of acyclovir will inhibit Epstein-Barr virus, but it is inactive in vitro against cytomegalovirus (CMV).

   1. Indications. Acyclovir is effective for treatment of primary genital herpes and severe herpes stomatitis in normal hosts. In immunocompromised hosts, acyclovir is also effective for therapy and prophylaxis of HSV infections and in the therapy of herpes zoster. Acyclovir can also be used for severe varicella (chickenpox) infections but must be given in much higher doses than those used for HSV infections.

   2. Pharmacokinetics. Acyclovir is distributed throughout the ECF; CSF levels are about 50% of plasma. Acyclovir is excreted by the kidney and its dosage must be reduced in renal failure. Each infusion of acyclovir should be given over 1 hour to minimize the risk of crystalline nephropathy.

   3. Dosage. For severe systemic infections the dosage is 5 mg/kg IV q8h for HSV and 10 mg/kg IV q8h for VZV. The oral dosage is 200 mg PO 5 times a day for HSV infection and 800 mg PO 5 times a day for localized herpes zoster infections.

   4. Adverse effects are uncommon. Reversible crystalline nephropathy may occur; preexisting renal failure, dehydration, and bolus infusion enhance the risk of nephrotoxicity. Elevation of serum transaminases and phlebitis also occur. CNS toxicity (delirium, tremors) has been reported, particularly with high dosages or in renal failure.

B. Ganciclovir (deoxyguanosine, DHPG) has antiviral activity against CMV and other herpesviruses.

   1. Indications. Ganciclovir is indicated for therapy of sight-threatening CMV retinitis. Uncontrolled studies show that ganciclovir may also be beneficial in CMV pneumonitis, esophagitis, colitis, and hepatitis in patients with AIDS. Bone-marrow and solid organ transplant patients with CMV disease may also benefit from ganciclovir therapy, but data are limited. Cytomegalovirus disease may progress despite ganciclovir therapy, and ganciclovir resistance has been reported. Patients whose conditions worsen on therapy sometimes respond to increased dosages of ganciclovir. However, even when patients respond to therapy, the relapse rate is extremely high when it is discontinued. Indefinite maintenance therapy may be required to suppress CMV in patients with AIDS.

   2. Administration. Initial **induction therapy** is 5 mg/kg bid for 10–21 days. The usual **maintenance therapy** is 5–6 mg/kg/day for 5 days every week. Ganciclovir is available only as an IV preparation and should be given as a one-hour infusion. It is widely distributed in body tissues and CSF. The dosage must be reduced for patients with renal dysfunction (see Appendix D).

   3. Adverse effects include reversible neutropenia and thrombocytopenia, which may require dosage reduction. Bone-marrow suppression is particularly severe when ganciclovir is used in conjunction with zidovudine, and few patients tolerate concurrent use of both drugs. Rash, confusion, CNS toxicity, and GI side effects have also been reported.

C. Foscarnet (trisodium phosphonoformate) has antiviral activity against herpes viruses and HIV.

1. Indications. Foscarnet is indicated for CMV retinitis in patients with AIDS. Its safety and efficacy have not been established for CMV infection at other sites, nor for infections caused by other viruses. Foscarnet is an alternative for immunocompromised patients with CMV infections in whom ganciclovir therapy is ineffective or who cannot tolerate ganciclovir. Foscarnet may also be useful in patients with serious infections due to acyclovir-resistant herpes simplex or varicella zoster. Like ganciclovir, foscarnet is virustatic, making maintenance therapy necessary for AIDS patients with CMV retinitis.

2. Administration. Initial induction therapy for CMV retinitis infection in patients with AIDS is 60 mg/kg IV over 1 hour q8h for 2–3 weeks depending on the clinical response. The recommended maintenance dose is 90–120 mg/kg-/day IV over 2 hours. For acyclovir-resistant herpes infections, a dose of 40 mg/kg IV q8h can be used. **The dosage should be carefully adjusted for the patient's renal function according to manufacturer's instructions.** To minimize nephrotoxicity, patients should also be given normal saline prior to and during the infusion, and an infusion pump should be used to control the rate of infusion. The concomitant use of other nephrotoxic agents (e.g., aminoglycosides, amphotericin, pentamidine) should be avoided.

3. Adverse effects. Nephrotoxicity can occur in up to 30% of patients treated with foscarnet. Nausea is also common. Other complications include disturbances of calcium, magnesium, and phosphorus levels, as well as seizures. A possible drug interaction with IV pentamidine has been described, resulting in severe hypocalcemia.

D. Zidovudine (ZDV; azidothymidine, AZT)

1. Indications. Zidovudine is indicated for therapy of human immunodeficiency virus (HIV) infection in patients with CD4 lymphocyte counts less than 500 cells/μl. Patients with higher CD4 lymphocyte counts may also benefit, but controlled data are lacking.

2. Administration. The recommended dosage of ZDV is 100 mg PO q4h, although dosages of 200 mg q8h are widely used. Zidovudine, 100 mg q8h, has also been shown to have antiviral activity (*N. Engl. J. Med.* 323:1009, 1990), but the long-term clinical efficacy of this dosage remains unproven.

3. Adverse effects. Nausea, myalgias, insomnia, and severe headaches are common side effects but are usually temporary. A mild macrocytic anemia is common. More severe marrow hypoplasia with anemia or neutropenia can also occur, especially in patients with advanced HIV disease. The anemia may respond to erythropoietin. In patients with recurrent bone-marrow suppression, lower dosages of ZDV (100 mg PO q8h) may be effective and less toxic. Proximal myopathy with muscle wasting or myositis may occur with long-term (greater than 1 year) use of ZDV.

E. Dideoxyinosine (ddI) is a nucleoside analog currently available for treatment of AIDS and advanced AIDS-related complex (ARC) in patients who cannot tolerate or are deteriorating on ZDV. Clinical data are extremely limited, but some zidovudine-resistant strains of HIV are susceptible to ddI in vitro. Uncontrolled trials suggest that ddI may increase CD4 cells, decrease viremia and symptoms, and improve immunologic response. The optimal dosage and clinical effectiveness against zidovudine-resistant strains are unknown. With low dosages, the most common adverse effects are headache, insomnia, and increased serum uric acid concentrations. Increased liver enzymes, pancreatitis, rash, thrombocytopenia, diarrhea, and confusion have also been reported. Dideoxyinosine appears to be minimally toxic to bone marrow.

F. Dideoxycytidine (ddC) is more active than ddI against HIV in vitro. Although data suggest clinical efficacy as well, severe peripheral neuropathy limits its use.

Antifungal Agents

I. **Amphotericin B** is a polyene antibiotic that disrupts the fungal cell by binding to ergosterol in the plasma membrane. It is indicated for most systemic mycoses except *Pseudallescheria boydii* infections.

   A. **Pharmacokinetics.** Amphotericin B is poorly absorbed and must be administered intravenously. **Low concentrations are obtained in the CSF.** Although the metabolism and excretion of amphotericin B are poorly defined, its dosage is not reduced in patients with preexisting renal failure, because only a small percentage of the administered dose is excreted by the kidneys.

   B. **Administration**

      1. **Intravenous infusion.** The drug must be suspended at a concentration less than 0.1 mg/ml in 5% dextrose in water (D/W). The dosage of amphotericin B is usually increased slowly to minimize toxicity. **A 1-mg test dose** should be given over 30 minutes and, if tolerated, can be followed by infusion of 0.2 mg/kg over 1 hour on the first day. The dosage is then increased by 0.1–0.2 mg/kg/day until a therapeutic or maximum tolerated dosage is reached, usually 0.5–1.0 mg/kg/day over 3–4 hours in adults and 1.0–1.5 mg/kg/day in children. Larger dosages may increase toxicity without improving efficacy. In patients with fulminant disease, the 1-mg test dose can be followed by 0.25 mg/kg on the first day and by full adult therapeutic doses (0.5–1.0 mg/kg) 24 hours later. The maintenance dosage can be doubled and given on alternate days, but a single dose should not exceed 1.5 mg/kg. This alternate-day regimen may reduce patient discomfort and decrease renal toxicity.

      2. **Intraventricular infusion** of amphotericin B is occasionally used in the treatment of fungal meningitis but often produces significant toxicity. This route of administration should only be used with expert consultation.

      3. **Bladder irrigation** may be useful in the treatment of fungal cystitis, but data are limited. Instillation of 5–15 mg amphotericin B in sterile water into the bladder with retention for 20–30 minutes q6–8h for 3–5 days appears to be effective. Less frequent instillation may be as effective, and continuous bladder irrigation with 50 mg amphotericin B in 1 liter sterile water administered at a rate of 1 liter/day for 3–5 days also appears to be effective.

   C. **Adverse effects.** Acute side effects, including fever, chills, headache, nausea, and vomiting, often occur but can be reduced by **premedicating** the patient with aspirin or acetaminophen, and diphenhydramine, 25–50 mg PO or IV, or with meperidine, 20–50 mg IV. The addition of hydrocortisone sodium succinate, 25–50 mg, to the infusion may also be useful. Patients often become tolerant to these adverse effects and may not require premedication after the first few weeks of therapy. **Thrombophlebitis** may be reduced by adding heparin, 1000 units, to the infusion. **Nephrotoxicity** develops in most patients treated with amphotericin B and is manifested by distal renal tubular acidosis, hypokalemia, hypomagnesemia, and impairment of glomerular filtration rate. Permanent renal damage is usually not significant unless underlying renal disease is present or the cumulative dose exceeds 3–4 g. Patients with serious renal dysfunction due to amphotericin B generally require a reduction in dosage or temporary cessation of therapy. If interrupted for more than 7 days, treatment should be restarted at 0.25 mg/kg/day and increased gradually. If possible, other nephrotoxic drugs should be avoided during therapy with amphotericin B. **Other toxicities** include anemia, as well as neuritis and arachnoiditis, which may occur with intrathecal administration.

II. **Flucytosine (5-FC),** 37.5 mg/kg PO q6h, is effective orally against some isolates of *Candida* and *Cryptococcus neoformans*. If used alone, resistance to 5-FC develops during prolonged treatment. Flucytosine is used in combination with amphotericin B in the treatment of cryptococcal meningitis or alone in short courses for persistent candidal UTI.

   A. **Pharmacokinetics.** Flucytosine is well absorbed from the gastrointestinal tract and reaches therapeutic levels in the CSF. The drug is excreted by the kidney, and the dosage must be reduced in renal insufficiency. Serum levels of 5-FC should be monitored during therapy.

   B. Adverse effects. Bone-marrow suppression is dose related and associated with serum levels greater than 100 μg/ml. Other adverse effects include gastrointestinal toxicity ranging from nausea and diarrhea to colitis with intestinal perforation.

III. Azoles. Most azoles are metabolized by the liver and do not require dosage reduction in renal insufficiency.

   A. Ketoconazole (200–600 mg PO qd) is an orally active imidazole effective in treating chronic mucocutaneous candidiasis, esophageal candidiasis, localized pulmonary histoplasmosis, blastomycosis, and paracoccidioidomycosis. It is inactive against *Aspergillus* spp. **Cerebrospinal fluid penetration is unreliable.** Ketoconazole should not be used for rapidly progressive or severe fungal infections in immunosuppressed patients.

   1. Administration. Absorption depends on gastric acidity and may be impaired in patients with achlorhydria or those taking antacids or H_2-receptor antagonists. A serum level should be obtained 2 hours after a dose to ensure adequate absorption.

   2. Adverse effects include nausea and fever, and effects due to decreased testosterone levels such as oligospermia, gynecomastia, decreased libido, and impotence. Inhibition of adrenal sterol synthesis may occur with prolonged use. Hepatotoxicity has been reported. Ketoconazole may increase cyclosporine (CSA) levels and should be used with caution in patients receiving this agent (see Appendix B).

   B. Fluconazole is more reliably absorbed than ketoconazole, even with achlorhydria. It is available both as oral and IV preparations. Fluconazole is widely distributed in the body and **penetrates readily into the CSF.** The dosage should be reduced in patients with renal dysfunction. Fluconazole may interfere with metabolism of phenytoin (Dilantin), CSA, and warfarin (Coumadin). Concurrent therapy with rifampin lowers fluconazole levels (see Appendix B).

   1. Administration. Fluconazole (200-mg load, 100 mg/day PO or IV) is useful for oropharyngeal and esophageal candidiasis, and as maintenance therapy for cryptococcal meningitis in patients with AIDS. Higher doses (400-mg load, 200–400 mg/day PO or IV) are recommended for therapy of cryptococcal meningitis. Its role in the treatment of other fungal infections, especially systemic candidiasis, is unclear.

   2. Adverse effects. Headache, GI side effects, elevated serum transaminases, and rashes have been reported most frequently. Stevens-Johnson syndrome and hepatic necrosis have been infrequently reported.

   C. Miconazole is a second-line antifungal agent. It is the drug of choice for *Pseudallescheria* infection. Miconazole has some efficacy in the treatment of coccidioidomycosis and systemic candidiasis but is ineffective against *Aspergillus* and *Histoplasma* spp. Cerebrospinal penetration is poor. A **test dose** of 200 mg is recommended, followed by gradual escalation of the dosage up to 400–1200 mg IV q8h as tolerated. **Adverse effects** include phlebitis, pruritus, nausea and vomiting, fever, rash, and CNS abnormalities. Transient decreases in hematocrit and serum sodium have been reported with IV infusion. Rare but serious toxicities include anaphylaxis and cardiac arrhythmias.

Treatment of Infectious Diseases

Thomas C. Bailey and
William G. Powderly

Principles of Therapy

I. **General principles of therapy.** In addition to the selection of antimicrobials, several aspects of care are important in the treatment of patients with infectious diseases.

A. **Treatment of protected sites** of infection involves the removal of foreign bodies, drainage of purulent material, and relief of obstruction.

B. **Predisposing conditions,** such as diabetes mellitus, uremia, heart failure, hepatic coma, and adrenal insufficiency should be treated. Iatrogenic immunosuppression should be minimized.

C. **Age,** renal function, and hepatic function should be considered before therapy since dosages may need to be adjusted.

D. **Supportive care** should include the maintenance of circulation, oxygenation, electrolyte balance, and provision of adequate nutrition.

E. **Passive immunization** is indicated for rabies, tetanus, and diphtheria (see Appendix E) and may also be useful in patients with immunoglobulin deficiency.

F. **Treatment of fever** is not required unless (1) complications of fever are present, (2) there is a significant probability of cardiac or respiratory insufficiency, or (3) there is a possibility of CNS damage. Care must be taken not to obscure fever due to inadequate therapy or emerging complications of infection. **Antipyretics should not be administered indiscriminately.**

G. **Isolation techniques.** Communicable diseases may be asymptomatic or undiagnosed (e.g., human immunodeficiency virus, herpes simplex virus, or hepatitis); body fluids from all patients should be considered potentially infectious. **Body substance isolation (BSI)** involves the use of barrier protection (e.g., gloves, mask, goggles) whenever direct contact with any body fluid is anticipated and should be employed for all patients (see Appendix F). Patients with diseases that are transmitted by the airborne route need respiratory precautions in addition to BSI.

II. **Assessment of therapy.** Some infections respond slowly, even when optimal therapy is employed. A premature change in therapy in such cases may confound the care of the patient. However, **when the expected response to treatment does not occur, the following questions should be asked:** (1) Is the isolated organism really the etiologic agent? (2) Is adequate antimicrobial therapy being given (i.e., the appropriate drug, dosage, and route)? (3) Is the antimicrobial penetrating to the site of infection (e.g., is drainage necessary)? (4) Have resistant or superinfecting pathogens emerged? (5) Is a persistent fever due to an underlying disease, an iatrogenic complication (e.g., phlebitis), a drug reaction, or another process?

III. **Upper respiratory infections**

A. **Pharyngitis.** Most cases of pharyngitis are viral. Treatable nonviral etiologies include group A *Streptococcus, Neisseria gonorrhoeae, Corynebacterium diphtheriae,* group C and G streptococci, *Haemophilus influenzae, Corynebacterium hemolyticum, Mycoplasma pneumoniae,* and *Chlamydia pneumoniae.* Noninfectious causes include pemphigus and systemic lupus erythematosus. Viral and bacterial pharyngitis may be indistinguishable on clinical grounds.

1. **Diagnosis**

a. **Throat cultures** are used to identify group A beta-hemolytic streptococcus, which requires therapy to prevent acute pyogenic complications or rheumatic fever. Throat culture in adults can be reserved for patients with a previous history of rheumatic fever, symptomatic patients exposed to a patient with streptococcal pharyngitis, and patients with significant infection (i.e., fever, pharyngeal exudate, and cervical adenopathy). Patients who fail to clear a pharyngeal infection despite symptomatic therapy should also be cultured. Cultures for *N. gonorrhoeae* should be performed if indicated by history. If diphtheria is suspected, specific culture techniques are required.

   b. Streptococcal antigen detection tests. Although specific, these tests vary in sensitivity. A positive test permits early diagnosis and treatment, but a negative test does not safely exclude group A streptococcal disease, making a culture necessary. Thus, the cost-effectiveness of rapid antigen detection tests is yet to be proven.

   c. Serology for infectious mononucleosis (e.g., a monospot test for heterophil agglutinin) and differential white blood cell count to detect atypical lymphocytes should be performed when infectious mononucleosis is suspected. Pharyngitis, atypical lymphocytosis, and a negative heterophil test should suggest the possibility of primary cytomegalovirus (CMV) or human immunodeficiency virus (HIV).

2. Treatment. Most cases of pharyngitis are self-limited and do not require antibiotic therapy. (For treatment of gonococcal pharyngitis, see Sexually Transmitted Diseases.)

   a. Treatment for group A beta-hemolytic streptococcus should be given (1) for a positive culture or antigen detection test, (2) if the patient is at high risk for development of rheumatic fever, or (3) if the diagnosis is strongly suspected, pending the results of culture. **Treatment schedules** include penicillin VK, 250 mg PO qid for 10 days; erythromycin, 250 mg PO qid for 10 days; or benzathine penicillin, 1.2 million units IM.

   b. Hospitalization and parenteral therapy are indicated when the patient is unable to take oral fluids or airway obstruction is present. Surgical treatment may be necessary in the latter case.

3. Prophylaxis against streptococcal infection is indicated for the prevention of **recurrent rheumatic fever** in the following situations: patients at high risk of streptococcal infection (children, parents of young children, school teachers, medical and military personnel, patients in crowded living conditions) and those who have had rheumatic fever within the previous 5 years. Prophylaxis can be provided by several regimens (*Circulation* 70:118A, 1984).

   a. Benzathine penicillin G, 1.2 million units IM q4 weeks, is the regimen of choice.

   b. Penicillin V, 125–250 mg PO bid, can also be used but compliance should be monitored.

   c. Sulfadiazine, 1 g PO qd, for adults with normal renal function is effective in patients with penicillin allergy.

   d. Erythromycin, 250 mg PO bid, may also be effective.

B. Epiglottitis should be considered in the febrile, toxic patient who complains of severe sore throat and dysphagia but has minimal findings on inspection of the pharynx.

1. Diagnosis. If epiglottitis is suspected, a lateral soft-tissue radiograph of the neck is indicated. Throat and blood cultures should be obtained.

2. Treatment. Hospitalization and early ENT consultation are suggested in all suspected cases. Antibacterial therapy should include an agent that is active against *H. influenzae,* such as ampicillin, 1–2 g IV q4–6h, or, in areas of ampicillin resistance, ceftriaxone, 1–2 g IV q12–24h; cefotaxime, 1–2 g q4–6h; or cefuroxime, 0.75–1.5 g IV q8h.

C. Influenza infection presents during the winter months with abrupt onset of high fever, severe myalgias, and a nonproductive cough. The elderly may have a more subtle presentation. Hospitalized patients with suspected influenza should be placed in respiratory isolation to prevent nosocomial transmission.

1. **Diagnosis** is usually clinical. If necessary, viral culture of a nasopharyngeal or pharyngeal swab can be performed.
2. **Treatment.** Amantadine, 200 mg PO followed by 100 mg PO bid for 5 days, given within 24–48 hours of initial symptoms may shorten the course of influenza A. The dose of amantadine should be reduced in patients over 65 years of age and in patients with renal insufficiency. Treatment is otherwise supportive. Vigilance for complications such as primary influenza pneumonia, secondary bacterial pneumonia, and rhabdomyolysis should be maintained.

IV. **Pneumonia** accounts for about 10% of admissions to medical wards and remains a common cause of death. Although *Streptococcus pneumoniae* is the most common etiologic agent, many bacteria, viruses, and fungi can cause pneumonia. A nonproductive cough is characteristic of *Mycoplasma, C. pneumoniae,* influenza, *Legionella,* and *P. carinii.*

A. **Diagnosis**
1. **Sputum examination. Specimens containing more than 10 epithelial cells/low-power field on a Gram's stain represent oral rather than pulmonary secretions and are not satisfactory.** Inducing sputum with inhalation of a warmed saline aerosol or nasotracheal suction can be helpful. At experienced centers, induced sputum examination is also appropriate in cases of suspected *Pneumocystis* pneumonia.
2. **Cultures.** In patients with a productive cough, **sputum** should always be cultured and results compared with those of a simultaneous Gram's stain. Sputum should not be cultured anaerobically, because contaminating pharyngeal organisms may produce misleading results. **Blood cultures** are often positive in patients with pneumococcal pneumonia. **Pleural fluid cultures** may also be helpful when a significant effusion is present.
3. **Invasive procedures,** such as transtracheal aspiration, transthoracic needle aspiration, bronchial brushings, bronchoalveolar lavage, transbronchial biopsy, and open lung biopsy may be required to diagnose severe pneumonias, especially in patients who (1) are immunocompromised, (2) fail to respond to therapy, or (3) are likely to have a nonbacterial etiology for their infiltrate (see Chap. 10).
4. **Leukocyte count.** Neutrophilia suggests bacterial infection. The leukocyte count may be low or normal in the elderly, in immunocompromised patients, and in patients with overwhelming infections.
5. **A chest radiograph** is helpful in confirming the diagnosis of pneumonia, although it is not specific. It is particularly valuable in detecting parapneumonic effusions, abscesses, and cavities.

B. **Therapeutic measures.** Adequate **hydration** is essential. **Oxygen** should be administered when indicated; occasionally, intubation and mechanical ventilation are required (see Chap. 9). **Antitussives** are unnecessary unless continued coughing exhausts the patient. **Control of pleuritic** pain may be achieved with anti-inflammatory agents, analgesics, or intercostal nerve block.

C. **Antimicrobial therapy.** Initial therapy of pneumonia is usually empiric, but a properly performed Gram's stain may allow more specific therapy. If a specific etiologic agent is subsequently identified, antimicrobial therapy can be adjusted accordingly. The otherwise healthy patient with community-acquired pneumonia will usually have subjective improvement and resolution of fever 1–3 days after initiation of therapy. **Delayed clearing of the chest radiograph** should not be cause for concern in a patient who is improving clinically (*N. Engl. J. Med.* 293:798, 1975).
1. **Empiric treatment** for suspected bacterial infection should be directed against the most likely pathogens and should be started promptly after appropriate cultures are obtained. If a diagnostic Gram's stain cannot be obtained, the following guidelines apply.
    a. **Community-acquired pneumonia in an otherwise healthy person** is usually due to *Strep. pneumoniae* or *M. pneumoniae.* Seriously ill patients should be treated for presumed pneumococcal disease with penicillin G,

6–12 million units/day IV. Vancomycin, 1 g IV q12h, is a reasonable alternative for patients with serious penicillin allergy. Erythromycin, 500 mg PO or IV qid, is effective for both *Strep. pneumoniae* and *M. pneumoniae,* and can be used in less severely ill patients. If outpatient therapy is instituted, careful follow-up study, including regular (initially daily) assessment of the patient, is necessary.

b. **Pneumonia complicating chronic obstructive pulmonary disease** (COPD) can be treated with amoxicillin, 500 mg PO q8h, or ampicillin, 1–2 g IV q6h, depending on the severity of illness. In regions where the incidence of ampicillin-resistant *H. influenzae* is high, trimethoprim/sulfamethoxazole (TMP/SMZ), 160 mg/800 mg PO bid; cefuroxime, 1.5 g IV q8h; ceftriaxone, 1–2 g IV q12–24h; cefotaxime, 1–2 g IV q4–6h; or cefamandole, 2 g IV q6h, are alternatives.

c. **Alcoholics and other debilitated patients** are at higher risk for gram-negative bacillary pneumonia than are other persons. *Legionella* should also be considered. **Neutropenic** patients are particularly susceptible to pneumonia with gram-negative organisms (especially *Pseudomonas aeruginosa*) (see sec. **IV.C.3**). **Diabetics and patients who have recently recovered from influenza** are at increased risk for *Staphylococcus aureus* pneumonia (see sec. **IV.C.2.b**).

d. **Nosocomial pneumonia.** Gram-negative and, less frequently, staphylococcal organisms are important considerations in the hospitalized patient. *Legionella* is also a nosocomial pathogen in some locations. In most patients, a combination of a broad-spectrum beta-lactam antibiotic with gram-positive activity (e.g., ceftriaxone) and an aminoglycoside is effective. If *P. aeruginosa* or other resistant gram-negative organisms are of particular concern, such as in an intensive care unit (ICU) setting or in an immunocompromised host, an antipseudomonal beta-lactam antibiotic (e.g., mezlocillin or ceftazidime) plus an aminoglycoside should be used.

e. **Aspiration pneumonia** (see Chap. 10). Alcoholism, neurologic disorders affecting airway protection, and abnormalities of deglutition or esophageal motility predispose patients to aspiration. In most cases of community-acquired aspiration pneumonia, penicillin (PCN) G, 1–2 million units IV q4h, is effective; clindamycin is an appropriate alternative. Hospitalized patients, nursing home residents, and persons receiving antibiotics are frequently colonized with gram-negative organisms; treatment should also include antimicrobials with activity against these organisms.

2. **Pneumonias caused by gram-positive bacteria**

a. *Streptococcus pneumoniae* **(pneumococcus).** In uncomplicated infection, procaine penicillin G, 600,000 units IM tid, is effective. After initial improvement, oral agents can be used (e.g., penicillin VK, 250–500 mg PO q6h) for a total of 10–14 days. Seriously ill patients should be treated with penicillin G, 1–2 million units IV q4h. Erythromycin, 500 mg PO or IV q6h, can be used in patients allergic to PCN, but vancomycin, 1000 mg IV q12h, may be preferable in seriously ill or immunocompromised patients. Multiply resistant *Strep. pneumoniae* has not been endemic in the United States and has been uniformly susceptible to vancomycin.

b. *Staphylococcus aureus.* Diabetics, patients with a recent history of influenza, and institutionalized or hospitalized patients are at increased risk. A beta-lactamase–resistant PCN (e.g., oxacillin, 6–12 g/day IV) or, where the risk of methicillin-resistant organisms is high, vancomycin should be used initially. Abscess formation and bacteremic spread are important complications. Treatment of staphylococcal pneumonia should usually be continued for a minimum of 3–4 weeks.

3. **Gram-negative pneumonias** usually result from aspiration in elderly, immunosuppressed, or otherwise debilitated patients, or in hospitalized patients. If the infecting species is unknown, two agents should be used initially (e.g., a third-generation cephalosporin and an aminoglycoside). The regimen can

then be adjusted according to the results of culture and susceptibility testing.

   a. *Klebsiella pneumoniae* causes a virulent, necrotizing pneumonia often seen in alcoholic or otherwise debilitated patients. Abscess formation is common. Third-generation cephalosporins (e.g., ceftriaxone, 1–2 g IV q12–24h) are the drugs of choice.

   b. *Haemophilus influenzae* pneumonia should be treated with ampicillin, 1–2 g IV q6h, if the pathogen is beta-lactamase negative. Second- and third-generation cephalosporins, TMP/SMZ, and chloramphenicol can be used for beta-lactamase–positive organisms.

   c. *Pseudomonas aeruginosa* pneumonia is a severe necrotizing infection requiring intensive parenteral therapy with a combination of an aminoglycoside and an antipseudomonal beta-lactam agent (see Chap. 12). **Combination therapy** should be used for synergy and because of potential bacterial resistance with single-agent therapy. The choice of individual agents should be made according to the local antimicrobial susceptibility patterns of *P. aeruginosa*. Empyema is common in this disease.

   d. *Moraxella (Branhamella) catarrhalis* is a gram-negative diplococcus that typically causes pneumonia in patients with underlying lung disease and can be treated with TMP/SMZ, amoxicillin-clavulanate, or erythromycin.

  4. *Mycoplasma pneumoniae.* The treatment of choice is erythromycin, 500 mg PO q6h, for 14–21 days. Tetracycline, 500 mg PO q6h, is an effective alternative.

  5. **Legionnaire's disease** (*Legionella pneumophila* and other Legionellaceae) occurs in debilitated and immunocompromised hosts. Extrapulmonary manifestations, including diarrhea, renal failure, and CNS dysfunction, should suggest the diagnosis. It is treated with erythromycin, 500 mg PO q6h for mild cases and 1000 mg IV q6h for severe cases. Therapy is continued for 21 days. Critically ill patients should be given high-dose IV therapy initially. The addition of rifampin, 600 mg PO qd, may be synergistic.

  6. **Plague and tularemia.** Severe infections with *Yersinia pestis* (plague) and *Francisella tularensis* (tularemia) produce pneumonia.

   a. **Plague** is enzootic among many small mammals in the southwestern United States. Human infection is acquired primarily by contact with infected animals or their carcasses. The treatment of choice is streptomycin, 7.5 mg/kg IM q6h. Doxycycline IV may be an effective alternative.

   b. **Tularemia** may be acquired by contact with infected animals (especially rabbits) or by a tick bite. Streptomycin, 7.5 mg/kg IM q6h for 10 days, is the treatment of choice. Tetracycline, 500 mg PO q6h for 14 days, and chloramphenicol, 0.5–1.0 g PO or IV q6h for 14 days, are alternatives.

  7. *Pneumocystis carinii* (see Human Immunodeficiency Virus Infection and AIDS, sec. **II.E**).

 D. **Complications** of pneumonia include effusion, empyema, abscess formation, purulent pericarditis, and the adult respiratory distress syndrome (ARDS). Significant pleural effusions should be tapped to exclude an empyema. Empyema requires chest tube drainage. Drainage by repeated thoracenteses has been associated with a significant failure rate and is not recommended. See Chap. 10 for the management of lung abscess and ARDS.

V. **Urinary tract infections.** Urinary tract infections can be classified as lower UTI (urethritis or cystitis) or upper UTI (pyelonephritis). **Lower UTI** is characterized by pyuria, often with dysuria, urgency, or frequency. A rapid, presumptive diagnosis can be made by microscopic examination of an **unspun, clean-voided urine specimen.** A urine Gram's stain can be helpful in guiding initial antibiotic choices. Bacteriuria (more than one organism/oil-immersion field) or pyuria (more than 8 leukocytes/high-power field) correlates well with the presence of infection. Quantitative culture usually yields greater than 10^4–10^5 bacteria/ml. Colony counts of less than 10^4 coliforms/ml may also indicate infection in women with acute dysuria. **Upper UTI** (pyelonephritis) represents infection of the renal parenchyma. Presenting symptoms include fever and flank pain, as well as lower tract symptoms. Urine specimens characteristically demonstrate significant bacteriuria, pyuria, and occasional leukocyte casts. Other sites of infection in the genitourinary tract (e.g., epididymis, prostate, perinephric areas) are often associated with less than 10^3 bacteria/ml and have different clinical manifestations. Special techniques, such as quantitative cultures before and after prostatic massage, may be necessary to demonstrate these infections.

A. **Acute urethral syndrome (AUS)** is a term used in women with lower UTI symptoms and pyuria who have fewer than 10^5 bacteria/ml of urine. These patients may have bacterial cystitis, or urethritis caused by *Chlamydia trachomatis, Ureaplasma urealyticum,* or, less frequently, *N. gonorrhoeae.* Specific cultures for *N. gonorrhoeae* should be performed. Vaginitis and genital herpes should be excluded. If no specific etiology is found, tetracycline, 500 mg PO qid, or doxycycline, 100 mg PO bid, should be given for at least 7 days. Erythromycin should be used for pregnant women with nongonococcal urethritis.

B. **Lower UTI** usually occurs in women and the incidence increases linearly with age. The significance of asymptomatic bacteriuria in the nonobstructed adult is controversial; it should be documented with at least two cultures if treatment is being considered. Infections in men younger than 50 years of age are uncommon and suggest anatomic or functional abnormalities of the genitourinary tract. Men should have a complete genitourinary evaluation after their first infection; women should be evaluated after more than two recurrences within 1 year. Recurrent UTI may be associated with sexual activity. Chronic UTI is usually related to bladder instrumentation or catheterization, or to significant urine residual produced by obstruction or neurogenic bladder dysfunction. The usual urinary pathogen in community-acquired UTI is *Escherichia coli. Staphylococcus saprophyticus* is a frequent pathogen in sexually active young women. Chronic, complicated infections may be due to *E. coli* but are also frequently caused by *Klebsiella, Enterobacter, Proteus, Enterococcus* spp, and *P. aeruginosa.*

   1. **Antibiotic therapy.** Single-dose oral regimens are sufficient for symptomatic, nonpregnant women with no known anatomic or functional abnormalities and no underlying illness. A follow-up urine culture should be obtained 7–14 days after therapy. **Single-dose failures** due to susceptible organisms should generally be treated with a 14-day regimen, and urologic evaluation may be appropriate. More prolonged oral regimens (7–10 days) should be given to symptomatic men, pregnant women, patients with symptoms of upper UTI, and patients with underlying renal disease or obstruction. Children and pregnant women with asymptomatic bacteriuria should also be treated for 7–10 days.

      a. **Single-dose regimens** include (1) amoxicillin, 3 g PO; (2) sulfisoxazole, 2 g PO; or (3) TMP/SMZ, 320 mg/1600 mg PO.

      b. **Seven- to fourteen-day therapy regimens** include (1) sulfisoxazole, 2 g PO initially, then 1–2 g PO qid; (2) TMP/SMZ, 160 mg/800 mg PO bid; (3) amoxicillin, 250 mg PO q8h; (4) ampicillin, 250–500 mg PO qid; and (5) cephalexin, 500 mg PO qid. Indanyl carbenicillin, 0.5–1.0 g PO qid; norfloxacin, 400 mg PO bid; or ciprofloxacin, 250 mg PO bid, can be used for UTI caused by *Pseudomonas* spp or other highly resistant gram-negative organisms.

   2. **Adjunctive measures** such as hydration and analgesia with phenazopyridine, 200 mg PO tid, may provide symptomatic relief during the first 24–48 hours. Analgesia should not be given for longer periods because it may obscure persistent infection.

   3. **Failure of therapy** for an infection due to a susceptible organism suggests an anatomic or functional genitourinary abnormality, or persistent renal infection.

   4. **Prophylaxis** may be helpful for patients with frequent lower UTI. Sterilization of the urine with a standard treatment regimen is necessary before prophylaxis is initiated. Then, TMP/SMZ, 40 mg/200 mg qd or qod, is usually sufficient. For women with relapses that correlate with sexual intercourse, ampicillin, 250 mg, or TMP/SMZ, 80 mg/400 mg after coitus, may provide adequate prophylaxis.

5. **Bladder catheters** may be indispensable for patient care but should be used only when absolutely necessary. Indwelling catheters should be inserted with aseptic technique and should not be irrigated unless obstruction is suspected. A closed urinary drainage system should be used. Catheters should be removed as soon as possible, and, after removal, a urine culture should be obtained within 1–2 days and bacteriuria treated. With **chronic indwelling catheters,** the development of bacteriuria is inevitable, and long-term antimicrobial suppression simply selects for multiply resistant bacteria. Such patients should be treated with systemic antimicrobials only if symptomatic infection is evident. Condom catheters may be associated with less frequent UTI in cooperative or paralyzed patients where patency of the outflow can be ensured (*J.A.M.A.* 242:340, 1979).

C. **Upper UTI** is usually associated with the same pathogens responsible for lower UTI. **Acute, nonobstructive pyelonephritis** should respond to antimicrobials and hydration without sequelae. TMP/SMZ, 160 mg/800 mg PO bid for 14 days, is the treatment of choice for mild infections (*Ann. Intern. Med.* 106:341, 1987). If hospitalization is required, antibiotic choices should be determined by the local pattern of susceptibility. Ampicillin, 1–2 g IV q6h, is appropriate initial therapy in community-acquired disease in areas where *E. coli* remains susceptible. Alternatively, a cephalosporin such as cefazolin, 1–2 g IV q8h, can be used. Ampicillin is preferred if enterococcal infection is suspected. An aminoglycoside should also be given to seriously ill patients until sensitivity data are available. Broad-spectrum beta-lactam agents and ciprofloxacin are useful for patients with infection caused by highly resistant organisms. Therapy is usually given for 14 days, but patients with severe infections or acute obstructive pyelonephritis may require more prolonged therapy. Relief of obstruction is critical for long-term cure in the latter case.

D. **Prostatitis** is usually caused by enteric gram-negative bacilli. TMP/SMZ, 160 mg/800 mg PO bid for 14 days, is the treatment of choice for acute infections. Norfloxacin and ciprofloxacin are useful alternatives. Patients with chronic bacterial prostatitis should receive prolonged therapy (for at least 1 month with the quinolones or 3 months with TMP/SMZ).

E. **Epididymitis** is usually caused by *N. gonorrhoeae* or *C. trachomatis* in sexually active young men and by gram-negative enteric organisms in older men. Diagnosis and therapy should be directed accordingly (see Sexually Transmitted Diseases).

VI. **Central nervous system infections**

A. **Acute bacterial meningitis is a medical emergency. The prognosis in bacterial meningitis depends on the interval between the onset of disease and the initiation of antimicrobial therapy.** Therefore, when bacterial meningitis is suspected, diagnostic procedures (e.g., lumbar puncture) should be completed and therapy instituted **within 1 hour** of presentation. **Adjunctive radiographic studies,** such as sinus x-rays and CT of the brain, can be performed electively **after the initiation of antimicrobial therapy.** Meningitis should be considered in any patient with fever and neurologic symptoms, especially if there is a history of other infection (e.g., pneumonia) or head trauma. Cerebrospinal fluid (CSF) pleocytosis with negative cultures may be associated with viral meningoencephalitis, parameningeal infection, neoplastic disease, subarachnoid hemorrhage, trauma, and partially treated bacterial meningitis. Chronic meningitis due to fungi or mycobacteria should be considered if initial culture for bacteria are negative. *Strep. pneumoniae* and *N. meningitidis* **are responsible for most adult bacterial meningitides.** *Haemophilus influenzae,* other gram-negative bacilli, streptococci, staphylococci, and *Listeria monocytogenes* are less frequent.

1. **Diagnostic measures.** In the absence of focal neurologic signs, a lumbar puncture should be performed immediately. Cerebrospinal fluid pressure should be measured and a CSF specimen should be obtained. Head CT, preferably with contrast, is indicated in the patient with focal neurologic signs or diminished level of consciousness. **However, in the seriously ill**

patient, antibiotic therapy should not be delayed for these procedures (including lumbar puncture) to be performed.

a. **Cultures.** Cerebrospinal fluid specimens should be taken immediately to the laboratory. Blood, nasal swabs, and aspirates of skin lesions should be handled similarly. If viral meningitis is a possibility, CSF specimens should be cultured promptly. If this is not possible, CSF and serum should be frozen at $-70°C$ for subsequent viral culture and serologic investigation; viral cultures of the throat and stool may provide additional evidence.

b. **Cerebrospinal fluid examination** should include cell counts with differential and gram-stained smears of the centrifuged sediment. Neutrophilic pleocytosis is usually seen in bacterial meningitis but may also be present early in viral meningitis (*N. Engl. J. Med.* 289:571, 1973). In very early bacterial meningitis, pleocytosis may be absent. **India ink preparations and acid-fast** stains should be examined if the Gram's stain does not yield a diagnosis. A wet-mount examination of the sediment may reveal motile amoebas in amoebic meningoencephalitis.

c. **Cerebrospinal fluid protein and glucose.** The CSF protein is commonly elevated (> 100 mg/dl) and glucose decreased (< 45 mg/dl or < 50–66% of blood glucose) in bacterial meningitis, as well as tuberculous and fungal meningitis.

d. **Detection of capsular polysaccharide antigens** is possible for *Strep. pneumoniae, H. influenzae* type B, *Neisseria meningitidis* (groups A and C), and group B streptococcus. Because false positives and false negatives may occur, these tests should not be the sole basis on which to guide initial antimicrobial therapy. In contrast, the detection of capsular polysaccharide of *Cryptococcus neoformans* in CSF by latex agglutination is sensitive and specific. The microbiology or serology laboratory should be consulted to determine which tests and specimens are appropriate for particular pathogens.

2. **Supportive measures** include maintenance of electrolyte balance and airway patency. Fluid intake should be restricted to 1000 ml/m^2/day. Comatose patients may require intubation. Treatment of associated seizures is discussed in Chap. 25.

3. **Initial antimicrobial therapy. When bacterial meningitis is suspected,** high-dose parenteral antibiotic therapy should be administered. Antimicrobial combinations are reasonable if the pathogen is unknown or if polymicrobial infection (e.g., brain abscess) is suspected. Aqueous penicillin G, 2 million units IV q2h, will usually provide effective initial therapy. However, if the cause of the meningitis is unclear, additional antimicrobials should be chosen on the basis of the clinical setting and the CSF Gram's stain. If no organisms are seen on Gram's stain, addition of a third-generation cephalosporin (e.g., ceftriaxone, 2 g IV q12h) is prudent while awaiting culture results. Antistaphylococcal coverage is also important in the appropriate clinical setting.

4. **Therapy for specific infections**

a. ***Streptococcus pneumoniae.*** Penicillin G, 2 million units IV q2h for 10–14 days, is appropriate in most cases. Patients allergic to PCN can be treated with chloramphenicol, 1.0–1.5 g IV q6h.

b. ***Neisseria meningitidis.*** Penicillin G, 2 million units IV q2h, should be continued for at least 5 days after the patient has become afebrile. Patients allergic to PCN can be treated with chloramphenicol, 1.0–1.5 g IV q6h. **Patients with meningococcal meningitis** should be placed in a private room on respiratory isolation for at least the first 24 hours of treatment. **Close contacts and family members should receive prophylaxis** with rifampin, 600 mg PO bid for 2 days, or, if the pathogen is susceptible, with sulfadiazine, 1 g PO bid for 2 days. Terminal component complement deficiency should be ruled out in patients with recurrent infections.

c. ***Haemophilus influenzae.*** *Haemophilus influenzae* is a rare cause of meningitis in adults. Cefotaxime, 2 g IV q4h, or ceftriaxone, 2 g IV q12h, is effective as initial therapy. Chloramphenicol, 1.0–1.5 g IV q6h, is the preferred alternative for patients who are allergic to penicillins and cephalosporins. Ampicillin, 2 g IV q4h, is the drug of choice for beta-lactamase-negative strains. Treatment should be continued for a minimum of 10 days.

d. *Staphylococcus aureus* is a rare cause of meningitis and produces high mortality despite treatment. It may result from high-grade staphylococcal bacteremia, direct extension from a parameningeal focus, a neurosurgical procedure, or skull trauma. **Initially, nafcillin or oxacillin, 2 g IV q4h, should be given.** First-generation cephalosporins should not be used because they do not enter the CSF. Vancomycin, 1000 mg IV q12h, is the drug of choice for PCN-allergic patients and when methicillin resistance is likely or is confirmed by culture. Documentation of adequate CSF levels may be prudent, particularly in patients who respond poorly to therapy. Rifampin may be beneficial in cases of methicillin-resistant *Staph. aureus* (MRSA) meningitis not responding to vancomycin alone.

e. *Staphylococcus epidermidis* meningitis is usually secondary to an infected ventricular shunt. Vancomycin, 1000 mg IV q12h, is the drug of choice. Intraventricular vancomycin, 10 mg qd–qod, may be a useful adjunct. A combination of rifampin and vancomycin has not shown superiority over vancomycin alone. Removal of an infected shunt is often necessary for cure.

f. **Gram-negative bacillary meningitis** occurs in the setting of head trauma and neurosurgical procedures and is also seen in neonates, the elderly, and debilitated patients (e.g., alcoholics). Third-generation cephalosporins such as cefotaxime, 2 g IV q4h, or ceftriaxone, 2 g IV q12h, are indicated for susceptible pathogens. TMP/SMZ, chloramphenicol, and ampicillin are alternatives. Ceftazidime, 2 g IV q8h, has been used effectively for *P. aeruginosa* meningitis but should probably be combined with IV aminoglycoside therapy.

g. *Listeria monocytogenes* is an important cause of meningitis in immunosuppressed adults. The treatment of choice is ampicillin, 2 g IV q4h (or penicillin G, 2 million units IV q2h), in combination with a systemically administered aminoglycoside. Treatment should be continued for at least 3–4 weeks.

B. **Brain abscess** may result from spread from a contiguous focus (e.g., mastoiditis, sinusitis), by hematogenous spread from a distant site (e.g., lung abscess, endocarditis), or by reactivation of a latent infection (e.g., toxoplasmosis).

1. **Clinical features.** The presentation is often subacute to chronic and is usually that of an expanding mass lesion with neurologic signs or symptoms. Fever may be absent. Hematogenous abscesses or abscesses that rupture into the ventricles may present more acutely, suggesting bacterial meningitis.

2. **Diagnosis.** Patients with a compatible clinical picture should undergo a head CT with contrast, which typically reveals ring-enhancing lesions, often with associated edema. MRI may be more sensitive in detecting small lesions or lesions in the posterior fossa. Lumbar puncture is unlikely to be helpful and is contraindicated in some patients. In patients with AIDS, multiple brain abscesses usually represent *Toxoplasma* encephalitis (see Human Immunodeficiency Virus and AIDS). The presence of pulmonary or skin lesions should suggest the possibility of nocardiosis, tuberculosis, or, in endemic areas, blastomycosis.

3. **Therapy.** Most patients will require either needle aspiration or surgical drainage for microbiologic diagnosis and therapy. In the immunologically normal host, a reasonable empiric combination while awaiting bacteriologic confirmation is intravenous penicillin G, 12–24 million units IV daily; a third-generation cephalosporin (e.g., ceftriaxone, 2 g IV q12h); and metronidazole, 500 mg IV tid–qid. If *Staph. aureus* is suspected, a penicillinase-resistant penicillin (e.g., oxacillin or nafcillin) should be used. Chloram-

phenicol, 1 g IV q6h, is suitable for the penicillin-allergic patient. Antibiotics should be continued for 3–4 weeks after drainage.

C. Herpes encephalitis. This is the most common cause of acute sporadic encephalitis. Successful treatment depends on a high degree of suspicion and early institution of therapy.

    1. Clinical features. The diagnosis should be suspected in any patient who presents with the abrupt onset of fever and behavioral changes, alteration of consciousness, focal neurologic findings, or seizures, particularly if such manifestations are out of proportion to CSF abnormalities.

    2. Diagnosis. Cerebrospinal fluid findings are nonspecific and may be minimal or absent. Technetium brain scan may show increased uptake in the involved temporal lobe. Computed tomography with contrast may demonstrate localized temporal lobe edema, mass effect, hemorrhage, and patchy contrast enhancement. MRI may be more sensitive than CT scan for detecting subtle abnormalities. Brain biopsy is occasionally required but is no longer considered imperative.

    3. Therapy. In suspected cases, treatment should be instituted without delay with acyclovir, 10 mg/kg IV q8h for 10 days.

VII. Infective endocarditis (IE) is usually caused by gram-positive cocci. Parenteral drug abusers and patients with catheter-associated sepsis have an increased risk of staphylococcal disease. Gram-negative and fungal endocarditis are infrequent and usually occur in drug addicts or in patients with prosthetic valves. **The clinical features of IE are influenced by the causative organism.** However, while viridans streptococci classically produce the clinical picture of subacute bacterial endocarditis (SBE), and *Staph. aureus* endocarditis produces acute bacterial endocarditis (ABE), either organism may cause either syndrome. Patients with ABE are typically ill for a short time (3–10 days) and present critically ill. In contrast, patients with SBE are often chronically ill, with symptoms of fatigue, weight loss, low-grade fever, immune complex disease (nephritis, arthralgias, petechiae, Osler's nodes, Janeway lesions), and emboli (renal, splenic, and cerebral infarcts). A deformed or previously damaged valve is the usual focus of infection in SBE. Left-sided endocarditis, involving the aortic or mitral valves, occurs most commonly in middle-aged and older patients with preexisting valvular disease. Dental procedures, instrumentation of the genitourinary or gastrointestinal tract, and bacteremia from distant foci of infection are frequent seeding events. Right-sided endocarditis, involving the tricuspid or pulmonic valves, is seen most frequently in parenteral drug abusers and in hospitalized patients with vascular catheters.

A. Diagnosis. The most reliable criterion is continuous bacteremia in a compatible clinical setting.

    1. Blood cultures are positive in more than 90% of patients. Three sets of blood cultures taken over a 24-hour period are usually adequate in patients with SBE; however, the yield may be reduced significantly if the patient has received antimicrobial therapy within 1–2 weeks. **Because ABE is a medical emergency,** three cultures should be taken from separate sites over a 1-hour period before empiric therapy is begun. Cultures should be incubated for 4 weeks if fastidious organisms are suspected.

    2. Echocardiography. Patients with IE and vegetations seen by conventional echocardiography are at higher risk of embolism, heart failure, and valvular disruption. A normal echocardiogram does not exclude the diagnosis of IE, and false-positive findings occur with myxomatous valvular degeneration, ruptured chordae tendineae, and atrial myxomas. Transesophageal echocardiography may be more sensitive than M-mode or two-dimensional techniques. Visualization of vegetations alone does not mandate surgical intervention. Vegetations visualized by echocardiography may persist unchanged for at least 3 years after clinical cure.

B. Treatment of bacterial endocarditis on native valves requires high doses of antimicrobials for extended periods. Quantitative susceptibility testing (minimal inhibitory concentrations and minimal lethal concentrations), the measurement of serum drug levels and serum bactericidal activity, and serial erythrocyte sedimentation rates help assess the adequacy of therapy (see Chap. 12).

1. **Streptococci** cause most cases of SBE. These organisms are susceptible to PCN, which produces a recovery rate of more than 90%. *Streptococcus bovis* bacteremia and endocarditis are associated with lower gastrointestinal disease, including neoplasms. Group B streptococcal endocarditis may also be associated with lower intestinal pathology.

    a. **Penicillin G,** 2 million units IV q4h for 4 weeks, is effective for PCN-susceptible strains (minimal inhibitory concentration ≤ 0.1 μg/ml). Therapy with parenteral PCN and an aminoglycoside for 2 weeks is an alternative, but extended aminoglycoside treatment should be avoided in the elderly and in patients who could not tolerate the potential nephrotoxicity or ototoxicity. If the minimal inhibitory concentration (MIC) of PCN is greater than 0.1 μg/ml but less than 1.0 μg/ml, the addition of streptomycin or gentamicin may be appropriate for the first 2 weeks of therapy, followed by PCN alone for 2 weeks. Patients with endocarditis caused by streptococci with PCN MICs greater than 1.0 μg/ml may require combination therapy similar to that given for enterococcal IE.

    b. **Patients allergic to PCN.** Penicillin skin testing and desensitization should be considered. Vancomycin is an acceptable alternative.

    c. *Streptococcus pyogenes* **(group A) and** *Strep. pneumoniae* typically cause ABE and should be treated with penicillin G, 2–4 million units IV q4h, for 4–6 weeks.

2. *Enterococcus* **spp** cause 10–20% of cases of SBE. High-level aminoglycoside resistance (MIC > 2000 μg/ml), vancomycin resistance, and beta-lactamase production occur and should be screened for in patients with enterococcal endocarditis. **The combination of a penicillin plus an aminoglycoside** (in the absence of beta-lactamase production and high-level aminoglycoside resistance) produces synergism against these bacteria and is the treatment of choice. Penicillin alone is often ineffective. Recommended doses are ampicillin, 2 g IV q4h, or penicillin G, 2–3 million units IV q4h, in combination with gentamicin, 1.0–1.5 mg/kg IV q8h for 6 weeks. Streptomycin can be used instead of gentamicin for susceptible strains. In susceptible strains, **vancomycin** in combination with an aminoglycoside is effective against enterococci and should be used for **PCN-allergic patients or patients with beta-lactamase–producing strains.** Aminoglycoside and vancomycin levels should be monitored. Weekly audiometry is also recommended. Serum bactericidal activity should be determined to optimize therapy. Enterococci with high-level aminoglycoside resistance are resistant to synergism with a PCN plus that specific aminoglycoside. The optimal management of IE due to enterococci with high-level resistance to all aminoglycosides is unclear.

3. *Staphylococcus aureus* endocarditis should be treated with oxacillin or nafcillin, 2 g IV q4h, although PCN is effective against sensitive strains. An aminoglycoside can be added during the initial 7–14 days of therapy or in patients who fail to respond to beta-lactam therapy alone. Antimicrobials should be continued for 6 weeks in most cases. The prognosis is better in young parenteral drug abusers with right-sided endocarditis; treatment with oxacillin or nafcillin alone for 4 weeks is usually sufficient and surgery is rarely required. A 2-week course of nafcillin plus an aminoglycoside has also been advocated as treatment for purely right-sided disease in parenteral drug abusers (*Ann. Intern. Med.* 109:619, 1988). Older patients with aortic valve infection have a high mortality and often require surgical intervention. For IE caused by MRSA, vancomycin is the drug of choice. Cephalosporins should not be used in such cases, even if the isolate is sensitive in vitro.

4. *Staphylococcus epidermidis* is an increasingly frequent cause of IE, particularly after cardiac surgery. These organisms are often resistant to PCN, semisynthetic penicillins, and the cephalosporins. Pending susceptibility studies, the treatment of choice is vancomycin, 1 g IV q12h, in combination with rifampin, 300 mg PO q12h, and gentamicin. Cephalosporins should not

be used to treat methicillin-resistant strains, even if the isolate is sensitive in vitro. Treatment should be continued for at least 6 weeks.

5. **Acute bacterial endocarditis** requires empiric antimicrobial treatment before culture results become available. *Staphylococcus aureus* and gram-negative bacilli are the most likely pathogens. Treatment should include oxacillin or nafcillin, 2 g IV q4h, plus gentamicin or tobramycin, 1.5–2.0 mg/kg IV q8h.

6. **Culture-negative endocarditis.** If the diagnosis of IE is well established on clinical grounds, therapy should be initiated despite negative cultures. Treatment usually includes penicillin G, 2–3 million units IV q4h, or ampicillin, 2 g IV q4h, plus an aminoglycoside. This regimen should be continued for 4–6 weeks.

C. **Prosthetic valve endocarditis (PVE)** occurs in 1–4% of patients after valve replacement. **Early infections** (within 2 months of surgery) are commonly caused by *Staph. aureus, Staph. epidermidis,* gram-negative bacilli, *Candida* spp, and other opportunistic organisms. The diagnosis is difficult, because fever and transient bacteremia often occur in the postoperative period; however, endocarditis must be considered in any patient with sustained bacteremia after valve surgery. Treatment should continue for at least 6 weeks and should be guided by the results of MIC and serum bactericidal studies. **Late prosthetic valve endocarditis** (i.e., > 2 months after surgery) is usually caused by organisms similar to those seen in SBE on native valves. Treatment should be continued for at least 6 weeks.

D. **Role of surgery.** Indications for urgent cardiac surgery include (1) uncontrolled infection as manifested by sustained bacteremia, (2) refractory heart failure, or (3) in PVE, an unstable prosthesis or valve obstruction. Surgical intervention may also be necessary when native valve endocarditis is complicated by recurrent systemic emboli, mycotic aneurysm, persistent conduction defects, chordae tendineae or papillary muscle rupture, or early closure of the mitral valve on echocardiography, or when PVE is complicated by a periprosthetic leak. In addition, **fungal endocarditis** is usually refractory to medical therapy and requires surgery. Endocarditis due to gram-negative bacilli may also be refractory to antimicrobials alone. Although 10 days of preoperative antibiotics is desirable, surgery must not be delayed in patients whose condition is deteriorating.

E. **Response to antimicrobial therapy.** Appropriate antimicrobial therapy in IE frequently leads to clinical improvement within 3–10 days. Persistent or recurrent fever usually represents extensive cardiac infection but may also be due to septic emboli or drug hypersensitivity. Such fever seldom represents the development of antibiotic resistance, and drug therapy should be altered only if there is clear evidence of another infection or drug hypersensitivity (*Lancet* 1:1341, 1986).

F. **Prophylaxis** (Table 13-1) should be provided for those at increased risk for IE, including patients with a previous history of IE, rheumatic heart disease, most forms of congenital heart disease, calcific aortic stenosis, hypertrophic obstructive cardiomyopathy, prosthetic valves and other intravascular prostheses, and mitral valve prolapse with mitral insufficiency. Parenteral prophylaxis for oral procedures is not required for high-risk patients (e.g., those with prosthetic valves) but may still be preferred by some physicians. For high-risk patients undergoing genitourinary or gastrointestinal procedures, parenteral prophylaxis is recommended (*J.A.M.A.* 264:2919, 1990).

VIII. **Enteric infections** are among the most common infections worldwide. They usually present with gastrointestinal symptoms but may also present as enteric fever or septicemia. Most cases of enteritis, including those caused by viruses and many bacterial pathogens, are self-limited and do not require specific therapy in the normal host. **Fluid replacement** is often the only treatment needed. Usually, oral replacement is satisfactory, but IV fluids may be required if the illness is protracted or if dehydration is severe. **Antidiarrheal agents** (see Chap. 15) may provide symptomatic relief but should generally be avoided if fever or symptoms of dysentery are present. **Diagnostic studies** are not cost-effective in acute illness of

Table 13-1. Endocarditis prophylaxis

Drug	Dosage
Dental procedures	
Standard regimens	
1. Amoxicillin	3.0 g PO 1 hour before procedure and 1.5 g PO 6 hours after initial dose
or (if PCN allergy is present)	
2. Erythromycin	Erythromycin ethyl succinate, 800 mg, or erythromycin stearate, 1.0 g, PO 2 hours before procedure; then half the dose 6 hours after the initial dose
or	
3. Clindamycin	300 mg PO 1 hour before procedure and 150 mg PO 6 hours after initial dose
Alternate regimens	
4. Ampicillin	2 g IM or IV 30 minutes before procedure; then ampicillin, 1 g IM or IV, or amoxicillin, 1.5 g PO, 6 hours after initial dose
or	
5. Clindamycin	300 mg IV 30 minutes before procedure; then 150 mg IV or PO 6 hours after initial dose
For high-risk patients who are not candidates for standard regimen	
1. Ampicillin, plus	2 g IM or IV 30 minutes before procedure
Gentamicin, plus	1.5 mg/kg (maximum 80 mg) IM or IV 30 minutes before procedure
Amoxicillin	1.5 g PO 6 hours after ampicillin plus gentamicin; alternatively, the parenteral regimen can be repeated 8 hours after the initial doses
or (if PCN allergy is present)	
2. Vancomycin	1 g IV over 1 hour beginning 1 hour before procedure
Lower gastrointestinal and genitourinary procedures	
Standard regimen	
1. Ampicillin, plus	2 g IM or IV 30 minutes before procedure
Gentamicin, plus	1.5 mg/kg (maximum 80 mg) 30 minutes before procedure
Amoxicillin	1.5 g PO 6 hours after ampicillin plus gentamicin
or (if PCN allergy is present)	
2. Vancomycin, plus	1 g IV over 1 hour beginning 1 hour before the procedure
Gentamicin	1.5 mg/kg (maximum 80 mg) IM or IV 1 hour before the procedure; can be repeated once 8 hours after the initial dose
Alternate regimen for low-risk patients	
3. Amoxicillin	3 g PO 1 hour before the procedure and 1.5 g PO 6 hours after the initial dose

mild to moderate severity. Fever, symptoms of dysentery, a prolonged course, or an unusual exposure history should prompt further evaluation. **A detailed history, methylene blue stain** of the stool to look for **fecal leukocytes** suggesting an invasive process, stool examination for **ova and parasites,** and **sigmoidoscopy** to exclude the characteristic pseudomembranes associated with *Clostridium difficile* toxin–induced enterocolitis may be useful. **Stool cultures** may reveal many common pathogens, but the microbiology laboratory should be notified if specific pathogens are anticipated to ensure optimal processing.

A. *Salmonella* infections may present as enteric fever, septicemia, or enterocolitis. The usual sources of nontyphoidal salmonella are contaminated meat and poultry products.

1. *Salmonella typhi* **is the classic cause of enteric fever,** but other species may present similarly and are more common in the United States. Multiple drug resistance has been a problem with *S. typhi*, particularly among strains acquired in Mexico. **Chloramphenicol,** 500 mg IV or PO q4h, is the initial treatment of choice. The dosage can be reduced as the patient's condition improves. Therapy should be continued for up to 21 days; ampicillin, 1–2 g IV q6h; TMP/SMZ, 160 mg/800 mg PO q12h; ciprofloxacin; and third-generation cephalosporins are alternatives. **Carriers** (patients who continue to excrete the organism in the stool for more than 3 months after recovery) are the reservoir of disease. Ampicillin, 2 g PO qid; amoxicillin, 2 g PO tid; or TMP/SMZ, 160 mg/800 mg bid, for at least 4 weeks, can eliminate the carrier state in patients with normal gallbladder function. Ciprofloxacin, 750 mg PO bid, may also be effective. Patients with cholelithiasis often need cholecystectomy to eradicate the carriage of *S. typhi.*

2. **Septicemia** caused by nontyphoidal salmonella frequently presents as fever without gastroenteritis. Uncomplicated septicemia should be treated (see sec. **VIII.A.1**) for a minimum of 14 days. Treatment of complications (e.g., intravascular infection, osteomyelitis) warrants prolonged antimicrobial therapy. Patients with AIDS may have recurrent, disseminated salmonella infections despite therapy (see Human Immunodeficiency Virus Infections and AIDS, sec. **II.B.1**).

3. **Enterocolitis** is the most common form of salmonellosis. Blood cultures are usually negative. Supportive therapy is adequate in the normal host, although antibiotics (see sec. **VIII.A.1**) may be useful in compromised hosts, the very young, and the elderly.

B. *Shigella* **infections.** Bacillary dysentery primarily affects children and is transmitted by the fecal–oral route. The infection is also prevalent in male homosexuals. Diagnosis is generally made by stool culture. The majority of patients with shigellosis recover spontaneously within 1 week and require only supportive therapy. Antibiotics may hasten recovery in more seriously ill patients. TMP/SMZ, 160 mg/800 mg PO or IV q12h for 5 days, or ampicillin, 500 mg IV or PO q6h for 5–7 days, is effective for susceptible strains. Norfloxacin, 400 mg PO bid, or ciprofloxacin, 500 mg PO bid, is the treatment of choice for resistant strains. Amoxicillin is less effective and should not be used. **Antidiarrheal agents should be avoided, if possible,** since they may increase the duration of symptoms and the risk of bacteremia.

C. *Campylobacter* **enteritis** usually presents as an acute dysenteric illness with spontaneous recovery within 4–5 days. Prolonged infections may be confused with inflammatory bowel disease. The diagnosis is confirmed by a positive stool culture. When treatment is necessary, the drug of choice is erythromycin, 0.5–1.0 g PO qid. Serious infections require 3–4 weeks of therapy to prevent relapse. Tetracycline and the quinolones are also active against *Campylobacter* spp.

D. *Yersinia* **spp** may cause enterocolitis, mesenteric adenitis, or septicemia. Childhood infection with *Y. enterocolitica* may present as an inflammatory enterocolitis. Infection in older children and adults may mimic acute appendicitis. Isolation of the pathogen requires special techniques and should be discussed with the microbiology laboratory. Enterocolitis and mesenteric aden-

itis are usually self-limited and require only supportive care. Septicemia is rare.
E. **Aeromonas hydrophila, Vibrio parahaemolyticus, and Pleisiomonas shigel-loides** have all been associated with self-limited, sporadic, or epidemic diarrhea. Treatment is rarely required.
F. **Traveler's diarrhea** results from ingestion of contaminated water and food in areas of poor hygiene. It is frequently caused by enterotoxigenic *E. coli* and less often by other bacteria and viruses. Treatment begun promptly with the onset of symptoms with TMP/SMZ, 160 mg/800 mg PO bid for 3–5 days; ciprofloxacin, 500 mg PO bid for 5 days; or norfloxacin, 400 mg PO bid for 5 days, is effective in decreasing the severity and length of the illness. **Prophylactic antimicrobial therapy** is effective in reducing the incidence of traveler's diarrhea, but the risk of toxicity outweighs the benefit for most people (*Rev. Infect. Dis.* 8 [suppl 2]:S227, 1986).
G. **Pseudomembranous enterocolitis** is caused by a toxin produced by *C. difficile,* an anaerobe that may proliferate when antimicrobials or other factors alter the normal bowel flora. The extended-spectrum PCNs (e.g., ampicillin), cephalo-sporins, and clindamycin are the most common offenders, but it has been reported with most antibiotics. Effective therapies include vancomycin, 125 mg PO qid; metronidazole, 500 mg PO or IV bid; and bacitracin, 25,000 units PO qid for 7–10 days. In patients who are unable to take oral medication, parenteral metronidazole is effective. Relapses usually respond to another course with the same agent.
H. **Protozoal infections**
   1. *Giardia lamblia* may cause acute or chronic gastrointestinal symptoms in sporadic cases or epidemics due to the ingestion of contaminated water. Patients with hypogammaglobulinemia and achlorhydria are predisposed to giardiasis. Diagnosis can often be made by stool examination, but duodenal aspiration or small-bowel biopsy may be required. **Treatment** with quinacrine hydrochloride, 100 mg PO tid after meals for 5 days, is effective. Metronida-zole, 250 mg tid PO for 5 days, and furazolidone, 100 mg qid PO for 7–10 days, are also effective.
   2. *Entamoeba histolytica* **infection (amebiasis)** is acquired by ingestion of contaminated food or water. Typical symptoms include crampy abdominal pain with dysentery; systemic symptoms are less common and imply more extensive disease. Complications include peritonitis, toxic megacolon, and hepatic abscess formation. Conversion to an asymptomatic carrier state occurs. The **treatment of choice** for intestinal disease and hepatic abscess is metronidazole, 750 mg PO tid for 10 days, followed by iodoquinol, 650 mg PO tid for 20 days. Asymptomatic carriage can be treated with iodoquinol, 650 mg PO tid for 20 days.
   3. *Cryptosporidium* **spp and** *Isospora belli* are related protozoa that cause acute self-limited diarrhea in normal hosts but may produce severe, chronic, watery, noninflammatory diarrhea in immunocompromised hosts such as those with AIDS. Therapy is usually unnecessary in immunologically com-petent patients (see Human Immunodeficiency Virus Infection and AIDS, sec. **II.F.2**).
IX. **Intra-abdominal infections**
   A. **Peritonitis**
      1. **Primary or spontaneous bacterial peritonitis** usually occurs in patients with cirrhosis and ascites. *Escherichia coli, Strep. pneumoniae,* and other strepto-cocci and Enterobacteriaceae account for the majority of infections, although anaerobic bacteria and *M. tuberculosis* may occasionally be responsible. Initial therapy with a third-generation cephalosporin with good activity against streptococci (e.g., cefotaxime or ceftriaxone) is appropriate (see Chap. 16).
      2. **Secondary peritonitis.** The causes of secondary peritonitis are numerous, including traumatic or disease-induced perforation of the gastrointestinal tract and contiguous spread from a visceral disease or abscess. Enterobacte-riaceae, obligate anaerobes, and enterococci are common pathogens, but

staphylococci, *M. tuberculosis,* and *N. gonorrhoeae* are also seen. Empiric antimicrobial therapy should include broad-spectrum coverage while awaiting culture results. **For peritonitis from a presumed gastrointestinal source,** a variety of regimens appear effective. These include (1) ampicillin or mezlocillin, an aminoglycoside, and either clindamycin or metronidazole; and (2) an aminoglycoside plus cefoxitin, clindamycin, or chloramphenicol. Cefoxitin alone may be adequate for community-acquired disease. Imipenem provides effective coverage and is used when more resistant organisms are likely to be present and aminoglycoside therapy is contraindicated. **Abscess formation is common and requires surgical or percutaneous drainage in the majority of cases.** Peritonitis complicating peritoneal dialysis is discussed in Chap. 11.

  B. **Visceral infections.** There is no evidence that antimicrobial therapy is of benefit in **uncomplicated cholecystitis or pancreatitis,** but broad-spectrum therapy is appropriate if there is evidence of sepsis, secondary peritonitis, or abscess formation (see sec. **IX.A.2** and Chap. 16).

X. **Infectious diseases with cutaneous manifestations**

  A. **Erysipelas and cellulitis. Erysipelas** is a superficial, erythematous, edematous, sharply demarcated lesion almost always caused by group A streptococcus (*Strep. pyogenes*). **Cellulitis** is typically more deep-seated with less distinct margins and, in normal hosts, is usually caused by group A streptococcus or *Staph. aureus,* which are indistinguishable on clinical grounds. If staphylococcal disease cannot be excluded, initial therapy with oxacillin or nafcillin, 4.0–8.0 g/day, or cefazolin, 1.0–2.0 g IV q8h, can be used. The treatment of choice for documented streptococcal disease is penicillin VK, 0.5–1.0 g PO qid; procaine penicillin G, 600,000 units IM bid; or penicillin G, 2–6 million units/day IV, depending on the severity of illness. In patients allergic to PCN, erythromycin, 500 mg PO qid, or vancomycin, 1 g IV q12h, is an alternative. Broad-spectrum treatment, such as oxacillin or cefazolin, plus an aminoglycoside, is indicated for cellulitis in immunocompromised or diabetic patients. **Lower extremity cellulitis associated with cutaneous ulcers in diabetic patients** is commonly polymicrobial in origin. Agents with activity against anaerobes (e.g., metronidazole or clindamycin) should be included when treating cellulitis in this setting. Alternatively, ticarcillin/clavulanic acid, 3.1 g IV q4–6h, or cefoxitin, 1–2 g IV q8h, can be used as single-agent therapy for these patients.

  B. **Petechial, purpuric, and macular skin eruptions** are associated with several important systemic infections.

    1. **Neisseria meningitidis septicemia (meningococcemia)** should be considered in any febrile patient with a petechial, purpuric, or macular rash because of its high mortality and potentially rapid course. The diagnosis can frequently be made from a Gram's stain of a peripheral blood buffy coat specimen or petechial scrapings. As in meningococcal meningitis, the treatment of choice is penicillin G, 2.0 million units IV q2h.

    2. **Encapsulated bacteria such as Strep. pneumoniae and H. influenzae** may produce a picture similar to that of meningococcemia in asplenic patients (see sec. **XII.A.2**).

    3. **Rocky Mountain spotted fever** due to *Rickettsia rickettsii* typically begins with fever, chills, headache, and myalgias, with the development of the characteristic macular rash 1–5 days later. With time, the rash may become petechial. The diagnosis should be suspected in patients with a compatible clinical picture and potential tick exposure. The treatment of choice is doxycycline, 100 mg IV or PO q12h. Chloramphenicol, 1.0 g IV or PO q6h, is also effective.

    4. **Other infections** associated with macular, maculopapular, or petechial rashes, including typhoid fever (rose spots), endocarditis, disseminated gonorrhea, and disseminated candidiasis in the neutropenic host, are discussed elsewhere in this chapter.

  C. **Toxic shock syndrome** is due to an exotoxin produced by *Staph. aureus.* It occurs most commonly in menstruating women using tampons but may also complicate staphylococcal colonization in surgical wounds. The diagnosis is based on the clinical presentation of fever, a diffuse macular erythroderma involving the palms and soles that often desquamates 1–2 weeks after the illness, hypotension, conjunctivitis, vomiting, and diarrhea. **Supportive care is the mainstay of acute therapy.** Antistaphylococcal therapy does not appear to affect the acute illness but may prevent progression of local infection and decrease the rate of relapse. Discontinuation of tampon use may also reduce recurrences.

D. **Lyme disease** is due to infection with the tick-borne spirochete *Borrelia burgdorferi*. The characteristic erythematous annular lesion known as **erythema chronicum migrans (ECM)** begins as a macular lesion at the site of the tick bite and is often accompanied by fever, fatigue, arthralgias, headache, and neck stiffness. Sequelae are common in untreated patients and include recurrent oligoarticular arthritis, CNS abnormalities (meningitis and cranial and peripheral neuropathies), and cardiac involvement (myopericarditis and heart block). **Treatment** of early Lyme disease with **tetracycline,** 250–500 mg PO qid for 10–21 days, shortens the duration of symptoms and usually prevents major sequelae. Penicillin VK, 500 mg PO qid, is also effective but may be associated with a higher incidence of sequelae. Established Lyme arthritis and neurologic complications have both been successfully treated with high-dose penicillin G, 20 million units/day IV; however, ceftriaxone may be more effective (*Lancet* 1:1191, 1988). The role of antibiotic therapy in patients with cardiac complications is unclear.

XI. **Osteomyelitis** should be considered in patients with localized bone pain who are febrile or septic. The **diagnosis** is made by **culturing the pathogen from bone.** An early bone biopsy is essential for management. The radiographic changes of soft-tissue swelling, periosteal elevation, bone lysis, and sclerosis may lag several weeks behind the clinical presentation. Abnormalities on technetium bone scan are often apparent before radiographic changes and biopsy of suspicious lesions may yield an early diagnosis. Conditions that predispose to osteomyelitis include (1) vascular insufficiency (e.g., diabetes mellitus), (2) soft-tissue infection contiguous with bone (e.g., a decubitus ulcer), (3) bacteremia, (4) hemoglobinopathy, and (5) recurrent urinary tract infection (UTI). In the absence of vascular insufficiency or a foreign body, acute osteomyelitis can usually be treated successfully with antimicrobial therapy alone. The appropriate antimicrobial agent depends on the results of culture and susceptibility testing. If a causative organism is not identified, antimicrobial therapy should be based on the most likely pathogens. Cure typically requires **at least 6 weeks of therapy** with high dosages of appropriate antimicrobials. Parenteral therapy should be given initially, but oral antibiotics can be considered after 2–3 weeks provided that the causative organism is susceptible and adequate bactericidal levels can be demonstrated.

A. **Acute hematogenous osteomyelitis** is most frequently caused by *Staph. aureus,* and blood cultures are often positive. Vertebral osteomyelitis may be due to *Staph. aureus* or gram-negative bacilli and may be associated with UTI, presumably arising by dissemination via communicating veins.

B. **Osteomyelitis associated with contiguous foci of infection** (e.g., postsurgical infections) may be due to *Staph. aureus* as well as gram-negative bacilli.

C. **Osteomyelitis in the presence of internal fixation devices** cannot usually be eradicated by antimicrobials alone. Cure typically requires the removal of the foreign material.

D. **Osteomyelitis associated with vascular insufficiency** (e.g., in diabetic patients) is seldom cured by drug therapy alone; revascularization, debridement, or amputation is often required.

E. **Osteomyelitis in patients with hemoglobinopathies** is usually caused by *Staph. aureus* but may also be caused by *Salmonella* spp.

F. **Chronic osteomyelitis** is usually associated with the presence of dead and sclerotic bone (i.e., a sequestrum) that serves as a nidus for persistent infection. Eradication requires a combined medical and surgical approach, with excision of the sequestrum. Suppressive antimicrobial therapy can be used if surgery is not feasible.

XII. Sepsis of unknown origin

A. **Early bactericidal treatment** is essential in the therapy of septicemia. If a probable source of infection is evident, antimicrobials can be selected to treat the most likely pathogens originating from that site. If no obvious source is uncovered, antibiotic selection is more empiric and should be based on the clinical situation. Before therapy is initiated, specimens of potentially infected body fluids (e.g., CSF, pleural fluid) should be examined and cultured, and several sets of blood cultures should be obtained from separate venipuncture sites. The broadest coverage is usually provided by a beta-lactam antibiotic plus an aminoglycoside, such as gentamicin or tobramycin, although amikacin can be used when resistance is suspected. Single-agent therapy with third-generation cephalosporins or imipenem has been studied less extensively, particularly in the treatment of immunocompromised patients. However, imipenem can be used when aminoglycosides are contraindicated.

1. **Community acquired with no obvious underlying disease.** A first-generation cephalosporin plus an aminoglycoside will cover most potential pathogens in this setting.

2. **Postsplenectomy patients or those with congenital or functional asplenia** (e.g., sickle cell anemia patients) are at particular risk for fulminant sepsis with encapsulated organisms such as *Strep. pneumoniae, H. influenzae,* and *N. meningitidis.* Penicillin G, 2 million units IV q2h, plus a third-generation cephalosporin (e.g., ceftriaxone, 2 g IV q12h) should be emergently administered. A Gram's stain of a buffy coat specimen can subsequently be performed and will sometimes reveal a probable diagnosis.

3. **Nosocomial septicemia in patients with intravascular catheters** is usually due to *Staph. aureus,* coagulase-negative staphylococci, aerobic gram-negative bacilli, or enterococci. Vancomycin plus an aminoglycoside is appropriate therapy.

4. **Neutropenic or otherwise immunocompromised patients,** in whom *P. aeruginosa* sepsis may be likely, are usually treated with an antipseudomonal beta-lactam antibiotic plus an aminoglycoside. The addition of an anti-staphylococcal agent such as vancomycin may be warranted in patients with **indwelling central venous catheters.**

B. **Septic shock** is usually caused by bacteremia, although it may complicate fungemia or viremia. Early recognition of bacteremic shock is critical, since delays in instituting therapy increase mortality. Cardiovascular collapse occurs in approximately 40% of gram-negative bacillary bacteremias and has an overall mortality of 40% (*Am. J. Med.* 68:344, 1980). Clinically, there may be two stages of bacteremic shock. In the early, hyperdynamic phase (warm shock), the cardiac output is elevated, peripheral vascular resistance is decreased, and the patient is warm, diaphoretic, and peripherally vasodilated. A second hypodynamic phase (cold shock) is manifested by normal or increased peripheral vascular resistance and cool, vasoconstricted skin. Ultimately decreased cardiac output may occur. Evaluation and treatment should address the underlying infection as well as the manifestations of circulatory compromise.

1. **Stabilization of the cardiovascular system** (see Chap. 26). Crystalloid fluids should be administered initially to achieve normal blood pressure; if this is unsuccessful, vasopressor drugs should be used. The placement of a Swan-Ganz catheter may be necessary for hemodynamic monitoring and fluid management. Because of the risk of catheter sepsis, these catheters should be replaced within 72 hours of insertion, especially if they were placed in emergency conditions.

2. **Electrolyte and acid-base disturbances** must be corrected, and adequate ventilation must be ensured.

3. **Disseminated intravascular coagulation (DIC).** Laboratory evidence of DIC may occur, but restoration of blood pressure and appropriate antimicrobials are usually adequate to reverse this problem. Other modes of treatment (e.g., heparin, fresh frozen plasma) are rarely necessary (see Chap. 17).

4. **The underlying infection** should be treated with antibiotics appropriate to the clinical situation.

5. There is **little evidence that steroids,** even in high dosages and early in the course of infection, significantly **alter the ultimate outcome** (*N. Engl. J. Med.* 311:1137, 1984).

6. **Antilipopolysaccharide antibody preparations** have shown some promise in early clinical trials, but their precise role is yet to be determined (*N. Engl. J. Med.* 324:429, 1991).

Sexually Transmitted Diseases

Sexually transmitted diseases (STDs) may be caused by bacterial, viral, and protozoal pathogens. Nevertheless, common principles should be applied when caring for any patient with a presumed STD. The patient's sexual practices may help identify risk factors for particular infections. The **physical examination and microbiologic studies** should be directed toward the oropharyngeal, rectal, and urogenital areas.

Because infection with multiple organisms is common, studies for gonorrhea and syphilis should be included when evaluating these patients. In addition, HIV testing and counseling are recommended by the U.S. Public Health Services (USPHS). When possible, cultures should also be obtained from **sexual contacts,** as treatment of asymptomatic carriers may prevent the spread of infection. Empiric treatment of sexual contacts is indicated in cases of primary and secondary syphilis. **Follow-up** cultures or serologic studies should be obtained after completion of therapy to document cure. An STD apparently refractory to treatment may represent reinfection, a concomitant previously undiagnosed STD, or antimicrobial resistance. Patients with STDs should be reported to the local health department. Most of the following guidelines are based on those from the USPHS (*M.M.W.R.* 38:1, 1989). The Centers for Disease Control (CDC) maintain a hot line to answer specific questions regarding STDs: 1-800-227-8922.

I. **Gonorrhea** usually presents as purulent urethritis in men and as urethritis or cervicitis in women after an incubation period of 2–8 days. Humans are the only reservoir. Both sexes, but women in particular, may be asymptomatic carriers.

A. **Diagnosis.** Gram's stain of a urethral discharge showing gram-negative intracellular diplococci is the best immediate diagnostic aid in men. In women, cervical and urethral saprophytic *Neisseria* spp may occasionally cause false-positive smears and are less sensitive than in symptomatic men. Cultures for *N. gonorrhoeae* should be obtained with noninhibitory swabs (e.g., calcium alginate) of the urethral discharge in men, and of the cervix and rectum of women; specimens should be plated **immediately on warm chocolate agar** (preferably inhibitory media—e.g., Thayer-Martin medium) and incubated in a carbon dioxide incubator.

B. **Resistance** has appeared in increasing numbers of isolates over the last decade. Currently, *N. gonorrhoeae* with **plasmid-mediated penicillinase production (PPNG)** account for the majority of clinically significant resistant isolates, although less important **plasmid-mediated high-level tetracycline resistance (TRNG)** also occurs. In 1988, approximately 4.5% of all *N. gonorrhoeae* isolates in the United States were PPNG, and 3% were TRNG. Other strains may have **chromosomally mediated antibiotic resistance (CMRNG)** to PCN and other commonly used antibiotics. Although the prevalence of CMRNG is greater than previously recognized, treatment failures due to these organisms are uncommon, probably because of the standard use of dual therapy for gonorrhea (see sec. **I.C.1**). PPNG strains are usually susceptible to spectinomycin; ceftriaxone resistance has not been reported. Other third-generation cephalosporins and the quinolones are also active against these isolates, but clinical experience with these agents is more limited. Ideally, all *N. gonorrhoeae* isolates should be tested for penicillinase production. In addition, all "post-treatment" isolates and isolates from patients with disseminated gonococcal infections or gonococcal ophthalmia should be tested for TRNG and CMRNG.

C. **Treatment**

1. **Uncomplicated urethral and endocervical gonorrhea.** Because coexistent *Chlamydia trachomatis* occurs in up to 40% of women and 25% of heterosexual men with gonorrhea, regimens that will treat both infections are recommended. **Ceftriaxone,** 250 mg IM, is the therapy of choice for all patients with gonorrhea, unless the strain is either known or highly likely to be susceptible to penicillin. Penicillin-sensitive isolates can be treated with a single dose of (1) amoxicillin, 3 g PO; (2) ampicillin, 3.5 g PO; or (3) procaine penicillin G, 4.8 million units IM distributed to two injection sites. Probenecid, 1 g PO, should accompany each of these regimens. Cefotaxime, 1 g IM, or ceftizoxime, 500 mg IM, may also be effective, although experience with these agents is limited. Other alternatives useful in patients allergic to beta-lactam antibiotics are spectinomycin, 2 g IM; ciprofloxacin, 500 mg PO; or ofloxacin, 400 mg PO, as a single dose. All these regimens should be followed by **doxycycline,** 100 mg PO bid for 7 days, or, for pregnant patients or those unable to tolerate tetracyclines, **erythromycin,** 500 mg PO qid for 7 days.

2. **Anorectal disease** in women can be treated with any of the above regimens. Oral penicillin regimens are less effective for anorectal infections in homosexual men, however.

3. **Pharyngitis.** Patients with pharyngitis should be treated with ceftriaxone or procaine penicillin G (see sec. **I.C.1**). Patients allergic to beta-lactam antibiotics can be treated with ciprofloxacin, 500 mg PO, or ofloxacin, 400 mg PO, although efficacy data are limited. Ampicillin, amoxicillin, and spectinomycin are relatively ineffective for pharyngeal infections.

4. **Acute salpingitis.** Gonococcal and nongonococcal salpingitis are clinically indistinguishable. Although first episodes are usually due to *N. gonorrhoeae* or *C. trachomatis,* subsequent infections often involve other pathogens, including gram-negative bacilli and anaerobes. The treatment of choice is not established. The USPHS currently recommends several antimicrobial combinations; however, data to assess the relative efficacy of these combinations are not available.

   a. **Inpatient antimicrobial therapy** is recommended when (1) the diagnosis is unclear, (2) potential surgical emergencies cannot be excluded (e.g., appendicitis), or (3) a pelvic abscess is suspected, or when the patient (4) is pregnant, (5) is severely ill, (6) is unwilling or unable to follow an outpatient regimen, (7) is a prepubertal child, (8) has not responded to outpatient therapy, or (9) cannot return for follow-up within 72 hours. Treatment should be given intravenously for at least 4 days, including at least 2 days after fever resolves. This should be followed by oral therapy for a total of 10–14 days. Suggested regimens include (1) doxycycline, 100 mg IV q12h, plus cefoxitin, 2 g IV q6h, or cefotetan, 2 g IV q12h, followed by doxycycline, 100 mg PO bid; or (2) clindamycin, 900 mg IV q8h, plus gentamicin, 2.0 mg/kg IV followed by 1.5 mg/kg IV q8h, followed by doxycycline, 100 mg PO bid, or clindamycin, 450 mg PO qid.

   b. **Outpatient treatment** can be attempted in reliable patients with none of the indications for hospitalization listed previously. The therapy of choice is ceftriaxone, 250 mg IM, followed by doxycycline, 100 mg PO bid for 10–14 days.

5. **Disseminated gonococcal infections (DGI).** Gonococcal bacteremia is often associated with fever, characteristic skin lesions, polyarthralgias, and tenosynovitis. Purulent monoarticular or occasionally polyarticular arthritis may follow and often requires joint aspiration (see Chap. 24). Patients with DGI should receive IV therapy for at least 3 days or until improvement occurs, followed by oral antibiotics to complete a minimum of 7 days of therapy. Ceftriaxone, 1 g IV qd for 7 days, is the treatment of choice, unless the organism is known to be sensitive to penicillin. For patients who respond rapidly, therapy can be completed with cefuroxime axetil, 500 mg PO bid;

ciprofloxacin, 500 mg PO bid; or ofloxacin, 400 mg PO bid, although definitive data with these regimens are lacking. DGI due to penicillin-susceptible strains can be treated with aqueous penicillin G, 2 million units IV q4h, followed by amoxicillin (or ampicillin), 500 mg PO qid, to complete 7 days of treatment. Patients with DGI should also be treated for concomitant chlamydial infection with doxycycline or erythromycin (see sec. **I.C.1**).

6. **Meningitis and endocarditis** may occur in patients with DGI. Therapy with ceftriaxone, 2 g IV/day, or, for susceptible isolates, with penicillin G, at least 10 million units/day, is effective and should be continued at least 10 days in meningitis and 3–4 weeks in endocarditis.

II. **Nongonococcal urethritis (NGU)** refers to urethral inflammation in men that is not attributable to *N. gonorrhoeae*. It cannot be differentiated from gonorrhea on the basis of symptoms. *C. trachomatis* is responsible for up to 40% of NGU seen in the United States and Western Europe. The cause in the remaining cases is unclear, although *U. urealyticum* may have a role. Neither of these organisms is reliably susceptible to the PCNs. Persistent urethritis in a patient treated for gonorrhea (postgonococcal urethritis) may represent coinfection with these organisms.

A. **Diagnosis.** NGU should be diagnosed if Gram's stain for *N. gonorrhoeae* and subsequent culture, if available, are negative in a man with urethritis, or if urethritis persists despite treatment for gonorrhea. A specific chlamydial diagnosis can be made by direct testing of urethral secretions for chlamydia or chlamydial antigens (culture requires special techniques). Therapy of NGU is usually initiated on the basis of a negative Gram's stain and a compatible history without waiting for a negative *N. gonorrhoeae* culture.

B. **Treatment** of nongonococcal and postgonococcal urethritis is doxycycline, 100 mg PO bid, for at least 7 days; erythromycin, 500 mg PO qid for 7 days, may be less effective and is inadequate for *N. gonorrhoeae*. Routine treatment of female sexual partners of men with NGU is recommended.

III. **Lymphogranuloma venereum (LGV)** is due to strains of *C. trachomatis* antigenetically distinct from those causing NGU. The primary lesion is an often trivial genital ulceration followed 1–2 weeks later by inguinal adenopathy and constitutional symptoms. In women and homosexual males, symptoms in the anal and rectal areas are common. LGV is treated with the same drugs as NGU, but for 21 days. Fluctuant nodes should be aspirated to decrease the chance of spontaneous drainage with scarring.

IV. **Syphilis** may present in primary (chancre), secondary (disseminated), or tertiary forms. Commonly, however, infection is discovered through serologic screening tests in the latent stages (early, within one year of infection, or late, one or more years following infection). The incubation period for the primary lesion is usually 2–6 weeks. Manifestations of secondary syphilis usually appear 2–12 weeks later and may occur several times during subsequent years. Both primary and moist secondary lesions are infectious. Diagnosis can be made by dark-field microscopy of the primary or moist secondary lesions, or by serologic testing.

A. **Serologic tests** are of major importance in diagnosis but present difficulties in interpretation, because false-positive nontreponemal tests occur in many nonsyphilitic conditions.

1. **Nontreponemal tests** (e.g., VDRL, RPR) are useful for screening. They require a minimum of 1–3 weeks from the onset of infection to turn positive, are usually positive in primary syphilis, and are invariably positive in secondary syphilis. However, they are nonspecific; biologic false-positive tests (usually ≤ 1:8) occur in intravenous drug users, in many acute infections (e.g., infectious mononucleosis, mycoplasma infection), in a variety of chronic disorders (e.g., systemic lupus erythematosus) (see Chap. 24), and possibly pregnancy.

2. **Treponemal tests** (e.g., FTA, TPHA) are specific. Their greatest value is in distinguishing false-positive from true-positive reagin tests, and in diagnosing late syphilis when blood and CSF reagin tests may be negative.

3. **Serologic response to therapy.** The nontreponemal test titers should decrease by at least two dilutions within three months of adequate treatment of

primary or secondary disease, and within six months following therapy of early latent disease. The CSF titer should also diminish with adequate therapy of neurosyphilis. However, the serum nontreponemal test titer may not change in patients with late latent syphilis. The FTA test is not useful in monitoring response to therapy because titers remain positive for life.

B. Treatment (see also Human Immunodeficiency Virus and AIDS)

1. **Early syphilis. Benzathine penicillin G,** 2.4 million units IM, is the recommended treatment for primary and secondary syphilis, latent syphilis of less than 1 year's duration, and case contacts. Penicillin-allergic patients can be treated with doxycycline, 100 mg PO bid, for 14 days.

2. **Syphilis exceeding 1 year's duration.** For latent syphilis of more than 1 year in duration, and for cardiovascular syphilis, recommended therapy is benzathine penicillin G, 2.4 million units IM weekly for 3 successive weeks. In patients allergic to PCN, doxycycline, 100 mg PO bid for 28 days, can be given. The treatment of neurosyphilis has not been well studied. Potentially effective regimens include (1) aqueous penicillin G, 2–4 million units IV q4h for 10 days, or (2) procaine penicillin G, 2.4 million units IM qd, plus probenecid, 500 mg PO qd, for 10 days, each followed by benzathine penicillin, 2.4 million units IM, weekly for 3 weeks. The efficacy of benzathine penicillin G, 2.4 million units IM weekly for 3 weeks, alone is uncertain because only very low CSF levels are achieved (*Arch. Intern. Med.* 140:1117, 1980).

3. **Syphilis during pregnancy** can be managed with one of the preceding penicillin regimens. The optimal treatment for PCN-allergic patients is controversial. Doxycycline should be avoided because of its potential adverse effects on both the mother and fetus. Penicillin skin testing and, if necessary, desensitization are therefore recommended for such patients (see Chap. 12).

V. Chancroid is due to *Haemophilus ducreyi*. The typical lesion is a painful, nonindurated, ulcerative lesion, often associated with tender inguinal adenopathy. Recommended regimens include (1) ceftriaxone, 250 mg IM as a single dose; (2) erythromycin, 500 mg PO qid for 7 days; (3) TMP/SMZ, 160 mg/800 mg PO bid for 7 days; and (4) ciprofloxacin, 500 mg PO bid for 3 days. As with LGV, aspiration of fluctuant nodes is recommended. HIV-infected patients may not respond as well to the one- to three-day regimens.

VI. Genital herpes simplex infection (primarily type II) usually presents with painful vesicles or shallow ulcerations (unroofed vesicles) involving the vulva, labia, or cervix in women, or the penis in men. Primary infection (first episode) may be associated with fever and inguinal adenopathy, whereas recurrent disease rarely produces constitutional symptoms. **Acyclovir,** 200 mg PO 5 times a day for 7–10 days, or, for severely ill patients, 5 mg/kg IV q8h, is effective treatment for primary disease. Patients with greater than 6 recurrences per year may have a marked decrease in the rate of recurrence when given prophylactic acyclovir, 200 mg PO 2–3 times a day. Less frequent recurrences are usually treated symptomatically. Pain can be treated with analgesics and topical anesthetics (e.g., benzocaine spray); sitting in a warm bath to urinate may relieve the severe dysuria frequent in women. Pregnant women with active genital lesions at the time of delivery should be delivered by cesarean section to reduce the likelihood of neonatal transmission.

VII. Vaginitis presents as a vaginal discharge, often with a musty or foul odor, and often associated with dysuria, burning, or pruritus. The most common etiologic organisms are *Trichomonas vaginalis* and *C. albicans. Gardnerella* (formerly, *Haemophilus*) *vaginalis,* in combination with anaerobic organisms, is responsible for bacterial vaginosis, previously known as nonspecific vaginitis. Trichomoniasis is usually venereally transmitted, but nonvenereal transmission has been described. *Candida* vaginitis and bacterial vaginosis are not venereally transmitted, and therefore treatment of sexual partners is not indicated.

A. Diagnosis. Although gross appearance of the discharge may be characteristic, diagnosis requires microscopic verification. Wet-mount examination of a drop of discharge mixed in a few drops of isotonic saline under high–dry magnification should demonstrate pear-shaped, motile *T. vaginalis.* A drop of 10% potassium hydroxide, added to lyse epithelial cells, may enhance visualization of *Candida* budding yeast forms, with or without *Candida* pseudohyphae. A diagnosis of bacterial vaginosis is usually based on three of the following four criteria: (1) a vaginal discharge, (2) malodor, often intensified after the addition of 10% KOH to a wet-mount slide, (3) clue cells (vaginal epithelial cells with overlying clumps of bacteria), or (4) a vaginal pH > 4.5.

B. Therapy

1. ***Trichomonas vaginalis* infection** in nonpregnant women is treated with single-dose metronidazole, 2 g PO. Sexual partners should also be treated. Pregnant women may obtain symptomatic relief and are sometimes cured with clotrimazole, 100 mg intravaginally qhs for 7 nights.

2. ***Candida albicans* vaginitis** responds to local therapy with miconazole or clotrimazole vaginal cream or suppositories, 100 mg intravaginally qhs for 7 days or 200 mg qhs for 3 days. The response may be better with longer regimens or a higher total dose. Nystatin vaginal suppositories, 100,000 units qhs for 14 days, are also effective. In patients who do not respond to topical therapy, ketoconazole, 200 mg PO, or fluconazole, 100 mg PO qd for 5–10 days, may be effective.

3. **Bacterial vaginosis** is treated with metronidazole, 500 mg PO bid for 7 days. Clindamycin, 300 mg PO bid for 7 days, is an alternative for **pregnant women** and those unable to tolerate metronidazole.

Mycobacterial Infections

I. **Tuberculosis** is a systemic disease caused by *M. tuberculosis*. Pulmonary disease is the most frequent clinical presentation. Lymphatic involvement, genitourinary disease, osteomyelitis, and miliary dissemination may occur, as well as meningitis, peritonitis, and pericarditis. Tuberculosis is more common among debilitated and otherwise immunocompromised patients (e.g., alcoholics and patients with AIDS). The prevalence of tuberculosis is increased among American Indians and immigrants from Southeast Asia, the Indian subcontinent, and Central America. Mycobacteria resistant to primary agents are also more common in these patients.

A. **Diagnosis** of tuberculosis is established by culturing the organism. Positive fluorochrome or acid-fast smears are presumptive evidence of active tuberculosis, although nontuberculous mycobacteria and some *Nocardia* spp may give positive results with these techniques.

B. **Treatment** of tuberculosis includes hospitalization to initiate therapy, patient education, and respiratory isolation for patients with pulmonary disease. The local health department should be notified of all cases of tuberculosis, so that contacts can be identified.

1. **Chemotherapy.** Antituberculous therapy is based on two principles: (1) At least two drugs to which the organism is susceptible must be used because of the high incidence of primary drug resistance to a single drug (roughly 1 in 10^6 tubercle bacilli), and (2) extended therapy is necessary because of the prolonged generation time of mycobacteria (> 20 hours). Treatment recommendations follow those of the American Thoracic Society and the USPHS (*Am. Rev. Respir. Dis.* 134:355, 1986).

   a. **Uncomplicated pulmonary infection** (including cavitary disease) can be treated with the following regimens:

      (1) Isoniazid (INH), 300 mg qd, and rifampin, 600 mg qd, for 6 months, plus PZA, 1.5–2.0 g qd, for the first 2 months with susceptible isolates. The final 4 months of therapy can be given twice a week: INH, 15 mg/kg (maximum of 900 mg), and rifampin, 600 mg each visit.

      (2) Isoniazid, 300 mg qd, and rifampin, 600 mg qd, for 9 months. After an initial clinical response for 4–8 weeks, treatment can be given twice a week (see sec. I.B.1.a(1)).

   b. **Drug resistance.** If drug resistance is suspected, **ethambutol**, 15 mg/kg/day, should be added until susceptibility results are available. Isolates with documented resistance to INH should be treated with rifampin and ethambutol for a minimum of 12 months. The addition of PZA for the first 2 months of therapy may be beneficial.

   c. **Extrapulmonary disease** can be treated in the same manner as pulmonary disease; bone and joint disease may require more prolonged therapy (*Ann. Intern. Med.* 104:7, 1986). If a third agent is needed for meningitis, PZA is recommended over ethambutol because of superior CNS penetration (*Chest* 87:117S, 1985).

   d. **Immunosuppressed patients** should be treated with INH and rifampin for 12 months, supplemented initially by ethambutol, PZA, or streptomycin (see also Human Immunodeficiency Virus Infection and AIDS).

   e. **Pregnant patients** should be treated in the standard fashion, but PZA and streptomycin should be avoided.

   2. **Corticosteroid administration** in tuberculosis is controversial. Prednisone, 1 mg/kg PO qd initially, has been used in combination with primary antituberculous drugs for life-threatening complications such as meningitis and pericarditis.

C. **Chemoprophylaxis.** In up to 5% of individuals whose intermediate-strength purified protein derivative (PPD) skin tests convert from negative to positive, active disease will develop within 1 year of conversion if left untreated. Although adequate prophylaxis will reduce this risk, the potential for drug toxicity must be considered in these individuals. Criteria for a positive PPD are 5-mm induration for patients with HIV infection or other defect in cell-mediated immunity; contacts of a known case or patients with chest radiographs typical for tuberculosis; 10-mm induration for immigrants from endemic areas, prisoners, the homeless, parenteral drug abusers, nursing home residents, and patients with chronic medical illnesses; and 15-mm induration for individuals who are not in a high prevalence group (*M.M.W.R.* 38:313, 1989). Prophylactic INH, 300 mg PO qd (adult dosage) for 1 year, should be considered for (1) persons in whom a tuberculin skin test conversion develops within 2 years of a previously negative PPD; (2) persons with a history of untreated tuberculosis or a positive PPD and chest radiographic evidence of previous infection; (3) PPD reactors younger than 35 years of age; (4) persons with a positive PPD who are at high risk for development of active disease, including patients with silicosis, diabetes mellitus, AIDS, end-stage renal disease, hematologic or lymphoreticular malignancy, and conditions associated with rapid weight loss or chronic malnutrition, and patients receiving immunosuppressive therapy; and (5) household members and other close contacts of patients with active disease, with a reactive PPD and no history of reactivity in the past. Contacts with a negative PPD who are at high risk for tuberculosis should also be treated, but treatment can be stopped if a repeat PPD at 3 months is negative. Untreated contacts with a nonreactive PPD should have a repeat PPD after 3 months.

II. **Nontuberculous mycobacteria** are generally more resistant to chemotherapy than *M. tuberculosis,* and multiple drug combinations are frequently used. Susceptibility testing should always be obtained to guide treatment.

   A. **Primary infection** with these organisms is seen occasionally (e.g., cervical adenitis in children caused by *M. kansasii* and *M. scrofulaceum*, skin lesions associated with *M. marianum*). Diagnosis in these cases is usually made by biopsy.

   B. **Patients with underlying chronic pulmonary disease.** *Mycobacterium avium-intracellulare (MAI)* and *M. kansasii* may be cultured from the sputum of these patients, but the distinction between colonization and infection is often difficult. Empiric therapy should be considered in symptomatic patients, especially if deterioration in pulmonary function occurs. The optimal treatment for MAI infection remains unclear; typical regimens utilize 4–6 drugs for prolonged periods (e.g., INH, rifampin, and ethambutol for 24 months, plus streptomycin or amikacin for the first 3 months).

   C. **Patients with disorders affecting cell-mediated immunity** may develop opportunistic infections with nontuberculous mycobacteria. Disseminated MAI infection is common in patients with AIDS (see Human Immunodeficiency Virus Infection and AIDS).

III. Rapidly growing mycobacteria. *Mycobacterium fortuitum* and *M. chelonei* account for the majority of cases and have been responsible for surgical wound and prosthetic implant infections (including endocarditis), pulmonary disease, lymphadenitis, and disseminated disease with skin lesions and positive blood cultures (*Rev. Infect. Dis.* 5:657, 1983). Treatment consists of surgical debridement combined with amikacin plus cefoxitin, doxycycline, or rifampin for at least 4–6 weeks after clinical response.

Actinomycotic Infections

I. Actinomycosis. Penicillin is the drug of choice for actinomycosis. Penicillin G, 1.5–3.0 million units IV q4h, should be given for at least 6 weeks, followed by 6–12 months of oral penicillin VK, 2–4 g/day, to prevent relapse. Tetracycline is an alternative in the PCN-allergic patient. Surgical drainage of localized lesions may be helpful.

II. Nocardiosis. Most infections require a prolonged course of therapy. Sulfadiazine or sulfisoxazole, given in amounts sufficient to produce peak serum levels of 120–150 µg/ml (e.g., 2 g IV or PO q6h), is the therapy of choice. Alternatives for patients with sulfonamide sensitivity include minocycline or the combination of ampicillin plus erythromycin. Therapy should be given for a minimum of 6 weeks.

Systemic Mycoses

The major fungal pathogens of North America are *Histoplasma capsulatum, Coccidioides immitis, Blastomyces dermatitidis,* and *Sporothrix schenckii.* The most common opportunistic fungal pathogens are *Cryptococcus neoformans, Candida* spp, *Torulopsis glabrata, Aspergillus* spp, and *Rhizopus* spp. Treatment schedules for most mycoses are based on clinical experience. Therefore, the recommendations that follow are general guidelines.

I. Cryptococcosis. Pulmonary cryptococcosis in a normal host is generally a self-limited disease that requires no specific treatment. **Meningeal infection** should always be excluded by a lumbar puncture; CSF should be examined for the presence of organisms (India ink preparation) and for the presence of cryptococcal antigen. Localized disease in an immunocompromised patient, or disseminated disease, including meningitis, always requires therapy. The **treatment** of choice for meningitis in patients without AIDS is amphotericin B, 0.3 mg/kg/day IV, and flucytosine, 37.5 mg/kg PO q6h, for a total duration of 6 weeks in most patients. Selected patients without underlying disease or immunosuppression can be treated with 4 weeks of therapy if (1) meningitis is diagnosed early and is not complicated by neurologic abnormalities; (2) the pretreatment CSF has greater than 20 leukocytes/µl; (3) the pretreatment serum cryptococcal antigen titer is less than 1:32; and, after 4 weeks of therapy, (4) a CSF India ink preparation reveals no yeast and (5) the CSF and serum cryptococcal antigen titers are less than 1:8 (*N. Engl. J. Med.* 317:334, 1987). Pulmonary disease in immunocompromised patients can be treated with the same regimen. Fluconazole, 200–400 mg PO qd, is effective against *C. neoformans,* but its role in patients without AIDS has not been evaluated.

II. Blastomycosis rarely demonstrates spontaneous remission; therefore, treatment is indicated. Amphotericin B, 2 g total dose, is most effective. Ketoconazole, 200–400 mg PO qd for 3–6 months, is effective in patients who are not immunocompromised.

III. Histoplasmosis. Treatment is indicated for chronic fibronodular and cavitary pulmonary disease, disseminated disease, and infection in immunocompromised hosts. The treatment of choice is amphotericin B, usually with a 1.5–2.5 g total dose. Ketoconazole, 200–400 mg PO qd for 3–6 months, is an alternative in nonimmunocompromised patients.

IV. Coccidioidomycosis. The majority of primary infections with *C. immitis* resolve without specific treatment. Black, Asian, pregnant, debilitated, and immunocompromised patients are at increased risk for dissemination, as are those with severe primary infections (e.g., complement fixation titers > 1:32, progressive pulmonary disease, persistent symptoms > 6 weeks in duration, negative skin test, or persisting serum precipitins). Such patients should be treated with amphotericin B, with a total dose of 0.5–1.5 g depending on the clinical response. Patients with chronic pulmonary disease should be given a total dose of 1–3 g. A lumbar puncture should always be performed to rule out meningeal involvement. Ketoconazole, 400–800 mg/day for prolonged periods, has been successful in suppressing or curing disease in some patients, but its precise role in therapy remains unclear. Fluconazole, 200–400 mg/day, may have a role in the treatment of meningitis (see Chap. 12).

V. Invasive aspergillosis usually presents with pulmonary infiltrates, sinusitis, or skin nodules in granulocytopenic or otherwise severely immunocompromised patients. Treatment of this life-threatening infection requires amphotericin B, 1 mg/kg/day, with a 2.0–2.5 g total dose. The investigational drug itraconazole has activity against aspergillus, but its role in therapy has not been established.

VI. *Candida* spp and *T. glabrata*. Oropharyngeal candidiasis occurs in both normal and immunocompromised hosts, including patients using oral contraceptives or being treated with inhaled or systemic steroids, antimicrobials, or chemotherapeutic agents, and patients with AIDS. Systemic infections with these organisms usually occur in immunocompromised patients, particularly those receiving broad-spectrum antimicrobials or parenteral hyperalimentation.

A. Oral and esophageal candidiasis. Oral disease can be treated with nystatin or clotrimazole (e.g., clotrimazole troches, 10 mg dissolved slowly in the mouth 5 times/day). Esophageal disease responds to ketoconazole, 200–400 mg PO qd; fluconazole, 100–200 mg PO or IV qd; or low-dose amphotericin B, 10–20 mg IV qd for 7–14 days.

B. Catheter-related fungemia with these organisms is a common nosocomial infection. Such infections may clear spontaneously with removal of the catheter and modification of other risk factors (e.g., discontinuation of antibiotics). However, in an unknown number of patients complications develop, including endophthalmitis, osteomyelitis, and other visceral involvement. Treatment is therefore recommended for most patients. In nonimmunocompromised patients without evidence of dissemination, a brief course of 200 mg amphotericin B may be adequate provided that fungemia resolves promptly with removal of the catheter. Other patients should receive therapy for disseminated disease.

C. Disseminated disease is treated with amphotericin B, 0.5 mg/kg/day, with a 0.5–1.5 g total dose. Fluconazole, 200–400 mg IV or PO, is an alternative for nonneutropenic patients unable to tolerate amphotericin B.

VII. Sporotrichosis. Cutaneous and subcutaneous disease is best treated with local heat and **oral iodides** (satured solution of potassium iodide, SSKI). The dose of SSKI is begun at 1 drop tid in milk or juice and is increased slowly until a maximum of 8 drops tid is attained or drug intolerance develops. Treatment should be continued for 1–2 months after all lesions have cleared. Toxicities include increased lacrimation and salivation, an unpleasant taste, gastric irritation, and diarrhea. Amphotericin B, with a 1.5- to 2.5-g total dose, should be used for patients with disseminated disease and for those unable to tolerate SSKI.

Malaria

Malaria is caused by protozoa of the genus *Plasmodium*. It is endemic to most of the tropical and subtropical world. Malaria begins as a nonspecific illness characterized by fever and chills, headache, myalgias, arthralgia, nausea, vomiting, or diarrhea. Left untreated, the illness may progress to severe anemia, thrombocytopenia, pulmonary edema, hypoglycemia, encephalopathy, and death. Malaria should be suspected when illness occurs in a patient who has recently visited an endemic area. **Diagnosis** is made by identification of the parasites in a blood smear stained with Giemsa stain. Current information on the incidence of resistance in various regions of the world, prophylaxis, and treatment issues can be obtained from the CDC, 404-332-4555.

I. **Plasmodium falciparum malaria,** the most severe form of the disease, is a potential medical emergency. Chloroquine resistance is widespread. To date the only areas of the world where there has been no documented chloroquine resistance are Central America, Haiti, the Dominican Republic, and Egypt. Fansidar (sulfadoxine-pyrimethamine) resistance occurs in Southeast Asia and the Amazon (CDC, *Health Information for International Travel,* 1991). **Chloroquine resistance should be presumed in patients in whom P. falciparum malaria develops unless a careful history reveals travel only to areas where resistance does not occur. Chloroquine resistance should also be presumed in patients with severe infections (i.e., parasitemia greater than 5% or mental status changes) and those in whom malaria develops despite chloroquine prophylaxis.**

A. **Plasmodium falciparum malaria,** which is presumed to be **chloroquine resistant,** should be treated with two drugs: quinine sulfate, 650 mg PO tid for 3 days, and tetracycline, 250 mg PO qid for 7 days. Fansidar, 3 tablets PO as a single dose, can be substituted for tetracycline, unless the disease is acquired in an area of Fansidar resistance. Patients who acquire *P. falciparum* in Thailand or surrounding countries should receive a 7-day course of quinine and tetracycline. **Severe P. falciparum infection requires parenteral therapy** with quinidine gluconate, 10 mg/kg IV over 1–2 hours, followed by 0.02 mg/kg/minute as a continuous infusion (*N. Engl. J. Med.* 321:65, 1989) and doxycycline, 100 mg IV q12h, or tetracycline, 250 mg PO qid. Patients requiring quinidine intravenously should be monitored for hypotension and arrhythmias in an intensive care setting (see Chap. 7). When the level of parasitemia falls to less than 1% and the patient is able to take oral medication, quinine sulfate can be substituted to complete a total of 3 days of quinidine/quinine. Tetracycline should be given orally to complete a 7-day course of tetracycline therapy. For parasitemias greater than 10%, exchange transfusion should be considered.

B. **Plasmodium falciparum malaria** acquired in areas where chloroquine resistance does not occur can be treated with **chloroquine base,** 600 mg (1000 mg chloroquine phosphate) PO, followed in 6 hours by 300 mg PO, and an additional 300 mg PO qd for 2 days. Severe infections should be treated as in sec. **I.A.**

II. **Nonfalciparum malaria** is less severe and usually responds to oral chloroquine (see sec. **I.B**). Patients with *Plasmodium vivax* or *P. ovale* infection may relapse several months after their initial illness because of the persistence of dormant forms (hypnozoites) in the liver. Therefore, after screening for glucose 6-phosphate dehydrogenase (G-6-PD) deficiency, patients should also be treated with primaquine, 15 mg of base PO qd for 14 days. Relapses should be treated with chloroquine and primaquine.

Human Immunodeficiency Virus Infection and AIDS

Human immunodeficiency virus–type 1 (HIV-1) is a human retrovirus that infects lymphocytes and other cells bearing the CD4 surface marker. Infection leads to lymphopenia, CD4 lymphocyte deficiency and dysfunction, impaired cell-mediated immune response, and polyclonal B-cell activation with impaired B-cell response to new antigens. This immune derangement gives rise to **AIDS,** which is characterized by opportunistic infections and unusual malignancies. The time from infection with HIV to onset of overt AIDS ranges from months to many years, with a median incubation period of about 10 years. The virus is transmitted primarily by sexual and parenteral routes. **Major risk groups** include sexual contacts of infected persons (in the United States, 60% of patients with AIDS are male homosexuals), IV drug users, recipients of infected blood products, and children born to HIV-infected mothers. Treatment of AIDS includes specific antiretroviral therapy and treatment of infectious and neoplastic complications.

Table 13-2. Immunologic monitoring of the HIV-positive patient

CD4 lymphocyte count	Recommendation
> 600 cells/mm^3	Repeat CD4 count every 6 months
500–600 cells/mm^3	Repeat CD4 count every 3 months
< 500 cells/mm^3	Repeat CD4 count in 1 week: **if < 500, recommend zidovudine therapy**
300–500 cells/mm^3	Repeat CD4 count every 6 months
200–300 cells/mm^3	Repeat CD4 count every 2–3 months
< 200 cells/mm^3 or < 20% of total lymphocytes	**Institute PCP prophylaxis;** no further need for regular CD4 testing

I. **Management of the HIV-positive patient.** Patients with HIV infection may present acutely near the time of seroconversion or at a late stage with an AIDS-defining complication. Initial assessment of patients should include assessment of the need for initiation of antiretroviral therapy and of prophylactic therapy against *P. carinii* pneumonia (PCP).

   A. **Primary HIV infection.** Initial infection with HIV-1 is usually asymptomatic but may be associated with a mononucleosis-like syndrome; treatment is supportive. HIV infection is also associated with aseptic meningitis, spinal vacuolar myelopathy, peripheral neuropathy, and subacute encephalitis.

   B. **Initial assessment.** Most patients are asymptomatic initially. In some, recurrent oral candidiasis, lymphadenopathy, weight loss, fevers, night sweats, and chronic diarrhea (**AIDS-related complex [ARC]**) may develop. Abnormal laboratory findings may include anemia, thrombocytopenia, and leukopenia. The most important initial laboratory test is measurement of the CD4 (T4) lymphocyte count. The normal range for adults is 600–1500 cells/mm^3. Counts less than 500 cells/mm^3 usually indicate HIV-associated immunodeficiency. The recommended frequency of measurement of the CD4 count in HIV-positive patients is shown in Table 13-2.

   C. **Antiretroviral therapy.** Zidovudine (ZDV) therapy is indicated for HIV-infected patients with a CD4 lymphocyte count less than 500 cells. The initial dosage is 200 mg PO q8h. Hematologic toxicity may require temporary discontinuation or dose reduction. However, the effectiveness of lower doses has not been definitively established (see Chap. 12). Dideoxyinosine (ddI) and dideoxycytidine (ddC) are available as alternative therapy in patients who are intolerant of or are failing zidovudine. Pancreatitis and a painful sensory neuropathy are the major side effects of these agents.

   D. **Prophylactic measures.** Because tuberculosis is an important complication of HIV infection, screening is warranted at the time of initial assessment (see sec. **II.C.1**). Patients often become anergic as the degree of immunodeficiency progresses. In such patients, chest radiography should be performed. **Immunizations** such as annual influenza vaccine, pneumococcal vaccine, and, for hepatitis B–seronegative patients, hepatitis B vaccine, can also be offered. **Prophylaxis against PCP** (see sec. **II.E**) is indicated when the CD4 count is less than 200 cells/mm^3 or when the percentage of CD4 lymphocytes is less than 20% of the total lymphocyte count.

II. **Complications of HIV infection**

   A. **Viral infections**

      1. **Cytomegalovirus infection** is common in patients with AIDS. Manifestations include viremia with fever and constitutional symptoms, chorioretinitis, esophagitis, gastritis, enterocolitis, pancreatitis, acalculous cholecystitis, bone-marrow suppression, necrotizing adrenalitis, and upper and lower respiratory tract infections. Therapy with **ganciclovir (DHPG)** is effective for chorioretinitis and gastrointestinal disease but is associated with significant

hematologic toxicity (see Chap. 12). **Relapse** after discontinuation of the drug is common, usually necessitating maintenance therapy. It is usually necessary to discontinue zidovudine when systemic ganciclovir is given. Concomitant granulocyte macrophage colony-stimulating factor (GM–CSF) can be used as a possible means of ameliorating ganciclovir myelotoxicity. Patients with retinitis who are intolerant of systemic ganciclovir may benefit from intravitreal administration of the drug by an experienced ophthalmologist. **Foscarnet** is indicated for patients who have a documented ganciclovir-resistant CMV strain or who are failing ganciclovir therapy.

2. **Other herpetoviradae. Herpes simplex virus** infection has been associated with esophagitis, proctitis, pulmonary disease, and large, atypical, persistent, cutaneous ulcerations. **Intravenous acyclovir** is usually effective for these problems, but relapses are frequent. **Varicella-zoster virus** may cause typical dermatomal lesions or may disseminate. Recurrent disease, meningoencephalitis, and cranial neuritis have been reported. Acyclovir is the treatment of choice. Evidence of **Epstein-Barr virus** infection is common in patients with AIDS, particularly hairy leukoplakia. Oral acyclovir may be effective but should be reserved for symptomatic cases.

3. **JC virus** is a papovavirus associated with **progressive multifocal leukoencephalopathy (PML).** PML is characterized by altered mental status, visual loss, weakness, and abnormalities of gait. Nonenhancing, hypodense lesions are seen on CT of the head, but MRI is probably more sensitive. No effective therapy has been identified.

B. **Bacterial infections** are common in patients with AIDS and often recur or follow an atypical or aggressive course despite adequate therapy. Intense initial therapy followed by prolonged suppression is often necessary.

1. **Nontyphoidal salmonellae** (especially *S. typhimurium*) are associated with invasive disease that often recurs or persists despite the use of appropriate antibiotics. Initial IV therapy with ampicillin, ceftriaxone, or TMP/SMZ should be followed by long-term oral suppressive therapy based on susceptibility testing (e.g., amoxicillin, 500 mg PO tid); even then, relapse may occur as soon as therapy is discontinued.

2. **Syphilis.** The natural history of syphilis may be altered by HIV infection. Reactivation of previously treated disease, active disease with negative serology, asymptomatic neurosyphilis, and relapse after standard therapy have all been reported. The optimal management of syphilis in this setting remains unclear. Lumbar puncture of seropositive patients, IV penicillin G for any suspected infections, and long-term maintenance therapy are all potentially necessary measures.

3. **Bacterial pneumonias** occur with increased frequency and are usually due to *Strep. pneumoniae, H. influenzae,* or group B streptococcus. Pneumonia due to gram-negative enteric organisms occurs in advanced HIV disease. Chest radiographs may reveal typical lobar pneumonia, but diffuse interstitial infiltrates similar to *P. carinii* pneumonia have been reported. These infections usually respond to specific antibiotic therapy, but relapses are not uncommon.

C. **Mycobacterial infections**

1. **Mycobacterium tuberculosis. Tuberculosis** occurs with increased frequency in patients with AIDS, particularly IV drug users and Haitian immigrants. Atypical radiographic patterns and extrapulmonary disease are quite common; apical cavitary disease is rare. **Antituberculous therapy** should be initiated whenever acid-fast bacilli are discovered in a specimen from a patient with AIDS. Standard INH and rifampin therapy (see Mycobacterial Infections) plus pyrazinamide, 20–30 mg/kg PO qd, for the first 2 months of treatment is recommended (*Am. Rev. Respir. Dis.* 136:492, 1987). Ethambutol should be added if INH resistance is suspected. Treatment should be continued for 9 months and at least 6 months after the last positive culture. If either INH or rifampin cannot be used, a minimum of 18 months of treatment (e.g., INH plus ethambutol or rifampin plus ethambutol) with at

least 12 months following the last positive culture is suggested. Prophylaxis with INH for 12 months should be considered in any HIV-positive patient with a reactive (5-mm induration) PPD skin test. Whether these patients or patients with AIDS who are treated for active tuberculosis should receive lifelong prophylaxis is unclear.

2. *Mycobacterium avium-intracellulare* is one of the most frequent opportunistic pathogens in patients with AIDS. Generalized infection and gastrointestinal disease are the most common manifestations. No clearly effective treatment regimen has been identified, although multiple-drug regimens, including rifampin, clofazimine, ethambutol, amikacin, ciprofloxacin, and virtually all standard antituberculous agents have been used and may result in symptomatic benefit. The new macrolide antibiotic clarithromycin offers promise as alternate therapy.

D. Fungal infections (see also Systemic Mycoses)

1. **Candidiasis.** Persistent oral, esophageal, and vaginal infections are common, but dissemination is rare in the absence of other risk factors such as IV catheters. The severity and frequency of mucocutaneous candidiasis increases with declining immune function.

2. *Cryptococcus neoformans* is the most common cause of fungal CNS disease in patients with AIDS. Symptoms may be mild, so the threshold for performing a lumbar puncture should be low. Initial treatment is with amphotericin B and flucytosine (see Systemic Mycoses) for 2–3 weeks, followed by fluconazole, 400 mg qd for 8–10 weeks. Following acute treatment, lifelong maintenance therapy is required with fluconazole, 200 mg qd. Response is usually monitored clinically and is usually slow. Repeat lumbar puncture is indicated for clinical deterioration. In addition to routine CSF chemistries, cell count, cryptococcal antigen, and culture, the CSF opening pressure should be measured to assess the possibility of intracranial hypertension as a complication.

3. *Histoplasma capsulatum* is an important pathogen in patients with AIDS from endemic areas and may cause disseminated disease and septicemia. Pancytopenia may result from bone-marrow involvement. Amphotericin B (total dose 1.5–2.0 g) has been used successfully, but relapses are common. Maintenance therapy with weekly amphotericin B appears justified, but experience is limited. Itraconazole is a promising investigational agent.

4. *Coccidioides immitis* also occurs in patients with AIDS from endemic areas. Extensive pulmonary disease with extrapulmonary spread is common. Amphotericin B therapy (total dose 1.5–2.0 g) is appropriate, and, as with histoplasmosis, lifetime maintenance therapy is probably indicated. Coccidioidal meningitis requires intracisternal or intraventricular therapy with amphotericin B (see Chap. 12). Fluconazole, 400 mg qd, is a promising agent for the treatment of coccidioidal meningitis and may alleviate the need for intraventricular therapy.

E. *Pneumocystis carinii* **pneumonia** remains the most common opportunistic infection in patients with AIDS and is a leading cause of mortality. Previously thought to be a protozoan, it is now believed to be a fungus. Extrapulmonary disease has also been described, particularly in patients receiving aerosolized pentamidine for prophylaxis. The **treatment** of choice for PCP is TMP/SMZ, 5 mg/25 mg per kg PO or IV q6–8h for 21 days. Serum levels of SMZ or TMP should be measured. Peak serum levels of 100–151 μg/ml SMZ may be necessary for therapeutic efficacy. Rashes are common in patients with AIDS treated with TMP/SMZ but do not usually require a change in therapy (*Ann. Intern. Med.* 109:280, 1988). Pentamidine, 4 mg/kg infused over 2 hours IV qd for 21 days, is also effective and is used in patients who cannot tolerate TMP/SMZ or fail to respond during the first 5–7 days of TMP/SMZ therapy. Dapsone/trimethoprim and clindamycin/primaquine are promising alternatives, but experience is limited. **Prophylactic therapy** (TMP/SMZ, 160 mg/800 mg [one double-strength tablet] PO qd; dapsone, 50 mg PO daily; or pentamidine, 300 mg each month by aerosol) is indicated for patients who recover from PCP and for HIV-infected

patients with CD4 lymphocyte counts less than 200 cells/mm^3. In patients with
well-documented PCP and moderate to severe disease (PaO$_2$ < 75 mm Hg on
room air), prevention of respiratory failure and survival benefit have been
demonstrated with adjunctive use of steroids (*N. Engl. J. Med.* 323:1451, 1990).
Prednisone (or equivalent parenteral methylprednisolone), 40 mg PO bid for 5
days, followed by 40 mg PO qd for 5 days, followed by 20 mg PO qd for the
duration of anti-*Pneumocystis* therapy, is recommended.

F. Protozoal infections

   1. *Toxoplasma gondii* typically causes multiple CNS lesions with encephalopathy and focal neurologic findings. Treatment with sulfadiazine, 25 mg/kg PO
   q6h, plus pyrimethamine, 100–150 mg PO on day 1, then 50–75 mg PO qd,
   often results in improvement, but indefinite therapy is needed to prevent
   relapse. Folinic acid, 5–10 mg PO qd, can be added to minimize hematologic
   toxicity. For patients who are intolerant of sulfonamides, clindamycin, 600
   mg PO qid, can be substituted for sulfadiazine. Corticosteroid therapy may
   also be useful for treating increased intracranial pressure (see also Central
   Nervous System Infections, sec. **VI.B.2**).

   2. *Cryptosporidium* and *Isospora belli* may cause protozoal enteric infections in
   patients with AIDS. *Isospora belli* infection can be treated with TMP/SMZ,
   160 mg/800 mg PO qid for 10 days, and then bid for 3 weeks (*N. Engl. J. Med.*
   315:87, 1986). Relapses are not uncommon. Shorter courses of TMP/SMZ
   therapy followed by prophylaxis with pyrimethamine/sulfadoxine may also
   be effective (*J. Infect. Dis.* 157:225, 1988). No therapy has proved to be
   effective for cryptosporidiosis.

G. Neoplasms associated with AIDS include non-Hodgkin's lymphomas and Kaposi's sarcoma. Primary CNS lymphomas are common and may be multicentric.

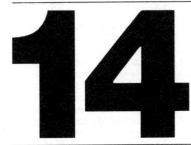

Gastrointestinal
Bleeding

Steven A. Edmundowicz and
Gary R. Zuckerman

Management

Acute gastrointestinal bleeding may result from a number of sources and with varying severity depending on the rate of blood loss. **The key to successful management of acute gastrointestinal bleeding is maintaining adequate circulatory volume while localizing the bleeding site and providing definitive therapy.** Risk factors for increased morbidity and mortality from gastrointestinal bleeding include (1) age greater than 60 years, (2) more than one co-morbid illness, (3) severe blood loss (> 5 units), (4) shock on admission, and (5) recurrent hemorrhage (within 72 hours).

I. **Evaluation and treatment of the unstable patient**
   A. **Initial evaluation.** A rapid assessment to identify patients with indications for immediate intervention should be performed as soon as the patient presents with bleeding. The extent of the initial evaluation is dictated by the patient's condition. **The general appearance** of the patient should be noted. Signs of distress (including confusion, obtundation, diaphoresis, clammy or mottled skin, and pain) indicate the need for urgent intervention. **In the hemodynamically compromised patient, resuscitative measures should be instituted concomitantly.**
      1. **Intravascular volume** and hemodynamic status should be assessed immediately. **Vital signs** (heart rate, blood pressure, and their postural changes) are of paramount importance in the evaluation and management of significant bleeding; they must be obtained reliably and frequently. A sudden increase in pulse rate is often the only early indication of recurrent bleeding. The physician must be aware of medications (e.g., beta-adrenergic antagonists) and medical conditions (e.g., autonomic dysfunction) that may alter interpretation of hemodynamic data. **Postural hypotension** (supine to upright fall in systolic blood pressure of > 10 mm Hg or increase in heart rate of > 20 beats/minute) is indicative of moderate blood loss (10–20% of circulatory volume). **Supine hypotension** suggests more severe blood loss (usually > 20% of the circulatory volume). Further loss in circulatory volume results in **shock** and is evidenced by hypotension, tachycardia, peripheral vasoconstriction, diaphoresis, and **ischemic organ dysfunction** (e.g., myocardial ischemia, confusion, or decreased urine output). Rapid restoration of circulatory volume is essential in this setting (see sec. **I.B.1** and Chap. 26). **Evidence of continued blood loss,** including recurrent hematemesis, hematochezia, melena, or changing vital signs, requires rapid initiation of therapy and close monitoring to assess the response to treatment.
      2. **Laboratory evaluation.** Blood specimens for typing and cross-matching, CBC, platelet count, prothrombin time (PT), partial thromboplastin time (PTT), and chemistries should be obtained (see sec. **II.C**). The hemoglobin and hematocrit are poor indicators of acute blood loss; these parameters may be normal initially despite significant blood loss and may take hours to reflect the actual degree of hemorrhage.
   B. **Emergent therapy** should be instituted as soon as a hemodynamically compromised patient is identified.
      1. **Restoration of intravascular volume.** Rapid restoration of the circulatory

volume with saline-containing solutions and blood products is the primary goal. **Two large-bore IV lines** should be established with short, No. 14- to 18-gauge catheters in large peripheral veins. Central venous catheterization offers no advantage over good peripheral access and may delay volume infusion. When possible, blood should be used to replace volume in patients with hemorrhagic shock. Isotonic saline, lactated Ringer's solution, or 5% hetastarch (Hespan) can be used until blood products are available. **The rate of volume infusion** should be guided by the patient's condition, the degree of volume loss suspected, and the rate of active bleeding. Patients in shock may require fluids or blood to be "pumped" or hand-infused using large syringes and stopcocks. The blood bank must be notified of the potential demand for blood products. Six units of packed red blood cells (PRBCs) should be held available at all times until the patient's condition has stabilized. In some situations, non–cross-matched O-negative blood, simultaneous multiple-unit infusions, or transient IV pressor therapy may be warranted (see Chap. 26).

2. **Transfusion therapy** (see Chap. 18). Blood transfusion should be utilized as soon as it is evident that the patient's bleeding is massive, ongoing, or to such a degree that colloid replacement alone will not result in adequate circulatory volume and tissue oxygenation. Packed RBC transfusion should be continued until the patient is hemodynamically stable and the hematocrit remains at 25% or greater. **Patients with cardiac or pulmonary disease** may require transfusion to a higher hematocrit (30% or greater) to prevent ischemia. If active bleeding is present, transfusion therapy must continue to keep pace with ongoing losses until hemostasis is obtained. **Coagulopathy** should be corrected with fresh frozen plasma (FFP) or other factor therapy (see Chap. 17). Initially, 4 units of FFP can be given. Further therapy should be based on clinical assessment. **Thrombocytopenia** with platelet counts of less than 50,000/μl should be corrected with platelet transfusions (see Chap. 18) or with therapy directed at the cause of thrombocytopenia. When large volume transfusions are needed (i.e., > 5 units), dilution of clotting factors or hypocalcemia due to chelating agents in the transfused blood may occur. Monitoring for these complications is appropriate and, if necessary, replacement therapy should be instituted.

3. **Hemodynamic monitoring** during resuscitation may be necessary for patients with known or suspected cardiovascular disease. However, placement of central venous or Swan-Ganz catheters should not interfere with the primary objective of restoring circulatory volume.

4. **Airway management. Prophylactic endotracheal intubation** to prevent aspiration should be considered in any patient with a diminished mental status due to shock or hepatic encephalopathy, massive bleeding with hematemesis, or active variceal hemorrhage.

5. **Early consultations** with a gastroenterologist, surgeon, or invasive radiologist are appropriate when significant hemorrhage, continued instability, or active bleeding occurs.

II. **Evaluation of the stabilized patient** is indicated to identify the source of bleeding, provide specific therapy, and detect risk factors for further bleeding.

A. **History.** Symptoms at presentation may help differentiate upper from lower gastrointestinal bleeding and may also suggest a particular diagnosis. **Hematemesis** virtually ensures an upper gastrointestinal source of bleeding. Pain may also help localize a bleeding source or suggest other diagnostic considerations (e.g., hematobilia, bowel infarction). Pertinent past medical history should be noted, including (1) prior bleeding episodes, (2) excessive alcohol use, (3) liver disease, (4) coagulation abnormalities or bleeding tendencies, (5) systemic disease associated with gastrointestinal lesions, (6) abdominal surgery, (7) trauma, or (8) previous aortic vascular surgery. Medications that may exacerbate or cause gastrointestinal bleeding (e.g., aspirin and aspirin-containing preparations, nonsteroidal anti-inflammatory agents [NSAIDs], and glucocorticoids) should also be noted.

B. **Physical examination** may help identify the source of blood loss. A naso-pharyngeal source should be excluded in all patients with hematemesis. Evidence of portal hypertension (e.g., splenomegaly, ascites, and dilated abdominal wall collateral vessels) should be noted. **The rectal examination** should include a careful digital examination for masses and hemorrhoids, inspection of stool for gross blood, and testing of stool for the presence of occult blood. Often the color and consistency of the stool will help direct further evaluation. **Melena,** a black, sticky stool with a characteristic odor, usually indicates bleeding proximal to the cecum. **Maroon stool** may be passed when the bleeding site is located in the distal small bowel or right colon. **Bright red blood** passed per rectum without a change in vital signs or hematocrit is suggestive of an anorectal or left colonic source of blood loss. However, brisk upper tract bleeding with rapid intestinal transit may present with passage of bright red blood per rectum.

C. **Laboratory testing** is appropriate in all patients with significant gastrointestinal bleeding.
   1. **Complete blood count.** The hemoglobin and hematocrit may not accurately reflect the degree of blood loss in acute and rapid bleeding because of the delay in equilibration. It is essential to follow these parameters in hospitalized individuals to assess the need for and the response to transfusion therapy. In general the hematocrit should increase approximately 3% for each unit of packed RBCs transfused. The hemoglobin and hematocrit are also used to monitor for continued bleeding and as an end point for transfusion therapy in the stabilized patient. Frequent monitoring of the hematocrit (e.g., q6h) is reasonable in the actively bleeding patient.
   2. **Platelet counts** should be measured in all patients with gastrointestinal bleeding. Patients with active bleeding and a platelet count of less than 50,000/μl should receive platelet transfusion or other therapy to increase the platelet count (see Chap. 18).
   3. **The prothrombin time and partial thromboplastin time** should be measured in all patients. Patients with active bleeding and a prolonged PT or PTT should receive FFP to correct the defect (see Chap. 17). In the stable patient, correction of a prolonged PT can be attempted with parenteral aqueous vitamin K (menadiol, 10 mg IV or SQ qd, or phytonadione, 10 mg SQ qd, for 3 days).

D. **Nasogastric (NG) tube placement.** Hematemesis or a bloody gastric aspirate obtained through an NG tube indicates upper gastrointestinal bleeding proximal to the jejunum.
   1. **Gastric aspirate.** A gastric aspirate should be considered positive only if it contains a significant amount of fresh blood (not the small amount common with tube trauma) or is very dark and strongly positive for occult blood. A positive gastric aspirate is usually associated with an identifiable upper tract bleeding site. False-negative aspirates are uncommon but may occur if the tube is coiled in the fundus of the stomach, the bleeding is intermittent, or there is a lack of reflux of blood through the pylorus from a bleeding site in the duodenum.
   2. **Gastric lavage** with room temperature water (or saline) can be used to clear the stomach of clots before endoscopy or to assess the rate of blood loss in a patient with bright red blood return on NG tube placement. **The use of iced saline for lavage is of no benefit** and may disrupt local hemostatic mechanisms and cause hypothermia. Unless the patient is obstructed or is suffering from protracted nausea and vomiting, the NG tube can be removed after a diagnostic aspirate is performed. Recurrent bleeding can be detected by following vital signs, stool appearance, and hematocrit. In addition, an indwelling tube can lead to mucosal damage, promote reflux esophagitis, and increase the risk of aspiration.

Upper Gastrointestinal Bleeding

I. **Diagnosis.** The approach to the patient with upper gastrointestinal (UGI) bleeding is dependent on patient stability, the rate of blood loss, procedural availability, and local expertise at the patient's hospital. Numerous lesions can lead to upper gastrointestinal tract blood loss (Table 14-1). Frequent assessment of the patient and treatment of blood loss must continue uninterrupted during the diagnostic evaluation.

A. **Esophagogastroduodenoscopy** is the preferred method of examination of patients with UGI bleeding. Endoscopy can be performed at the bedside and offers high diagnostic accuracy, low morbidity, the ability to recognize potential bleeding sites even when active bleeding is not occurring, and the opportunity for rapid therapeutic intervention. To effectively diagnose patients, endoscopy should be performed as soon as is reasonably possible (e.g., within 24 hours). Although early diagnostic endoscopy has not been shown to improve mortality, therapeutic endoscopy may reduce transfusion requirements, length of hospitalization, and the need for emergent surgery (*N. Engl. J. Med.* 316:1613, 1987). Endoscopy may be most helpful in determining which of several potential lesions are actually bleeding and which patients have lesions with an increased risk of recurrent bleeding. Endoscopy is also indicated for precise identification of the site of bleeding before the implementation of potentially hazardous therapy such as esophageal balloon tamponade (see sec. **II.B.3**).

B. **Arteriography.** When bleeding is so brisk that the GI tract cannot be adequately cleared for complete examination by endoscopy, selective abdominal angiography may localize the site of hemorrhage. However, diagnostic success is likely only when the rate of bleeding is greater than 0.5 ml/minute at the time of the study. Arteriography may also be both diagnostic and therapeutic (see sec. **II.A.3**).

C. **Upper gastrointestinal barium radiography** has no role in the initial evaluation of active gastrointestinal bleeding when endoscopy is available. Barium studies may identify mucosal lesions but cannot confirm active bleeding from a site. Furthermore, barium contrast may subsequently interfere with both endoscopic and arteriographic studies.

II. **Therapy of specific lesions.** Results of therapeutic trials in UGI bleeding must be interpreted with caution since up to 85% of bleeding episodes will resolve with supportive therapy alone.

A. **Peptic ulcers** remain the most common cause of UGI bleeding.

1. **Therapeutic endoscopy.** Injection therapy, monopolar and bipolar electrocoagulation, heater probe therapy, and laser coagulation are useful in obtaining hemostasis. These modalities, when available, offer the advantage of immediate treatment at the time of diagnosis. Endoscopic electrocoagulation treatment of active UGI bleeding has been shown to decrease transfusion requirements, length of hospital stay, and the need for surgical intervention (*N. Engl. J. Med.* 316:1613, 1987 and 318:186, 1988).

2. **Surgery** is considered the therapy of choice for intractable or recurrent bleeding from peptic ulcer disease. In the patient with exsanguinating hemorrhage, it may be necessary to proceed directly to the operating suite, with resuscitation and endoscopy being completed in this setting. Surgical consultation should be obtained early in the management of patients with active gastrointestinal bleeding. Surgical therapy for peptic ulcer disease should be considered in the following situations:

a. **Severe hemorrhage** that requires a high rate of blood transfusion (e.g., > 5 units in 24 hours) with continued circulatory instability. The overall assessment of the patient and an inability to maintain hemodynamic stability are of greater concern than is exceeding an arbitrary number of transfused units.

Table 14-1. Diagnosis at endoscopy for upper gastrointestinal bleeding in 482 patients

Diagnosis[*]	Patients (No.)	Prevalence (%)
Duodenal ulcer	99	21
Gastric ulcer	96	20
Erosive gastritis	63	13
Esophageal varices	50	10
Angiodysplasia (gastric and duodenal)	34	7
Erosive esophagitis	30	6
Mallory-Weiss tear	26	5
Pyloric channel ulcer	10	2
Gastric tumor	9	2
Erosive duodenitis	7	1
Anastomotic ulcer	4	0.8
Aortoenteric fistula	2	0.4
Metastatic tumor, duodenum	2	0.4
Gastric polyps	1	0.2
Schönlein-Henoch syndrome	1	0.2
Rendu-Osler-Weber syndrome	1	0.2
Blood seen but no lesion identified	15	3
No potential bleeding lesion seen or normal examination findings	50	10

*Some patients had more than one diagnosis.
Source: Reproduced with permission, from: G. R. Zuckerman et al. Upper gastrointestinal bleeding in patients with chronic renal failure. *Ann. Intern. Med.* 1985; 102:588.

  b. Recurrent bleeding after nonsurgical management that requires additional transfusion during the same hospitalization.
  c. Difficulty in obtaining adequate amounts of compatible blood.
  3. Arterial angiotherapy can be used to control massive gastrointestinal bleeding in patients with peptic ulcer disease who are considered at high risk for surgical complications. These radiographic procedures require a skilled angiographer who can perform selective arterial catheterization.
  a. Arterial vasopressin produces cessation of bleeding in some patients with gastric or duodenal ulcers. This therapy requires selective catheterization of the bleeding artery and continuous infusion of vasopressin. The infusion is titrated to control bleeding while minimizing side effects such as bradycardia, myocardial ischemia, and abdominal pain. Patients with known coronary artery disease are at increased risk for complications from the systemic effects of vasopressin.
  b. Arterial embolization can be performed after selective catheterization of a bleeding artery. Absorbable gelatin sponge (Gelfoam) particles, metal coil springs, or other agents can be placed in the bleeding vessel to produce immediate occlusions and allow healing of the lesion. The success rate for hemostasis is variable and related to the location and type of lesion (*Gastroenterology* 86:876, 1984). Most complications occur in patients with previous gastric surgery or mesenteric vascular disease.
  4. H_2 antagonists have a well-defined role in the therapy of peptic ulcer disease and in the prevention of bleeding from stress ulceration (see Chap. 15). They are not effective in stopping active UGI bleeding. The efficacy of these agents in reducing the incidence of recurrent hemorrhage during the hospitalization of patients with gastrointestinal bleeding remains unproved (*Am. J. Med.* 76:361, 1984).

B. **Esophageal varices** develop most commonly in patients with portal hypertension. Hemorrhage from esophageal varices is a medical emergency associated with high morbidity and mortality (*N. Engl. J. Med.* 320:1393 and 1469, 1989). As many as one third of patients die during their initial hospitalization (*Gastroenterology* 80:800, 1981). There is no ideal therapy for variceal hemorrhage, and all of the available therapeutic options are associated with significant complication rates. The etiology and severity of the patient's portal hypertension are the major determinants of long-term survival. **Intensive care unit** (ICU) admission should be considered for all patients with known or suspected varices who have active gastrointestinal bleeding. **Endotracheal intubation** to protect the airway and prevent aspiration may be necessary. Following stabilization, **early endoscopy** should be performed to confirm the bleeding site before the initiation of specific, potentially hazardous therapies. If the diagnosis of variceal hemorrhage is confirmed and active bleeding persists, the following therapeutic options exist.

1. **Endoscopic sclerotherapy** can be provided at the bedside as soon as the diagnosis of variceal bleeding is confirmed. Sclerotherapy is effective in controlling primary hemorrhage and for the obliteration of varices after the initial bleeding episode (*Am. J. Gastroenterol.* 82:813, 1987). Sclerotherapy is associated with significant complications (*Am. J. Gastroenterol.* 82:823, 1987). **Recurrent bleeding** occurs in up to 50% of patients undergoing a course of sclerotherapy. Usually, this bleeding is not massive and can be controlled with further sclerotherapy. Patients who cannot be controlled with repeat injections should be managed with another form of therapy. **Other complications** include ulcerations, stricture formation, perforation, and sepsis. **Fever** occurs in up to 40% of patients in the first 48 hours after sclerotherapy. Patients with persistent fever after 2 days should be carefully evaluated, as bacteremia frequently occurs during the procedure. **Pulmonary complications** are also common and range from mildly abnormal chest radiographs to pleural effusions and adult respiratory distress syndrome (ARDS). Sclerotherapy of esophageal varices may be most helpful in (1) actively bleeding patients as primary therapy or as a stabilizing measure before shunt or transplant surgery, (2) patients who are not surgical candidates, and (3) patients in whom other forms of therapy have failed. Varices have also been successfully sclerosed by the percutaneous transhepatic approach.

2. **Intravenous vasopressin** has been the standard therapy for variceal hemorrhage for many years, but data regarding its efficacy are conflicting (*N. Engl. J. Med.* 320:1393, 1989). Nevertheless, ready availability, ease of administration, and the potential for success make it a reasonable alternative when other therapies cannot be implemented. **A standard formulation** is 100 units of vasopressin in 250 ml of 5% dextrose in water (D/W; 0.4 units/ml) delivered by a microdrip infusion pump into a central or peripheral vein (with good blood return) on the following schedule: 0.3 units/minute for 30 minutes, followed by increments of 0.3 units/minute every 30 minutes until hemostasis is achieved, side effects develop, or the maximum dosage of 0.9 units/minute is reached (*Gastroenterology* 77:540, 1979). Once bleeding is controlled, the infusion rate should be gradually reduced. Intravenous vasopressin is as effective as the intra-arterial approach and has fewer side effects. **Significant complications of vasopressin therapy** include myocardial ischemia and infarction, ventricular arrhythmias, cardiac arrest, mesenteric ischemia and infarction, and cutaneous ischemic necrosis. Vasopressin therapy should be used with extreme caution in patients with vascular disease or coronary artery disease. All patients should be admitted to an ICU and have cardiac monitoring. The infusion should be reduced or terminated if chest pain, abdominal pain, or arrhythmias develop. **Concomitant IV infusion of nitroglycerin** reduces undesirable cardiovascular side effects and may improve efficacy of vasopressin therapy (*Hepatology* 6:523, 1986); its use should be considered in all patients with a history of coronary artery or vascular disease. Nitroglycerin is administered only if the systolic blood pressure is greater than 100 mm Hg. A reasonable dose is 10 μg/minute IV, increased by 10 μg/minute every 10–15

minutes until the systolic blood pressure falls to 100 mm Hg or a maximum dosage of 400 µg/minute is reached (*Hepatology* 6:410, 1986).

3. **Balloon tamponade** of varices allows direct pressure to be applied to the bleeding varix or to the gastric cardia in an attempt to achieve hemostasis. Several different types of tubes are available: The **Sengstaken-Blakemore** tube has both a gastric and esophageal balloon, the **Linton** tube has a large-volume gastric balloon without an esophageal balloon, and the **Minnesota** tube has a large-volume gastric balloon plus an esophageal balloon. **These tubes should be used according to the manufacturer's specific directions** for placement, traction, and balloon volume, and with the aid of personnel experienced in the use of such equipment. Although balloon tamponade has been shown to be effective in controlling hemorrhage, there is a high incidence of major complications and a significant mortality due to tube displacement (*Dig. Dis. Sci.* 34:913, 1989). In addition, although temporary hemostasis can frequently be obtained, **permanent control of bleeding is much less common.** In patients bleeding from gastric varices, the Linton tube may offer better control of hemorrhage than the Sengstaken-Blakemore tube. The following are guidelines for the use of balloon tamponade:

   a. **Intensive care unit admission** is necessary to ensure careful monitoring and a rapid response to changes in the patient's condition.

   b. **Prophylactic endotracheal intubation** is often necessary, as aspiration and asphyxiation are major causes of mortality related to balloon tamponade.

   c. **The site of bleeding** should be confirmed by endoscopy, and tube selection made with respect to the bleeding site.

   d. **Modification of the Sengstaken-Blakemore tube** by the attachment of an NG tube above the esophageal balloon should be completed before insertion (*Gastroenterology* 61:291, 1971). This NG tube is connected to high intermittent suction to remove secretions from the posterior pharynx and upper esophagus in an attempt to prevent aspiration of oropharyngeal secretions. It should be clearly labeled and should not be lavaged.

   e. **Gastric balloon position** should be confirmed by radiography. Inflating the gastric balloon in the esophagus can result in esophageal rupture.

   f. **All balloon tube outlets** should be clearly labeled, and inflation tubes should be clamped to prevent leakage and tube migration. Scissors must be kept at the bedside so that the tube can be immediately transected and withdrawn if necessary.

   g. **Mucosal ulceration** and necrosis may occur rapidly, especially if large balloon volumes, high pressure, or traction are necessary to control bleeding. Balloon pressure should be reduced intermittently as detailed in the manufacturer's instructions and when bleeding has been controlled. The tube with its balloon deflated can be left in place so that pressure can again be applied if bleeding resumes.

4. **Shunt surgery** (portacaval or distal splenorenal shunt [DSRS]) controls variceal bleeding in 95% of patients. However, operative and hospital mortality are substantial (approximately 12%), and there is a significant incidence of severe encephalopathy. The results of surgical therapy for portal hypertension and variceal bleeding depend on the degree of liver decompensation as measured by the Child's classification (*Hepatology* 1:673, 1981). The patient's underlying liver disease remains the major factor limiting survival. **In individuals with good hepatic reserve,** shunt therapy should be considered if the patient (1) fails sclerotherapy, (2) is unable to return for follow-up visits, (3) lives a great distance from medical care, or (4) is at great risk from recurrent bleeding because of cardiac disease or difficulty in obtaining blood products. Sclerotherapy followed by shunt surgery for failures manifested by significant recurrent hemorrhage may be superior to DSRS alone (*Ann. Intern. Med.* 112:262, 1990).

5. **Hepatic transplantation** has become an accepted and available therapy for patients with end-stage liver disease. Successful hepatic transplantation

results in a reversal of portal hypertension and resolution of esophageal and gastric variceal hemorrhage.

6. **Other therapies. Intravenous somatostatin infusion** has been used to reduce portal hypertension in patients with acute variceal hemorrhage. In limited clinical trials it offers similar efficacy to vasopressin infusion with fewer side effects (*Am. J. Gastroenterol.* 85:804, 1990). **Endoscopic elastic banding to ligate varices** may prove to be as effective as sclerotherapy with fewer complications (*Gastrointest. Endosc.* 35:431, 1989). **Transjugular intrahepatic portacaval shunt (TIPS)** using expandable vascular stents inserted through the jugular vein creates an intrahepatic shunt between the venous and portal circulation that effectively reduces portal pressure and prevents recurrent variceal hemorrhage (*Radiology* 174:1027, 1990). **Other aggressive surgical procedures,** such as transection of the esophagus, have occasionally been successful when all other attempts to arrest variceal hemorrhage fail. Oral propranolol has not been used in acute variceal bleeding but may be effective for long-term management of patients with a history of variceal bleeding.

C. **Mallory-Weiss tear** is a mucosal tear at the gastroesophageal junction. Patients often have a history of retching or emesis (which induces the tear) followed by hematemesis. Most patients with a Mallory-Weiss tear will stop bleeding spontaneously and seldom have recurrent bleeding. For some patients, hemostasis has been achieved with therapeutic endoscopic techniques (see sec. **II.A.1**) or arterial angiotherapy (see sec. **II.A.3**).

D. **Aortoenteric fistula** is an uncommon but particularly lethal cause of UGI bleeding that occurs almost exclusively in patients with prior aortic graft surgery (*Surgery* 94:1, 1983). Over half of all cases reported presented with some form of **"herald" bleeding** before massive gastrointestinal hemorrhage. Recognition of this syndrome is essential, as undiagnosed aortoenteric fistulas almost always result in death. Patients may present with aortoenteric fistula 2 months to 8 years after surgery, with the average onset of symptoms occurring at just over 4 years. The fistula is aortoduodenal in over 90% of cases. **Endoscopy should be performed** as soon as bleeding is detected, including examination to the fourth portion of the duodenum. If bleeding is massive the procedure can be performed in the operating suite. While angiography or CT of the abdomen may be helpful by demonstrating leakage at the graft site or evidence of prosthesis infection, all patients with prior aortic graft surgery and gastrointestinal bleeding should be considered to have aortoenteric fistula until another actively bleeding lesion is documented. Awareness of this diagnostic possibility and expedient surgical correction are necessary to prevent a catastrophe.

E. **Stress ulceration** is a common cause of gastrointestinal bleeding in the intensive care unit patient. **Patients at risk** include those with head injuries, burns, major trauma, shock, sepsis, prolonged mechanical ventilation, and CNS disease requiring intensive care. **Prophylactic therapy** should be provided for all patients at risk. H_2 antagonists are as effective as antacid therapy in preventing significant bleeding (*Ann. Intern. Med.* 106:562, 1987). Sucralfate (in a slurry form) is also effective for prophylaxis of stress ulcer bleeding (*N. Engl. J. Med.* 317:1376, 1987).

F. **Angiodysplasia** (arteriovenous malformation) of the stomach or small intestine is an uncommon source of gastrointestinal bleeding in the general population, but is the most frequent source of UGI bleeding in patients with chronic renal failure (*Ann. Intern. Med.* 102:588, 1985). These very small mucosal lesions are frequently multiple. Some patients have associated colonic angiodysplasia. The lesions of the upper gastrointestinal tract are most commonly diagnosed by endoscopy. Actively bleeding lesions can be treated by coagulation or injection therapy. Limited data suggest that combined estrogen and progesterone therapy may decrease bleeding episodes in patients with and without renal failure (*Ann. Intern. Med.* 105:371, 1986; *Lancet* 335:953, 1990). Although the natural history of this lesion is one of recurrent bleeding and high transfusion requirements over time, the mortality from bleeding angiodysplasia is low.

G. **Other causes** of UGI bleeding include gastritis, esophagitis (peptic and infectious), and malignancies. **Hematobilia** (bleeding into the biliary tree) is an uncommon cause of gastrointestinal bleeding that is often associated with jaundice or biliary colic at the time of active bleeding.

Lower Gastrointestinal Bleeding

Common causes of lower gastrointestinal bleeding include diverticulosis, angiodysplasia, neoplasm, inflammatory bowel disease, ischemic colitis, infectious colitis, and anorectal diseases. Brisk UGI or small intestinal bleeding can occasionally mimic lower gastrointestinal bleeding. As with UGI bleeding, lower gastrointestinal hemorrhage will stop spontaneously in most cases and can be managed with supportive care alone. Initially, patients with lower gastrointestinal bleeding should be stabilized and supported while diagnostic studies are performed.

I. **Diagnosis**
  A. **Rectal examination** and anoscopy or sigmoidoscopy should be performed to search for a rectal source of bleeding. However, a rectal source can be diagnosed with certainty only if an actively bleeding lesion is identified.
  B. **Technetium-99m labeled red blood cell scanning** (^{99m}Tc RBC scan) should be performed in patients thought to be actively bleeding since bleeding rates as low as 0.1 ml/minute can be detected. If positive, further localization and therapy with arteriography may be helpful; if negative, the patient should undergo colonoscopy. Delayed images can be obtained if recurrent bleeding is suspected.
  C. **Arteriography** is the best initial test if bleeding is so rapid that hemodynamic stability is difficult to maintain. It allows rapid localization and potential treatment of the bleeding lesions.
  D. **Colonoscopy** should be utilized in all patients who can be prepared adequately for endoscopic examination with standard oral lavage. Patients in whom ^{99m}Tc RBC scanning or arteriography is negative should undergo colonoscopy for definitive evaluation. Colonoscopy allows identification of lesions that are not actively bleeding at the time of the study. In addition, tissue can be obtained for diagnosis of mass lesions and therapeutic intervention with electrocautery, heater probe, or laser therapy of active bleeding sites can be performed.
  E. **Patients** with suspected lower gastrointestinal bleeding who have no site of blood loss identified on initial studies should be further evaluated. Sources of blood loss in the upper gastrointestinal tract and small bowel should be considered. If gastrointestinal bleeding has ceased and an evaluation, including ^{99m}Tc RBC scan, upper and lower endoscopy, and small-bowel radiographs or endoscopy, does not reveal a potential bleeding site, the patient can be discharged with specific instructions to report to the hospital as soon as bleeding is again noticed. At that time, an immediate ^{99m}Tc RBC scan may localize a bleeding site.

II. **Therapy of specific lesions**
  A. **Diverticular hemorrhage** is the most common cause of major lower GI bleeding in the western world, but occurs in less than 5% of patients with diverticulosis. Bleeding persists in 20% of patients, and recurrent bleeding is also common. In patients with persistent bleeding, selective arterial vasopressin is often effective. Surgery may be necessary in patients (1) with recurrent bleeding, (2) who fail vasopressin therapy because of continued bleeding or complications (e.g., myocardial ischemia), or (3) with extremely rapid bleeding.
  B. **Angiodysplasia** (arteriovenous malformation) of the colon may cause acute or chronic lower gastrointestinal bleeding. The lower intestinal lesions are usually found in the cecum and right colon. Bleeding lesions can be treated with endoscopic coagulation or heater probe therapy, laser photocoagulation, intra-arterial vasopressin, or surgical resection. Angiodysplasia of the colon is a common finding in elderly patients without gastrointestinal bleeding.
  C. **Other causes** of lower gastrointestinal bleeding are discussed in Chap. 15.

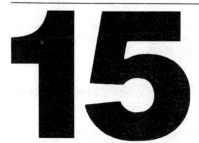

Gastroenterologic Diseases

Deborah C. Rubin

Nausea and Vomiting

Nausea and vomiting may result from systemic illnesses, CNS disorders, and primary gastrointestinal diseases and as side effects of medications. **Pregnancy** should be ruled out when relevant; treatment of nausea and vomiting in pregnant patients should be directed by an obstetrician. In otherwise healthy individuals, the most common cause is a **viral illness. Intestinal obstruction** can cause nausea and vomiting and can be diagnosed radiographically. Hospitalized patients frequently demonstrate toxicities from **medications** such as theophylline and digoxin. Specific therapy can often be initiated once an etiology is established.

I. **Supportive measures.** The patient should be NPO or on a clear liquid diet if tolerated. Many patients with self-limited illnesses will require no further therapy. Nasogastric decompression may be beneficial for patients with protracted nausea and vomiting. Parenteral fluid resuscitation is necessary for patients with significant intravascular volume depletion.

II. **Pharmacotherapy**

A. **Centrally acting antiemetics** include the phenothiazines and other related agents. Prochlorperazine, 5–10 mg PO tid–qid, 10 mg IM q4h (maximum IM dose is 40 mg/day), or 25 mg PR bid; promethazine, 12.5–25 mg PO, IM, or PR q4–6h; trimethobenzamide, 250 mg PO tid–qid, 200 mg IM tid–qid, or 200 mg PR tid–qid; and thiethylperazine, 10 mg PO, IM, or PR qd–tid are effective. Drowsiness is a common side effect, and acute dystonic reactions may occur with these agents.

B. **Metoclopramide** is a prokinetic agent useful in the treatment of vomiting associated with diabetic gastroparesis. The standard dosage is 10 mg PO 30 minutes ac and hs. High-dose IV metoclopramide is often used in chemotherapy-induced nausea and vomiting (see Chap. 19 and Table 19-2). Drowsiness and extrapyramidal reactions may occur.

Diarrhea

The approach to the patient with diarrhea consists of (1) identification and treatment of the specific underlying disease, (2) correction of fluid and electrolyte disturbances (see Chap. 3), and (3) occasional use of nonspecific antidiarrheal agents.

I. **Acute diarrhea.** Infectious agents (viral, bacterial, and parasitic), toxins, poisons, and drugs are the major causes of acute diarrhea. Inflammatory bowel disease may also have an acute presentation. **In hospitalized patients** common causes include lactose intolerance unmasked by hospital diets, antibiotic-associated diarrhea (including pseudomembranous colitis), drug-induced diarrhea, and fecal impaction.

A. **Viral and bacterial infections.** The most common causes of diarrhea in the United States include viral enteritis and bacterial infections with organisms such as enterotoxigenic *Escherichia coli, Shigella, Salmonella, Campylobacter,* and *Yersinia* spp (see Chap. 13). **Evaluation** with stool cultures, methylene blue stain for fecal leukocytes, stool ova and parasite examination, and flexible sigmoidoscopy may be warranted in patients with bloody diarrhea, a prolonged course, or dysenteric symptoms. Most acute diarrheal episodes of viral or bacterial origin are self-limited and do not require specific therapy (see Chap. 13 for the role of antimicrobial agents).

B. Parasitic infections

1. **Amebiasis** may cause acute diarrhea (it occurs most often in travelers and homosexual men and in areas with poor sanitation). The diagnosis may be made at sigmoidoscopy or by demonstration of trophozoites or cysts of *Entamoeba histolytica* in stool. **Treatment** for asymptomatic intestinal infection is iodoquinol, 650 mg PO tid for 20 days. Treatment for symptomatic disease is metronidazole, 750 mg PO tid for 10 days, followed by iodoquinol, 650 mg PO tid for 20 days.

2. **Giardiasis** commonly presents as acute or chronic diarrhea. The diagnosis can be made by identification of *Giardia lamblia* trophozoites in the stool, from a duodenal aspirate, or on a small-bowel biopsy. Quinacrine, 100 mg PO tid, or metronidazole, 250 mg PO tid, for 7 days is usually effective. More prolonged therapy may be required in the immunodeficient patient.

C. Drugs are a frequent cause of diarrhea. Common offending agents include laxatives, antacids, cardiac medications (e.g., digitalis and quinidine), colchicine, and antimicrobial agents. Antimicrobials may produce diarrhea by causing nonspecific alteration of enteric flora or by causing **pseudomembranous colitis,** which requires specific therapy (see Chap. 13). Antibiotic-associated diarrhea without evidence of pseudomembranous colitis usually responds to cessation of the offending agent.

II. Chronic diarrhea may be a sign of serious illness or a functional symptom.

A. History. Frequent small-volume stools associated with urgency and tenesmus suggest the site of the underlying disorder is most likely the distal colon. Stools that are bulky and large in volume often indicate small bowel disease. Symptoms of steatorrhea suggest small-bowel or pancreatic disease.

B. Classification of chronic diarrhea. In many diarrheal illnesses, there is both an osmotic and a secretory component. Response to feeding and fasting as well as calculation of stool osmolality may help distinguish between them.

1. **Osmotic diarrhea** is caused by the accumulation of poorly absorbed solutes in the intestine. It usually stops with fasting. Causes include ingestion of lactose (in lactase deficiency) and osmotic laxatives such as milk of magnesia.

2. **Secretory diarrhea** is caused by abnormal secretion of water and electrolytes into the intestinal lumen. Typically, the diarrhea persists despite fasting. Secretory diarrhea may be caused by bacterial enterotoxins, secretory hormones (e.g., gastrin or vasoactive intestinal peptide), some laxatives, dihydroxy bile acids, and fatty acids.

3. **Mucosal injury.** Diarrhea with both osmotic and secretory components may result from mucosal diseases such as inflammatory bowel disease, celiac sprue, lymphoma, or ischemic bowel injury.

4. **Deranged intestinal motility,** which occurs in irritable bowel syndrome, can also cause diarrhea.

III. Diarrhea in patients with AIDS. Diarrhea is a common symptom in homosexual men with or without a preexisting diagnosis of AIDS. Frequently, one or more pathogens can be isolated. Specific infections associated with the "gay bowel" syndrome include both venereal infections (syphilis, gonorrhea, chlamydiosis, herpes simplex infection) and nonvenereal infections (amebiasis, giardiasis, salmonellosis, shigellosis). In patients with AIDS, **opportunistic agents** including *Cryptosporidium, Isospora,* cytomegalovirus (CMV), and *Mycobacterium avium-intracellulare* (MAI) and tumors such as Kaposi's sarcoma and lymphoma also occur (see Chap. 13).

A. Watery diarrhea is commonly caused by giardiasis, cryptosporidiosis, or MAI infection. Stool examination for ova and parasites as well as acid-fast stains are necessary. Small-bowel biopsy may also be helpful in diagnosis. Giardiasis tends to be recurrent and difficult to treat (see Chap. 13). No clearly effective treatment is currently available for *Cryptosporidium* or MAI infection.

B. Dysenteric symptoms are commonly associated with bacterial pathogens (see

Chap. 13), CMV (see Esophageal Disease, sec **II.D**), and amebiasis (see sec. **I.B.1**).

C. **Anorectal symptoms** should prompt careful physical examination and proctoscopy with swabs for gonorrhea and herpes simplex virus culture and dark-field examination for syphilis. For treatment of these entities, see Chap. 13.

IV. **Nonspecific antidiarrheals** are generally overused. In most cases of acute diarrhea, they are unnecessary. In chronic diarrhea, they are not a substitute for treatment of the underlying illnesses. In *Salmonella* and *Shigella* infections, they may prolong the illness. Antiperistaltic drugs (diphenoxylate, paregoric, loperamide) may precipitate toxic megacolon in patients with invasive bacterial infection.

A. **Bulk-forming agents** (see Constipation, sec. **II.B.2**).

B. **Absorbents** (e.g., Kaopectate, 60–120 ml of regular strength or 45–90 ml of concentrate PO after every loose bowel movement).

C. **Opioid agents** should be used cautiously in patients with asthma, chronic lung disease, benign prostatic hypertrophy, and acute angle-closure glaucoma. Their potential for abuse should be recognized (see Chap. 1).

1. **Paregoric** (camphorated tincture of opium), 4–8 ml PO qid, or 4–8 ml PO after each liquid stool, not to exceed 32 ml/day.

2. **Deodorized tincture of opium,** 0.3–1.0 ml PO qid (maximum 6 ml/day).

3. **Opium and belladonna,** 25 mg of powdered opium and 15 mg of belladonna, one capsule PO tid–qid.

4. **Codeine,** 30–60 mg PO bid–qid.

5. **Diphenoxylate hydrochloride** (Lomotil), a meperidine congener, effectively inhibits excessive gastrointestinal motility. Side effects are uncommon. It is contraindicated in patients with advanced liver disease. Respiratory depression will occur with overdose and may be potentiated by phenothiazine derivatives, barbiturates, and tricyclic antidepressants. Each diphenoxylate tablet or 5 ml of liquid contains 2.5 mg of diphenoxylate hydrochloride and 0.025 mg of atropine sulfate (a subtherapeutic amount added to discourage deliberate overdose). The dosage is 5 mg PO qid until initial control of diarrhea is achieved, followed by the lowest effective dose.

6. **Loperamide hydrochloride** 2–4 mg PO after each loose stool, is another effective synthetic opioid antidiarrheal. The maximum dose is 8 mg/day.

Constipation

I. **Etiology.** Many drugs induce constipation, including narcotics, aluminum hydroxide antacids, anticholinergics, iron supplements, and some antihypertensive agents. Conditions that predispose to constipation include lack of exercise, disorders that cause pain on defecation (e.g., thrombosed external hemorrhoids, anal fissures, and anal strictures), and systemic diseases such as diabetes, hypothyroidism, and hyperparathyroidism. When constipation develops in a middle-aged or elderly person, colon cancer should be excluded. Constipation in hospitalized patients is a common problem, often due to prolonged immobilization, barium sulfate, and many medications. In addition, when straining at stool is especially undesirable (e.g., patients with recent myocardial infarction or recent abdominal surgery), avoidance and treatment of constipation are particularly important.

II. **Therapy.** Treatment of the underlying disease and correction of other predisposing factors are the most important aspects of therapy of constipation. However, many patients require additional therapy.

A. **Fiber.** Patients who are chronically constipated, with no underlying illness, frequently benefit from an increase in the insoluble fiber content of the diet or from treatment with bulk-forming agents. Dietary fiber can be increased with wheat bran flakes or unprocessed bran, 2 tablespoons/day. Fiber supplements in wafer and tablet form are available.

B. **Laxatives** should be used judiciously because of their potential for abuse. Contraindications to laxative use include undiagnosed abdominal pain and intestinal obstruction.

1. **Emollient laxatives.** Docusate sodium, 50–200 mg PO qd, and docusate calcium USP, 240 mg PO qd, soften the stool by allowing water and fat to penetrate the fecal mass. Emollient laxatives promote the intestinal absorption of mineral oil and so should not be used concurrently with mineral oil.
2. **Bulk-forming agents** include psyllium derivatives (e.g., Metamucil), 1–2 teaspoons in 8 ounces of water PO qd–tid, or methylcellulose, 1.0–1.5 g PO bid–tid.
3. **Stimulant cathartics**
   a. **Castor oil,** 15 ml PO, acts on the large intestine, producing prompt evacuation. A dose of 15–60 ml is used in bowel preparation for radiologic examination.
   b. **Bisacodyl** stimulates peristalsis in the colon. It may be administered PO or as a suppository. The dosage is 10–15 mg PO hs; 10-mg rectal suppositories are available and act in 15–60 minutes.
   c. **Extract of cascara and extract of senna** stimulate the colon and usually produce a single bowel evacuation 6–10 hours after administration. The dosage of cascara is 2–6 ml PO qd; 1 tablet of extract of senna is given PO qd–bid. Chronic use of these agents should be avoided because they can cause colonic denervation with atony.
4. **Osmotic cathartics** are relatively nonabsorbable salts or carbohydrates that osmotically retain water in the lumen of the colon. Standard preparations and dosages are as follows:
   a. **Milk of magnesia,** 15–30 ml PO.
   b. **Magnesium citrate solution,** 200 ml PO of a standard solution.
   c. **Lactulose,** 15–30 ml of standard syrup PO (often used in the elderly).
   d. **Lavage solutions** containing nonabsorbable sulfate and polyethylene glycol (e.g., GoLYTELY, Colyte) are effective for rapidly clearing the colon in preparation for endoscopic examination or surgery. The dosage is 4–6 liters PO over 3–4 hours (e.g., 8 ounces ingested q10min).

Esophageal Disease

I. **Reflux esophagitis.** The lower esophageal sphincter (LES) is the major physiologic barrier to reflux of gastric contents into the esophagus. Abnormally low LES pressure may lead to "pathologic" reflux manifested by esophageal inflammation, ulceration, and heartburn. **Complications** of reflux esophagitis include esophageal stricture, Barrett's esophagus, pulmonary aspiration, and bleeding. Hiatal hernias can often be seen on radiographs of patients with reflux esophagitis; however, the competency of the sphincter, not the presence of the hernia, determines whether acid will enter the esophagus. Medical therapy is aimed mainly at reducing the quantity and acidity of the gastric contents available for reflux and, to a lesser extent, at pharmacologic elevation of LES pressure (*Gastro. Clin. North Am.* 18:293, 1989).

A. **Nonpharmacologic measures** often significantly improve symptoms in patients with reflux.
   1. **Bed blocks.** Drainage of the esophagus can be enhanced by placing 4- to 6-inch blocks under the head of the bed. Propping the patient's head up with pillows increases intraabdominal pressure and may exacerbate reflux.
   2. **Diet.** Eating or drinking before retiring should be discouraged. Alcohol, mints, chocolate, and coffee should be avoided, since they lower LES pressure. The obese patient may achieve a reduction in reflux symptoms by losing weight.
   3. **Cigarette smoking should be avoided.**

B. **Medical therapy** is useful in patients who have persistent symptoms despite nonpharmacologic measures. A barium swallow or upper endoscopy may be indicated to exclude infectious esophagitis, an esophageal stricture, or tumor.
   1. H_2-receptor antagonists (Table 15-1) are highly effective in improving symptoms and healing esophageal inflammation. However, prolonged ther-

Table 15-1. H_2-receptor antagonist and omeprazole dosing regimens

	Oral therapy				Parenteral therapy
	DU (acute therapy)	DU (maintenance therapy)	GU	GERD	
Cimetidine	300 mg qid 400 mg bid 800 mg hs	400 mg hs	300 mg qid	300 mg qid	300 mg q6h
Ranitidine	150 mg bid 300 mg hs	150 mg hs	150 mg bid	150 mg bid	50 mg q8h
Famotidine	40 mg hs	20 mg hs	40 mg hs		20 mg q12h
Nizatidine	300 mg hs 150 mg bid	150 mg hs			
Omeprazole	20 mg qd			20–40 mg qd	

Key: DU = duodenal ulcer; GU = gastric ulcer; GERD = gastroesophageal reflux disease.

apy (up to 12 weeks) may be required to achieve these goals, and relapse when treatment is discontinued is common.

2. **Antacids.** For patients whose symptoms are only mild or intermittent, 2 tablespoons of a high-potency liquid antacid at bedtime or with heartburn may be sufficient (Table 15-2).

3. **Metoclopramide** improves gastric emptying and increases LES pressure. Doses ranging from 5–15 mg PO qid may improve symptoms (*Ann. Intern. Med.* 104:21, 1986), yet side effects are common (see Nausea and Vomiting, sec. II.B). It is currently approved for short-term use (up to 4 weeks).

4. **Omeprazole** decreases gastric acid secretion by blocking parietal cell hydrogen-potassium adenosine triphosphatase (ATPase). This drug is presently approved for the short-term treatment of severe erosive esophagitis refractory to therapy with H_2-receptor antagonists (see Table 15-1) (*Gastroenterology* 95:903, 1988). **Side effects** include diarrhea, nausea, dizziness, and headaches. The potential risk of carcinoid tumors associated with long-term use still needs to be clarified. If treatment with H_2 antagonists has been unsuccessful, an upper endoscopy should be considered prior to use of omeprazole to rule out other esophageal lesions.

5. **Anticholinergics** should not be used in patients with reflux because they decrease LES pressure.

C. **Surgery** should be considered in patients with aspiration, bleeding, strictures not readily managed with peroral dilatation, or intractable esophagitis despite aggressive medical therapy. Before surgery is recommended, the existence of significant esophagitis should be documented by endoscopy and biopsy, and adequate peristalsis should be confirmed by manometry.

II. **Infectious esophagitis** usually presents with odynophagia and dysphagia and is most common in patients with malignancy, diabetes, or other causes of impaired immunity. Major pathogens include *Candida albicans,* herpes simplex virus, and CMV. The presence of typical oral lesions (thrush, herpetic vesicles) may suggest an etiologic agent. Endoscopy with biopsy and brush cytology is frequently diagnostic for a specific pathogen.

A. **General measures.** Transient symptomatic relief for patients with severe odynophagia can be achieved using viscous lidocaine (2%) swish and swallows, 15 ml PO q3–4h prn.

B. **Candida esophagitis.** Mild disease can be treated with nystatin oral suspension,

Table 15-2. Antacid preparations

Antacid	Buffering capacity (mEq/15 ml)	Buffering capacity (ml/100 mEq)	Sodium content (mEq/15 ml)
Al(OH)$_3$			
Amphojel	30	50	0.30
Basaljel	34.5	43	0.39
Basaljel Extra Strength	66	23	3.00
Al(OH)$_3$ + Mg(OH)$_2$			
Maalox TC	82	18	0.09
Maalox Plus[a]	40	37.5	0.18
Mylanta[a]	37.5	40	0.10
Mylanta-II[a]	75	20	0.15
Riopan	45	33	0.04
Gelusil[a]	36	42	0.10
CaCO$_3$			
Tums tablets	19.5[b]		0.125[b]
Titralac	33	45	0.00
Al(OH)$_3$ + Mg(OH)$_2$ + CaCO$_3$			
Camalox	54	26	0.15

[a]Contains simethicone.
[b]Per 2 tablets.

500,000 units in water PO qid, or oral lozenges, 5 times daily for 2 weeks. Ketoconazole, 200 mg PO qd–bid, should be used in more severe disease. For unresponsive disease, especially in immunocompromised patients, a short course of parenteral amphotericin B should be considered. Amphotericin B is the treatment of choice for neutropenic patients (see Chap. 13).

  C. Herpes simplex esophagitis in immunocompromised patients may be treated with parenteral acyclovir, 5 mg/kg IV q8h for 7 days. The dosing interval should be increased in the presence of impaired renal function. In healthy patients, this infection is usually self-limited and treatment is supportive.

  D. CMV esophagitis. Ganciclovir (DHPG) may be effective for a variety of gastrointestinal CMV infections in immunocompromised hosts, including esophagitis (*Ann. Intern. Med.* 113:589, 1990).

  III. Esophageal motility disorders may cause noncardiac chest pain or intermittent dysphagia to both liquids and solids. If a barium swallow or upper endoscopy is unrevealing, esophageal manometry studies can be performed to demonstrate spastic disorders and reproduce symptoms. Optimal treatment is not defined, although a variety of agents, including long-acting nitrates, calcium channel blockers, and psychoactive agents such as trazodone, 50 mg PO bid–tid (*Gastroenterology* 92:1027, 1987), have been used. Gastroenterologic consultation is recommended for advice regarding diagnosis and therapy.

Peptic Ulcer Disease

Peptic ulcer is ulceration of the gastroduodenal mucosa typically extending through the muscularis mucosa. About 5–10% of the general population will have a peptic ulcer during a lifetime. At least half of these patients will have a recurrence within 5 years.

  I. Management considerations. The goals of ulcer therapy include relief of symptoms and prevention of recurrences and complications. Although most clinical studies have focused on ulcer healing as the major goal of therapy and as the basis of comparison of therapeutic efficacy, the practitioner should be more concerned with patient symptoms and, in the case of **duodenal** ulcer, should not feel compelled to demonstrate ulcer healing. Young, otherwise healthy individuals presenting with ulcer-like symptoms can often be treated with short-term empiric therapy. Nonresponders or older patients, with atypical or recurrent symptoms, should undergo diagnostic testing with radiographs or endoscopy (*Ann. Intern. Med.* 102:266, 1985).

A. Gastric ulcers are malignant in about 5% of cases. Therefore, endoscopic biopsy of gastric ulcers at the time of initial diagnosis is generally recommended. Patients with a gastric ulcer should have a follow-up upper gastrointestinal (UGI) series or endoscopy after 6–8 weeks of medical therapy. If the lesion has not changed in size, upper endoscopy with additional biopsies should be performed. If the lesion is smaller but not fully healed, another UGI series or endoscopy should be performed after an additional 6 weeks of therapy. Longer follow-up periods may be necessary to demonstrate healing of large gastric ulcers that are benign by biopsy (*Arch. Intern. Med.* 143:264, 1983). Surgical therapy should be considered for nonhealing gastric ulcers.

B. Duodenal ulcers are almost never malignant, and many heal even in the absence of therapy. However, H_2-receptor antagonists, sucralfate, and high-dose antacids have been demonstrated to increase the rate of healing and the percentage of ulcers that heal. Each is associated with a 70–85% incidence of ulcer healing at 4–6 weeks, compared with 40–50% with placebo.

II. Treatment. Reduction of stomach acidity remains the cornerstone of therapy in peptic ulcer disease. Gastric acid may be effectively neutralized with antacids, H_2-receptor antagonists, or omeprazole.

A. H_2-receptor antagonists (see Table 15-1)

1. Duodenal ulcer

a. Acute therapy. Cimetidine, ranitidine, famotidine, and nizatidine are all effective as short-term therapy for acute duodenal ulcer. Once or twice daily dosage regimens may improve patient compliance. Dosage intervals should be prolonged in the presence of renal insufficiency (see Appendix D). Parenteral therapy should be reserved for patients unable to tolerate oral medications.

b. Maintenance therapy. Recurrence rates may be as high as 80% within 1 year after acute ulcer healing. Maintenance therapy reduces the relapse rate to 10–15% at 1 year. Maintenance therapy is justified in patients with frequent and/or severe recurrences, a history of complications (see sec. **III**), or other serious medical problems that would make them poor surgical candidates. Patients with mild, infrequent, symptomatic recurrences can be managed with a 6-week course of full-dose therapy when symptoms recur (*Ann. Intern. Med.* 105:757, 1986).

2. Benign gastric ulcer. Cimetidine, ranitidine, and famotidine are effective in healing benign gastric ulcer. Gastric ulcers should be followed until completely healed to ensure that they are not malignant (see sec. **I.A**). Dosage schedules are the same as those for duodenal ulcer. Experience with nizatidine is limited.

3. Adverse reactions and drug interactions. Short-term therapy with these agents is remarkably well tolerated by most patients.

a. Cimetidine. Reversible impotence has been reported with long-term, high-dose cimetidine for Zollinger-Ellison syndrome. Gynecomastia and reduced sperm counts are more common in patients receiving higher than conventional dosages. Elderly patients and patients with impaired hepatic or renal function occasionally develop mental status abnormalities. Leukopenia and thrombocytopenia occur rarely. **Cimetidine impairs metabolism of warfarin anticoagulants, theophylline, and phenytoin** (see Appendix B).

b. Ranitidine, famotidine, and nizatidine have been in use for shorter periods of time than cimetidine, and their toxicity profiles are therefore less well established. Experience with nizatidine is particularly limited, and the effects of long-term therapy with this agent are unknown. Impotence, gynecomastia, and confusion have been reported less frequently with these drugs than with cimetidine. In addition, these agents appear to cause little or no interference with the hepatic microsomal enzyme system. Reversible drug-induced hepatitis has been reported with all the H_2 antagonists and may occur more frequently with ranitidine (*Am. J. Gastroenterol.* 82:987, 1987).

B. Sucralfate, 1 g PO qid (1 hour ac and hs) or 2 g bid, is as effective as H_2-receptor antagonists or high-dose antacids in the healing of duodenal ulcers. Sucralfate does not block acid secretion but appears to act locally at the mucosal surface; very little is absorbed. The associated side effects are minimal, the most frequent complaint being constipation in up to 2% of patients. **The absorption of cimetidine, phenytoin, and tetracycline may be reduced if given concomitantly with sucralfate.** Sucralfate may also be useful for the treatment of gastric ulcer and the prevention of peptic ulcer recurrence. Its efficacy in the treatment of peptic esophagitis is not established.

C. Antacids (see Table 15-2). Because alternative therapies require less frequent dosing and are more palatable, antacids are best used as supplemental therapy for pain relief. The choice of antacid is determined by buffering capacity, sodium content, and side effects. In general, liquid antacids are more effective than tablets. **Typically,** 30 ml of a high-potency liquid antacid is effective for symptomatic relief. Magnesium hydroxide is a potent antacid, but large or frequent doses can cause severe osmotic diarrhea. Therefore, magnesium hydroxide is combined with aluminum hydroxide in most popular preparations. For patients who have diarrhea while taking a magnesium hydroxide–aluminum hydroxide mixture, use of a constipating antacid such as pure aluminum hydroxide in alternating doses may be helpful. However, aluminum hydroxide binds phosphate in the intestinal lumen and may cause hypophosphatemia. It also binds a number of drugs, including tetracycline, thyroxine, and chlorpromazine, and may decrease absorption of these agents. Aluminum hydroxide is often used in patients with renal failure, since oral ingestion of magnesium-containing antacids should be avoided. Calcium carbonate is an effective and well-tolerated antacid, but high doses may cause hypercalcemia and hypercalciuria.

D. Omeprazole is a potent inhibitor of the hydrogen-potassium ATPase that profoundly decreases gastric acid secretion (see Esophageal Disease, sec. **I.B.4**). A dosage of 20 mg/day is effective in the acute treatment of duodenal ulcer.

E. Other therapeutic measures

  1. Diet. There is no evidence that a bland diet improves symptoms or promotes ulcer healing. Patients should be instructed to avoid foods that are reproducibly associated with dyspeptic symptoms. Late evening snacks should also be avoided, since they stimulate gastric acid production at a time when the patient is asleep and unable to take antacids.

  2. Hospitalization. Short-term hospitalization may be necessary in rare refractory cases.

  3. Cessation of cigarette smoking should be strongly encouraged because cigarette use is associated with an increased risk of peptic ulcer development, delayed ulcer healing, a decreased overall rate of ulcer healing, and an increased rate of ulcer recurrence (*N. Engl. J. Med.* 311:689, 1984).

  4. Aspirin and nonsteroidal anti-inflammatory drugs (NSAIDs) should be avoided in patients with peptic ulcer disease. High-dose aspirin ingestion is associated with an increased incidence of gastritis and gastric ulcer. Enteric coating or concomitant anti-ulcer therapy may reduce mucosal damage from aspirin. NSAIDs are toxic to the gastric mucosa and are associated with dyspepsia and mucosal ulcerations. Concomitant therapy with H_2-receptor antagonists or sucralfate may ameliorate some of these symptoms in patients who have strong indications for continued use of NSAIDs. Misoprostol (a synthetic prostaglandin E derivative), 200 μg PO qid, can help prevent NSAID-associated gastric ulcer and inflammation (*Gastroenterology* 96:675,

1989). Side effects of misoprostol include abdominal pain, self-limited diarrhea, and abortifacient activity.

5. **Alcohol,** in high concentrations, damages the gastric mucosal barrier and is associated with gastritis. However, there is no evidence that alcohol induces recurrence in peptic ulcer disease.

III. Complications of peptic ulcer disease

A. **Gastrointestinal bleeding** (see Chap. 14)

B. **Gastric outlet obstruction** occurs in about 5% of patients with peptic ulcer disease and is more likely to occur with ulcers situated close to the pyloric channel. Severe nausea and vomiting suggest obstruction. Plain abdominal radiographs often show a dilated stomach with an air-fluid level. If obstruction is present, nasogastric suction should be maintained for at least 72 hours to decompress the stomach. Dehydration, metabolic alkalosis, and hypokalemia should be corrected. Many patients respond to medical management alone, but the problem tends to recur; endoscopic dilatation or surgical intervention may be required.

C. **Perforation** occurs in a small percentage of ulcer patients and usually necessitates emergency surgery. In some patients, perforation occurs in the absence of previous symptoms of peptic ulcer disease. A plain upright radiograph of the abdomen may aid diagnosis by showing the presence of free air under the diaphragm.

D. **Penetration into the pancreas,** when it occurs, is most often associated with ulcers in the posterior wall of the duodenal bulb. The onset of penetration is often characterized by a change in symptoms. The pain becomes severe and continuous, radiates to the back, and is no longer relieved by antacids. Serum amylase is often elevated. These patients frequently require surgery.

E. **Intractability.** Since the advent of newer medical therapies, the frequency of ulcer operations for intractability has declined dramatically. An active ulcer must be documented radiographically or endoscopically before an operation is performed. The preoperative evaluation of a patient's ulcer should include a fasting gastrin determination and a search for potential reversible factors (e.g., ulcerogenic drugs, cigarette smoking). The physician should be aware that significant problems can occur following gastric surgery (see sec. **IV**). Surgical options vary depending on the location of the ulcer (gastric versus duodenal) and the presence of associated complications.

IV. Morbidity following gastrectomy and vagotomy

A. **Abdominal complaints.** The most common complaint after gastric surgery is abdominal discomfort or vomiting after meals. Some patients may have recurrent ulcer, afferent loop obstruction, bile reflux gastritis, gastric outlet obstruction, or stump carcinoma (a late complication). In most postgastrectomy patients with these complaints, however, no surgically correctable lesion exists. Their symptoms are often due to the **dumping syndrome,** which is caused by rapid gastric emptying of a large osmotic load into the upper small intestine. The discomfort and vomiting may be accompanied by vasomotor symptoms (palpitations, sweating, dizziness). Changing the patient's diet to six small meals each day that are relatively high in protein and low in refined carbohydrate often decreases these symptoms. Liquids with meals should be avoided. Anticholinergics may also be useful in the relief of these complaints.

B. **Malabsorption.** Mild steatorrhea can occur after gastric surgery and is probably related to decreased intestinal transit time and inadequate mixing of food with bile and pancreatic secretions. Rarely, bacterial overgrowth secondary to afferent loop stasis may lead to steatorrhea. Chronic malabsorption of calcium and vitamin D may be significant. **Metabolic bone disease,** usually osteomalacia, will develop in at least 30% of patients with a Billroth II anastomosis. Calcium and vitamin D supplementation should be given (see Chap. 23).

C. **Anemia.** Postgastrectomy anemia typically develops slowly and may be secondary to deficiencies of folate, vitamin B_{12}, or, most commonly, iron. Iron-deficiency anemia is usually a result of dietary iron malabsorption, but blood loss from gastritis or a marginal ulcer may also contribute. When the cause of anemia is identified, appropriate replacement should be given.

D. Diarrhea. Mild diarrhea is a common problem following vagotomy. The patient should be evaluated for treatable conditions (lactase deficiency or fat malabsorption). If none is found, a trial of symptomatic therapy with diphenoxylate or tincture of opium is appropriate (see Diarrhea, sec. **IV.C**).

V. Zollinger-Ellison syndrome is caused by a gastrin-secreting, non-beta islet cell tumor of the pancreas or duodenum that results in marked gastric acid hypersecretion (*N. Engl. J. Med.* 317:1200, 1987). Approximately two-thirds of Zollinger-Ellison tumors are malignant. Multiple endocrine neoplasia type I (MEN-I) is associated in 25% of patients. **The most common presentation** is a simple duodenal bulb ulcer, but large or multiple ulcers in the distal duodenum or jejunum, or recurrent ulceration after an adequate ulcer operation, should alert the physician to the possibility of this disease. Diarrhea is a common symptom. With currently available H_2-receptor antagonists and omeprazole, the major morbidity and mortality of this syndrome have shifted from the effects of uncontrolled acid hypersecretion to long-term effects of tumor growth. Control of acid hypersecretion with H_2-receptor antagonists and omeprazole (initial dose 60 mg/day) requires much higher doses than used to treat peptic ulcer disease. Careful dose titration with measurement of acid secretion rates by gastric analysis is necessary. Identification of tumors for possible curative resection and detection of metastases to avoid unnecessary surgery is recommended in many cases.

VI. *Helicobacter* **(formerly** *Campylobacter***)** *pylori* is a spiral gram-negative organism that can be demonstrated histologically and by culture in gastric mucosal biopsies in some patients with gastritis, peptic ulcer disease, and nonulcer dyspepsia. Although *H. pylori* is associated with chronic gastritis, its role in the pathogenesis of peptic disease is unclear (*Arch. Intern. Med.* 150:951, 1990). The efficacy of treatment with bismuth compounds alone or in conjunction with antibiotics such as amoxicillin and metronidazole in an attempt to eradicate this organism is still being evaluated.

VII. Nonulcer dyspepsia is a common syndrome of persistent ulcer-like symptoms in the absence of radiographic and endoscopic abnormalities. Motor abnormalities, microscopic inflammation, *H. pylori*–associated gastritis, and associated psychiatric disease have been proposed to explain this syndrome. Therapy remains largely empiric. Although some patients appear to respond to H_2-receptor antagonists, these agents have not been shown to be effective in double-blind placebo-controlled studies (*N. Engl. J. Med.* 314:339, 1986). Some patients may benefit from psychoactive agents such as alprazolam, 0.25–0.50 mg PO bid, or tricyclic antidepressants, including amitriptyline, 25–50 mg PO hs.

Gastroparesis

I. Etiology. Delayed gastric emptying occurs with a wide variety of acute and chronic disorders and metabolic derangements (hypokalemia, hyper- or hypocalcemia, or acute hyperglycemia) or due to the ingestion of medications (e.g., tricyclic antidepressants, narcotics, and anticholinergic agents). **Chronic gastric retention** is frequently associated with diabetes mellitus, scleroderma, and previous gastric surgery or atrophic gastritis but may also be idiopathic. **Mechanical** obstruction from a duodenal ulcer or pyloric stenosis should be ruled out. Many other chronic metabolic, endocrine, and collagen vascular diseases can be associated with gastric motor dysfunction. Treatment of chronic gastric emptying disorders is often difficult.

II. Diagnosis. Symptoms include nausea, bloating, early satiety, and vomiting. Delayed gastric emptying can be diagnosed by ingestion of a radiolabeled solid meal followed by scintigraphic analysis to determine rates of emptying.

III. Therapy. Patients should avoid high-fat, high-fiber meals. In more severe cases, high-calorie, liquid iso-osmotic meals may be used. Prokinetic agents such as metoclopramide, domperidone, and cisapride have been used with some success.

Metoclopramide, the only approved agent, can be used in doses of up to 10 mg PO qid. Its efficacy in chronic gastroparesis is variable, and side effects, including dyskinesias and drowsiness, are common. Erythromycin, a macrolide antibiotic, has been used in PO (250 mg tid) and IV (200 mg) forms to stimulate gastric motility (*N. Engl. J. Med.* 322:1028, 1990), but its efficacy remains to be established.

Malabsorption and Maldigestion

I. **Diagnosis.** Malabsorption of macronutrients (especially fat) should be considered in patients with unexplained weight loss, steatorrhea, or biochemical abnormalities consistent with malabsorption. Fat malabsorption is suggested by clinical history and qualitative stool fat determination by Sudan black staining and is confirmed by quantitative 72-hour fecal fat determination. For an accurate 72-hour fecal fat measurement, the patient should be placed on a fixed fat (usually 100 g/day) diet beginning 24 hours **before** the stool collection starts. More than 6 g of fat in the stool is consistent with malabsorption. The D-xylose and bentiromide (Chymex) tests are screening studies for the presence of diffuse small bowel mucosal disease (malabsorption) and pancreatic exocrine insufficiency (maldigestion) (see Pancreatitis, sec. **II.B**), respectively. Serum calcium and magnesium levels should be measured. In diseases of the ileum, bile acids and vitamin B_{12} are not absorbed normally. Malabsorption of fat-soluble vitamins may also occur, requiring replacement therapy (Table 15-3).

II. **Specific disorders.** Once the presence of malabsorption is established, the underlying cause should be sought. Barium radiographs of the small bowel may be abnormal in Crohn's disease, celiac sprue, blind loop syndrome, amyloidosis, and multiple jejunal diverticulosis. **Small-bowel biopsy** is a valuable test in many kinds of diffuse small intestinal disease, including celiac sprue, giardiasis, Whipple's disease, and lymphangiectasia.

A. **Celiac sprue** (gluten-sensitive enteropathy). Patients with celiac disease are sensitive to gluten, a group of proteins present in wheat, barley, rye, and possibly oats. The diagnosis is made by biopsy of the small intestine, which characteristically reveals complete absence of villi, and by the favorable clinical and histologic response to a gluten-free diet (see M. N. Wood, *Gourmet Food on a Wheat-Free Diet.* Springfield, IL: Thomas, 1972). Because of the implications of lifelong therapy, diagnosis should always be confirmed by biopsy. Careful dietary instruction is important, since gluten is present in many different types of food. Patients with sprue also frequently have **secondary lactase deficiency** and should be on a lactose-free diet until the small bowel recovers. Patients may require iron, folate, calcium, or vitamin supplementation (see Table 15-3). In severely symptomatic or refractory cases, a trial of prednisone, 20 mg PO qd, may be effective. The most common cause of continued or worsening symptoms in celiac disease is dietary indiscretion. Sprue is associated with an increased incidence of small bowel lymphoma; patients who decompensate despite adherence to dietary restriction should be evaluated by barium study or abdominal computed tomography (CT).

B. **Lactose intolerance** is a common disorder due to a selective deficiency of lactase. It is present in 70–90% of adult blacks, Asians, and American Indians and in 10% of people of Western European ancestry. Undigested lactose in the bowel lumen results in an osmotic diarrhea. Symptoms consist of abdominal cramps, flatulence, and diarrhea associated with ingestion of dairy products. Temporary lactase deficiency may occur due to other small bowel illnesses such as viral and bacterial enteritis and Crohn's disease. Dietary restriction of milk products is usually sufficient for both diagnosis and treatment. Rarely, the diagnosis will need to be confirmed with a lactose tolerance test. The patient ingests 50–100 g of lactose with blood glucose determinations at 0, 15, 30, 60, and 120 minutes. A positive test is indicated by the onset of cramps and diarrhea and failure of the

Table 15-3. Representative dosages for agents used in the management of patients with malabsorption syndromes

Calcium: Normal replacement is 1–2 g/day; calcium carbonate may be given as Titralac (400 mg Ca^{2+}/5 ml) or Os-Cal (250 or 500 mg Ca^{2+}/tablet).

Magnesium: Magnesium gluconate, 500 mg qid (each tablet contains 29 mg of magnesium).

Iron: Ferrous sulfate, one 325-mg tablet qid; each tablet contains 64 mg of iron.

Fat-soluble vitamins

Vitamin A: 25,000-unit tablets; for severe deficiency, 25,000–100,000 units/day; maintenance is 3000–5000 units/day.

Vitamin D: Initial dose is 50,000 units 2–3 times weekly; dosage varies considerably based on response as determined by serum and urine calcium.

Vitamin K: Vitamin K_1 (water miscible), 10 mg PO or IM qd, or vitamin K_3 Water-soluble vitamins (menadione), 10 mg PO qd.

Folic acid: 1–5 mg PO qd for 4–5 weeks is adequate to replenish stores and correct anemia; maintenance dosage is 1 mg PO qd.

Vitamin B_{12}: 100–1000 µg/day IM for 2 weeks as a loading dose (if required); maintenance dosage is 1000 µg/month.

Vitamin B complex: Any multivitamin preparation that contains daily requirements (thiamine 1.6 mg, riboflavin 1.8 mg, niacin 20 mg) should be administered twice daily.

---

blood glucose to rise more than 20 mg/dl over baseline. Some patients retain enough lactase to tolerate small amounts of dietary lactose (as in highly processed cheese such as cheddar, parmesan, and roquefort). Yogurt is a low-lactose dairy product that is generally well tolerated (*N. Engl. J. Med.* 310:1, 1984). Enzyme replacement therapy with products such as Lactaid liquid or tablets or Lactrase capsules is available.

C. Bacterial overgrowth of the small intestine can result from any condition that causes intestinal stasis (i.e., jejunal diverticulosis, scleroderma, afferent loop obstruction of a Billroth II anastomosis, or partial small bowel obstruction secondary to adhesions or to Crohn's disease). Deconjugation of bile salts by the excess bacteria causes fat malabsorption. The bacteria may also have a direct toxic effect on the mucosa itself and can compete for available vitamin B_{12} in the intestine, leading to megaloblastic anemia. The diagnosis of small bowel bacterial overgrowth is usually made by history and radiography. **Treatment** consists of administration of broad-spectrum antimicrobials such as tetracycline, 250 mg PO qid. For long-term therapy, it is usually advisable to give antimicrobials intermittently (e.g., for 2 weeks out of each month). Surgical correction of the intestinal abnormality may be performed if possible.

D. Ileal resection. Bile salts and vitamin B_{12} are absorbed in the terminal ileum. Loss of more than 50 cm of this portion of intestine (as in Crohn's disease) will lead to malabsorption of bile salts; a greater loss may result in malabsorption of vitamin B_{12}. Unabsorbed bile salts pass into the colon, where they produce a secretory diarrhea (see Diarrhea, sec. **II.B.2**).

1. Cholestyramine, 4 g PO qid, controls diarrhea in these patients by binding bile salts in the intestinal lumen. However, patients who have had more than 100 cm of ileum resected will lose enough bile salts to result in fat malabsorption. The diarrhea in these cases may be due to the irritant effect of hydroxy fatty acids on the colonic mucosa and may be aggravated by cholestyramine; it will improve with a low-fat diet.

2. Low-fat diets containing 50–75 g/day of fat will often reduce steatorrhea in patients with ileal resections of greater than 100 cm and provide a tolerable diet. Diets containing less than 40 g/day of fat, however, are unpalatable and make it difficult for patients to maintain adequate caloric intake. Medium-chain triglycerides (MCTs), which do not require solubilization by bile salts, can be used as an additional source of fat in patients with significant fat malabsorption. Although MCT oil is relatively unpalatable, recipe books are available that include it in many different dishes. About 3–4 tablespoons/day (14 g of fat/tbs) can be ingested as MCTs. Larger amounts of MCTs cause diarrhea. Patients with ileal resection and fat malabsorption often require fat-soluble vitamin and calcium supplementation in addition to parenteral vitamin B_{12} (see Table 15-3).

E. Giardiasis rarely leads to malabsorption in immunocompetent persons but is often present in the intestine of hypogammaglobulinemic patients and is a cause of malabsorption in this group (see Diarrhea, sec. **I.B.2**).

Inflammatory Bowel Disease

I. Ulcerative colitis is an idiopathic chronic inflammatory disease of the colon and rectum characterized by remissions and exacerbations. The predominant symptom of ulcerative colitis is **bloody diarrhea.** Proctoscopy is the most important examination for establishing the diagnosis and following the course of therapy, as rectal involvement is essentially universal. In newly diagnosed cases, stool culture for enteric pathogens and examination for ova and parasites should be obtained. A barium enema is useful in determining the extent of involvement but can exacerbate the disease and should never be performed during an acute or relapsing phase of the illness. Most patients can be treated medically as outpatients, but in a small proportion, the disease runs a severe course and can be life-threatening. Treated patients with frequent relapses or fulminant disease will often require surgery. Total proctocolectomy is curative. One of the major risks of long-standing ulcerative colitis is the development of **colon cancer;** surgical intervention may be required in this circumstance as well.

A. Medical therapy

   1. Sulfasalazine is useful for treatment of mild acute exacerbations and as maintenance therapy for prolonging the length of remission. The intact drug reaches the colon, where bacteria metabolize it to a sulfapyridine moiety (responsible for most of this drug's toxicity) and 5-aminosalicylate (5-ASA), the active component.

   a. Dosage. For patients with active disease, the recommended starting dosage is 0.5 g PO bid, slowly advancing as tolerated to 0.5–1.0 g PO qid. The usual maintenance dosage is 1 g PO bid.

   b. Side effects

   (1) Toxic reactions include headache, nausea, vomiting, and abdominal pain. These effects are dose-related and are more common in patients treated with 4 g/day or more. Patients suffering toxic side effects should have the drug stopped for 1–2 weeks but may be restarted on a dosage of 0.125–0.25 g/day for a week with increases of 0.125 g/day each week until a dosage of 2 g/day is achieved (*Ann. Intern. Med.* 101:377, 1984).

   (2) Hypersensitivity reactions occur less frequently and include skin rash, fever, agranulocytosis, hepatotoxicity, and aplastic anemia. Reintroduction at a lower dosage, as described previously, may be considered for patients with skin rash, but the drug should not be restarted in patients with more serious hypersensitivity reactions. Rarely, paradoxic exacerbations of colitis have been reported with sulfasalazine.

   2. 5-Aminosalicylate (5-ASA) lacks the sulfa moiety of sulfasalazine and is associated with a decreased incidence of side effects. It is available in oral form (olsalazine), in which two molecules of 5-ASA are coupled by a diazo bond, facilitating its delivery to the colon. Olsalazine is approved for use in maintenance of remission in patients with ulcerative colitis who have demonstrated hypersensitivity reactions to sulfasalazine. It is also available in enema form (mesalamine); 4 g (60 ml) given qhs is effective in the treatment of left-sided colitis (*Gastroenterology* 92:1984, 1987).

3. **Glucocorticoids** are beneficial in producing remission in patients with moderate or severe colonic disease and may be given in conjunction with sulfasalazine. **Extracolonic manifestations,** such as ocular lesions, skin disease, and peripheral arthritis, whose activity often parallels (although it may precede or follow) that of the colonic disease, also usually respond to glucocorticoids. Disease limited to the rectum (**ulcerative proctitis**) is effectively treated with glucocorticoid enemas (100 mg of hydrocortisone or 20 mg of methylprednisolone qd). More extensive disease should be treated with oral prednisone, 20–40 mg/day, for several weeks. When symptoms lessen and improvement is noted on proctoscopic examination, prednisone can be tapered over 2–3 months and then discontinued. If symptoms are refractory to outpatient management, the patient should be hospitalized and given initial therapy with hydrocortisone, 50–100 mg IV q6h. Colectomy should be considered if the patient requires more than 15 mg of prednisone daily over a period of many months to keep the disease under control. There is no evidence that glucocorticoids are beneficial in maintaining remission. When relapse occurs during sulfasalazine maintenance, glucocorticoids in full doses should again be used and gradually tapered when remission is achieved.

4. **Immunosuppressive agents** such as azathioprine and 6-mercaptopurine (up to 1.5 mg/kg/day PO) have a limited role in the management of ulcerative colitis but may be used in patients unresponsive to conventional medical management who are not surgical candidates. Azathioprine may also be used to reduce the maintenance dosage of glucocorticoids in patients who are not surgical candidates.

5. **Anticholinergic and antidiarrheal drugs** are often beneficial in decreasing abdominal pain and diarrhea. Such drugs include tincture of belladonna, tincture of opium, diphenoxylate, and codeine (see Diarrhea, sec. **IV.C**). They are contraindicated in severe exacerbations of disease.

B. **Diet.** Patients in remission have no specific dietary restrictions. Occasionally, lactose intolerance may develop. A low-roughage diet often provides symptomatic improvement for patients in relapse. Elemental diets may also be useful during acute phases of the disease (see Chap. 2).

C. **Fulminant disease and toxic megacolon.** An acute fulminant phase occurs in 5–10% of ulcerative colitis patients and presents with severe diarrhea, abdominal pain, hemorrhage, hypoalbuminemia, fever, sepsis, electrolyte disturbances, and dehydration. **Toxic megacolon,** in which the colon becomes atonic and dilates, develops in 1–2% of patients with ulcerative colitis. The diagnosis of toxic megacolon is made when the colon is dilated to a diameter of 6 cm or more (measured radiographically at the midtransverse colon) and systemic toxicity is present. Treatment includes the following:

1. **Nasogastric suction** should be started to prevent further bowel distention, and the patient should be given nothing by mouth. Total parenteral nutrition is sometimes necessary during this period (see Chap. 2).

2. **Dehydration and electrolyte disturbances** should be vigorously treated. Hypokalemia is common, and up to 200 mEq/day of K^+ supplementation may be required.

3. **Parenteral broad-spectrum antimicrobials** for intraabdominal sepsis should be administered (see Chap. 13).

4. **Parenteral glucocorticoids** such as hydrocortisone, 100 mg IV q6h, should be given.

5. **Total colectomy** must be considered for acutely ill patients not responding to intensive medical therapy within 48 hours. Early surgical consultation is necessary in severely ill patients.

6. **Anticholinergic and opioid drugs should not be used** because they can precipitate or aggravate toxic megacolon.

D. **Cancer in ulcerative colitis.** Patients with ulcerative colitis have a tenfold greater incidence of adenocarcinoma of the colon than the general population.

The incidence of cancer increases with the duration of disease (at 15 years, the cumulative risk is 5–8%; at 25 years, 25%); cancer risk increases with the extent of the disease. Surveillance endoscopic examinations with multiple biopsies are recommended after approximately 8–10 years, especially in patients with pancolitis.

II. **Crohn's disease.** Like ulcerative colitis, Crohn's disease is marked by remissions and exacerbations. Common presenting symptoms include diarrhea, abdominal pain, and weight loss. In contrast to ulcerative colitis, Crohn's disease can affect any portion of the tubular gastrointestinal tract and therefore cannot be cured with surgical resection. The clinical course of Crohn's disease is frequently complicated by fistulae, perianal disease, and strictures. Therapy is directed toward symptomatic relief and treatment of specific complications.

A. **Medical therapy of uncomplicated Crohn's disease**

1. **Antidiarrheal agents** may be useful as primary therapy in selected patients with mild exacerbations of symptoms or postresection diarrhea.

2. **Glucocorticoids,** such as prednisone, 20–40 mg PO qd, are beneficial in acute exacerbations. In more fulminant disease, glucocorticoids should be given parenterally at a dosage equivalent to hydrocortisone, 50–100 mg IV q6h. Corticosteroids have no proven benefit in maintenance of remissions in Crohn's disease. As in ulcerative colitis, extraintestinal manifestations (eye, skin, and joint disease) often parallel colonic activity and respond to glucocorticoids.

3. **Sulfasalazine,** 0.5 g PO bid, slowly increased as tolerated to 0.5–1.0 g PO qid, is effective in the treatment of mild to moderate acute exacerbations of colonic or ileocolic disease, but not in the treatment of disease confined to the ileum. Sulfasalazine is not effective in maintenance of remission in Crohn's disease.

4. **Immunosuppressive agents** such as 6-mercaptopurine (6-MP) and azathioprine have a controversial role in the management of active Crohn's disease. They may be used when corticosteroids have failed or in an attempt to decrease steroid requirements in patients with major steroid-induced side effects (*N. Engl. J. Med.* 302:981, 1980). Significant side effects include bone marrow suppression and pancreatitis. These drugs should be administered only by persons with experience in taking care of complicated Crohn's disease patients; careful monitoring for toxicity with frequent complete blood counts and physical examinations is mandatory. Cyclosporine has been used in severe acute exacerbations of Crohn's disease unresponsive to standard intensive therapy, but this treatment remains experimental.

5. **Metronidazole,** 250 mg PO tid, although not commonly used as primary therapy for colitis, has been shown to be as effective as sulfasalazine in colonic Crohn's disease and may be beneficial in selected patients unable to tolerate, or unresponsive to, other agents (*Gastroenterology* 83:550, 1982). It is contraindicated in pregnancy.

6. **Maintenance of adequate nutrition** is essential. Patients with ileitis frequently need parenteral vitamin B_{12} therapy. In patients with bile salt deficiency due to ileal disease, substitution of MCTs for dietary fat will result in better absorption and diminished steatorrhea. Specific oral replacement of calcium, magnesium, folate, iron, vitamin D, and other micronutrients may be necessary. In patients with ileal resection or extensive small bowel Crohn's disease, oxalate nephrolithiasis may occur; treatment consists of a low-fat, low-oxalate, high-calcium diet. In some cases, elemental formulas or parenteral nutrition will be necessary to support the patient through a severe phase of the illness (see Chap. 2).

B. **Medical therapy of complications of Crohn's disease**

1. **Perianal disease.** In conjunction with surgical drainage of obvious collections of pus, metronidazole, 250 mg PO or IV tid, is useful in healing active Crohn's perianal disease (*Gastroenterology* 79:357, 1980). Significant toxicities include possible teratogenicity and peripheral neuropathy with chronic use (see Chap. 12).

2. **Fistulae** (enterocutaneous, enterovesicular, enterovaginal). Medical management with (1) total parenteral nutrition (TPN) and bowel rest, (2) metronidazole, or (3) 6-MP may be useful in specific circumstances in conjunction with surgical consultation.

3. **Intestinal obstruction** may occur due to stricture formation. Acutely, decompression with a nasoenteral tube, parenteral hydration, and corticosteroids may allow edema and spasm to subside, avoiding the need for surgical resection. Patients with intermittent obstructive symptoms should be cautioned to avoid highly indigestible foods such as nuts, popcorn, and hardskinned fruits, which may precipitate obstruction.

C. Other therapeutic measures. Most uncomplicated cases of Crohn's disease can be managed medically. Surgery is generally reserved for patients with fistulae, obstruction, abscess, perforation, and bleeding, and rarely for medically refractory disease. Percutaneous abscess drainage and endoscopic balloon dilatation can be useful in selected patients. Efforts should be made to avoid multiple resections due to the risk of producing short bowel syndrome.

Diverticular Disease

I. **Diverticulosis.** The occurrence of diverticula increases markedly with age. Diverticulosis occurs more frequently in developed nations than in Third World countries, due to ingestion of a highly refined diet that is low in dietary fiber. Most diverticula are asymptomatic and do not require treatment; however, they can be the cause of profuse **lower gastrointestinal bleeding,** which in most cases resolves spontaneously. Some of these patients may also suffer from symptoms of irritable bowel syndrome and should be treated accordingly (see Irritable Bowel Syndrome).

II. **Diverticulitis** is a complication of diverticular disease in which perforation of a diverticulum occurs. Left lower quadrant pain accompanied by fever and chills, alteration of bowel habit, and laboratory evidence of inflammation are the most common manifestations of acute diverticulitis. Occasionally, a left lower quadrant mass may be present. Rarely, fistulas to the bladder, vagina, or skin may form from the diseased colon. Patients ill enough to require hospitalization should be given nothing by mouth. IV fluid replacement is necessary. Nasogastric suction should be instituted if there are signs of bowel obstruction. Outpatients should be given a clear liquid diet until the initial symptoms subside. The choice of antimicrobials depends on the severity of the clinical condition. When the inflammatory response is localized, a course of oral ampicillin, a cephalosporin, or a tetracycline derivative may be used. If the patient is systemically ill, broad-spectrum parenteral antibiotic coverage appropriate for intraabdominal sepsis is required (see Chap. 13). Surgical consultation is advisable in hospitalized patients, since operative intervention may be required if complications arise. After the acute episode has subsided, dietary bulk supplementation may help to prevent recurrence.

Irritable Bowel Syndrome

Irritable bowel syndrome (IBS) is the most common gastrointestinal problem seen by physicians. Typically, patients present with long-standing symptoms of crampy abdominal pain, bloating, excessive flatulence, diarrhea, constipation, or alternating diarrhea and constipation. Lactose intolerance should be excluded, as it may have a similar presentation and the two disorders can coexist (see Malabsorption and Maldigestion, sec. **II.B**). Although IBS is ultimately a diagnosis of exclusion, certain features, including stable weight, chronic gastrointestinal symptoms, and an unrevealing physical examination often allow a presumptive diagnosis to be made and treatment initiated without extensive diagnostic testing. Associated psychiatric symptoms are frequently seen. Patients with new onset symptoms or those who fail an initial therapeutic trial should undergo further evaluation. Some patients respond to dietary bulk supplementation as the sole therapeutic maneuver (see Constipation). Anticholinergics are frequently prescribed for patients with IBS, although there is no documentation of their efficacy. Tincture of belladonna, 5–10 drops PO tid ac; hyoscyamine, 0.125 mg SL prn or 0.375 mg PO bid; and dicyclomine, 20 mg PO qid, are commonly used agents. In patients unresponsive to these measures or in those with associated psychiatric symptoms, tricyclic antidepressants in low dosage such as amitriptyline, 10–50 mg PO hs, doxepin, 10–50 mg PO hs, or desipramine, 50 mg PO hs (*Dig. Dis. Sci.* 32:257, 1987), can be helpful.

Common Anorectal Problems

I. **Hemorrhoids**
  A. **External thrombosed hemorrhoids** present with sudden onset of pain. On physical examination, they appear as tense, bluish lumps covered with skin. If pain is severe, prompt relief can be obtained by excision of the thrombosed vein under local anesthesia. If pain is mild or has already started to resolve, the patient can be given oral analgesics, sitz baths, stool softeners, and topical emollients (see sec. **I.B**).
  B. **Internal hemorrhoids** commonly present with either bleeding or a prolapsing mass that may or may not be reducible. Pain is usually not a prominent feature. Prolapsed internal hemorrhoids appear as masses separated by radial folds. The upper portions are covered with red mucosa. Treatment includes the following:
    1. **Bulk–forming agents** are useful in preventing straining at stool (see Constipation, sec. **II.B.2**).
    2. **Sitz baths** (sitting in a tub of warm water) taken for 15 minutes twice daily are useful for relief of inflammation and for hygiene. Tucks Pads (cotton soaked in witch hazel) also give symptomatic relief.
    3. **Ointments and suppositories** containing various analgesics, emollients, astringents, and hydrocortisone (e.g., Anusol HC suppositories, one PR bid for 7–10 days) can be effective for symptomatic treatment of internal hemorrhoids. Steroid-containing suppositories should not be used for long-term therapy.
    4. **Surgery** is indicated if medical management fails.
II. **Anal fissures** present with acute onset of pain during defecation and are commonly caused by the passage of a hard stool. Physical examination and anoscopy reveal an elliptical tear in the skin of the anus, usually in the posterior midline. Acute fissures usually heal in 2–3 weeks with stool softeners, analgesics, and sitz baths. Chronic fissures require surgical therapy.
III. **Perirectal abscess** commonly presents as painful induration in the perianal area. High-risk groups for development of a perirectal abscess include diabetics, immunocompromised patients, and patients with inflammatory bowel disease. Because of potentially serious morbidity with delayed treatment, prompt drainage is of the utmost importance. Antimicrobials directed against bowel flora should be administered to patients with significant associated cellulitis or systemic toxicity and to diabetic or immunocompromised patients.

Pancreatitis

I. **Acute pancreatitis** is frequently associated with excessive alcohol consumption or gallstones. Less common causes include hypercalcemia, hypertriglyceridemia, and a variety of drugs. The **Ranson criteria** provide useful prognostic information. Severe illness and increased mortality are associated with age over 55, WBC greater than 16,000/mm^3, glucose greater than 200 mg/dl, serum LDH greater than 350 IU/liter, SGOT greater than 250 IU/liter, hematocrit drop of greater than 10%, rise in BUN greater than 5 mg/dl, arterial PO$_2$ less than 60 mm Hg, base deficit greater than 4 mEq/liter, serum calcium less than 8.0 mg/dl, and estimated fluid sequestration greater than 6 liters. Therapy is largely supportive. Specific therapy is reserved for complications.

A. Supportive treatment. Narcotic analgesics are necessary for pain relief. Meperidine is most commonly used, as it has no significant effect on the sphincter of Oddi. Patients should be kept NPO until free of pain and nausea. Nasogastric suction is needed only in patients with protracted nausea and vomiting. **Aggressive volume repletion** with parenteral fluids is necessary with careful monitoring of input/output and awareness of the potential for significant fluid sequestration within the abdomen. Serum calcium, magnesium, and glucose as well as hematocrit should be monitored and abnormalities corrected as necessary. There is no clear role for prophylactic antibiotic therapy in acute pancreatitis. Although H_2-receptor antagonists have no proven beneficial effects in the therapy of acute pancreatitis, they may be necessary in severely ill patients with significant risk factors for stress ulcer bleeding (see Chap. 14).

B. Management of specific complications

1. **Infection.** There are many potential sources of fever in patients with acute pancreatitis, including pancreatic necrosis, abscess, infected pseudocyst, and aspiration pneumonia. In severely ill, febrile patients, culture material should be obtained and broad-spectrum antibiotics appropriate for bowel flora should be started (see Chap. 13). The development of fever 2 or more weeks into the course of acute pancreatitis suggests pancreatic abscess formation. CT scan of the abdomen may be helpful in this setting.

2. **Pseudocyst formation.** Persistent pain or hyperamylasemia suggests that a pseudocyst may have formed. Prolonged bowel rest and parenteral nutrition may allow pseudocysts to resolve or develop a mature wall, making surgical or percutaneous drainage safe. Pseudocysts that fail to resolve spontaneously after 4–6 weeks of conservative therapy should be treated definitively because of the risks of infection, hemorrhage, and perforation (*Am. J. Surg.* 137:135, 1979).

3. **Pulmonary complications,** including atelectasis, pleural effusion, pneumonia, and the adult respiratory distress syndrome, can develop in severely ill patients (see Chap. 10).

4. **Acute renal failure** due to severe intravascular volume depletion or acute tubular necrosis can develop. Occasionally, patients may require acute dialysis (see Chap. 11).

5. **Surgical therapy** may be required for severe hemorrhagic or necrotizing pancreatitis, pancreatic abscess, persistent pseudocyst, and, rarely, common bile duct or duodenal obstruction.

II. Chronic pancreatitis is usually associated with chronic alcoholism. Major complications requiring therapy include chronic pain and exocrine and endocrine insufficiency. The presence of a calcified pancreas on plain abdominal film is diagnostic of chronic pancreatitis.

A. Pain. Many patients with chronic pancreatitis have severe pain as the major manifestation of their illness. Narcotics are often required for analgesia, and addiction is common. In patients with chronic alcoholic pancreatitis and mild to moderate exocrine insufficiency, oral pancreatic enzyme supplements may be beneficial for pain control (*Gastroenterology* 87:44, 1984). Patients with intractable pain may be candidates for surgical management.

B. Exocrine insufficiency. Weight loss and steatorrhea in a patient with prior history of acute pancreatitis suggest pancreatic exocrine insufficiency.

1. **Diagnosis.** The **bentiromide (Chymex) test** is a simple screening study (*Gastroenterology* 89:685, 1985). After an overnight fast, 500 mg of bentiromide is given, followed by 250 mg of water PO initially and after 3 hours. Urine is collected for 6 hours. If less than 50% of the administered dose is found in the urine as arylamines, there is probably severe pancreatic exocrine insufficiency. The more invasive and less widely available secretin test is a direct measure of pancreatic secretion. Alternatively, an empiric trial of pancreatic enzyme replacement may be attempted.

2. **Therapy.** Most patients can be managed with a low-fat diet (< 50 g/day) and

oral pancreatic enzyme supplements. Supplements should be administered 20–30 minutes before meals and snacks. Non-enteric-coated preparations such as Viokase or Cotazym, 2–4 tablets, can be given in conjunction with H_2-receptor antagonists to prevent degradation by gastric acid. Enteric-coated preparations such as Pancrease or Creon, 1–2 capsules with meals, are used more commonly and are associated with fewer gastrointestinal side effects. They should not be given with H_2-receptor antagonists. Fat-soluble vitamin supplementation may be necessary (see Malabsorption and Maldigestion).

C. **Endocrine insufficiency.** Many patients with chronic pancreatitis will have abnormalities of glucose tolerance due to destruction of islet cells and may require supplemental insulin therapy (see Chap. 20).

Gallstones

I. **Cholelithiasis.** Asymptomatic cholelithiasis is a common incidental finding for which no specific therapy is generally necessary. The spectrum of symptomatic cholelithiasis includes a history of prior episodes of biliary colic, the acute onset of right upper quadrant pain, fever, nausea and vomiting (cholecystitis), or gallstone pancreatitis.

A. **Cholecystectomy.** The best therapy for symptomatic cholelithiasis remains cholecystectomy. **Laparoscopic** techniques have recently been introduced.

B. **Medical therapy.** A small, select group of patients with cholesterol stones who have uncomplicated biliary colic or who are at high risk for complications from surgical therapy may qualify for prolonged medical therapy with **chenodeoxycholic acid,** 13–16 mg/kg/day PO in two divided doses, or **ursodeoxycholic acid,** 8–10 mg/kg/day PO. Selection criteria include the presence of small (< 20 mm in diameter) radiolucent stones in a functioning gallbladder as judged by oral cholecystography. Total dissolution of stones occurs in approximately 30% of carefully selected patients after 1 year of therapy. **Side effects** include diarrhea and reversible elevations in serum transaminase levels, although the frequency of such problems appears to be lower with ursodeoxycholic acid.

C. **Other nonsurgical therapies** include percutaneous instillation of contact solvents such as methyl-tertiary-butyl ether (*N. Engl. J. Med.* 320:633, 1989) into the gallbladder and extracorporeal shock wave lithotripsy (*N. Engl. J. Med* 314:818, 1986) alone or in combination. However, experience with these therapies is limited, and neither is necessarily definitive, as the underlying abnormal gallbladder remains in place. Concomitant adjuvant therapy with an oral dissolution agent may be necessary.

II. **Cholecystitis.** Acute cholecystitis is most often caused by obstruction of the cystic duct by gallstones, but acalculous cholecystitis can occur especially in hospitalized patients. Surgical removal of the gallbladder is the mainstay of treatment. Intravenous fluid resuscitation is usually necessary, and broad-spectrum antimicrobial agents may be indicated, especially if sepsis, peritonitis or abscess is suspected. Severely ill patients who are not surgical candidates can undergo drainage by percutaneous cholecystostomy.

III. **Complications** of cholelithiasis/cholecystitis include choledocholithiasis with common bile duct obstruction and cholangitis, pancreatitis, ileus, gallbladder empyema, and perforation. In patients who have undergone cholecystectomy, **retained common bile duct stones** may complicate the postoperative course. Patients with **ascending cholangitis** due to choledocholithiasis present with right upper quadrant pain, fever, and jaundice (**Charcot's triad**). Therapy consists of parenteral broad-spectrum antimicrobials and drainage of the biliary tree. Ampicillin plus an aminoglycoside usually provides adequate initial therapy, although in severe cases anaerobic coverage may be added. Endoscopic retrograde cholangiopancreatography (ERCP) with sphincterotomy and stone removal or placement of a nasobiliary cannula is often performed, as is surgical or radiologic decompression.

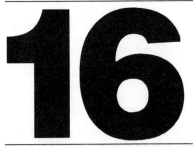

Hepatic Diseases

Heather M. White

Gastroenterologists frequently refer to liver disease as acute or chronic. Acute liver disease refers to abnormalities present for less than 6 months, and chronic liver disease refers to abnormalities present greater than 6 months. Fulminant hepatic failure specifically implies progression from onset of liver disease to liver failure in less than 4 weeks and therefore only occurs in acute disease.

Evaluation of Liver Function

I. **Laboratory evaluation** usually includes several screening tests of liver function. The biochemical tests may include (1) serum enzymes, including the aminotransferases, alkaline phosphatase, and 5'-nucleotidase; (2) excretory products, such as bilirubin, bile acids, and ammonia; and (3) synthetic products such as albumin, coagulation factors, and cholesterol.

   A. **Serum enzymes.** Hepatic disorders associated with predominant elevations in aspartate aminotransferase (AST) and alanine aminotransferase (ALT) are referred to as hepatocellular; hepatic disorders with predominant elevations in alkaline phosphatase (AP) and 5'-nucleotidase are referred to as cholestatic.

      1. **The aminotransferases** are **AST (SGOT)** and **ALT (SGPT).** Markedly elevated levels (> 500 units/liter) typically occur with acute hepatocellular injury (e.g., viral, drug-induced, ischemic hepatitis), whereas modest elevation (< 300 units/liter) may be seen in a variety of conditions (e.g., acute or chronic hepatocellular injury, infiltrative diseases, biliary obstruction). ALT is generally more sensitive than AST for detecting viral hepatitis. In alcoholic liver disease, AST is elevated in excess of ALT, typically by a factor of two or more (*Dig. Dis. Sci.* 24:835, 1979).

      2. **Alkaline phosphatase (AP)** is an enzyme present in a variety of body tissues including bone, intestine, and liver. Heat fractionation can be used to distinguish the source of serum AP, but more frequently the elevation of other hepatic enzymes is helpful in establishing the hepatic origin of AP. Serum AP levels are most frequently elevated in biliary obstruction or cholestasis or in the setting of space-occupying lesions or infiltrative diseases of the liver.

      3. **5'-Nucleotidase** is an enzyme elevated in a similar spectrum of diseases as AP and GGT (see sec. **I.A.4**). 5'-Nucleotidase is comparable in sensitivity to AP in detecting biliary obstruction, cholestasis, or infiltrative hepatobiliary diseases.

      4. **Gamma-glutamyl transpeptidase (GGT)** is an enzyme also present in a variety of tissues. Increases in GGT and AP tend to occur in similar hepatic diseases. The utility of GGT is limited by high sensitivity and predictable elevation in patients ingesting agents known to stimulate the hepatic microsomal mixed-function oxidase system (e.g., barbiturates, phenytoin, alcohol).

   B. **Excretory products**

      1. **Bilirubin** is a degradation product of heme. Serum bilirubin concentration represents a balance between bilirubin production and excretion; levels may

be elevated as a consequence of either increased bilirubin production or impaired hepatic excretion. Bilirubin concentration is composed of both **direct** (conjugated) and **indirect** (unconjugated) fractions. Predominantly indirect bilirubin elevations can occur as a result of excessive bilirubin production (hemolysis or ineffective erythropoiesis), impaired bilirubin conjugation (Gilbert's or Crigler-Najjar syndromes), or reduced hepatic bilirubin uptake (heart failure, portal-systemic shunting). Direct bilirubin elevations usually occur as a result of either hepatocellular dysfunction or biliary tract obstruction.

2. **Bile acids** are produced in the liver and secreted into bile, where they are required for lipid digestion and absorption. Under normal circumstances, bile acids undergo enterohepatic recirculation. Minor degrees of hepatic dysfunction can result in elevations of serum bile acids.

3. **Serum ammonia** may be elevated with hepatic dysfunction due to disturbances in the urea cycle. However, absolute levels do not correlate directly with clinical findings.

C. **Synthetic products**

1. **Serum albumin.** Depressed levels of albumin are most frequently seen with chronic liver disease. However, malnutrition and renal disease may also be associated with hypoalbuminemia. The half-life of albumin is relatively long, so levels are frequently preserved in acute liver disease.

2. **Coagulation factors.** All coagulation factors except factor VIII are synthesized by the liver, and most have half-lives measured in hours or days. Synthesis of factors II, VII, IX, and X is vitamin K–dependent. Hepatic synthetic function can be estimated by the **prothrombin time** (PT), which determines the interaction of factors II, V, VII, and X (see Chap. 17). PT prolongation occurs as a consequence of either impaired factor synthesis or vitamin K deficiency. Improvement in the PT following administration of vitamin K indicates vitamin K deficiency.

3. **Cholesterol and cholesterol-derived hormones** are synthesized in the liver. Thus, patients with advanced liver disease may have very low cholesterol levels and decreased levels of certain hormones (e.g., testosterone).

II. **Radiographic evaluation**

A. **Ultrasound (USG)** is best utilized as a screening tool for visualization of biliary tree dilation and gallstones but can also be used to detect parenchymal disease. USG is particularly operator dependent. USG with color-flow Doppler can assess patency of blood vessels and direction of flow.

B. **CT with intravenous contrast** is best utilized for evaluation of parenchymal liver disease but can also be used to assess biliary tree dilation and has the added features of contrast enhancement to assess space-occupying lesions such as abscess and tumor.

C. **MRI** has similar utility to CT but allows visualization of vessels without contrast dye. However, MRI requires a cooperative patient, and MRI may not be readily available.

D. **Liver-spleen scanning (LS)** is an older modality used primarily to detect colloid shift, which is present in hepatocellular dysfunction.

E. **Percutaneous transhepatic cholangiography (PTC) and endoscopic retrograde cholangiopancreatography (ERCP)** place contrast dye in the biliary tree and are most useful after preliminary screening by USG, CT, or MRI reveals biliary tree abnormalities.

Hepatotrophic Viruses

I. **Viral agents** include the hepatotrophic viruses hepatitis A, hepatitis B, hepatitis C, hepatitis D, hepatitis E, and non-A, non-B (NANB) hepatitis (Table 16-1).

A. **Hepatitis A (HAV).** Infection with HAV is usually transmitted via the fecal-oral route, and large-scale outbreaks due to contamination of food and drinking water can occur (*Semin. Liver Dis.* 6:42, 1986). The period of greatest infectivity is during the 2 weeks prior to the onset of clinical illness; however, stool precautions are indicated during the first 2–3 weeks of clinical illness. Although the period of viremia is brief, the disease can be transmitted in blood products.

B. **Hepatitis B (HBV).** The complete agent, or Dane particle, consists of an outer viral envelope protein (which contains the hepatitis B surface antigen [HBsAg]) and the viral nucleocapsid (which contains the hepatitis B core antigen [HBcAg]). **HBsAg** is detectable in serum in almost all cases of acute and chronic HBV infection. **HBcAg** does not freely circulate but can be detected in liver cells when there is active viral replication. Hepatitis B e antigen (**HBeAg**) appears to be a component of the HBcAg; it can usually be detected in serum when there is active viral replication. Circulating antibodies against the various viral antigens develop in response to infection, and these antibodies can be readily detected by serology. Antibody against HBsAg (**anti-HBs**) appears following HBV infection or vaccination; its presence confers immunity (except in rare cases of chronic HBV infection when low titers of heterotypic anti-HBs are detectable). **Hepatitis B core antibody** can be detected in two fractions: the hepatitis B core IgM (anti-HBcIgM) and the hepatitis B core total (anti-HBcTotal). Anti-HBcIgM is usually present in acute infection but occasionally can be detected during periods of high viral replication in chronic disease. Anti-HBcTotal includes IgM and IgG fractions and is positive in acute disease (due to the presence of IgM), in chronic disease (due to predominantly IgG), and in patients who have recovered from infection (due to IgG). Infection with HBV is usually spread via either apparent (e.g., needlestick) or inapparent (e.g., sexual contact) parenteral transmission. Although blood is the most effective vehicle for transmission, HBsAg is present in other body fluids (e.g., saliva, semen), which can also transmit the infection. HBsAg is rarely present in feces or urine. **Patients with HBV infection should avoid intimate contact (e.g., sharing razors, toothbrushes) with other household members since they are infectious until seroconversion occurs** (*Semin. Liver Dis.* 6:1, 1986; *Semin. Liver Dis.* 6:11, 1986) **or until household contacts have completed vaccination.**

C. **Hepatitis C (HCV)** has an incubation period that may be as short as 2 weeks but is usually 6 weeks to 6 months. The only serologic test currently available is hepatitis C antibody (HCVAb). **The presence of HCVAb suggests chronic infection with HCV, and the antibody does not confer immunity.** HCVAb is frequently negative in acute infection (60–90% of patients) and may take up to 12 months to become positive after acute infection. It may be positive in 60–80% of patients with chronic infection (*Science* 244:362, 1989; *N. Engl. J. Med.* 321:1494, 1989). Confirmatory assays and additional antigen/antibody detection systems are under investigation. The primary established transmission route is blood exposure (e.g., transfusion, intravenous drug use), but up to 60% of patients have no exposure history. Data regarding sexual transmission are conflicting but suggest that HCV may be transmitted sexually, though at a much lower frequency than HBV (*J.A.M.A.* 262:1201, 1989; *Ann. Intern. Med.* 112:544, 1990). Perinatal transmission has not been clearly documented, although the HCVAb (an IgG antibody) crosses the placenta. Therefore, isolation guidelines are controversial; at a minimum, blood and body fluids should be considered infectious.

D. **Hepatitis D (HDV), or delta agent, requires the presence of HBV for infection and replication to occur.** HDV infection can only occur if an individual with chronic HBV is subsequently exposed to HDV (superinfection) or if an individual is simultaneously infected with both HBV and HDV (co-infection). Although HDV is found throughout the world, it is endemic to the Mediterranean basin, the Middle East, and portions of South America; outside of these areas, infections occur primarily in multiply transfused individuals and, in the United States, in intravenous drug abusers. Fulminant disease is more common in HDV, and chronic disease occurs in most patients (*Semin. Liver Dis.* 6:28, 1986). Acute HDV is diagnosed by the presence of HDVAg and anti-HDVIgM in serum.

E. **Hepatitis E (HEV)** has an incubation period of 2–6 weeks. Transmission closely resembles HAV. HEV has been implicated in epidemics in such areas as India,

Table 16-1. Comparison of hepatotrophic viruses—clinical and epidemiologic features

Organism	Hepatitis A	Hepatitis B	Hepatitis C	Hepatitis D	Hepatitis E	NANB
Incubation	2–6 wk	1–6 mo	2 wk–6 mo	3 wk–3 mo	3–6 wk	2 wk–6 mo
Transmission	Fecal/oral Rarely blood or sexual	Blood Sexual Perinatal	Sporadic Blood ?Sexual—report with multiple partners ?Perinatal—none reported	Blood Sexual	Fecal/oral Food contamination	Sporadic Blood ?Sexual ?Perinatal
Risk groups	Military Day care	IV drug abusers Homosexuals Native Asians Health care workers Transfused patients	IV drug abusers Health care workers Transfused patients	IV drug abusers (high risk in U.S.) Anyone with hepatitis B	Travelers to endemic areas	IV drug abusers Health care workers Transfused patients
Fever	Common	Uncommon	Uncommon	Uncommon	Common	Uncommon
Nausea/vomiting	Common	Common	Common	Common	Common	Common
Immune complex disease	Uncommon	Common	Common	Common	Uncommon	Unknown
Severity	Mild	Mild to moderate	Mild to moderate	Moderate to severe	Mild to moderate	Mild to moderate
Diagnosis Acute	Anti-HAVIgM	Anti-HBcIgM HBsAg	Clinical	Anti-HDVIgM HDVAg	Clinical	Diagnosis of exclusion in the appropriate clinical setting
Chronic		Anti-HBcTotal HBsAg ±HBeAg	HCVAb	HDVAg		

Sequelae						
Fulminant	0.1–0.2%	<5%	<5%	5–20%	1–2% 10–30% in pregnant women	<5%
Carrier	No	Yes	Unknown	Yes	No	Unknown
Chronic hepatitis	No	Yes	Yes	Yes	No	Yes
Prophylaxis						
Adults	ISG[a]	HBIG[b] + Vaccine[c]	?ISG[a]	None available	None available	?ISG[a]
Perinatal	ISG[a]	HBIG[d] + Vaccine[e]	?ISG[a]			?ISG[a]

[a] Immune serum globulin, 0.02 ml/kg IM. Use in NANB and HCV unsubstantiated.
[b] Hepatitis B immunoglobulin, 5 ml IM.
[c] Vaccine is either Heptavax B, 20 μg IM, or Recombivax, 10 μg IM at 0, 1, and 6 months.
[d] Hepatitis B immunoglobulin, 0.5 ml IM within 12 hours of birth.
[e] Vaccine is either Heptavax B, 10 μg IM, or Recombivax, 5 μg IM at 0, 1, and 6 months.
Note: Immune serum globulin may be substituted (0.12 ml/kg) if HBIG is not available.

Southeast Asia, Africa, and Mexico. The only reported cases in the United States have been in travelers to endemic areas. Diagnostic testing methods are under investigation. HEV is associated with high fatality rates in pregnant women.

F. Non-A, Non-B (NANB) is the exclusionary category of hepatotrophic viruses that remain when serologic tests for other viruses are negative. Previously, HCV comprised a significant proportion of this group. NANB occurs sporadically and following blood exposure. Transmission and isolation recommendations are similar to those for HCV.

II. Management of viral hepatitis includes prophylaxis of close contacts and therapy based on the severity and chronicity of the disease.

A. Pre-exposure prophylaxis is important but rarely considered. Pre-exposure prophylaxis for HAV should be given to travelers to endemic areas. For trips lasting up to 2 months, immune serum globulin (ISG), 0.02 ml/kg IM, should be administered; for longer travel, ISG, 0.06 ml/kg IM, should be given every five months. Pre-exposure prophylaxis for HBV and HDV should be considered in patients with anticipated multiple transfusions (e.g., transplant recipients), health care workers, IV drug abusers, household contacts of HBsAg carriers, homosexuals, heterosexual contacts of HBsAg carriers, institutionalized mentally retarded people, and Alaskan Eskimos (*Semin. Liver Dis.* 6:23, 1986). Prevaccination screening for previous exposure or infection is recommended in the high-risk groups to avoid vaccinating recovered individuals or those with chronic infection. Pre-exposure prophylaxis for HBV is HBV vaccine at 0, 1, and 6 months. Two vaccines are available; the plasma-derived vaccine dose is 20 μg (1 ml), and the recombinant vaccine dose is 10 μg or 20 μg (1 ml) (depending on the product used) IM in the deltoid. In hemodialysis and other immunosuppressed patients, three 40-μg doses of the plasma-derived vaccine are recommended, using the same schedule (*Ann. Intern. Med.* 107:353, 1987). Revaccination is not generally recommended for individuals who fail to respond to the initial series of vaccinations (*N. Engl. J. Med.* 315:209, 1986). The need for and timing of booster doses has not yet been determined. There is no specific vaccine for HDV. Patients vaccinated against HBV are immune to HDV. Pre-exposure prophylaxis for HCV and NANB is not available. Pre-exposure prophylaxis for HEV is not available (ISG is not protective).

B. Postexposure prophylaxis (Table 16-1). Of special importance is the postexposure prophylaxis of HBV in the perinatal period. All infants of infected mothers should receive HBIG and a series of vaccinations within 24 hours of birth, as they are at very high risk for chronic infection.

C. Therapy of viral hepatitis is largely supportive. Dietary therapy usually has little role in acute hepatitis. A clear liquid diet may be helpful in those patients with nausea or vomiting. Fat intake should be restricted in individuals with diarrhea, nausea, or vomiting. **Rarely, patients may require hospitalization for hydration.** Alcohol should be avoided. Multivitamin supplements may be appropriate in malnourished or severely anorectic patients. Activity restrictions are recommended if a clinical or biochemical relapse occurs with full ambulation. **Management of acute hepatitis is predominantly on an outpatient basis; liver enzymes (AST, ALT), bilirubin, and synthetic function (albumin, PT) should be monitored to assess recovery.** In a small group of patients (see Table 16–1) fulminant hepatic failure occurs, reflected by falling transaminases, falling albumin, rising bilirubin, and rising prothrombin time.

D. Fulminant hepatic failure (FHF) may occur as a result of viral hepatitis, drugs, ischemia, toxin exposure, acute fatty liver of pregnancy, Wilson's disease, or Reye's syndrome. Viral hepatitis is the most common setting, but the clinical description and medical management apply to all cases of fulminant hepatic failure. **Manifestations** may include encephalopathy, deepening jaundice, gastrointestinal bleeding, sepsis, coagulopathy, hypoglycemia, renal failure, and electrolyte abnormalities. **Supportive therapy in the inpatient setting is essential.** Caloric intake should be maintained with dextrose-containing IV solutions. Serum glucose should be monitored q4h and more often if glucose is less than 60 mg/dl. Vitamin supplements (including vitamin K) should be given.

Antacids or H$_2$-receptor antagonists, in a dose sufficient to keep gastric pH greater than 5.0, may prevent upper gastrointestinal hemorrhage (*Lancet* 1:617, 1989). **Fresh frozen plasma** (FFP) and blood should be administered when there is evidence of active hemorrhage. However, prophylactic administration of FFP is not recommended, as it may lead to volume overload and makes assessment of residual synthetic function difficult. In patients with signs suggestive of elevated intracranial pressure (see Chap. 25) or stage III or IV hepatic coma, an intracranial pressure monitor should be placed and IV mannitol (1 g/kg) may be given. Hyperventilation to lower the PCO$_2$ to less than 30 mm Hg should be reserved for management of acute rises in intracranial pressure, as the brain adapts to chronic hyperventilation. Glucocorticoids seem to have little effect on the cerebral edema associated with FHF, and controlled trials have failed to demonstrate the efficacy of glucocorticoids in this disease (*N. Engl. J. Med.* 294:681, 1976; *Gastroenterology* 75:992, 1978; *Gastroenterology* 76:1297, 1979; *Gut* 23:625, 1982). In patients with stage IV hepatic coma, mortality exceeds 80% and transplantation should be considered (see Hepatic Transplantation). Death ensues from progressive liver failure, gastrointestinal bleeding, cerebral edema, sepsis, or arrhythmias.

E. **Chronic viral hepatitis** is defined as the presence of liver inflammation that persists for a period of at least 6 months and is associated with HBV, HCV, HDV, and NANB. Chronic viral hepatitis is subdivided into (1) the **carrier state,** characterized by normal enzymes and no inflammation on biopsy but persistent circulating viral particles, (2) **chronic persistent hepatitis (CPH),** characterized by the presence of chronic inflammation limited to the portal tracts, and (3) **chronic active hepatitis (CAH),** characterized by the presence of chronic inflammation involving the portal tracts and periportal parenchyma. Both CPH and CAH may progress to cirrhosis. A chronic carrier state has long been known in HBV, where patients express the HBsAg in the serum and virus is present on tissue immunostaining of the liver. HDV can also exist in the carrier state, although by definition the patient must also have HBV. It is unknown if HCV or NANB have a carrier state, but it is likely. Although many agents have been tried in viral CPH and CAH, the best results to date are with alpha interferon. Experimentally, in hepatitis B, alpha interferon administered over a 4-month period appears to result in sustained loss of viral replication as well as biochemical and histologic remission in approximately one-third of patients, with loss of HBsAg in approximately 10% (*N. Engl. J. Med.* 323:295, 1990). In hepatitis C, alpha interferon therapy administered over 6–12 months has a response rate of approximately 50%, but a relatively high relapse rate has also been observed (*Semin. Liver Dis.* 9:259, 1989). Intron A (interferon alpha-2b) is approved for hepatitis C/NANB therapy at a dose of 3 million units (1 ml) SQ three times a week for 6 months. Therapy is appropriate only in selected patients due to significant toxicity and side effects. The success of alpha interferon in hepatitis D patients is quite limited, and years of treatment with high doses are required to effect any response (*Semin. Liver Dis.* 9:264, 1989). Hepatic transplantation may be indicated in advanced disease, but disease recurrence has been documented in HBV, HCV, and HDV.

Toxic and Drug-Related Liver Disease

I. **Intrinsic hepatotoxins** include **direct hepatotoxins** (e.g., carbon tetrachloride, phosphorus), which cause predictable damage to liver cells by direct physicochemical attack, and **indirect hepatotoxins** (e.g., tetracycline, methotrexate, 6-mercaptopurine, acetaminophen, *Amanita phalloides* [mushroom toxin], and alkylated anabolic steroids), which may interfere with hepatocyte metabolic pathways or secretory mechanisms. Oral contraceptives may cause mild abnormalities in liver enzymes, but overt cholestatic jaundice is unusual. Associated liver disorders with oral contraceptives include hepatic adenomas and Budd-Chiari

Table 16-2. Some drugs associated with chronic hepatitis or cirrhosis[*]

Acetaminophen	Isoniazid
Amiodarone	Methyldopa
Chlorpromazine	Nitrofurantoin
Dantrolene	Oxyphenisatin
Ethanol	Propylthiouracil
Halothane	Sulfonamides

[*]These drugs should be used carefully or avoided, if possible, in patients with chronic liver disease.

syndrome. Treatment for all intrinsic hepatotoxins is withdrawal of the offending drug and institution of supportive measures. An attempt to remove the agent from the gastrointestinal tract should be made in most cases using lavage or cathartics (see Chap. 26). Except for acetaminophen (see Chap. 26) and methotrexate (see Chap. 19) ingestion, no specific therapy is available in most cases.

II. **Idiosyncratic hepatotoxins** may present with either hypersensitivity reactions or idiosyncratic metabolic reactions.

  A. **Hypersensitivity reactions** are characterized by a sensitization period of 1–5 weeks and prompt recurrence of the liver injury in response to a repeat challenge. Associated signs and symptoms include fever, rash, and eosinophilia. The presence of eosinophilic or granulomatous inflammation is a typical histologic finding. Responsible drugs include sulfonamides, nitrofurantoin, para-aminosalicyclic acid, phenytoin, and halothane.

  B. **Metabolic idiosyncrasy** in susceptible patients occurs as a result of altered drug clearance or accelerated production of hepatotoxic metabolites (e.g, isoniazid, methyldopa, perhaps halothane) (H. Zimmerman, *Hepatotoxicity: The Adverse Effects of Drugs and other Chemicals on the Liver.* New York: Appleton-Century-Crofts, 1978). See Table 16-2 for a list of drugs commonly associated with chronic hepatitis and cirrhosis.

III. **Alcohol.** Alcohol-induced hepatic injury is a significant problem in the United States. Although current evidence suggests that alcohol exerts a direct toxic effect on the liver, only 10–20% of chronic alcoholics develop significant liver damage. Thus, additional factors (e.g., genetic, nutritional, environmental) may be important in the pathogenesis of alcoholic liver disease. The spectrum of alcoholic liver disease is broad and a single patient may be affected by more than one entity.

  A. **Fatty liver** is the most common abnormality observed in chronic alcoholics. If fat alone is present, patients are usually asymptomatic. Clinical findings include hepatomegaly and mild liver enzyme abnormalities (usually elevated AP). The disorder is believed to be reversible if alcohol intake is stopped and a nutritious diet is ingested.

  B. **Alcoholic hepatitis** may be clinically silent or severe enough to lead to rapid hepatic failure and death. Clinical features include fever, abdominal pain, anorexia, nausea, vomiting, and weight loss; in patients with underlying cirrhosis, manifestations of portal hypertension may predominate. Laboratory features typically demonstrate elevations in AST, ALT, and AP, with AST characteristically higher than ALT; hyperbilirubinemia and prolonged PT may also be seen. Although clinical presentation is helpful, liver biopsy is required for definitive diagnosis and demonstrates characteristic polymorphonuclear infiltrate, necrosis, Mallory bodies, and intrasinusoidal collagen deposition. Features associated with a **poor prognosis** include prolongation of PT that does not correct with vitamin K, marked elevation of total bilirubin, leukocytosis, and an elevated blood urea nitrogen (BUN) or serum creatinine (Cr).

  C. **Alcoholic or Laennec's cirrhosis** is the most common cause of cirrhosis in the United States. Diagnosis can only be made by liver biopsy.

  D. **Therapy of alcoholic liver disease** is directed at abstinence from alcohol as well as vitamin and nutritional support. Glucocorticoids, anabolic steroids, and propylthiouracil may improve survival and biochemical parameters in some patients treated with these agents; however, their use is controversial and their role is not determined. In severe cholestatic alcoholic hepatitis, particularly in association with encephalopathy, glucocorticoids may have a role (*Ann. Intern. Med.* 110:685, 1989).

   E. Drug interactions between alcohol and a variety of pharmaceuticals are known. Alcohol may potentiate the effects or alter the metabolism of a number of medications. Potentially dangerous interactions between alcohol and sedative-hypnotics, anticoagulants, and acetaminophen (even in the absence of alcoholic liver disease) may occur in clinical practice due to shared metabolic pathways (*Ann. Intern. Med.* 104:399, 1986).

IV. Acetaminophen may cause significant hepatocellular injury in accidental or intentional overdosage. Toxic potentiation of alcohol in combination with even therapeutic doses of acetaminophen may cause significant hepatocellular injury. Management of acetaminophen overdose is covered elsewhere (see Chap. 26). Close observation for signs of fulminant hepatic failure is recommended.

Cholestatic Liver Disease

Cholestatic liver disease is characterized by predominant elevations in AP and bilirubin, although the bilirubin may appear normal until late in the course.

I. Primary biliary cirrhosis (PBC) is a progressive, cholestatic disorder of unknown cause that most often affects middle-aged women. The course is highly variable, and patients may be asymptomatic for many years. Pruritus is usually the most troublesome symptom. Typical clinical features are hyperpigmentation, xanthelasma, gallstones, and osteoporosis. Key laboratory features include elevated levels of AP, cholesterol, immunoglobulin M, and bile acids, associated with the presence of antimitochondrial antibodies (present in 95% of patients).

   A. Nutritional deficiencies. Patients are at risk for malnutrition secondary to fat malabsorption, and a low-fat diet, 40–60 g/day, may be helpful in patients with diarrhea. Fat-soluble vitamin deficiency (vitamins A, D, K) is seen in more advanced disease and in those patients with steatorrhea. Vitamin replacement doses include vitamin A, 5,000–25,000 IU PO daily; vitamin D, 50,000 IU PO 3–5 times weekly; vitamin K_1 (phytonadione), 10 mg SQ or IM weekly; or vitamin K tablets, 5–10 mg PO daily. PT and serum levels of vitamin A and 25-hydroxyvitamin D should be measured to judge the adequacy of replacement therapy. Vitamin A deficiency is the least common; large doses of vitamin A can be hepatotoxic and teratogenic so it should be administered with caution. Zinc deficiency may also occur in some patients, and zinc sulfate, 220 mg PO daily (50 mg of elemental zinc) for 4 weeks, will usually correct low serum zinc levels.

   B. Spontaneous fractures due to osteoporosis can occur, and oral calcium supplementation (1.0–1.5 g/day) should be given to all patients with PBC; vitamin D supplement may also be required (see Chap. 23). Dual energy radiography or bone densitometry of the wrist or spine should be performed in all patients.

   C. Pruritus in PBC and other cholestatic diseases is best treated with cholestyramine, a bile acid sequestrant resin. The drug is usually given as one packet (4 g of resin) mixed with water before the morning meal with additional doses added before meals if symptoms are not controlled. Cholestyramine should not be given concurrently with vitamins or other medications, since it may impair their absorption. Phenobarbital, 60–120 mg PO daily, can be added if cholestyramine alone is ineffective in controlling pruritus.

   D. Therapy for PBC. No specific therapy has clearly been shown to be effective in altering the course of PBC, but colchicine, cyclosporine, methotrexate, and ursodeoxycholic acid are currently under investigation. Hepatic transplantation may be required in advanced disease.

II. Primary sclerosing cholangitis (PSC) is an idiopathic chronic cholestatic disorder characterized by inflammation, fibrosis, and eventual obliteration of the extrahepatic and intrahepatic bile ducts. Most patients are middle-aged men, and there is a frequent association with inflammatory bowel disease. **ERCP or PTC** demonstrating strictures or irregularity of the intrahepatic and extrahepatic bile ducts confirms the diagnosis. Clinical manifestations typically include intermittent episodes of jaundice, hepatomegaly, pruritus, weight loss, and fatigue. Episodes of bacterial cholangitis primarily occur in patients who have had surgical biliary drainage procedures. Patients are at a substantially increased risk of developing cholangiocarcinoma. No specific therapy has proved to be successful; a number of experimental trials with cyclosporine, methotrexate, and ursodeoxycholic acid are ongoing. Supportive therapy is as outlined for PBC. **Cholangitis** episodes should be managed as described elsewhere (see Chap. 15). Hepatic transplantation should be reserved for advanced disease or recurrent cholangitis.

III. **Granulomatous hepatitis** presents primarily as a cholestatic disorder with many different etiologies. Patients typically present with fevers and abnormal liver enzymes (particularly AP) and may have hepatosplenomegaly. The major differential diagnosis includes mycobacterial disease, chronic fungal infections such as *Cryptococcus* or *Histoplasma,* sarcoidosis, drug-induced injury, and idiopathic granulomatous hepatitis. Specific therapy is directed at selected disease entities. If the clinical suspicion for tuberculosis is high, an empiric trial of antituberculous therapy may be warranted despite negative mycobacterial cultures. Steroids may be useful in selected noninfectious cases.

Metabolic Liver Disease

A number of treatable metabolic disorders may present with hepatocellular dysfunction. Disorders include Wilson's disease, hemochromatosis, and alpha$_1$-antitrypsin deficiency. Other rare disorders include glycogen storage disease, phospholipidoses, and Byler's syndrome.

I. **Wilson's disease** may present with fulminant hepatic failure but more typically presents with progressive hepatic dysfunction, which may be accompanied by neuropsychiatric disorders. Diagnosis is suggested by elevated serum copper, low serum ceruloplasmin, and elevated 24-hour urinary copper and is confirmed by quantitative copper on liver biopsy. Treatment is with copper chelating agents (penicillamine or trientine).

II. **Hemochromatosis** may present with slate-colored skin, diabetes, cardiomyopathy, arthritis, or hepatic dysfunction and usually is not diagnosed until middle age. Diagnosis is suggested by elevated serum iron levels and high transferrin saturation and confirmed by quantitative iron on liver biopsy. Therapy consists of phlebotomy and genetic counseling.

III. **Alpha$_1$-antitrypsin deficiency** may present with pulmonary, hepatic, or pancreatic manifestations. Diagnosis is suggested by abnormal alpha$_1$-antitrypsin levels and can be confirmed by liver biopsy. No specific medical therapy for hepatic disease is available; transplantation is curative.

Miscellaneous Disorders

I. **Vascular disease of the liver** is due to impaired arterial or venous blood flow.
   A. **Hepatic artery ischemia** may occur as a result of profound hypotension and can result in markedly elevated transaminases, which typically resolve over 24–48 hours if hypotension is treated. Hepatic artery thrombosis is rare except in liver transplant recipients or after surgery near the porta hepatis. The hepatic artery may be involved in systemic arteritis. Venous occlusion is a much more common vascular injury.
   B. **Hepatic vein thrombosis,** Budd-Chiari syndrome, is the most common vascular disease. Classically, Budd-Chiari presents with new onset ascites and tender hepatomegaly. It is seen in association with lymphoreticular malignancy or hypercoagulable states. In one-third of cases, no cause can be determined. There

is controversy about thrombolytics in the acute setting, but the prognosis is poor. Transplantation is recommended if no malignancy can be identified.

C. Veno-occlusive disease is an unusual syndrome of intrahepatic venous obliteration most typically seen following total body irradiation and high-dose chemotherapy in bone marrow transplant patients. Veno-occlusive disease has also been described in renal transplant patients who have not received irradiation but have been immunosuppressed with azathioprine and in association with ingestion of Jamaican bush teas.

D. Portal vein thrombosis is seen in a variety of clinical settings including cirrhosis (particularly with sudden decompensation), malignancy causing obstruction either by direct invasion of the portal vein or by compression secondary to portal adenopathy, or intraabdominal sepsis.

II. Hepatic abscess may be either pyogenic or amebic.

A. Pyogenic abscess most often occurs as a complication of either biliary tract disease or malignancy. Clinical features include fever, abdominal pain, and anorexia with tender hepatomegaly. Laboratory studies may demonstrate leukocytosis and elevated AP. Diagnosis is usually made by USG or CT. **Therapy** includes antibiotic treatment and percutaneous drainage; surgical drainage is required in selected cases. Attempts should be made to collect culture material before initiating antibiotic therapy. Combination therapy with ampicillin (or penicillin), an aminoglycoside, and an anti-anaerobic drug is recommended when cultures are pending or unavailable. In patients responding to treatment, parenteral therapy is recommended for 10–14 days, followed by 4–6 weeks of oral therapy (*Medicine* 66:472, 1987). Repeat imaging is recommended to document resolution.

B. Amebic abscess. Diagnosis of amebic abscess requires a high index of clinical suspicion and should be considered in patients from endemic areas. Ameba titers are helpful in establishing the diagnosis. Amebic abscesses should always be treated with metronidazole with or without chloroquine and should never be drained percutaneously or surgically.

III. Sepsis, due to a variety of organisms, has long been associated with liver function test abnormalities, which are typically mild, transient, and of no prognostic significance (*Arch. Intern. Med.* 149:2246, 1989). The most common abnormality reported is direct hyperbilirubinemia; however, mild elevations in AST, ALT, and AP have also been noted (usually less than threefold above normal).

IV. Autoimmune chronic active hepatitis occurs most often in females and frequently presents with cirrhosis in childhood or young adulthood. Autoimmune hepatitis is characterized by the presence of autoantibodies (antinuclear antibody and anti–smooth muscle antibody) and hypergammaglobulinemia. Improved life expectancy has been demonstrated in patients treated with glucocorticoids. Therapy is initiated with prednisone, 40–60 mg PO qd, which is then tapered to a maintenance dose of 7.5–10.0 mg PO daily as serum transaminase levels fall. Combination therapy with azathioprine, 1–2 mg/kg/day PO, and prednisone may also be used and is associated with fewer steroid-related side effects. Histologic remission occurs in as many as 80% of patients. Therapy should be discontinued in individuals who fail to demonstrate either a clinical, biochemical, or histologic improvement after 18 months of therapy (*Gastroenterology* 73:1422, 1977). Relapse may occur in greater than 50% of patients following cessation of therapy. Retreatment is effective in most cases but appears to be associated with more side effects (*N. Engl. J. Med.* 304:5, 1981). Many patients require lifelong low-dose therapy. Hepatic transplantation may be offered in end-stage disease.

Complications of Hepatic Insufficiency

I. Portal-systemic (or hepatic) encephalopathy (PSE) is the syndrome of disordered consciousness and altered neuromuscular activity seen in patients with hepatocellular failure or portal-systemic shunting. The normal liver protects the systemic circulation from ingested toxic agents and the by-products of intestinal bacterial metabolism. The specific toxins and their mechanisms are unclear, but ammonia, gamma-aminobutyric acid, other amino acids, mercaptans, and short-chain fatty acids have all been implicated.

A. Precipitating factors include azotemia from dehydration, diuretics, or renal failure; use of a tranquilizer, opioid, or sedative-hypnotic medication; gastrointestinal hemorrhage; hypokalemia and alkalosis; constipation; infection; high-protein diet; progressive hepatocellular dysfunction; and surgery (especially portal-systemic shunts).

B. Treatment should be initiated as soon as possible. Precipitants should be identified and treated or eliminated whenever possible. Dietary protein should initially be eliminated while adequate calories (25–30 kcal/kg) are administered by either the enteral or parenteral route. Once clinical improvement occurs, a 20–40 g/day protein diet may be administered with 10–20 g/day increases every 3–5 days. Vegetable-protein diets may be better tolerated by patients with PSE than diets containing meat protein (*Dig. Dis. Sci.* 27:1109, 1982). Branched-chain amino acid–enriched formulas are available in both oral and parenteral forms, but their use should be reserved for PSE that is difficult to manage or does not respond to usual measures.

C. Medical therapies include lactulose, neomycin, and metronidazole.

    1. Lactulose is a poorly absorbed, synthetic disaccharide. While its mechanism of action is not certain, lactulose appears to produce an osmotic diarrhea and alter intestinal flora, resulting in the production of acidic diarrhea.

        a. Oral lactulose can be given in doses of 15–45 ml PO bid–qid. Maintenance dosages should be adjusted to produce two to three soft stools per day. Hourly doses of 30–45 ml PO may be used to induce a rapid catharsis during the initial phases of treatment or in PSE associated with constipation or blood in the gastrointestinal tract. Oral lactulose should not be given to patients with an ileus or possible bowel obstruction. Excess usage can lead to dehydration, hypernatremia, and patient discomfort due to excessive diarrhea.

        b. Lactulose enemas, prepared with 300 ml of lactulose added to 700 ml of tap water, can be administered bid–qid. The enema is administered with the patient on his or her left side and in the Trendelenburg position; during retention, the patient should be rolled onto his or her right side, and the head should be elevated to promote filling of the proximal colon.

    2. Antibiotic preparations can be effective in treating PSE. Neomycin can be given PO or by nasogastric tube, 1 g q4–6h or by a retention enema, as a 1% solution (1–2 g in 100–200 ml of isotonic saline) bid–qid. Approximately 1–3% of the administered dose of neomycin is absorbed, with an attendant risk of ototoxicity and nephrotoxicity. The risk of toxicity is increased in patients with renal insufficiency. Because lactulose is as effective as neomycin in the treatment of PSE and is less toxic, lactulose is preferred for initial as well as chronic therapy (*Gastroenterology* 72:573, 1977).

    3. Combination therapy with lactulose plus neomycin should be considered in patients refractory to either agent alone.

    4. Metronidazole is useful for short-term therapy when neomycin is unavailable or poorly tolerated; a dosage of 250 mg PO q8h is generally effective and well tolerated.

II. Ascites and edema occur as a result of avid sodium retention by the kidney, decreased plasma oncotic pressure, increased splanchnic lymph flow, and elevated hydrostatic pressure in the hepatic sinusoids or portal vein. Treatment of ascites should be undertaken cautiously and gradually, since ascites itself is rarely life-threatening.

A. Salt restriction is the most important initial treatment measure; no more than 1,000 mg Na^+/day should be allowed. Rarely a more rigid restriction may be required; however, most patients find such diets unpalatable and very restricted in protein, so compliance is diminished. A more liberal sodium intake (1,000–2,000 mg/day) can be allowed when diuresis is effected. Low-sodium liquid formula diets may be useful in some patients.

B. Bed rest is occasionally helpful in mobilizing ascites in patients with refractory ascites. After diuresis is initiated, a gradual increase in activity can be allowed.

C. Diuretics should be considered in patients who fail to initiate a diuresis with salt restriction and bed rest. Under optimal conditions, the capacity to reabsorb ascitic fluid is no more than 700–900 ml/day; therefore, diuresis should proceed gradually. Diuretics should not be administered to individuals with an increasing serum creatinine. The goal of diuretic therapy should be a daily weight loss of 0.5–1.0 kg in patients with edema and approximately 0.25 kg in patients without edema. The dosage of medication may be increased every 3–5 days to initiate or maintain an adequate diuresis. Spironolactone is the diuretic of choice. The starting dosage is 25 mg PO bid; this may be increased to a maximum of 150 mg PO qid. Amiloride or triamterene is useful in patients who cannot tolerate spironolactone. Loop diuretics (furosemide, ethacrynic acid, bumetanide) may be added when spironolactone fails to initiate a diuresis. Furosemide, 20 mg PO qd, may be used initially, with the dosage increased every 3–5 days depending on the response. Such loop diuretic agents are potent and may be associated with serious side effects; patients receiving these drugs should be observed closely for signs of volume depletion, electrolyte disturbances, encephalopathy, and renal insufficiency. In selected situations, other agents such as metolazone or thiazides may be useful.

D. Water restriction is not routinely necessary. If dilutional hyponatremia occurs, a fluid restriction of 1,000–1,500 ml/day will usually suffice. A more stringent fluid restriction may be required in patients with severe hyponatremia or with renal failure and oliguria.

E. Paracentesis should be performed for diagnostic purposes (e.g., new onset ascites, suspicion of malignant ascites, spontaneous peritonitis) or when there is tense ascites causing respiratory compromise or impending peritoneal rupture. Up to 5 liters of ascitic fluid can be safely removed provided that (1) the patient has edema, (2) the fluid is removed slowly (over 30–90 minutes), and (3) a fluid restriction is instituted to avoid hyponatremia (*Hepatology* 5:403, 1985). Rarely, however, paracentesis of as little as 1,000 ml may lead to circulatory collapse, encephalopathy, and renal failure.

F. Peritoneovenous (LeVeen or Denver) shunts (PVS) may be useful in the 5–10% of patients with ascites that is refractory to all medical therapy (*Gastroenterology* 82:790, 1982). PVS may be associated with complications such as disseminated intravascular coagulation, shunt closure, and fever. The shunt should be ligated if overt bleeding occurs. PVS should not be used in patients with infected ascites, recent variceal hemorrhage, markedly elevated bilirubin, hepatorenal syndrome, or coagulopathy.

G. Other agents occasionally helpful in the management of ascites are salt-poor albumin and dopamine. Albumin is sometimes useful in patients with azotemia and intravascular volume depletion. Unfortunately, albumin rapidly leaves the intravascular space, is expensive, and appears to offer little advantage over the use of crystalloid solutions for volume expansion. Albumin infusion in conjunction with repeated paracentesis appears to be useful and safe in patients with tense ascites (*Gastroenterology* 93:234, 1987). Dopamine in vasodilator dosages (1–5 μg/kg/min) may be administered in an attempt to improve renal blood flow. Its value in ascites management is not clear.

III. Spontaneous bacterial peritonitis (SBP) occurs only in patients with preexisting ascites. The illness is typified by the presence of abdominal pain and distention, fever, decreased bowel sounds, and worsening of hepatic encephalopathy; however, the disease may be present in the absence of specific clinical signs. All cirrhotic patients with ascites and evidence of any clinical deterioration should undergo a diagnostic paracentesis to exclude SBP. The diagnosis can be made when the ascitic fluid contains greater than 250 polymorphonuclear leukocytes (PMN)/μl or when the clinical signs and symptoms are highly suggestive of SBP. A positive culture confirms the diagnosis. The highest yield cultures are derived from 10 ml of ascitic fluid inoculated into blood culture bottles; the most common organisms are *Escherichia coli,* pneumococcus, and *Streptococcus* (*Hepatology* 8:171, 1988). In suspected cases, empiric antibiotic therapy with a third-generation cephalosporin (ceftriaxone or cefotaxime) should be instituted. Aminoglycosides should be avoided, as they do not achieve adequate levels in ascitic fluid, are inactivated at an acid pH, and may precipitate renal failure. A repeat paracentesis should be performed 48–72 hours after initiation of therapy if no organism is grown or clinical deterioration on appropriate therapy is observed.

IV. **Portal hypertension** is a significant complication of cirrhosis typically manifest by gastrointestinal bleeding and hypersplenism. Gastrointestinal bleeding is usually due to varices or congested mucosa (see Chap. 14). Splenomegaly is usually associated with thrombocytopenia in advanced cases; occasionally, leukopenia or pancytopenia is seen.

V. **Coagulopathy** occurs as a result of impaired synthetic function in the liver, particularly vitamin K–dependent coagulation factors. Usually, patients have only a prolonged PT; in far-advanced disease, PTT may also be affected. The appropriate replacement for vitamin K deficiency is 5–10 mg PO qd, or 10 mg SQ qd (for patients unable to absorb oral vitamin K or for hospitalized patients).

VI. **Impaired drug clearance** can be a problem in chronic liver disease because the liver, along with the kidneys, is the primary organ involved in drug metabolism and excretion. In addition, drug availability may be increased in liver disease due to the presence of portal-systemic shunts or to decreased levels of drug binding to plasma proteins (e.g., albumin). In most cases, medication can be used safely in patients with liver disease, provided that (1) drug dosages are reduced when a medication that undergoes significant hepatic excretion or metabolism is used, (2) patients are followed closely for signs of toxicity and, when available, serum or blood levels are monitored, (3) alternative agents that do not undergo significant hepatic excretion or metabolism are used when available, and (4) drugs associated with the development of chronic liver disease are avoided.

Hepatic Transplantation

Hepatic transplantation is now the accepted therapy for irreversible fulminant hepatic failure and for complications of end-stage chronic liver disease. Timing of liver transplantation is complex. Patients with fulminant hepatic failure should be considered for transplantation if signs of advanced encephalopathy (stage III or IV), marked coagulopathy (PT > 20 seconds), or hypoglycemia are present. Patients with chronic liver disease should be considered for transplantation when complications, including refractory ascites, spontaneous bacterial peritonitis, encephalopathy, variceal bleeding, or severe impairment of synthetic function with coagulopathy or hypoalbuminemia, occur (*Ann. Intern. Med.* 104:377, 1986).

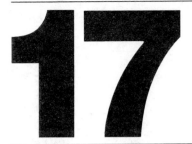

Disorders of Hemostasis

Steven R. Lentz

Evaluation of Hemostatic Function

I. **Regulation of hemostasis.** The integrity of blood vessels is maintained through a complex series of interactions between the vascular endothelium, subendothelial macromolecules, platelets, and plasma coagulation factors. Disruption of the normal balance between procoagulant and anticoagulant activities may result in hemorrhagic or thrombotic disorders.

A. **Primary hemostasis.** During the initial response to vessel injury, platelets adhere to the subendothelial matrix in a reaction that requires von Willebrand factor. Platelets subsequently aggregate to form a hemostatic plug and promote vasoconstriction through the release of thromboxane A_2.

B. **The coagulation cascade** (Fig. 17-1). Efficient activation of the coagulation cascade requires calcium, protein cofactors (factors Va, VIIIa, and tissue factor), and negatively charged phospholipid surfaces, which are provided by platelets at sites of primary hemostasis. Formation of a fibrin clot occurs when thrombin is generated from prothrombin. In addition to cleaving fibrinogen, thrombin provides positive feedback by activating factors V and VIII, as well as the fibrin cross-linking enzyme, factor XIII. The extrinsic pathway may be initiated by the exposure of blood to tissue factor, a membrane protein present in most extravascular tissues but normally absent from blood cells and intact endothelium. The pathologic expression of tissue factor may play a role in some cases of disseminated intravascular coagulation (DIC) (*N. Engl. J. Med.* 322:1622, 1990). The molecular events that trigger the intrinsic pathway are poorly understood. Although deficiencies of factor XII, prekallikrein, and high–molecular weight kininogen cause prolongation of the activated partial thromboplastin time (aPTT) in vitro, these deficiencies are not associated with clinical bleeding. In contrast, all of the other components of the intrinsic, extrinsic, and common pathways are required for normal hemostasis.

C. **Fibrinolysis** (Fig. 17-2). Fibrin is degraded by the proteolytic enzyme plasmin, which is generated selectively from fibrin-bound plasminogen by the action of tissue plasminogen activator (tPA). Plasminogen may also be activated by the administration of urokinase, a urinary tract enzyme, or streptokinase, a nonenzymatic activator produced by beta-hemolytic streptococci. Circulating alpha$_2$-antiplasmin and plasminogen activator inhibitors serve to limit fibrinolysis and prevent systemic fibrinogen degradation. Soluble fibrin degradation products (FDPs) produced by the action of plasmin on fibrin or fibrinogen can bind to fibrin monomers and inhibit coagulation.

D. **Natural anticoagulants** serve to restrict the coagulation process to sites of vascular injury and protect normal vessels from thrombosis.

1. **Prostacyclin (PGI$_2$)** synthesized by endothelial cells inhibits platelet aggregation and promotes vasodilation.

2. **Antithrombin III** inhibits thrombin and factors IXa, Xa, and XIa by forming irreversible complexes with these proteases. The inhibitory reaction is accelerated by endothelial surface proteoglycans or by exogenously administered heparin.

3. **Thrombomodulin,** a protein expressed on the luminal surface of endothelium,

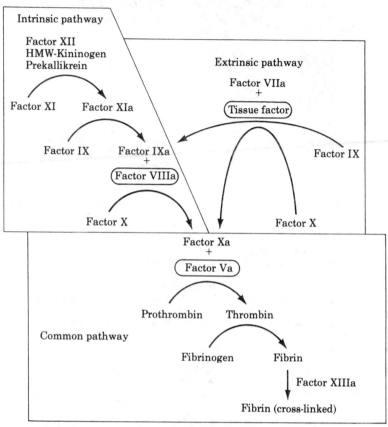

Fig. 17-1. Blood coagulation cascade. Plasma zymogens are sequentially converted to active proteases as depicted by the arrows. Nonenzymatic protein cofactors (*ovals*) are required at several stages of the cascade. Factors IX, X, and prothrombin are activated on phospholipid surfaces. Thrombin cleaves fibrinogen, yielding fibrin monomers that polymerize to form a clot. (HMW = high molecular weight.)

directly inhibits the procoagulant activities of thrombin and accelerates the activation of protein C by thrombin. In the presence of the cofactor protein S, activated protein C specifically degrades factors Va and VIIIa, resulting in further inhibition of coagulation.

II. **History and physical examination.** The cause of abnormal bleeding or thrombosis is often suggested by a careful history. Platelet abnormalities often lead to petechiae, ecchymoses at sites of minor trauma, and prolonged bleeding from superficial lacerations. A coagulation factor deficiency is suggested by the delayed appearance of hemarthroses or deep hematomas. Details of previous bleeding episodes, including duration and severity of bleeding, requirement for blood transfusions, and response to hemostatic stress (e.g., dental extractions, trauma, pregnancy, major and minor surgery), should be obtained. All recent prescription and nonprescription medications, including ethanol, aspirin or other nonsteroidal anti-inflammatory drugs (NSAIDs), oral contraceptives, and anticoagulants, should be identified. Any family history of bleeding or thrombosis should be thoroughly documented. Physical examination should include a careful inspection of the skin, oral mucosa, and joints and a search for evidence of liver disease, uremia, malnutrition, or malignancy.

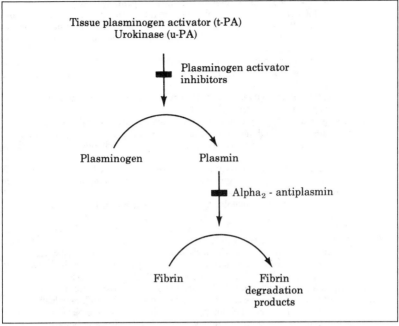

Fig. 17-2. Fibrinolysis. The protease plasmin is generated enzymatically from fibrin-bound plasminogen by tissue plasminogen activator, or independent of fibrin by urokinase. The bacterial cofactor streptokinase forms a nonenzymatic complex with plasminogen, resulting in the conversion of additional plasminogen to plasmin. Plasmin degrades fibrin clots, generating fibrin degradation products. Plasminogen activation and fibrin degradation are inhibited by plasminogen activator inhibitors and alpha$_2$-antiplasmin, respectively.

III. **Laboratory evaluation.** Many hemostatic disorders can be defined precisely on the basis of laboratory studies. Screening tests, including platelet count, prothrombin time (PT), aPTT, and bleeding time, are useful in evaluating patients with abnormal bleeding but may be normal in cases of mild platelet or coagulation factor disorders. None of these tests detect factor XIII deficiency, which can be established only by fibrin clot solubility assays. Therefore, additional evaluation is important in patients who have significant bleeding but normal screening tests.

A. **The peripheral blood smear** from all patients with abnormalities of hemostasis should be examined. Normally, about 10–20 platelets/oil-immersion field can be seen. However, smears prepared from finger sticks may exhibit an inhomogeneous platelet distribution. Quantitative or qualitative abnormalities of leukocytes or erythrocytes may suggest an underlying hematopoietic disorder. Fragmented erythrocytes suggesting microangiopathy are seen in thrombotic thrombocytopenic purpura (TTP), hemolytic uremic syndrome, and DIC.

B. **Evaluation of platelet function**

1. **The platelet count,** normally 150,000–400,000/μl, is determined as part of an automated blood count or by manual phase contrast microscopy. Pseudothrombocytopenia due to EDTA-induced platelet clumping is a rare artifact that can be excluded by careful examination of the peripheral blood smear or by repeating the platelet count on a citrated blood sample.

2. **The bleeding time** is a functional test of primary hemostasis. Normal values for the template bleeding time range from 2.5–9.5 minutes, but considerable individual variability can occur. The bleeding time may be

prolonged (> 10–15 minutes) in thrombocytopenia (platelet count less than 100,000/μl), qualitative platelet abnormalities, von Willebrand disease, and occasionally vascular disorders. Aspirin can prolong the bleeding time for up to 1 week after ingestion; other drugs may have transient effects (see Platelet Disorders, sec. **III**).

3. **Platelet aggregometry** is used primarily for the classification of congenital platelet disorders and is rarely helpful in the evaluation of acquired bleeding abnormalities.

C. **Evaluation of von Willebrand factor** (vWF) is appropriate when the bleeding time is prolonged, the platelet count is normal, and there is no apparent cause of acquired platelet dysfunction. vWF is synthesized by endothelial cells and megakaryocytes and forms multimers containing from 2 to more than 40 subunits. It is required for normal platelet adhesion and prolongs the half-life of factor VIII.

1. **Ristocetin cofactor** activity is based on the ability of ristocetin to enable vWF to interact with platelet glycoprotein Ib in vitro. It is reduced in most patients with von Willebrand disease.

2. **Ristocetin-induced platelet agglutination** is decreased in most types of von Willebrand disease except type IIB (see Inherited Bleeding Disorders, sec. **II.A**), in which agglutination occurs at very low concentrations of ristocetin.

3. **vWF antigen** (factor VIII–related antigen) can be measured by various immunoassays, and the size distribution of vWF multimers determined by crossed-immunoelectrophoresis or agarose gel electrophoresis. These tests are useful for the subclassification of von Willebrand disease.

D. **Evaluation of coagulation factor activity** is accomplished through functional assays that measure the time required for citrate-anticoagulated plasma to clot after the addition of calcium, phospholipids, and an appropriate activating agent. Clotting times can be prolonged by **factor deficiencies, heparin, FDPs, or acquired coagulation factor inhibitors.** The distinction between a coagulation factor deficiency and an acquired inhibitor can often be made by repeating the abnormal coagulation test using a 50:50 mixture of normal plasma with the patient's plasma (see sec. **III.D.7**). Improper collection or delay in processing of a blood sample can adversely affect the results of coagulation factor tests. Polycythemia can result in artifactually prolonged clotting times due to a disproportionately high ratio of anticoagulant to plasma in the sample.

1. **The prothrombin time (PT)** is the clotting time measured after addition of tissue thromboplastin (tissue factor and phospholipids) to recalcified plasma. The normal PT is approximately 11–14 seconds but may vary considerably. Therefore, a control PT using normal plasma should always be performed when determining the patient's PT. The PT measures the activity of the extrinsic and common pathways; it is most sensitive to deficiencies of factors VII and X but may also be prolonged in patients with deficiencies of factor V, prothrombin, or fibrinogen.

2. **The activated partial thromboplastin time (aPTT),** normally 22–36 seconds, is the clotting time measured after addition of phospholipid to recalcified plasma that has been preincubated with particulate material to initiate contact activation of the intrinsic pathway. Concentrations of factors VIII, IX, XI, or XII below 30% of normal are usually detected by prolongation of the aPTT.

3. **The thrombin time (TT)** is the time required for plasma to clot after the addition of thrombin. Normally 11–18 seconds, the TT may be prolonged in DIC, hypofibrinogenemia, or dysfibrinogenemia. Heparin also prolongs the TT but can be neutralized in the laboratory by the addition of protamine sulfate.

4. **Fibrinogen concentration** is frequently estimated from the clotting time of diluted plasma after addition of excess thrombin (Clauss method). This method may underestimate fibrinogen concentration in the presence of FDPs, paraproteins, or heparin. Therefore, hypofibrinogenemia (< 100 mg/dl) should be confirmed with an end-point turbidometric assay (Ellis method), which does not depend on the rate of fibrin polymerization.

5. **Fibrin degradation products (FDPs)** in serum are detected by agglutination of latex beads coated with antibodies to FDPs or fibrinogen. Increased levels of FDPs (> 8 μg/ml) occur in DIC, in thromboembolism, and during fibrinolytic therapy. Severe liver disease may cause mild elevation of FDPs, and a false-positive test may occur in patients with rheumatoid factor. The D-dimer test measures cross-linked FDPs and can help distinguish fibrinogenolytic from fibrinolytic processes.

6. **Individual factor** assays measure the ability of the patient's plasma to correct the clotting times of known factor-deficient plasmas. The results are expressed as a percentage of the activity in plasma pooled from normal donors. The normal range for coagulation factor activities is generally 60–160% but should be determined independently by each laboratory.

7. **Assays for acquired anticoagulants.** Prolongation of the PT or aPTT may be due to antibodies that inhibit coagulation factor activity. When an abnormal coagulation test is repeated using a 50:50 mixture of normal plasma with the patient's plasma, the clotting time will usually remain prolonged if an inhibitor is present but will correct to normal in the case of a coagulation factor deficiency. Less dilute mixtures of the patient's plasma with normal plasma may be required to detect inhibitors with weak affinity or those present in low concentration. Antibodies that react with certain individual coagulation factors (e.g., factors VIII or IX) are associated with abnormal bleeding. In contrast, **lupus anticoagulants** often predispose to arterial or venous thrombosis. Initially described in patients with systemic lupus erythematosus (SLE), these antibodies interfere with coagulation factor assays in vitro, probably by binding to phospholipids. The presence of a lupus anticoagulant can be confirmed by comparing the clotting time of the patient's plasma to control plasma in the presence of a dilute concentration of phospholipids. Assays for antibodies to cardiolipin are positive in some, but not all patients with lupus anticoagulants (*Semin. Thromb. Hemost.* 16:182, 1990).

Platelet Disorders

I. **Thrombocytopenia** is defined as a platelet count less than 150,000/μl. Although rare hereditary forms exist, most cases of thrombocytopenia are caused by acquired disorders. Thrombocytopenia can result from decreased platelet production, increased peripheral platelet destruction, or sequestration. This distinction is most reliably made by examination of a bone marrow aspirate, which normally contains 3–7 megakaryocytes/low-power field. Normal or increased numbers of megakaryocytes imply increased platelet destruction or sequestration; decreased numbers suggest decreased platelet production. In general, platelet counts in excess of 50,000/μl are not associated with significant bleeding, and severe spontaneous bleeding is unusual in patients with platelet counts higher than 20,000/μl in the absence of coagulation factor abnormalities or concomitant qualitative platelet dysfunction. All patients with thrombocytopenia should be instructed to avoid trauma and to seek early treatment if trauma occurs. **Intramuscular injections, rectal examinations and suppositories, and enemas should be avoided** if possible. Phlebotomy should be minimized, and pressure should be applied to venipuncture sites for 10 minutes. **Drugs known to inhibit platelet function (e.g., NSAIDs) should not be given.** Patients should be instructed not to use hard toothbrushes, dental floss, or metal razors. In acute thrombocytopenia, platelet transfusions are generally reserved for patients experiencing hemorrhage or anticipating major surgery. Prophylactic platelet transfusions may be of benefit in patients with chronic thrombocytopenic states such as aplastic anemia or chemotherapy-induced thrombocytopenia (see Chap. 18).

A. **Drug-induced thrombocytopenia** is diagnosed by noting temporal relationships between drug administration and the onset of thrombocytopenia. Decreased platelet production has been associated with thiazide diuretics, ethanol, estrogens, trimethoprim-sulfamethoxazole, and chemotherapeutic agents. Increased platelet destruction, presumably through immune mechanisms, can occur in patients receiving quinine, quinidine, heparin, gold salts, rifampin, or sulfonamides. Many other drugs have been implicated as rare causes of thrombocytopenia (Williams, et al., *Hematology* [4th ed.]. New York: McGraw-Hill, 1990. P. 1370). **All nonessential drugs should be discontinued in patients with thrombocytopenia of undetermined etiology.** Structurally unrelated drugs may be substituted when necessary. Thrombocytopenia usually resolves within days of discontinuing the offending drug but in some cases can persist for months because of slow excretion of the drug (e.g., gold). Prednisone, 1 mg/kg PO qd, may decrease the duration of thrombocytopenia in some cases. Platelet transfusions are often ineffective but should be administered in cases of profound drug-induced thrombocytopenia associated with serious hemorrhage.

B. **Autoimmune thrombocytopenia** results from accelerated platelet destruction mediated by antiplatelet antibodies. Most cases arise in previously healthy patients as idiopathic thrombocytopenic purpura (ITP), but similar syndromes occur in association with SLE, chronic lymphocytic leukemia, or lymphoma. Clinical manifestations include severe thrombocytopenia (platelet counts below 50,000/μl in most patients), normal erythrocyte and leukocyte morphology, and a normal or increased number of bone marrow megakaryocytes. Platelet-associated IgG can be detected in greater than 90% of patients with ITP but may also be present in other thrombocytopenic states (*Blood* 76:859, 1990). **Acute ITP** usually occurs in children 1–2 weeks following a viral infection and usually resolves spontaneously within 6 months. **Chronic ITP,** which includes the majority of adult patients with ITP, is not usually associated with an obvious initiating event. Spontaneous remissions of chronic ITP are rare; however, complete or partial remissions in response to treatment with glucocorticoids or splenectomy occur in most patients.

1. **Glucocorticoids.** Prednisone, 1–2 mg/kg PO qd, or its equivalent, should be administered at the time of diagnosis and as initial therapy in relapsing disease. Selected patients with severe thrombocytopenia and active bleeding may benefit from initial treatment with methylprednisolone, 1 g IV qd for 3 days, followed by prednisone, 1–2 mg/kg PO qd. Two weeks of glucocorticoid therapy may be required before an increase in the platelet count is observed. The prednisone dosage should be slowly tapered when the platelet count becomes greater than 100,000/μl. A minority of patients ($<$ 25%) achieve a complete remission after glucocorticoid therapy alone.

2. **Splenectomy** should be considered in patients who (1) fail to respond to glucocorticoids, (2) develop serious glucocorticoid toxicity, or (3) develop recurrent thrombocytopenia when glucocorticoids are tapered. A rapid increase in the platelet count usually occurs after splenectomy and may be lifesaving in the setting of serious hemorrhage. Pneumococcal vaccine should be administered to all patients prior to splenectomy. Glucocorticoids should be continued following splenectomy until the platelet count returns to normal and then gradually tapered. At least two-thirds of patients with chronic ITP will achieve sustained remissions following splenectomy. Some patients who relapse following splenectomy have accessory spleens, which may be detected by a variety of radiographic techniques. Accessory splenectomy may produce remission in such patients.

3. **Immunosuppressive therapy** should be considered in patients who remain profoundly thrombocytopenic following splenectomy. **Vincristine,** 1–2 mg IV weekly for 4–6 weeks, or **cyclophosphamide,** 1–2 mg/kg PO qd for 2–3 months, occasionally produces prolonged improvement in the platelet count. Many patients with chronic thrombocytopenia do not have significant bleeding despite platelet counts below 30,000/μl, however, and chronic treatment with immunosuppressive agents is rarely justified.

4. **Danazol,** 200 mg PO tid, produces a gradual improvement in the platelet count in some patients with chronic ITP. Several months of therapy may be necessary before improvement occurs, and responses are less frequent in patients less than 45 years of age (*Ann. Intern. Med.* 111:723, 1989).

5. **Platelet transfusions** have limited utility in ITP due to rapid destruction of transfused platelets. However, transfusions may be given in the setting of life-threatening bleeding.

6. **Immune globulin,** 0.4 g/kg IV qd for 5 days, or 1 g/kg IV qd for 2 days, produces a rapid but temporary increase in the platelet count in many patients with chronic ITP and may prolong the survival of transfused platelets. Immune globulin should be reserved for patients with severe hemorrhage or those undergoing surgical procedures.

C. **Pregnancy-associated thrombocytopenia.** Gestational thrombocytopenia occurs in 5–10% of pregnancies, usually without significant maternal or fetal morbidity. However, infants born to women with chronic ITP may develop severe thrombocytopenia and have an increased risk of intracranial hemorrhage. Studies suggest that isolated thrombocytopenia diagnosed for the first time during pregnancy is not associated with significant fetal thrombocytopenia and may be treated conservatively (*N. Engl. J. Med.* 323:264, 1990). Women with a previous history of ITP may benefit from glucocorticoids or immune globulin prior to delivery. Cesarean section may be unnecessary if the fetal platelet count is determined to be greater than 50,000/μl.

D. **Human immunodeficiency virus (HIV)–associated thrombocytopenia.** Thrombocytopenia is a common finding in patients seropositive for HIV and may be the presenting manifestation of HIV infection. Isolated thrombocytopenia similar to chronic ITP is most frequently observed, but impaired thrombopoiesis, drug-induced thrombocytopenia, or thrombotic thrombocytopenic purpura (TTP) may also occur. Treatment of isolated HIV-associated thrombocytopenia is similar to treatment of chronic ITP (see sec. **I.B**), with more limited use of glucocorticoids and immunosuppressive therapy because of the underlying immune deficiency. Zidovudine (AZT) therapy (see Chap. 12) may improve the platelet count in some patients.

E. **Transfusion-associated thrombocytopenia.** Acute thrombocytopenia may follow massive transfusion or extracorporeal circulation, due to dilution or mechanical removal of platelets. The thrombocytopenia lasts 3–5 days and may be treated with platelet transfusions. Posttransfusion purpura is a rare type of immune thrombocytopenia that occurs primarily, although not exclusively, in multiparous Pl^{A1} antigen-negative women. Onset occurs approximately 7 days after a blood transfusion. The thrombocytopenia is usually severe and may be associated with intracranial hemorrhage. Plasma exchange by plasmapheresis, or immune globulin, 0.4 mg/kg IV daily for 5 days, may produce a rapid improvement in the platelet count in some patients. Platelet transfusions are contraindicated in posttransfusion purpura, and glucocorticoids are of questionable benefit.

F. **Thrombotic thrombocytopenic purpura (TTP)** is a rare syndrome characterized by thrombocytopenia, microangiopathic hemolytic anemia, and fluctuating neurologic abnormalities, often accompanied by fever and renal dysfunction. The diagnosis is supported by microangiopathic findings (e.g., fragmented erythrocytes) on the peripheral blood smear, elevation of the reticulocyte count and serum lactate dehydrogenase, and the absence of laboratory evidence for DIC. The demonstration of characteristic microvascular occlusions in biopsies of skin, gingiva, or other tissues lends further support but is not required to make an initial diagnosis and begin treatment in most cases. The adult **hemolytic-uremic syndrome (HUS)** is a closely related disorder in which renal failure is the predominant manifestation. Thrombotic microangiopathy may also occur in association with pregnancy, SLE, carcinoma, or certain infections (e.g., HIV, *Escherichia coli* gastroenteritis) or after high-dose chemotherapy or transplantation. **TTP should be viewed as a medical emergency** and therapy should be instituted promptly, since rapid neurologic deterioration and death may ensue. Platelet transfusions should be avoided because of the potential for accelerated thrombosis.

1. **Initial therapy** should include daily total plasma exchange by **plasmapheresis** (PP) with fresh frozen plasma (FFP) as the replacement fluid. If PP is not

available, FFP, 2 units IV q6h, should be given. Plasma therapy should continue until the platelet count has risen to greater than $100,000/\mu l$ and then be gradually discontinued. Prednisone, 1 mg/kg PO qd, or methylprednisolone, 1 mg/kg IV qd, is usually included in the initial therapy of TTP, although responses to glucocorticoids alone are rare. Aspirin, 325 mg PO qd, and dipyridamole, 75 mg PO q6h, are often started at the time of diagnosis or added after partial improvement in the platelet count has occurred. Despite their common usage, the effectiveness of these antiplatelet agents in TTP remains uncertain. Because relapses may occur up to several years after an initial episode of TTP, patients should be followed closely and plasma therapy reinstituted promptly if relapse occurs.

2. Refractory patients who do not achieve a prompt hematologic remission or who require prolonged plasma therapy may benefit from **vincristine**, 1–2 mg IV at weekly intervals, or **immune globulin**, 0.4 g/kg IV qd for 5 days. Occasional refractory patients have been reported to respond to splenectomy.

G. **Hypersplenism** results in inappropriate splenic sequestration and destruction of blood cells. It occurs most often in patients with hepatic cirrhosis and portal hypertension and less frequently in association with splenomegaly of other causes. Anemia or leukopenia may be present in addition to thrombocytopenia, which is rarely severe enough to cause serious bleeding. Because of the increased risk of operative mortality in these patients, splenectomy should be considered only in the setting of unmanageable hemorrhage.

H. **Other causes of thrombocytopenia** include DIC, nutritional deficiencies of folic acid or vitamin B_{12}, bone marrow infiltration due to myelophthisic disease (e.g., tuberculosis, metastatic carcinoma, myelofibrosis), primary hematopoietic disorders (e.g., leukemia, aplastic anemia, myelodysplasia, multiple myeloma, paroxysmal nocturnal hemoglobinuria), and various viral, bacterial, and rickettsial infections. Specific therapy is directed at the underlying disorder.

II. **Thrombocytosis**, defined as a platelet count greater than $400,000/\mu l$, may arise as either a primary or secondary disorder.

A. **Primary thrombocytosis** occurs in myeloproliferative disorders, including polycythemia vera, chronic myelogenous leukemia, and idiopathic myelofibrosis. Essential thrombocythemia (ET) is a myeloproliferative disorder in which the platelet count is typically above $1,000,000/\mu l$ and is associated with both thrombotic and hemorrhagic complications. Although the risk of thrombosis or bleeding correlates poorly with platelet count, patients with ET may benefit from treatment with **hydroxyurea**, 15 mg/kg PO qd, to lower the platelet count below $600,000/\mu l$ (*Cancer* 66:549, 1990). Intermittent painful erythema and cyanosis of the distal extremities, or erythromelalgia, may respond to aspirin, 325 mg PO qd, or hydroxyurea. Patients with diffuse hemorrhage, extreme thrombocytosis, and no other underlying coagulation abnormalities may benefit from **platelet pheresis** to lower the platelet count acutely.

B. **Secondary thrombocytosis** may occur in response to splenectomy, iron deficiency, carcinoma, or chronic inflammatory disorders. Platelet counts are occasionally greater than $1,000,000/\mu l$, but there is little risk of thrombosis or hemorrhage, and specific treatment is usually unnecessary.

III. **Qualitative platelet disorders.** Congenital platelet disorders may produce a prolonged bleeding time and hemorrhage. In the majority of patients, however, abnormal platelet function results from acquired disorders, including uremia, liver disease, cardiopulmonary bypass surgery, paraproteinemia, myeloproliferative disorders, and drugs, especially aspirin, other NSAIDs, and certain beta-lactam antibiotics (*N. Engl. J. Med.* 324:27, 1991). Therapy is primarily directed toward the underlying disease. Patients with uremia may respond to hemodialysis.

A. **Desmopressin acetate** transiently shortens the bleeding time in many patients with acquired platelet dysfunction. It is administered in a single dose, 0.3 μg/kg IV or SQ, prior to surgical procedures.

B. **Conjugated estrogen**, 0.6 mg/kg IV qd for 5 days, may produce a more durable improvement in the bleeding time in some patients.

C. **Cryoprecipitate**, 1–2 bags/10 kg IV, may also improve hemostatic function in these patients, but its use is associated with the potential risk of viral transmission (see Inherited Bleeding Disorders, sec. **I.A.2**).

D. Platelet transfusions should be given during episodes of severe bleeding.

IV. **Vascular purpura** occurring in the setting of normal platelet function and normal coagulation studies may result from chronic glucocorticoid therapy, purpura simplex, senile purpura, Cushing's syndrome, connective tissue diseases, scurvy, cryoglobulinemia, multiple myeloma, amyloidosis, allergic purpura, certain infections, or factitious purpura. Therapy is directed toward the underlying condition.

Inherited Bleeding Disorders

I. **Hemophilia.** Inherited deficiencies of factors VIII (hemophilia A) and IX (hemophilia B) are X-linked disorders with similar clinical presentations. Severely affected patients with less than 1% of normal factor VIII or IX activity have frequent spontaneous hemarthroses and other bleeding. In moderate hemophilia (1–5% of normal activity), bleeding is usually associated with known trauma, but occasional spontaneous hemorrhage can occur. Patients with mild hemophilia (5–40% of normal activity) rarely experience hemorrhage in the absence of severe trauma or surgery; these patients may remain undiagnosed until adulthood. Patients with hemophilia characteristically have a prolonged aPTT, normal PT, and normal bleeding time. Hemorrhagic episodes are generally managed by factor replacement therapy, which should be instituted as early as possible to minimize long-term complications. Aspirin or NSAID-containing medications should not be administered to patients with hemophilia.

A. **Factor replacement therapy.** The dosage of replacement therapy is determined by the nature of the bleeding episode and the type of hemophilia. One unit of a coagulation factor is defined as the amount present in 1 ml of fresh plasma pooled from normal donors. Since the plasma volume can be estimated as approximately 50 ml/kg body weight, the following formula can be used to calculate the replacement dose of factor VIII needed to achieve a desired plasma concentration (expressed as % of normal):

Dose (units) = (desired % activity − initial % activity) × (weight in kg)/2

Because factor IX appears to have a significant extravascular distribution, the dose required to produce a desired plasma concentration is approximately *twice* that predicted by the formula. Treatment of patients with hemophilia requires an understanding of the potential infectious complications of factor replacement therapy. Prior to the routine use of viral inactivation procedures in the preparation of coagulation factor concentrates, more than 80% of patients with severe hemophilia became seropositive for hepatitis viruses B and C and for HIV. Donor screening, heat and chemical treatments, and immunoaffinity purification have markedly reduced, but not completely eliminated, the risks of viral transmission from currently used concentrates (*Blood* 73:2067, 1989; *J.A.M.A.* 261:3434, 1989). The development of recombinant coagulation factor concentrates may further reduce these risks.

1. **Fresh-frozen plasma (FFP)** contains all the coagulation factors in nearly normal concentrations. FFP can be used to treat patients with mild factor IX deficiency who require infrequent therapy; however, because FFP is not treated with viral inactivation procedures, prothrombin-complex concentrate is the preferred therapy for most patients with hemophilia B.

2. **Cryoprecipitate** contains factor VIII, vWF, and fibrinogen. The concentration of factor VIII is approximately 100 units/bag, so several bags must be pooled to obtain therapeutic levels of factor VIII in patients with hemophilia A. Each bag of cryoprecipitate is derived from a single donor and is not treated to inactivate viruses. Therefore, the use of cryoprecipitate is associated with a substantial risk of viral transmission.

3. **Lyophilized factor VIII** concentrate is purified from plasma pooled from 2,000–30,000 donors. In addition to factor VIII, variable amounts of functional vWF are present. All currently available factor VIII concentrates are viral inactivated, and recombinant preparations are being developed (*N. Engl. J. Med.* 323:1800, 1990). Factor VIII concentrate is the preferred therapy for most patients with severe hemophilia A.

4. **Prothrombin-complex concentrate** contains prothrombin, factor X, and factor IX, as well as variable amounts of factor VII. Prothrombin-complex concentrates are now heat treated, and the potential risks of viral transmission are similar to those for factor VIII concentrates. Prothrombin-complex concentrates are occasionally associated with thromboembolism or DIC, presumably due to the presence of activated coagulation factors. Prothrombin-complex concentrates should never be given by prolonged continuous infusion, and concurrent use of antifibrinolytic agents (e.g., epsilon-aminocaproic acid) should be avoided. Prothrombin-complex concentrates are used to treat patients with hemophilia B and patients with acquired antibodies to factors VIII or IX (see sec. **I.D**).

B. **Treatment of factor VIII deficiency** is governed by the severity of hemophilia A and the clinical indication.

1. **Minor bleeding,** such as superficial abrasions and ecchymoses, is managed with local measures and usually does not require factor replacement therapy. Desmopressin acetate, 0.3 μg/kg IV, increases the level of factor VIII up to fourfold in many patients with mild or moderate hemophilia A. This dose of desmopressin may be repeated at 12- to 24-hour intervals, although tachyphylaxis may occur (*Blood* 74:1997, 1989). Control of hemorrhagic episodes and preparation for surgery in patients with mild hemophilia A can sometimes be accomplished with this agent alone. Desmopressin cannot substitute for factor replacement therapy in patients with life-threatening bleeding or severe factor VIII deficiency.

2. **Major bleeding,** including complicated hemarthroses, expanding soft-tissue hematomas, and gastrointestinal hemorrhage, can be treated by giving a dose of factor VIII concentrate calculated to achieve a factor VIII activity approximately 50% of normal (see sec. **I.A**). The same dose should then be repeated q12h for 2–4 days. Life-threatening hemorrhage, potential airway obstruction, and major surgery require a dose of factor VIII that will achieve approximately 100% of the normal activity, followed by administration of one-half the initial dose q8h for 1–2 days. This dose should be continued q12h until 3–5 days after cessation of bleeding. Any head trauma serious enough to require medical attention should be treated with a 100% replacement dose of factor VIII, regardless of neurologic findings.

3. **Epsilon-aminocaproic acid** (EACA), an inhibitor of fibrinolysis, can be used to help control mucous membrane bleeding (e.g., from dental surgery) in patients with hemophilia A. EACA, 50–100 mg/kg PO q6h, is administered on the day prior to surgery and for 3–5 days afterward (maximum dosage 24 g/day) in conjunction with a single 50% replacement dose of factor VIII concentrate immediately prior to the procedure. **EACA should not be used in patients with hematuria or prior to infusion of prothrombin-complex concentrate.**

C. **Treatment of factor IX deficiency** is similar to that of factor VIII deficiency. Factor IX has a longer half-life (about 24 hours) than factor VIII (about 12 hours); therefore, the appropriate dosage interval for factor IX is 18–24 hours. Minor bleeding episodes may be treated with **FFP**, but severe bleeding should be treated with **prothrombin-complex concentrate.** Desmopressin is ineffective in hemophilia B.

D. **Inhibitory antibodies** to factors VIII or IX develop in 5–10% of patients with hemophilia A and in approximately 1% of patients with hemophilia B. Rare patients without a history of hemophilia may also acquire inhibitory antibodies (see Acquired Coagulation Factor Disorders, sec. **IV**). Patients with low inhibitor titers (< 10 Bethesda units/ml) can often be treated with factor VIII concentrate or prothrombin-complex concentrate but require higher doses than usual. In many patients, termed high-responders, the inhibitor titer rises dramatically after exposure to exogenous coagulation factors; such patients should not be treated with factor concentrates for episodes of minor bleeding. Hemorrhage in patients with high titers of factor VIII inhibitors is often difficult to treat but may respond to massive doses of factor VIII concentrate, prothrombin-complex concentrate, activated prothrombin-complex concentrate, or porcine factor VIII. Alternative approaches include extracorporeal immunoabsorption, plasmapheresis, and recombinant factor VIIa (*Blood* 75:1069, 1990). Reduction in the inhibitor titer may be achieved in some patients by frequent regular infusions of small doses of factor VIII (*Prog. Hemost. Thromb.* 9:57, 1989).

E. Hemarthrosis is the most frequently encountered problem in the adult patient with hemophilia. The duration of an episode and subsequent joint deformity may be minimized by prompt initiation of factor replacement therapy and immobilization of the joint for 2–3 days. Arthrocentesis should be considered only if (1) severe pain and swelling are present, (2) a postinfusion factor VIII or IX level is in the desired range, and (3) the affected joint is easily accessible.

II. von Willebrand disease (vWD) is an inherited autosomal disorder characterized by a prolonged bleeding time, decreased ristocetin cofactor activity, and a variable decrease in coagulation factor VIII activity that may be associated with prolongation of the aPTT. The clinical manifestations are similar to those of platelet dysfunction, although a patient with markedly decreased factor VIII activity may present with a hematoma or hemarthrosis.

A. Classification. Several subtypes of vWD are distinguished based on laboratory evaluation of the structure and activity of plasma vWF (see Evaluation of Hemostatic Function, sec. **III.C**). Patients with type I vWD, which accounts for approximately 70% of vWD, typically have mild decreases in ristocetin cofactor and factor VIII activities and a normal vWF multimer pattern. Type II vWD results from selective deficiency of the high–molecular weight multimers of vWF, due to qualitative abnormalities in the protein. In type IIB vWD, the interaction between vWF and platelets is enhanced, and accelerated clearance of platelet aggregates may result in thrombocytopenia. Patients with type III vWD have severe quantitative deficiencies of vWF, often resulting in clinically significant reduction in factor VIII activity.

B. Treatment. In general, bleeding episodes in patients with vWD are more easily controlled than those in patients with hemophilia. The choice of therapy depends on the type of vWD and the clinical setting.

1. **Desmopressin acetate** may be effective in patients with mild or moderate vWD (usually type I). Dosage and administration of desmopressin in vWD are the same as in factor VIII deficiency (see sec. **I.B.1**). **Desmopressin is contraindicated in patients with type IIB vWD** because of the potential for exacerbating thrombocytopenia. For this reason, the subtype of vWD should be established prior to the administration of desmopressin.

2. **Cryoprecipitate.** When replacement therapy is required, cryoprecipitate is the preferred blood product in all types of vWF. An infusion of 1–2 bags of cryoprecipitate/10 kg of body weight will usually produce prompt normalization of the factor VIII coagulant activity and bleeding time. A single infusion is sufficient to control most minor bleeding episodes; the infusion should be repeated q12–24 hours if bleeding continues. Treatment should be continued for 5–10 days following major surgery or trauma. Factor VIII concentrates contain variable amounts of functional vWF and are not reliable for the treatment of vWD.

III. Other inherited coagulation factor deficiencies. Patients with hemophilia A, hemophilia B, and vWD constitute more than 90% of all patients with severe inherited bleeding disorders. Deficiencies of other coagulation factors should be considered in patients with abnormal bleeding that is not explained by the more common hereditary or acquired coagulation disorders. In factor XI deficiency, bleeding is usually mild, but extensive postoperative hemorrhage can occur.

Treatment with FFP to achieve a factor XI level 30% of normal is adequate for normal hemostasis in most patients.

Acquired Coagulation Factor Disorders

I. **Vitamin K deficiency.** Vitamin K is a necessary cofactor for the hepatic gamma-carboxylation of certain glutamate residues in coagulation factors VII, IX, X, prothrombin, protein C, and protein S. The noncarboxylated forms of these proteins are inactive; thus, vitamin K deficiency results in abnormal blood coagulation and bleeding. The PT is usually prolonged but corrects to normal when a 50:50 mixture of normal plasma with the patient's plasma is used (see Evaluation of Hemostatic Function, sec. III.D.7). Conditions associated with vitamin K deficiency include biliary obstruction, malabsorption syndromes, antibiotic therapy, nutritional deficiency, and warfarin ingestion. Hospitalized patients who are unable to eat and are receiving antibiotics that suppress intestinal flora may become vitamin K deficient in 1–2 weeks without supplementation.

A. **Vitamin K preparations** include vitamin K_1 (phytonadione) and synthetic water-soluble derivatives of vitamin K_3 that require hepatic activation. Hospitalized patients at risk for the development of vitamin K deficiency should receive prophylactic treatment with either vitamin K_1 or vitamin K_3, 10 mg PO or SQ 3 times weekly. Mild deficiency can usually be corrected by administration of vitamin K_1 or synthetic vitamin K_3, 10–15 mg SQ or IV qd for 1–3 days. Severe deficiency due to overdosage of warfarin or other oral anticoagulants requires treatment with parenteral vitamin K_1 (see Antithrombotic Therapy, sec. I.C.3). Intravenous administration of vitamin K has been associated with anaphylaxis in rare patients; therefore, it should be given in a closely monitored setting.

B. **FFP,** 4 units IV, should be administered to patients with serious hemorrhage. Additional FFP, 2 units IV q8–12h, should be given if bleeding persists and the PT remains prolonged.

II. **Coagulopathies associated with liver disease.** Severe liver disease causes decreased synthesis of fibrinogen, prothrombin, and factors V, VII, IX, X, and XI. Acquired dysfibrinogenemia may result from the synthesis of abnormally glycosylated fibrinogen, and FDPs may be elevated because of reduced hepatic clearance. Thrombocytopenia due to hypersplenism may complicate the hemostatic defect. Bleeding in a patient with liver disease presents a difficult therapeutic problem. Empiric therapy with parenteral vitamin K_1, 10–15 mg SQ or IV qd for 3 days, may be administered, although the majority of patients will not respond. Replacement therapy with FFP will often transiently improve hemostatic function, and platelet transfusions may be considered if thrombocytopenia is present.

III. **Disseminated intravascular coagulation (DIC)** is the consequence of intravascular activation of both the coagulation and fibrinolytic systems. Laboratory findings in DIC often include thrombocytopenia, hypofibrinogenemia, increased FDPs, and prolongation of the TT and aPTT. Microangiopathic hemolysis may also occur. DIC varies greatly in clinical severity and may present with a predominance of either bleeding or thrombosis (microvascular or venous). DIC is often associated with malignant neoplasms (e.g., carcinoma of the prostate, lung, or other organs), infections (e.g., gram-negative sepsis, meningococcemia, Rocky Mountain spotted fever, certain viral infections), acute leukemia (especially promyelocytic leukemia), liver disease, snakebites, obstetric complications, connective tissue diseases, massive trauma, extensive burns, or shock. **Treatment of the underlying condition is the major therapeutic approach to DIC.** Supportive therapy is directed toward preventing hemodynamic compromise and hypoxemia. Both anticoagulant and factor replacement therapy are potentially dangerous in the setting of DIC and should be considered only if serious hemorrhagic or thrombotic complications are present. Platelet transfusions and infusions of FFP or cryoprecipitate may be given if bleeding is the major complication. Heparin may be beneficial in some patients;

however, its effectiveness remains largely unproved. When given for DIC, heparin should be initiated at a low dosage (e.g., 500 units/hour by continuous IV infusion) that may be slowly increased. The desired outcome is cessation of bleeding, increases in the plasma fibrinogen concentration and platelet count, and a decrease in FDPs. The utility of prophylactic heparin therapy during induction chemotherapy for acute promyelocytic leukemia is controversial (*Br. J. Haematol.* 68:283, 1988; *Blood* 75:2112, 1990).

IV. **Acquired anticoagulants** are substances, usually antibodies, that inhibit the function of specific coagulation factors, frequently factors VIII or IX, but occasionally factors V, XI, XIII, or vWF. The presence of an acquired anticoagulant should be suspected when a prolonged PT or aPTT fails to correct to normal with a 50:50 mixture of the patient's plasma with normal plasma (see Evaluation of Hemostatic Function, sec. **III.D.7**). Inhibitory antibodies may arise in patients with preexisting coagulation factor deficiencies, or in association with pregnancy, collagen-vascular diseases, or lymphoproliferative disorders. Rarely, inhibitors develop spontaneously in previously healthy patients or are induced by certain drugs, such as penicillins, sulfonamides, phenytoin, or isoniazid. Treatment of acute bleeding in patients with inhibitors of factors VIII or IX has been discussed (see Inherited Bleeding Disorders, sec. **I.D**). Immunosuppressive therapy with cyclophosphamide, vincristine, and prednisone may be effective in refractory patients (*Ann. Intern. Med.* 110:774, 1989). Acquired vWD may result either from the presence of circulating inhibitors of vWF activity or from rapid antibody-induced clearance of vWF. Lupus anticoagulants are antibodies that nonspecifically interfere with phospholipid-dependent coagulation assays but are associated with thrombosis, not bleeding (see Thromboembolic Disorders, sec. **I.B**).

Thromboembolic Disorders

I. **Predisposing conditions.** Although most cases of thromboembolic disease are idiopathic, several clinical conditions have been associated with an increased risk of thrombosis.
   A. **Inherited deficiencies of antithrombin III, protein C, and protein S** are found more frequently in patients with recurrent thrombosis than in the general population. However, many patients with reduced plasma levels of these proteins do not have a significantly increased risk for thromboembolism (*Semin. Thromb. Hemost.* 16:158, 1990). Laboratory assays for antithrombin III, protein C, and protein S may be unreliable in patients with acute thrombosis, liver disease, or DIC, in pregnancy, and during anticoagulant therapy. In general, the nature and duration of therapy in patients with thromboembolism are primarily determined by the clinical presentation (see sec. **IV.B.2**) and are unlikely to be altered by the identification of an inherited disorder. Therefore, screening for these disorders should probably be limited to patients with recurrent thromboembolism, unusual sites of thrombosis (e.g., axillary, mesenteric, or cerebral veins), or a positive family history of thromboembolism. Patients with antithrombin III deficiency who have a positive personal or family history of thrombosis should receive prophylactic low-dose heparin during pregnancy. Replacement therapy with antithrombin III concentrate may be considered for patients with known inherited antithrombin III deficiency in the setting of acute thrombosis, trauma, or surgery. Asymptomatic individuals with protein C or protein S deficiency are unlikely to benefit from chronic prophylactic antithrombotic therapy.
   B. **Lupus anticoagulants** occur in patients with SLE or other immunologic disorders, in patients with infections (e.g., HIV), or in association with certain drugs (e.g., chlorpromazine, procainamide, hydralazine). A subset of patients with lupus anticoagulants appear to have an increased risk for arterial and venous thrombosis and recurrent spontaneous abortions.
   C. **Other clinical conditions** that may predispose patients to thromboembolism include pregnancy, malignancy, immobilization, congestive heart failure, and

Table 17-1. Relative contraindications to anticoagulant therapy

Active bleeding (e.g., active peptic ulcer disease)
Bleeding tendency (e.g., hemophilia, thrombocytopenia)
Uncontrolled hypertension
Cerebrovascular hemorrhage
Recent surgery or invasive procedures (e.g., arterial or lumbar puncture)
Pericarditis or pericardial effusion
Severe trauma
Pregnancy (contraindications primarily relate to warfarin)
Patients prone to falling (e.g., elderly or debilitated patients)
Inadequate laboratory facilities
Unsatisfactory patient compliance

cigarette smoking. Thrombosis in patients with nephrotic syndrome may be related in part to acquired antithrombin III deficiency.

II. **Prophylactic therapy** for asymptomatic patients may be effective in preventing thrombosis in certain high-risk situations. Low-dose heparin, 5,000 units SQ q12h, has been shown to reduce the incidence of venous thrombosis in patients with acute myocardial infarction or congestive heart failure and may benefit patients undergoing major surgery or prolonged immobilization. Relative contraindications to heparin therapy should be taken into consideration (Table 17-1). Prophylactic warfarin therapy is appropriate for all patients with mechanical prosthetic heart valves and certain patients with valvular heart disease or atrial fibrillation (*Chest* 95[suppl.]:37S, 1989). Intermittent pneumatic leg compression may reduce thrombotic complications associated with certain surgical procedures.

III. **Acute arterial occlusion** is an urgent medical situation that necessitates early recognition and institution of treatment. Arterial occlusions frequently result from embolization of left atrial or ventricular thrombi or from atherosclerotic emboli arising in proximal arteries. Paradoxical arterial embolization from a venous thrombus can occur via an atrial septal defect or patent foramen ovale. Physical findings suggestive of peripheral arterial occlusion include an absent or diminished pulse and coolness or pain in an extremity. In addition to full-dose anticoagulation with **heparin** (see Antithrombotic Therapy, sec. **I.B.1**), most peripheral arterial thrombi require prompt **surgical embolectomy or angioplasty. Fibrinolytic therapy** should be considered in patients with surgically inaccessible peripheral arterial occlusions or early acute myocardial infarction (see Chap. 5).

IV. **Venous thrombosis** is a frequent occurrence in both ambulatory and hospitalized patients.

A. **Superficial thrombophlebitis** poses little risk for embolism and is generally controlled by supportive measures consisting of local heat, elevation of the affected extremity, and rest. Anti-inflammatory agents such as aspirin may also be given.

B. **Deep venous thrombosis (DVT)** presents a more difficult diagnostic and therapeutic problem and is associated with a significant risk of pulmonary embolism.

1. **Diagnosis.** Because clinical findings are notoriously unreliable in DVT, the diagnosis should always be established by an objective invasive or noninvasive test. Contrast **venography** remains the most reliable technique for the detection of DVT but is associated with postvenography phlebitis in 5–10% of patients (*Radiology* 165:113, 1987). **Impedance plethysmography** is a noninvasive technique with high sensitivity and specificity in the diagnosis of obstruction of the proximal veins (i.e., iliac, femoral, and popliteal), particularly in ambulatory patients (*Surg. Clin. North Am.* 70:143, 1990). **Realtime (duplex) ultrasonography** appears to be the most accurate noninvasive method for the diagnosis of proximal DVT but is less reliable in detecting

isolated calf vein thrombi (*Arch. Intern. Med.* 149:1731, 1989). Negative noninvasive studies should either be confirmed by contrast venography or repeated serially several times during the next 10–14 days. Contrast venography should be performed when the results of noninvasive testing are equivocal.

2. **Treatment.** Thrombosis confined to the calf veins carries a low risk of embolization, and anticoagulation therapy is usually unnecessary. However, approximately 20% of untreated calf vein thrombi eventually extend into the proximal veins. Therefore, noninvasive testing should be repeated 2–3 days after diagnosis and several additional times during the following 2 weeks if anticoagulation therapy is withheld. In general, patients with proximal DVT detected by either invasive or noninvasive methods should receive supportive measures (see sec. **IV.A**) plus anticoagulation with heparin, preferably administered by continuous IV infusion (see Antithrombotic Therapy, sec. **I.B.1**). Heparin should be continued until 48 hours after the PT reaches a therapeutic value (see Antithrombotic Therapy, sec. **I.C.1**), or for a minimum of 5 days (*N. Engl. J. Med.* 322:1260, 1990). Oral anticoagulation with warfarin should be started on day 1–3 of heparin therapy and continued for 3–6 months, depending on the estimated risks of recurrent thrombosis and hemorrhage in each individual patient. Adjusted-dose subcutaneous heparin is an effective alternative to warfarin for chronic anticoagulation during pregnancy or in situations in which close monitoring is impractical (*Ann. Intern. Med.* 107:441, 1987). Fibrinolytic therapy may accelerate thrombus dissolution, resulting in a reduction in the incidence of postphlebitic syndrome. However, because of uncertain long-term benefits and the increased risk of hemorrhagic complications, fibrinolytic agents are not recommended for routine use in patients with acute DVT (*Arch. Intern. Med.* 149:1841, 1989). Patients with recurrent DVT should receive warfarin therapy for an extended period of time, probably indefinitely (*Prog. Hemost. Thromb.* 9:1, 1989). Chronic anticoagulation with adjusted-dose subcutaneous heparin is occasionally required to prevent recurrent DVT in patients refractory to warfarin. Such patients often have an underlying malignancy or other predisposition to thrombosis.

C. **Pulmonary embolism (PE)** is a serious complication of DVT. The diagnosis and therapy of PE are discussed in Chapter 10.

Antithrombotic Therapy

I. **Anticoagulants.** The decision to use an anticoagulant always involves weighing the risk of anticoagulant-induced bleeding against the risk of thrombosis or embolism if therapy is withheld. Prior to the initiation of anticoagulant therapy, patients must be screened for the presence of relative contraindications to therapy (Table 17-1) because the failure to detect such contraindications could result in fatal hemorrhage. The final decision to utilize anticoagulant therapy must always be individualized.

A. **Precautions.** Patients receiving anticoagulants should be advised to report any signs of bleeding. Invasive procedures and intramuscular injections should be minimized and NSAID-containing medications avoided. It is advisable to measure the hematocrit periodically and to examine the stool for occult blood. If manifestations of bleeding are present, the PT, aPTT, hematocrit, and platelet count should be promptly determined. Bleeding that occurs in the setting of therapeutic anticoagulation may suggest a localized lesion (e.g., occult carcinoma) and should prompt further diagnostic evaluation.

B. **Heparin** is a naturally occurring glycosaminoglycan that acts by potentiating the activity of antithrombin III. Heparin is administered parenterally and produces immediate prolongation of the TT, the aPTT, and to a lesser extent, the PT. The half-life of heparin in the circulation is approximately 60–90 minutes but is prolonged in patients with severe liver disease. Heparin does not cross the placenta.

1. **Administration.** Heparin therapy is initiated with a loading dose of 5000 units IV as a bolus injection, followed by 1,000–2,000 units/hour delivered by continuous IV infusion. A convenient preparation consists of 25,000 units of heparin in 500 ml of D5W or normal saline; the amount of **heparin should not exceed 25,000 units/bag of IV fluid,** since mechanical pump failure during infusion could lead to massive overdosage. The aPTT should be measured prior to starting heparin therapy and q4–6h during adjustment of the infusion rate. A clotting time of 1.5–2.0 times the control aPTT (generally between 50–80 seconds) is considered therapeutic. In most patients, this can be achieved with infusion rates of 800–1600 units/hour. When given by adjusted-dose subcutaneous administration, the heparin dosage is adjusted to achieve a mid-dose aPTT (measured 6 hours after administration) of 1.5–2.0 times the control value. A dosage of 7,500–15,000 units SQ q12h is usually necessary to achieve this degree of anticoagulation.

2. **Heparin-associated thrombocytopenia.** Mild thrombocytopenia commonly occurs in patients 2–10 days after the initiation of heparin therapy; the platelet count usually remains greater than 100,000/µl, and heparin can be continued. Less frequently, severe thrombocytopenia apparently mediated by an immune mechanism occurs 6–14 days after starting intravenous or subcutaneous heparin therapy; patients who have been previously treated with heparin may develop severe thrombocytopenia within hours to days of re-exposure. Paradoxically, the severe form of heparin-associated thrombocytopenia may be associated with arterial thrombosis. Periodic platelet counts should be obtained in all patients on heparin therapy and heparin discontinued if severe thrombocytopenia occurs. Because of the potential for arterial thrombosis, platelet transfusions should be reserved for patients with serious bleeding (*Annu. Rev. Med.* 40:31, 1989).

3. **Reversal of heparin** anticoagulation generally occurs within hours after cessation of heparin infusion. In the rare instances in which anticoagulation must be reversed more rapidly, protamine sulfate can be given to neutralize heparin. Protamine sulfate should be administered by slow intravenous injection, in doses of no more than 50 mg over a 10-minute period. The dosage is calculated according to the estimated amount of heparin circulating at the time of administration of protamine sulfate. One milligram of protamine sulfate will neutralize approximately 100 units of heparin. If given 30–60 minutes after a bolus injection of heparin, approximately 0.5 mg of protamine sulfate will be required for every 100 units of heparin. If heparin is administered by continuous IV infusion, the dose of protamine sulfate should be calculated to neutralize approximately half of the preceding hourly dose of heparin. No more than 100 mg of protamine sulfate should be given except in extreme circumstances. The effect of protamine sulfate should be monitored by determining the aPTT immediately after administration. Rare life-threatening anaphylactic reactions to protamine sulfate may occur, particularly in diabetic patients receiving protamine-insulin preparations (*N. Engl. J. Med.* 320:886, 1989).

C. **Warfarin** interferes with hepatic vitamin K–dependent carboxylation (see Acquired Coagulation Disorders, sec. I). Although the onset of anticoagulation is less rapid than that produced by heparin, warfarin is more convenient for chronic outpatient therapy. After initiation of warfarin therapy, vitamin K–dependent clotting factor activities will decline with approximately the following half-lives: factor VII, 6 hours; factor IX, 24 hours; and factor X and prothrombin, 48 hours. The PT will usually become prolonged in less than 48 hours due to depletion of factor VII, but several more days of therapy may be required before therapeutic anticoagulation occurs. **Warfarin crosses the placenta and may produce fetal death.**

1. **Administration** is usually initiated with warfarin sodium, 10 mg PO qd for 2 days; subsequent daily doses are adjusted until the PT stabilizes in the

Table 17-2. Partial list of agents that interact with warfarin

Potentiate anticoagulation (increase prothrombin time)	Antagonize anticoagulation (decrease prothrombin time)
Alcohol*	Alcohol*
Allopurinol	Antacids
Amiodarone	Barbiturates
Anabolic steroids	Cholestyramine
Chloramphenicol	Glucocorticoids
Cimetidine	Griseofulvin
Clofibrate	Haloperidol
Levothyroxine	Oral contraceptives
Methyldopa	Ranitidine*
Metronidazole	Rifampin
Nonsteroidal anti-inflammatory drugs	
Phenytoin	
Phenothiazines	
Propylthiouracil	
Ranitidine*	
Quinidine	
Sulfonamides	
Sulfonylureas	
Tamoxifen	
Tricyclic antidepressants	

* May cause increased or decreased PT.

therapeutic range. The PT reflects the warfarin dose given 24–48 hours earlier. Because of variability in the PT, an international normalized ratio (INR) has been developed for standardization of warfarin anticoagulation. For most indications, an INR of 2.0–3.0, which usually corresponds to a PT value of 1.3–1.5 times control, is considered to be therapeutic (*Chest* 95[suppl.]:37S, 1989). In patients with mechanical prosthetic heart valves, a PT of 1.5 times control should be maintained (*N. Engl. J. Med.* 322:428, 1990). The required maintenance dosage is subject to wide individual variation but usually ranges from 2–15 mg PO qd. Once stabilization of the dosage has been achieved, the PT should be determined approximately every 2 weeks. In the setting of poor patient compliance, the PT should be determined more frequently.

2. **Drug interactions and toxicity.** Maintenance of warfarin anticoagulation may be affected by the dietary intake or absorption of vitamin K or by alterations in warfarin degradation by the liver. Certain drugs displace warfarin from albumin and thus increase its anticoagulant effect; other drugs induce hepatic microsomal enzymes, decreasing warfarin activity (Table 17-2). Any condition that affects liver function or the availability of vitamin K (e.g., alterations in intestinal bacteria or food intake) can affect hemostatic balance and may lead to fatal hemorrhagic or thrombotic complications. Therefore, medication or dietary changes should be accompanied by frequent PT determinations and the dosage of warfarin adjusted accordingly. Warfarin skin necrosis is an extremely rare complication in which a cutaneous microvascular thrombotic process develops 3–10 days after starting warfarin therapy. Several cases have been reported in patients with protein C deficiency (*Semin. Thromb. Hemost.* 16:169, 1990).

3. **Reversal of warfarin anticoagulation.** The PT will gradually return to normal several days following discontinuation of warfarin. This may be hastened by administration of vitamin K_1, 2.5–10.0 mg SQ or IV, which will usually return the PT to normal within 24 hours. Some patients may require a larger dose (e.g., 25–50 mg); this may make resumption of oral anticoagulation very difficult for several days thereafter. Intravenous vitamin K_1 should be administered slowly, at a rate not exceeding 1 mg/minute. Synthetic derivatives of vitamin K_3 (e.g., Synkayvite) are ineffective in reversing warfarin anticoagulation and should not be given. Patients with severe hemorrhage, who require immediate reversal of warfarin anticoagulation, should receive FFP, 2–4 units IV.

II. **Fibrinolytic therapy** with urokinase, streptokinase, or tPA may be indicated in selected patients with acute myocardial infarction, pulmonary embolism, proximal DVT, or peripheral arterial occlusion. Appropriate dosage and administration are determined by the specific indication and fibrinolytic agent used (*N. Engl. J. Med.* 318:1512, 1988). Contraindications to and use of fibrinolytic therapy in acute myocardial infarction and pulmonary embolism are discussed in Chaps. 5 and 10, respectively.

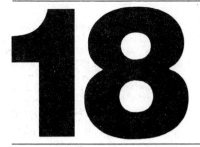

Anemia and Transfusion Therapy

David Gailani

Approach to the Anemic Patient

Anemia is a frequently encountered clinical condition that may be caused by a primary abnormality of the red blood cell (RBC) or bone marrow or may be a manifestation of an underlying systemic disorder. Anemia is defined as a decrease in the circulating RBC mass; the usual criteria are a hemoglobin (Hb) of less than 12 g/dl (hematocrit [Hct] < 36%) in women and less than 14 g/dl (Hct < 42%) in men.

I. **Clinical manifestations** of anemia vary depending on the etiology, degree, and rapidity of onset. Other underlying disorders such as cardiopulmonary disease contribute to the severity of symptoms. In general, patients with Hb less than 7 g/dl will have symptoms related to tissue hypoxia (fatigue, headache, dyspnea, light-headedness, angina). Pallor and compensatory tachycardia may signal severity. Even severe anemia may be well tolerated if it develops gradually.

II. **History and physical examination** are critical to the evaluation of the anemic patient because anemia is often an indicator of an underlying systemic process. One must look for a family history of anemia, drug exposure (including alcohol), or blood loss. Physical findings that aid in diagnosis include lymphadenopathy, hepatic or splenic enlargement, jaundice, bone tenderness, neurologic symptoms, and evidence of blood in the stool.

III. **Laboratory evaluation** is based on the Hb and Hct, reticulocyte count, mean corpuscular volume, and an examination of the peripheral blood smear.

A. **The hemoglobin (Hb) and hematocrit (Hct)** serve as an estimate of the RBC mass, but their interpretation must take into consideration the volume status of the patient. Immediately after acute blood loss, the Hb will be normal because compensatory mechanisms have not had time to restore normal plasma volume. In pregnancy, the Hb will be low despite a normal RBC mass due to an increase in plasma volume.

B. **The reticulocyte count** reflects the rate of production of RBCs and is an indicator of the bone marrow response to the anemia. The reticulocyte count is usually reported as reticulocytes/100 RBCs. The reticulocyte index (RI) corrects for the severity of the anemia and assesses the appropriateness of the bone marrow response.

$$RI = \frac{(\text{reticulocyte count} \times \text{patient Hct/normal Hct})}{2}$$

An RI greater than 2–3% indicates an adequate response, and a value less than this indicates that there is a hypoproliferative component to the anemia.

C. **The mean corpuscular volume (MCV)** is a measure of the average size of the RBCs and is often used in classifying anemia (microcytic, normocytic, and macrocytic for anemia with low, normal, and high MCV, respectively). The normal range for the MCV is 80–98 femtoliters. Proper use of the MCV in establishing a diagnosis depends on examination of the peripheral smear for the following reasons: (1) small and large cells may be present simultaneously, resulting in a normal MCV; (2) reticulocytes are larger than mature RBCs and will spuriously raise the MCV; and (3) abnormal cells may be present in numbers too small to affect the MCV.

The red cell distribution width (RDW) is a measure of anisocytosis (variation in RBC size) and may be useful in differentiating anemias sharing similar MCV ranges. For example, thalassemia and iron deficiency are both characterized by anemia with low MCV; the former usually has a normal RDW, while in the latter the RDW is often increased.

D. **Examination of the peripheral blood smear** is critical in evaluating the anemic patient. The smear must be free of preparative artifact. RBC morphology is best evaluated in a portion of the smear where the RBCs are just touching one another. Specific morphologic abnormalities (discussed under the individual anemias) should be sought as well as abnormalities in white blood cell and platelet morphology and number. Examination of the peripheral smear often reveals a single diagnosis or suggests a limited number of diagnoses, which may be investigated with specific tests.

E. **Special tests** to establish an exact diagnosis should be performed before administration of blood transfusions if possible.

IV. **Classification of anemias.** There are a number of classification schemes for the anemias. One such scheme is shown in Table 18-1. The RI determines which of the major categories the anemia falls into, and the MCV and peripheral smear further aid in establishing the diagnosis.

Anemia may be multifactorial in origin (e.g., alcoholism with gastrointestinal bleeding, nutritional deficiencies, and liver disease). A search for additional causes of anemia should be undertaken in a patient with a poor response to presumably adequate therapy or if a chronic stable anemia inexplicably worsens.

Management of Anemias Associated with Decreased RBC Production

A low reticulocyte index indicates either an underproduction of RBCs or ineffective erythropoiesis.

I. **Iron deficiency.** Iron deficiency is a common disorder. In the United States, 90% of cases occur in women. In the absence of menstrual bleeding, gastrointestinal blood loss is the presumed etiology in the adult patient; appropriate radiographic and endoscopic procedures should be performed to identify a source and to exclude occult malignancy. Decreased iron absorption (celiac disease, postgastrectomy) or increased iron requirements (pregnancy, lactation, infancy) can also lead to iron deficiency.

A. **History and physical examination.** Evidence for a source of blood loss (melena, menorrhagia) should be sought. In severe iron deficiency anemia, a history of pica (consumption of substances such as ice, starch, and clay) may be obtained. Splenomegaly is present in 5–10% of patients; koilonychia ("spoon nail") is a rare finding. Iron deficiency may also be associated with glossitis, dysphagia, and esophageal webs (Plummer-Vinson syndrome).

B. **Laboratory findings.** The MCV is usually normal in early iron deficiency. As the deficiency worsens, anisocytosis increases, hypochromic microcytic cells appear, followed by a decrease in the MCV and development of anemia. Other findings on the peripheral smear include "pencil cells" and occasional target cells. The platelet count may be increased. Diagnosis requires the documentation of low iron stores, which can be accomplished indirectly by measuring serum ferritin.

1. **A serum ferritin level** less than 12 µg/dl (normal 12–300 µg/dl) is indicative of low iron stores. Ferritin is an acute-phase reactant, and normal levels may be seen in inflammatory states, liver disease, or malignancy despite low iron stores. A ferritin level of greater than 200 µg/dl generally indicates adequate iron stores regardless of other underlying conditions. **Serum iron** is usually low (< 60 µg/dl) and **total iron binding capacity (TIBC)** is increased (> 360 µg/dl) in iron deficiency, but these values may fluctuate in a number of common clinical conditions and hence are less reliable indicators of iron stores.

Table 18-1. Classification of anemia based on red cell kinetics

I. Anemias associated with decreased RBC production (low reticulocyte index):
    A. Anemias with low mean corpuscular volume
        1. Iron deficiency
        2. Thalassemia
        3. Anemia of chronic disease
        4. Sideroblastic anemia
        5. Lead intoxication
    B. Anemias with high mean corpuscular volume
        1. Megaloblastic anemia
            a. Vitamin B_{12} deficiency
            b. Folic acid deficiency
            c. Drugs
        2. Alcoholism
        3. Myelodysplastic syndromes
        4. Hypothyroidism
    C. Anemias with normal mean corpuscular volume
        1. Aplastic anemia
        2. Anemia of chronic disease
        3. Anemia of chronic renal insufficiency
        4. Anemia associated with endocrine disorders
        5. Sideroblastic anemia
        6. Anemia associated with marrow infiltration (myelophthisis)

II. Anemia associated with increased RBC destruction (appropriate reticulocyte
        index):
    A. Bleeding
    B. Hereditary hemolytic anemias
        1. Hemoglobinopathies (e.g., sickle cell, HbSC disease)
        2. RBC enzyme deficiencies (e.g., glucose 6-phosphate dehydrogenase defi-
            ciency)
        3. RBC structural protein abnormalities (e.g., hereditary spherocytosis)
    C. Acquired hemolytic anemias
        1. Immune mediated
            a. Warm antibody
            b. Cold antibody
        2. Drug-induced
        3. Paroxysmal nocturnal hemoglobinuria
        4. Microangiopathic hemolytic anemia (MAHA)
        5. Traumatic hemolysis
        6. Liver disease
        7. Hypersplenism

---

    2. Erythrocyte protoporphyrin levels are generally increased in iron deficiency.

    3. Bone marrow biopsy with absent staining for iron is the definitive test for establishing iron deficiency but is rarely needed for diagnosis.

C. Therapy of iron deficiency anemia requires identifying the cause and repleting iron stores. The latter requires either oral or parenteral iron administration; normal dietary intake will only meet daily losses. With therapy, the reticulocyte count will peak in 5–10 days, and the Hb will rise over 1–2 months. The most common cause of poor response to therapy is noncompliance; other causes such as poor absorption, continued blood loss, or a multifactorial anemia must also be considered.

    1. Oral therapy with ferrous sulfate, 325 mg PO tid for 6 months, will usually correct the anemia and replace iron stores. Approximately 25% of patients will develop gastrointestinal side effects such as constipation, cramping, diarrhea, and nausea. These side effects can be decreased by initially administering the drug once a day or with meals. Ferrous gluconate and fumarate are alternative therapies. Sustained-release or enteric-coated preparations dissolve poorly and generally should not be recommended.

2. **Parenteral iron therapy** may be useful in patients with (1) very poor absorption (inflammatory bowel disease, malabsorption), (2) very high iron requirements that cannot be met with oral supplementation, or (3) intolerance of oral preparations. Parenteral iron will not generally correct anemia faster than oral preparations. Iron dextran (Imferon) is the preferred parenteral agent and may be administered intramuscularly or intravenously. The following formula may be used to calculate the amount required:

$$\text{Iron (mg)} = (\text{normal Hb} - \text{patient Hb}) \times \text{wt(kg)} \times 2.21 + 1000$$

This amount should restore RBC mass and provide 1,000 mg for iron stores. A typical dosing schedule is 1 ml (50 mg) IM in a large muscle on each side per day. The recommended intravenous dose is no more than 2 ml/day. The site of injection may be painful, and extravasation into subcutaneous tissue may cause staining of the skin; this can be avoided by injecting with a "Z" tract. "Total dose" intravenous infusion of iron dextran has been used without increased incidence of complications (*Int. J. Gynecol. Obstet.* 26:235, 1988). Intravenous administration may be complicated by phlebitis. Both intramuscular and intravenous therapy may rarely be complicated by anaphylaxis, and a 0.5-ml test dose should be administered prior to initiating therapy, with epinephrine and diphenhydramine readily available. Delayed reactions such as arthralgia, myalgia, fever, splenomegaly, and lymphadenopathy may rarely be seen 4–10 days after therapy.

II. **The megaloblastic anemias** are a group of disorders associated with altered morphology of bone marrow cells and other rapidly dividing cells due to abnormalities in DNA synthesis. While over 90% of cases are due to folic acid or vitamin B_{12} deficiency, drugs such as sulfa compounds, methotrexate, and hydroxyurea are causing an increasing number of cases. **Folic acid deficiency** may develop within a few months. Common causes include (1) decreased intake (alcoholism), (2) malabsorption, (3) oral contraceptives or anticonvulsant drugs, and (4) increased utilization (hemolytic anemia, pregnancy). **Vitamin B_{12} deficiency** takes years to develop because very little of the body's store is used each day. Causes of vitamin B_{12} deficiency include (1) pernicious anemia, (2) gastrectomy, (3) pancreatic insufficiency, (4) gastrointestinal bacterial overgrowth, (5) ileitis or ileal resection, and (6) intestinal parasites.

A. **History and physical examination.** Symptoms are primarily due to anemia, although glossitis, jaundice, and splenomegaly may be present. **Vitamin B_{12} deficiency** may cause decreased vibratory and positional sense, ataxia, paresthesias, confusion, and frank dementia. **Neurologic symptoms may occur in the absence of anemia and may not remit completely with treatment.**

B. **Laboratory.** The MCV and RDW are usually increased. Leukopenia and thrombocytopenia may occur. The peripheral smear may show anisocytosis, poikilocytosis, polymorphonuclear leukocytes with five or more nuclear lobes (hypersegmented), and macroovalocytes several months prior to the development of anemia. Serum lactate dehydrogenase (LDH) and bilirubin may be elevated, reflecting ineffective erythropoiesis.

1. **Serum vitamin B_{12} and folate levels** should both be measured. RBC folate may be a more accurate indicator of body folate stores than serum folate, particularly if folate therapy has been started. A vitamin B_{12} value (normal 200–900 pg/ml) of less than 100 pg/ml is almost always accompanied by clinical disease. Occasionally, symptomatic patients with values in the normal range will respond to therapy.

2. **Serum methylmalonic acid (MMA) and homocysteine** may be useful when the vitamin B_{12} or folate level is equivocal. Both MMA and homocysteine will be elevated in vitamin B_{12} deficiency; homocysteine will be elevated in folic acid deficiency.

3. **A Schilling test** may be useful in vitamin B_{12} deficiency to diagnose pernicious anemia.

4. **Bone marrow biopsy** may be necessary to rule out myelodysplastic syndromes and hematologic malignancy; these disorders may present with similar findings on peripheral smear.

C. **Therapy** is directed toward first identifying the underlying cause of the deficiency and then replacing the deficient factor.

1. **Folic acid** may be administered at 1 mg PO qd until the deficiency is corrected.

2. **Vitamin B$_{12}$** deficiency is corrected by administering cyanocobalamin. A typical schedule is 1,000 µg IM qd for 7 days, then weekly for 1–2 months. Long-term therapy is 1,000 µg/month.

   With therapy, the reticulocytosis should rise and peak in 1 week followed by a rising Hb over 6–8 weeks. Coexisting iron deficiency is present in one-third of patients and is a common cause for failure of therapy. **Megaloblastic anemia should not be treated empirically with folic acid** because the anemia of unrecognized vitamin B$_{12}$ deficiency may respond while the neurologic abnormalities progress.

III. **Anemia of chronic disease,** often seen in patients with inflammatory diseases, malignancies, autoimmune disorders, and chronic infections, usually develops a few months after the onset of disease. Abnormalities in mobilizing stored iron, inappropriately low erythropoietin levels, and decreased RBC survival have all been implicated in the pathogenesis.

A. **Laboratory.** A mild normocytic normochromic anemia is typical. The peripheral smear is usually normal, although microcytes may be seen.

1. **Serum iron and total iron binding capacity (TIBC)** are usually both decreased, with transferrin saturation greater than 10%.

2. **Ferritin** is usually normal but may be elevated, since it is an acute-phase reactant.

B. **Treatment** is directed at the underlying cause and at prevention of exacerbating factors such as nutritional deficiencies and marrow suppressive drugs. Erythropoietin is being investigated for use in the anemias of malignancy and inflammatory diseases.

IV. **Anemia of chronic renal insufficiency** results primarily from decreased erythropoietin production. Nutritional deficiencies, blood loss, hemolysis, and "uremic toxins" may also contribute.

A. **Laboratory.** The Hb is usually 5–8 g/dl. MCV is normal. The peripheral smear shows normocytic, normochromic cells with echinocytes (burr cells). The polymorphonuclear leukocytes may have hypersegmented nuclei.

B. **Treatment** of anemia of chronic renal insufficiency has been revolutionized by the availability of recombinant human erythropoietin (*Semin. Dialysis* 3:112, 1990). Therapy is indicated in both predialysis and end-stage patients who are symptomatic. Symptoms that respond to erythropoietin are fatigue, poor appetite, coldness, disordered sleep patterns, depression, and sexual disinterest. Patients with baseline Hct greater than 30% are less likely to benefit from therapy.

1. **Administration** may be intravenous (hemodialysis patients) or subcutaneous (predialysis or peritoneal dialysis patients). The initial dosage needed to raise the Hct to 30% is usually 50–150 units/kg 3 times/week. The average dosage required to maintain the Hct is 75 units/kg 3 times/week, although 10% of patients will require up to 200 units/kg. It may be possible to give subcutaneous therapy once a week. Iron deficiency and inflammatory processes may decrease the efficacy.

2. **Adverse effects associated with erythropoietin therapy**

a. **Iron deficiency** may occur due to the mobilization of large amounts of iron. Patients with pretherapy ferritin levels less than 100 µg/dl are at increased risk. Dietary supplementation with ferrous sulfate, 325 mg tid, is recommended. Intravenous iron dextran has also been used to supplement or restore iron stores.

b. **Hypertension** may develop or worsen when the Hct rises, particularly in patients with initial Hct below 20%. Twenty-five percent of patients require new or increased medication for hypertension. Seizures have been reported with erythropoietin therapy, often in association with the rise in Hct and blood pressure.

V. The thalassemias are inherited disorders characterized by underproduction of either the alpha or beta chains of the hemoglobin molecule. Individuals of Mediterranean, Middle Eastern, Indian, Chinese, and Southeast Asian descent are most commonly affected. In beta-thalassemia, there is a reduced production of beta-globin chains without a concomitant decrease in alpha-globin production. The excess alpha-globin chains form insoluble tetramers in the RBCs, causing membrane damage, ineffective erythropoiesis, and hemolytic anemia. In alpha-thalassemia, the beta tetramers that form are more soluble, and thus the clinical severity is milder.

A. Classification. Thalassemias have been classified by the degree of anemia, by associated symptoms, and by the abnormalities in the globin genes (there are four alpha- and two beta-globin genes in a normal cell).

1. **Thalassemia trait** is caused by decreased function of one or two alpha- or one beta-globin genes. Patients are asymptomatic with a mild hypochromic, microcytic anemia (Hb > 10 g/dl).

2. **Thalassemia intermedia** is associated with moderate dysfunction of three alpha-globin genes (Hb H disease) or both beta-globin genes. Clinical severity is intermediate (Hb 5–8 g/dl), and patients are usually not transfusion dependent.

3. **Thalassemia major** is caused by severe dysfunction of both beta-globin genes. Anemia is severe, and transfusions are required to sustain life. A loss of all four alpha-globin genes causes hydrops fetalis.

B. History and physical examination. A family history of anemia is the most important piece of information. Splenomegaly and bone abnormalities due to the expanded marrow are common in thalassemia major.

C. Laboratory. The MCV is low, and the RDW is normal. Microcytic, hypochromic cells with variation in shape (poikilocytosis), as well as target cells and nucleated RBCs may be present on the peripheral smear. Hb electrophoresis aids in diagnosis. **In thalassemia trait, the most important consideration is to avoid the incorrect diagnosis of iron deficiency anemia.**

D. Treatment is centered on transfusions adequate to sustain life, improve exercise tolerance, and prevent skeletal abnormalities. In severe thalassemia, the transfusions required will result in tissue iron overload. This may cause congestive heart failure, hepatic dysfunction, glucose intolerance, and secondary hypogonadism due to desposition of iron in the hypothalamus. Iron chelation therapy with deferoxamine mesylate may prevent these complications (see sec. **V.D.3**).

1. **Transfusions.** A Hb of 8 g/dl prevents skeletal deformities and can usually be achieved with 1 unit of packed RBCs every 2–3 weeks or 2 units every month. Transfusion-dependent patients should receive **packed RBCs** through a leukocyte filter (see Transfusion Therapy).

2. **Splenectomy** removes the primary site of extravascular hemolysis. It should not be performed before the age of 5–6 years because of the risk of sepsis. Pneumococcal vaccine should be administered 1 month before surgery. Patients should be advised to seek prompt medical attention for fevers and should have ampicillin, 250-mg tablets, for use when medical care is delayed. **Asplenic patients with fever should be treated with intravenous broad-spectrum antibiotics until culture results are obtained.**

3. **Iron chelation therapy** with deferoxamine mesylate (Desferal) is administered by continuous subcutaneous infusion for several hours a day. If started by about the age of 5 years, it helps prevent the complications of iron overload. It is uncertain whether deferoxamine can prevent death from cardiac hemochromatosis if started in adults. Therapy may be complicated by local irritation at the injection site, and pruritus and hypotension may occur if it is infused too rapidly. Long-term side effects, particularly with high-dose therapy, include optic neuropathy and sensorineural hearing loss. Patients

receiving deferoxamine should be followed at a center where thalassemics are regularly treated.

4. **Nutritional supplementation** with vitamin C increases iron excretion during chelation therapy. Large doses may cause massive release of iron, precipitating congestive heart failure, and should be avoided. Vitamin C, 100 mg PO, should be given 30 minutes after initiation of the deferoxamine infusion. Folic acid, 1 mg/day, and vitamin E, 200 units/day, are also recommended.

VI. **Refractory anemia** may be associated with the myelodysplastic syndromes (MDSs) or with myelofibrosis. Presentations range from mildly decreased peripheral blood counts without symptoms to severe pancytopenia. Progression to marrow failure or acute leukemia may occur. The MDSs are classified according to findings on bone marrow biopsy: (1) refractory anemia (RA), (2) RA with ringed sideroblasts (see sec. **VII**), (3) RA with excess blasts (RAEB), (4) RAEB in transformation, and (5) chronic myelomonocytic leukemia. MDS may be idiopathic or secondary to radiation, chemotherapy, or toxin exposure. Myelofibrosis may be idiopathic or occur in the setting of polycythemia vera, essential thrombocythemia, chronic myelogenous leukemia, or marrow invasion by carcinoma. Therapy is largely supportive, although in patients with a good prognosis, iron chelation therapy with deferoxamine mesylate should be considered after 50–100 units of packed RBCs have been transfused.

VII. **Sideroblastic anemias** are a heterogeneous group of disorders characterized by abnormal RBC iron metabolism. Sideroblastic anemias may be acquired or hereditary. Acquired sideroblastic anemia may be due to drugs (isoniazid, chloramphenicol, chemotherapy, alcohol), lead exposure, or neoplastic, endocrine, or inflammatory diseases. The acquired idiopathic disorder is considered a myelodysplastic syndrome.

A. **Laboratory.** Marked anisocytosis and poikilocytosis may be seen in the congenital and idiopathic forms. The peripheral smear may show two populations of RBCs (one normocytic and one microcytic); however, the MCV is usually normal or slightly elevated (MCV may be low in the congenital form). Basophilic stippling is usually present. Serum iron and transferrin are normal or elevated. Diagnosis is established by demonstrating increased or abnormal sideroblasts on iron stain of bone marrow.

B. **Therapy** is supportive. Myelosuppressive drugs should be stopped, and nutritional deficiencies should be corrected. Chronically transfused patients may require iron chelation.

1. **Pyridoxine,** 50–200 mg PO qd, may be tried empirically, although the response rate is low.

2. **Androgens** may rarely stimulate RBC production.

VIII. **Aplastic anemia** is usually an abnormality of bone marrow stem cells and is associated with leukopenia and thrombocytopenia. Most cases are idiopathic, although 10% are associated with toxic exposure (butazones, gold, anticonvulsants, chlorpromazine, chloramphenicol) and another 10% with viral illnesses (e.g., hepatitis, Epstein-Barr virus, cytomegalovirus). Twenty percent of patients with paroxysmal nocturnal hemoglobinuria will develop aplastic anemia. Presenting symptoms are usually related to anemia or thrombocytopenia, although some patients present with fever and leukopenia.

A. **Laboratory.** The red cell indices are normocytic. Bone marrow biopsy is necessary to demonstrate aplasia and to rule out myelodysplasia, leukemia, or infiltration with tumor or granulomas. Cytogenetic studies may also be useful.

B. **Therapy** is supportive. Potentially offending drugs should be discontinued and compounding factors corrected.

1. **Early referral** to a center experienced in managing aplastic anemia is recommended. In individuals less than 30–35 years of age, bone marrow transplantation has achieved a success rate of 80%.

2. **Transfusions** with packed RBCs and platelets to keep Hb at 7–8 g/dl and the platelet count above 10–20,000/μl are the usual recommendations. Transfusion with blood products from family members should be avoided if bone marrow transplantation is anticipated. RBCs should be given through leukocyte filters to prevent sensitization against HLA antigens.

3. **Infection.** Patients should be instructed to seek medical attention immediately in the event of fever over 38°C. When the neutrophil count is less than 500 PMNs/μl, some authors recommend prophylactic antibiotics.

Management of Anemias Associated with Increased RBC Destruction

Anemias associated with an adequate response by the bone marrow (i.e., an appropriate reticulocyte index) are due to bleeding or destruction of RBCs (hemolysis) that exceeds the capacity of the bone marrow to correct the Hct. **Bleeding is much more common than hemolysis.** The reticulocyte count will be elevated in both of these situations, although typically bilirubin and LDH will be normal in the bleeding patient and elevated in the patient with hemolysis. Hidden sites of bleeding (retroperitoneum, fractured hip) may result in laboratory findings that are similar to those seen in a hemolytic process. When an anemia associated with decreased RBC production, such as iron deficiency, is treated, the reticulocyte count may increase markedly prior to the correction of anemia and thus mimic a hemolytic anemia. All patients with suspected hemolysis should have a **direct Coombs' test** performed. This test detects the presence of IgG and the third component of complement (C3) on the surface of RBCs.

I. **Classification.** Hemolytic anemias can be classified by the predominant site of RBC destruction.
   A. **Intravascular hemolysis** may present with fever, chills, tachycardia, and backache. Serum haptoglobin levels will decrease as the protein binds with free hemoglobin. If hemolysis is severe, free hemoglobin may be measured in the plasma and urine. Renal failure may develop secondary to hemoglobinuria. Hemosiderin may be measured in the urine beginning 7 days after a hemolytic event.
   B. **Extravascular hemolysis** is characterized by RBC destruction in the reticuloendothelial system, primarily the spleen. Jaundice and splenomegaly may be present. Haptoglobin levels are normal or slightly reduced, and serum LDH may be elevated. Indirect hyperbilirubinemia may be present.

II. **Autoimmune hemolytic anemia (AHA)** is caused by antibodies to RBCs. In warm AHA, antibodies interact best with RBCs at 37°C, while in cold AHA, antibodies act best at lower temperatures. The direct Coombs' test is frequently positive in both forms of AHA.
   A. **Warm antibody autoimmune hemolytic anemia** is usually due to an IgG autoantibody. It may be idiopathic or associated with an underlying malignancy (lymphoma, chronic lymphocytic leukemia), collagen vascular disorder, drug use, or AIDS.
      1. **Clinical presentation** may include weakness, jaundice, and moderate splenomegaly. Severe hemolysis may be associated with fever, chest pain, syncope, and hemoglobinuria.
      2. **Laboratory** findings are those of extravascular hemolysis with a positive direct Coombs' test and decreased haptoglobin. The peripheral smear shows spherocytes.
      3. **Therapy** should be directed at the underlying cause. In some cases the hemolysis may need to be treated directly with glucocorticoids and/or splenectomy.
         a. **Glucocorticoids** are the initial treatment of choice. Prednisone, 1.0–1.5 mg/kg/day PO, is administered until the Hct stabilizes and then is tapered over 3–4 months. Up to 80% of patients will respond, but relapses are common. In severe cases, hydrocortisone, 100 mg IV q8h, may be used initially.
         b. **Splenectomy** is indicated in patients who do not respond to glucocorticoids or who require prolonged high doses. It is successful in 60% of patients

who have failed prednisone. Even if splenectomy does not normalize the Hct, it may reduce the glucocorticoid requirement.

   c. **Cytotoxic therapy** with azathioprine (125 mg/day) or cyclophosphamide (100 mg/day) with or without prednisone may produce responses in 40–50% of refractory patients. Vincristine and the androgen danazol have been used with occasional success.

   d. **Intravenous IgG** at 0.5–1.0 g/kg/day for 5 days may produce a sustained response in some patients.

   e. **Transfusions** may occasionally be necessary in severe hemolysis. The conventional cross-matching procedure will not be possible because the warm antibody is a panagglutinin. The major risk in this situation is failing to detect RBC alloantibodies, which may precipitate a transfusion reaction (see Transfusion Therapy).

B. **Cold antibody autoimmune hemolytic anemia** is associated with episodic cold-induced intra- or extravascular hemolysis and vasoocclusive events resulting in cyanosis of the ears, nose, and digits. Two general syndromes have been described:

   1. **Cold agglutinin disease** may be due to an idiopathic paraprotein or secondary to mycoplasma infection, mononucleosis, or lymphoma. IgM and C3 are found on the RBCs (the direct Coombs' test usually shows only the presence of C3).

   2. **Paroxysmal cold hemoglobinuria** is a rare disorder that may be idiopathic or associated with acute viral infections (mumps, measles) or tertiary syphilis. Avoidance of cold temperatures is of prime importance, and any transfused blood should be heated to 37°C to prevent exacerbation of hemolysis.

III. **Drug-induced hemolytic anemia** may be caused by several mechanisms. Treatment consists of discontinuing the offending agent.

A. **Drug-induced autoimmune hemolytic anemia** presents similarly to warm antibody AHA. Methyldopa is the most common cause. Up to 20% of patients taking this drug have a positive direct Coombs' test, and 1% have hemolytic anemia. A positive Coombs' test without hemolysis is not a contraindication to methyldopa use. Anemia usually resolves within a few weeks of stopping the drug.

B. **Haptens.** Penicillin (or other related antimicrobials) coats RBCs. If antibodies against penicillin are present and the patient receives the drug (particularly with high doses, i.e., 10–30 million units/day) a Coombs'-positive hemolytic anemia may result.

C. **Immune complexes.** IgM (occasionally IgG) antibodies may develop against drugs such as quinine, isoniazid, and phenacetin and form drug-antibody complexes that adhere to RBCs. Since the antibody involved is usually an IgM, the Coombs' test will be positive only for C3.

IV. **Sickle cell anemia** and other sickling syndromes are associated with structurally abnormal hemoglobin molecules that polymerize under reduced oxygen conditions. This results in deformed RBCs that increase blood viscosity and occlude the microcirculation. Eight percent of American blacks are heterozygous for sickle cell hemoglobin (HbAS), and 2–3% are heterozygous for HbC (HbAC). Sickle cell syndromes are associated with the homozygous HbS condition (HbSS) or with double heterozygous conditions (HbS–beta thalassemia, HbSC, HbSD).

A. **Clinical manifestations** vary widely. Signs of disease usually develop in infancy or childhood. Delayed growth and development and increased susceptibility to infections are common. Patients with sickle cell trait (heterozygous for HbS) are usually asymptomatic but may have an increased risk of sudden death with rigorous exercise. Sickle cell anemia (homozygous HbSS) has a spectrum of manifestation from mild disease to frequent pain crises and life-threatening illness (see sec. **IV.C.2**).

B. **Laboratory.** The Hb ranges from 5–10 g/dl in sickle cell anemia (it is nearly normal in sickle cell trait), and the MCV is often slightly elevated due to the increased reticulocyte count. Indirect hyperbilirubinemia is common, and chronic neutrophilia (10,000–20,000/μl, which may rise to 30,000–40,000/μl during pain crisis) is often present. Platelets may be increased. The peripheral smear will show the classic distorted sickled erythrocytes. Howell-Jolly bodies may be seen due to functional asplenism, which usually occurs by the age of 10 years. Target cells may be present, particularly in HbSC disease. A Hb electrophoresis will distinguish homozygous disease from sickle cell trait or other abnormal hemoglobins.

C. **Treatment** must address both the acute and chronic complications of the disease. Hydroxyurea has been shown to increase levels of fetal hemoglobin and decrease hemolysis in patients with sickle cell anemia (*N. Engl. J. Med.* 322:1037, 1990). This therapy is considered experimental and should only be used in ongoing clinical trials.

1. **General measures**
   a. **Avoid dehydration and hypoxia,** which may precipitate or exacerbate sickling.
   b. **Folic acid,** 1 mg PO qd, should be administered to any patient with a chronic hemolytic anemia.
   c. **Infection prophylaxis** with penicillin VK, 125–250 mg PO qd, should be given to children between the ages of 3 months and 5 years because of their high risk of infection. After age 3, a polyvalent pneumococcal vaccine should be administered. Antibiotic prophylaxis does not appear to be effective in adults. **Fever should be treated promptly because of the increased risk of sepsis with encapsulated organisms in asplenic patients.**
   d. **Regular yearly ophthalmologic examinations** are recommended because of a high incidence of proliferative retinopathy and retinal infarction, particularly in patients with HbSC disease. Monocular blindness can frequently be prevented with laser therapy.
   e. **Transfusion therapy** is indicated in the following situations:
      (1) Aplastic crisis.
      (2) After a cerebrovascular accident (CVA) (*Blood* 63:162, 1984). There is a greater than 90% recurrence rate of CVA within 5 years of the primary event. Regular transfusions to keep the HbS concentration less than 50% for 5 years will reduce the chances of recurrent CVA.
      (3) Severe recurrent pain crises, refractory to conventional therapy, that require frequent hospitalizations.
      Transfusions have also been used in preparation for major surgery, to treat chronic leg ulcers, and in the acute chest syndrome. Up to 40% of patients with sickle cell anemia may develop alloantibodies to RBC antigens, which may cause transfusion reactions and make it difficult to obtain compatible blood (*N. Engl. J. Med.* 322:1617, 1990); therefore transfusions must be used judiciously.

2. **Treatment of crises**
   a. **Pain crises** are the most common manifestation of sickle cell anemia. Pain is usually in the back, ribs, and limbs. The pattern of pain is usually consistent in any one patient from crisis to crisis. A deviation from the pattern may suggest another complication such as cholecystitis. Fever is unusual initially in adults but may develop with time. Pulmonary infiltrates may be present. Precipitating factors such as an infection should be sought. Oral or intravenous fluid sufficient to ensure good hydration should be given. Adequate analgesia is necessary (narcotics are usually required). As symptoms improve, the analgesics should be switched from parenteral to oral agents. The majority of patients will not require significant amounts of analgesic therapy between crises, although narcotics may be required by some. **Blood transfusions will NOT change the immediate course of an acute pain crisis.**
   b. **Aplastic crisis** is generally associated with a viral illness, usually parvovirus B19. A sudden decrease in Hb and reticulocytes suggests this diagnosis. Transfusions are the mainstay of therapy. The majority of patients will recover in 10–14 days. Folic acid deficiency should be ruled out.
   c. **Sequestration crisis** refers to loss of blood into the spleen and is associated

with sudden splenomegaly, hypotension, and shock. Hemodynamic support is required. This event usually occurs in patients with an intact spleen such as small children or those with HbSC or HbS–beta thalassemia disease.

  d. **Acute chest syndrome** is associated with chest pain, pulmonary infiltrates, leukocytosis, and hypoxia. It may be difficult to distinguish this problem from pneumonia or pulmonary infarction. Initial management should include oxygen therapy to correct hypoxia and empiric coverage with antibiotics. Transfusion support may be useful.

3. **Special situations**
  a. **Pregnancy** in sickle cell disease is associated with an increased incidence of premature delivery and fetal death. Prophylactic transfusions do not appear to change the outcome of the pregnancy but do decrease the risk of pain crisis during pregnancy (*N. Engl. J. Med.* 319:1447, 1988).
  b. **Surgery. Measures to avoid volume depletion and hypoxia are critical.** For major surgery, transfusion to decrease the HbS level to less than 50% may help prevent crises, but this point is controversial.

4. **Complications**
  a. **Osteomyelitis** (which may be multifocal) occurs with increased frequency in sickle cell anemia. Therapy should be directed by biopsy cultures. *Staphylococcus* and *Streptococcus* are the most common pathogens, but there is an increased incidence of *Salmonella* osteomyelitis.
  b. **Leg ulcers** should be treated with rest, leg elevation, and intensive local care. In cases where healing is poor, chronic transfusions, split-thickness skin grafts, or skin flap procedures may be necessary.
  c. **Priapism** may respond to rehydration; however, decompressive surgery may be necessary. Permanent impotence can occur.
  d. **Cholelithiasis,** primarily with bilirubin stones, is present in over 50% of patients. Cholecystitis usually requires cholecystectomy.
  e. **Other complications.** Renal tubular defects due to sickling in the anoxic hyperosmolar environment of the renal medulla lead to isosthenuria (the inability to concentrate urine) in sickle cell disease and trait. This predisposes patients to dehydration. Cardiomyopathy, pulmonary infarcts, and cerebral ischemic events occur more often. Aseptic necrosis of the femoral and humeral heads may cause significant mortality.

V. **Hereditary RBC structural protein abnormalities** may cause membrane defects that precipitate extravascular hemolysis. The classic example is **hereditary spherocytosis (HS),** which may be autosomal dominant or recessive. HS is associated with a microcytic anemia, splenomegaly, jaundice, cholelithiasis, and spherocytes on the peripheral smear. The **osmotic fragility test** is positive, and the direct Coombs' test is negative. If therapy is required, splenectomy will correct the anemia. Folic acid should be given chronically.

VI. **Hereditary RBC enzyme deficiencies** may be associated with chronic or episodic hemolysis. The most common disorder is **glucose 6-phosphate dehydrogenase (G-6PD) deficiency,** a sex-linked disorder that affects men of Mediterranean, African (about 10% of American blacks), and Chinese origin. The disease is rarely seen in women. The enzyme deficiency results in RBCs that are more susceptible to oxidant stress. Hemolytic episodes may be triggered by infections, drug exposure (particularly sulfonamides and quinine), or eating fava beans. The peripheral smear shows RBC inclusions called **Heinz bodies.** Diagnosis is based on measurements of enzyme levels. Senescent RBCs contain less G-6PD and are more easily destroyed. Thus, after a hemolytic episode, the G-6PD level may be normal, reflecting the younger population of cells in the circulation. Enzyme measurements should be made several weeks after a crisis, or the patient's family should be studied. Therapy consists of adequate hydration to protect renal function during hemolysis, avoidance of precipitating factors, and, if needed, transfusion.

Other enzyme deficiencies such as pyruvate kinase deficiency may cause hemolysis. Family history and measurement of enzyme levels will confirm the diagnosis.

VII. **Paroxysmal nocturnal hemoglobinuria (PNH)** is a rare acquired disorder of bone marrow stem cells characterized by intermittent episodes of intravascular hemolysis. Venous thromboses, particularly of the mesenteric, portal, and cerebral veins, are frequent and require anticoagulation. Twenty percent of patients with PNH will develop aplastic anemia. Diagnosis is made by a positive acid-hemolysis test (Ham test) or sucrose hemolysis test. Alternatively, **decay accelerating factor (DAF),** a membrane protein absent in PNH-affected cells, can be measured. Androgens (to stimulate erythropoiesis) and glucocorticoids (to decrease lysis) have been used. Iron replacement may be necessary to cover loss in the urine but may precipitate hemolysis. Transfusion of 2 units of packed RBCs prior to iron therapy may prevent hemolysis.

VIII. **Traumatic hemolytic anemia** refers to intravascular RBC destruction usually associated with a prosthetic aortic valve that is not functioning properly or that has developed a perivalvular leak. Porcine valves or valves in the mitral position are not as likely to cause significant hemolysis. This phenomenon has also been associated with synthetic arterial bypass grafts. The peripheral smear will show schistocytes and other RBC fragments (these findings may be present to a lesser degree in uncomplicated valve replacements). Plasma hemoglobin is increased, haptoglobin may be decreased or absent, and hemosiderinuria is usually present. Therapy involves correction of the mechanical abnormality.

IX. **Microangiopathic hemolytic anemia** is another syndrome of traumatic intravascular hemolysis, thought to be caused by deposition of fibrin strands in the lumen of small blood vessels. It may be seen in disseminated intravascular coagulation (DIC), thrombotic thrombocytopenic purpura (TTP), hemolytic-uremic syndrome (HUS), severe hypertension, vasculitis, eclampsia, and some disseminated malignancies. The peripheral smear will show fragmented RBCs (helmet cells, schistocytes) and may show thrombocytopenia. Management of DIC, TTP, and HUS is described in Chap. 17.

Transfusion Therapy

Advances in collection, preparation, and administration have allowed blood component transfusion to become useful in a wide variety of clinical situations. The administration of blood products exposes the patient to the risk of a number of adverse effects, some of which are life-threatening. The benefits and risks of transfusion therapy must be carefully weighed in each situation. This section will review the indications for transfusion of blood components as set forth by the National Blood Resources Education Program (NIH publication no. 89-2974a, 1989). These recommendations are meant to serve as guidelines. Certain clinical situations may necessitate deviation from these recommendations.

In each case, the need for transfusion must be carefully recorded in the medical record. It is generally agreed that, if possible, informed consent should be obtained for the administration of all blood products. In elective surgery, this may require informing the patient several weeks in advance of the procedure so that the options of autologous donation and directed donation may be explored.

I. **Indications for blood product transfusion**

A. **Red blood cell transfusion** is indicated to increase the oxygen-carrying capacity of blood in an anemic patient when the anemia is responsible for poor tissue oxygenation. Adequate tissue oxygenation can usually be attained with a Hb of 7–8 g/dl in a normovolemic patient. One unit of packed RBCs will increase the Hb by 1 g/dl (Hct 3%) in the average adult. Patient age, cause and severity of anemia, and coexisting disorders such as cardiopulmonary disease must be considered when determining the need for transfusion. If the cause of anemia is easily treatable (e.g., iron or folic acid deficiency), it is preferable to avoid transfusions. Red blood cells should not be used as volume expanders, to enhance wound healing, or to improve general "well-being" if symptoms are not related to anemia.

1. **The type and screen procedure** tests the recipient's RBCs for the A, B, and D (Rh) antigen and also screens the recipient's serum for antibodies against

other RBC antigens. This procedure allows the blood bank to respond rapidly when a blood product is required and allows for more efficient use of blood products than with cross-matching alone. Cross-matching tests the patient's serum for antibodies against antigens on the donor's RBCs and is performed prior to dispensing a specific unit of blood for a patient.

2. **Administration.** Patient and blood product identification procedures must be carefully followed, as clerical errors are the most common cause of transfusion reactions due to RBC incompatibility. The IV catheter should be at least 18-gauge to allow adequate flow. All blood products should be administered through a 170-μm filter to prevent infusion of macroaggregates, fibrin, and debris. Only 0.9% NaCl should be used with blood components to prevent cell lysis. Patients should be observed for the first 5–10 minutes of the transfusion for adverse side effects and at regular intervals thereafter.

3. **Chronically transfused patients** (e.g., thalassemia major, refractory anemia) should receive packed RBCs (not washed or frozen RBCs), as these units have the greatest RBC volume. The blood should be administered through a leukocyte filter, which decreases the incidence of alloimmunization and febrile reactions.

B. **Platelet transfusion** is indicated to control or prevent bleeding due to thrombocytopenia or platelet dysfunction. One unit of platelets should raise the platelet count at least 5,000/μl. Transfusion for chronic thrombocytopenia is probably not necessary in the absence of bleeding or other coagulation defects. Patients with temporary severe thrombocytopenia but normal platelet function (e.g., acute leukemia) may benefit from prophylactic transfusion to keep the platelet count greater than 10,000–20,000/μl. In general, if platelet function is normal and the platelet count is 50,000/μl or greater, it is unlikely that prophylactic transfusion will be beneficial for most invasive procedures. Higher platelet counts may be necessary for major surgery or in situations where additional coagulation defects, sepsis, or platelet dysfunction related to disease or medication is present. Platelet transfusion is not indicated in immune thrombocytopenic purpura (unless there is life-threatening bleeding), prophylactically with massive blood transfusion, or prophylactically following coronary artery bypass procedures.

C. **Fresh frozen plasma (FFP) transfusion** is indicated to increase the level of clotting factors in patients with a documented deficiency. Patients with thrombotic thrombocytopenic purpura and rare conditions such as congenital antithrombin III deficiency may also benefit from FFP. Specific indications are covered in Chap. 17. A unit of FFP will increase each clotting factor by 2–3%. Administration of FFP is generally not necessary if the prothrombin time and partial thromboplastin time are less than 1.5 times normal. FFP should not be used for volume expansion, as a nutritional supplement, prophylactically with massive blood transfusion, or prophylactically following coronary artery bypass surgery.

II. **Complications of transfusion therapy**

A. **Risks common to all blood components.** Infection and alloimmunization are the major complications of blood product transfusion. The risk of these complications rises with the number of units of blood products transfused.

1. **Infection.** Risk of transfusion-associated infection varies with geographic location. By far the most frequently transmitted agents are non-A, non-B hepatitis viruses, with an exposure risk of 1 in 100 units transfused. Previously hepatitis C virus (HCV) comprised a significant proportion of this group. A screening test for HCV has been routinely used since May 1990 and may reduce the incidence of transfusion-related non-A, non-B hepatitis. Screening for hepatitis B and human immunodeficiency virus (HIV) is performed on all blood products. The risk of transfusion-associated transmission of HIV is 1 in 40,000 to 1 in 1,000,000. Hepatitis B, HTLV-1, Epstein-Barr virus, cytomegalovirus, malaria, trypanosomiasis, babesiosis, and leishmaniasis have also been transmitted by transfusions.

2. **Hemolytic transfusion reactions** (see sec. **II.B**) are usually due to errors in

labelling units of RBCs or patient identification. Fatal reactions are almost always due to ABO incompatibility. The risk of a fatal hemolytic transfusion reaction is about 1 in 100,000 units transfused.

3. **Alloimmunization.** The recipient of any blood product may form antibodies against donor antigens. This may result in transfusion reaction of hemolytic or nonhemolytic types as well as poorer increments in blood counts with subsequent transfusions.

4. **Nonhemolytic transfusion reactions** are characterized by fevers, chills, urticaria, pruritus, and respiratory distress and are usually seen in previously transfused patients or multiparous women. Antibodies against donor plasma proteins or leukocyte antigens are thought to be the cause. Treatment of symptoms with acetaminophen for fever and diphenhydramine, 25–50 mg PO or IV, is usually sufficient. Rarely, epinephrine or glucocorticoids are required. Some patients may require premedication with acetaminophen, diphenhydramine, or steroids to prevent recurrence of symptoms with subsequent transfusions. Meperidine, 25–50 mg IV, is effective in preventing shaking chills. Leukocyte filters will prevent reactions due to sensitivity to donor WBCs. Anaphylactic reactions may be seen in patients who are IgA deficient (1 in 1,000 individuals) and are caused by anti-IgA antibodies in the recipient.

5. **Volume overload** with signs of congestive heart failure is often seen when patients with cardiovascular compromise are transfused. Slowing the rate of transfusion and judicious use of diuretics help prevent this complication.

6. **Noncardiogenic pulmonary edema** is caused by antileukocyte antibodies present in the donor's plasma. The donors are usually multiparous women and should not give further blood donations. Therapy is supportive.

B. **Complications of red cell transfusions**

1. **Acute hemolytic reactions** are usually caused by preformed antibodies in the recipient and are characterized by intravascular hemolysis of the transfused RBCs soon after the administration of the incompatible blood. Fever, chills, back pain, chest pain, nausea, vomiting, and symptoms related to hypotension may develop. Acute renal failure with hemoglobinuria may occur. In the unconscious patient, a decrease in blood pressure or increased bleeding may be the only manifestation. If a hemolytic transfusion reaction is suspected, the transfusion should be stopped immediately and all IV tubing should be replaced. Clotted and EDTA-treated samples of the patient's blood should be sent to the blood bank along with the remainder of the suspected unit for repeat of the cross-match. Serum bilirubin and tests for DIC should be obtained, and the plasma and freshly voided urine should be examined for free hemoglobin.

Management includes preservation of intravascular volume and protection of renal function. Urine output should be maintained at 100 ml/hour or greater with the use of IV fluids and diuretics or mannitol, if necessary. The excretion of free hemoglobin may be aided by alkalinization of the urine. Sodium bicarbonate may be added to IV fluids to increase the urinary pH to 7.5 or greater.

2. **Delayed hemolytic transfusion reactions** may occur from 1–25 days after transfusion and are caused by either an anamnestic response or a primary antibody response to RBC antigens. Many of these patients probably had antibodies to RBC antigens prior to the transfusion, but titers were too low to be detected by the screening procedures. Usually there is a fall in the Hb/Hct and the bilirubin rises. The direct Coombs' test may be positive, resulting in confusion with autoimmune hemolytic anemia. Delayed hemolytic transfusion reaction may at times be severe and in these cases should be treated similarly to acute transfusion reactions.

3. **Bleeding complications** due to dilution of platelets and plasma coagulation factors may be seen after administration of large amounts of packed RBCs. Correction of platelet and coagulation factor deficiencies should be based on laboratory monitoring rather than an empiric formula. Administration of

FFP generally is not necessary if the prothrombin time and partial thromboplastin time are less than 1.5 times normal.

4. **Transfusion-associated graft-versus-host disease (GVHD)** is usually seen in immunocompromised patients and is thought to result from the infusion of immunocompetent T lymphocytes (*N. Engl. J. Med.* 323:315, 1990). This entity has been reported in immunocompetent patients who share an HLA haplotype with HLA-homozygous blood donors (usually a relative or members of inbred populations). Rash, elevated liver function tests, and severe pancytopenia are seen. Mortality is greater than 80%. **It is recommended that direct-donated blood from first-degree relatives be irradiated to avoid this complication.** The chances of shared HLA haplotypes with a random blood donor is extremely low, so irradiation of nonrelated blood products is not indicated for the immunocompetent patient.

5. **Adverse effects due to massive transfusion.** Administration of a volume of RBCs or plasma in excess of the normal blood volume of the patient in a 24-hour period (massive transfusion) is associated with several complications in addition to those already outlined.

   a. **Hypothermia** due to chilled blood may cause cardiac dysrhythmias. A blood-warming device can prevent this problem.

   b. **Citrate intoxication** may cause hypocalcemia and resulting tetany, hypotension, and decreased cardiac output. This may be treated with calcium gluconate, 10 ml of a 10% solution IV.

   c. **Acidemia and hyperkalemia** may occur. Hyperkalemia is not usually significant unless the patient was hyperkalemic prior to transfusion. Twenty-four hours after massive transfusion, hypokalemia may occur as RBCs become more metabolically active and take up potassium from the plasma.

C. **Complications associated with platelet transfusions**

1. **Alloimmunization.** Fifty to 75% of patients who receive platelets on a regular basis will develop antibodies against platelet antigens. Clinically, this disorder is diagnosed when platelet transfusion produces little increase in platelet count. Inadequate platelet count response may also be caused by fever, increased platelet destruction (e.g., ITP), splenomegaly, and increased consumption (e.g., DIC). Patients who do not respond to random-donor platelets may benefit from single-donor products. In situations where multiple transfusions are foreseen (e.g., bone marrow transplantation), HLA typing will allow HLA-matched single-donor platelets to be used.

2. **Posttransfusion purpura** is a rare syndrome associated with thrombocytopenia, purpura, and bleeding that starts 7–10 days after exposure to blood products containing platelets. It is usually seen in previously transfused individuals or multiparous women who have antibodies against platelet antigen PI^{A1}. The process usually resolves within 10–20 days; however, bleeding may prove fatal during this period. Plasmapheresis (up to three treatments) on alternate days is usually effective in raising the platelet count. Intravenous immunoglobulin has been recommended as an alternative to plasmapheresis. Responses to glucocorticoids are rare. Platelet transfusions are ineffective in this disorder.

III. **Emergency blood transfusions** should be used only in situations where massive blood loss has resulted in cardiovascular compromise. Volume expansion with normal saline should be attempted initially. Blood typing can be performed in 10 minutes and cross-matching within 30 minutes in emergency situations. If unmatched blood must be used, it should be group O/Rh-negative type that has been previously screened for reactive antibodies. At the first sign of a transfusion reaction the infusion should be stopped.

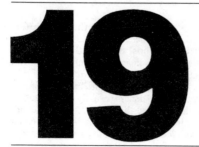

Medical Management of Malignant Disease

Joanne E. Mortimer,
Morey A. Blinder, and
Matthew A. Arquette

Approach to the Cancer Patient

I. **General principles in treating cancer.** Because of the emotional impact of the diagnosis of cancer, patients should be initially approached not only with the diagnosis but also with a plan for workup and treatment. Before initiating chemotherapy or radiation therapy, all patients should have a tissue diagnosis of cancer, and if possible, a clinical, biochemical, or radiographic marker of disease should be identified to assess the results of therapy.

A. **Stage and grade of tumor. Stage** is a clinical or pathologic assessment of tumor spread. The major roles of staging are to determine local and regional disease treatable by surgery and radiation therapy and to define the optimal therapy and prognosis in subsets of patients. The **grade** of a tumor defines its retention of characteristics compared to the cell of origin and is designated as low, moderate, or high as the tissue loses its normal appearance.

B. **Induction, consolidation, maintenance, and adjuvant therapy. Induction** is the chemotherapy used to achieve a complete remission. **Consolidation** chemotherapy is administered to patients who initially respond to treatment. **Maintenance** therapy refers to low-dose, outpatient treatment used to prolong remissions; its use has proved effective in a small number of malignancies. **Adjuvant** chemotherapy is given after complete eradication of a primary malignancy in an attempt to eliminate any presumed but unmeasurable metastatic disease.

C. **Response to treatment** may be defined by either clinical or pathologic criteria. **A complete response** (or remission) is achieved when all evidence of malignancy is eradicated. **A partial response** is defined as a decrease in tumor mass by greater than 50%.

D. **Palliative care and pain therapy.** Pain is present at diagnosis in 5–10% of patients with localized cancer and 60–90% of patients with metastases. Improved oral analgesics, widespread use of indwelling venous access devices, development of home nursing care agencies, and public acceptance of the hospice philosophy now allow patients to receive a large portion of their palliative treatment out of the hospital. Successful treatment of the underlying disease usually provides relief of pain; painful foci of disease refractory to systemic intervention may be controlled with local radiation therapy, regional nerve block, or an ablative surgical procedure. In many situations, however, analgesics are necessary (see Chap. 1). In general, nonopioid analgesics should be used initially, followed by opioid analgesics as needed. Most opioid analgesics have a short duration of action, requiring frequent doses. **Sustained-release morphine,** 30–60 mg PO q8–12h, is particularly efficacious in the management of chronic pain. Occasionally, infusions of morphine, 3–5 mg/hour IV, and increased by 2–4 mg/hour as needed, are necessary. When using a morphine drip, the patient must be monitored for respiratory depression, and **naloxone,** 2 ampules IV (0.4 mg/ampule), should be available at the bedside. Under supervision, morphine drips may be used in the home setting. While tolerance and physical dependency can develop with chronic narcotic administration, drug abuse and psychological dependency seldom occur in the setting of chronic pain from cancer. These concerns should not compromise the ability to achieve adequate analgesia.

II. **Therapy of selected solid tumors.** Recommendations regarding specific chemotherapeutic regimens are beyond the scope of this chapter. This section defines guidelines for a treatment plan, but **consultation with an oncologist should be obtained prior to drug and dosage selection.**

A. **Breast cancer**

1. **Approach to an undiagnosed lump in the breast.** Approximately 11% of women in the United States will develop breast cancer. A lump in a premenopausal woman is less likely to be cancer than in a postmenopausal woman. In a younger woman a mass should be observed for one month to identify any cyclic changes suggesting benign disease. When a mass is found, bilateral mammography should be performed. The accuracy of mammography to diagnose cancer in pre- and postmenopausal women is about 90%. Estrogen receptor and progesterone receptor levels should be measured on all newly diagnosed breast cancers.

2. **Surgical options.** Treatment is focused on local control and the risk of systemic spread. Local control with **tylectomy** (lumpectomy and axillary lymph node dissection) is as effective as a modified radical mastectomy. An axillary lymph node dissection should be included because it provides prognostic information and is of therapeutic value.

3. **Adjuvant chemotherapy.** The presence or absence of axillary lymph node metastases is the most important prognostic factor in breast cancer. **Premenopausal women** with axillary lymph node involvement should receive six cycles of adjuvant chemotherapy. In the absence of axillary lymph node involvement, chemotherapy is often recommended because it has been shown to improve the disease-free survival. In **postmenopausal women,** adjuvant therapy is administered according to estrogen receptor status. Tamoxifen increases the disease-free survival in both axillary lymph node–negative and –positive patients with estrogen receptor–positive disease. However, improved overall survival has been demonstrated only in lymph node–positive patients. In estrogen receptor–negative postmenopausal women with axillary nodal involvement, cytotoxic chemotherapy may be of benefit (*Cancer* 67:1744, 1991).

4. **Metastatic disease.** Initial treatment is dictated by menopausal status, hormone receptor status, and sites of metastatic disease. Estrogen receptor–negative breast cancer, lymphangitic lung disease, or liver metastasis will seldom respond to hormonal manipulation and should be treated with chemotherapy. In other metastatic sites, estrogen receptor–positive disease is treated by hormonal manipulation. Premenopausal women are treated with bilateral oophorectomy or hormonal agents; postmenopausal women are treated with hormonal agents. The various hormonal therapies produce similar response rates, but tamoxifen is most often used as initial treatment because it has few side effects. If the disease responds to hormonal therapy, subsequent progression may respond to further manipulations with other hormonal agents. Chemotherapy should be considered if there is no response to initial hormonal therapy or if there is progression during subsequent hormonal manipulations.

5. **Inflammatory and unresectable cancers.** Inflammatory breast cancer manifests as "peau d'orange" changes or erythema involving more than one-third of the chest wall. Because of the high likelihood of metastases at diagnosis, these patients and patients with inoperable primary breast cancers are initially treated with chemotherapy. Subsequently, surgery and radiation therapy are used for maximal local control.

6. **Radiation therapy** is indicated in patients treated with tylectomy and in some patients with multiple positive axillary lymph nodes. It is also used for palliation of painful or obstructing metastatic lesions.

B. **Gastrointestinal malignancies** commonly present with vague symptoms and are often advanced at the time of diagnosis.

1. **Esophageal cancers** are either squamous cell (associated with cigarette smoking and alcohol use) or, rarely, adenocarcinoma (arising in Barrett's

esophagus). Surgical resection of the esophagus is recommended whenever feasible. Local control of unresectable cancers can be achieved with combined chemotherapy and radiation therapy. Palliation of obstructive symptoms may be accomplished by radiation therapy, dilatation, prosthetic tube placement, or laser therapy.

2. **Gastric cancer** is usually adenocarcinoma and may be cured with surgery in the rare patient with localized disease. Chemotherapy has been ineffective as adjuvant therapy. Locally advanced but unresectable cancers may benefit from concomitant radiation therapy and chemotherapy. Chemotherapy may offer palliation for metastatic disease.

3. **Colon and rectal adenocarcinomas** are primarily treated by surgical resection. Data have shown prolonged survival in patients with colon cancer and regional lymph node involvement who receive adjuvant fluorouracil and levamisole for 6 months (*N. Engl. J. Med.* 322:352, 1990). Rectal cancer arising below the peritoneal reflection commonly recurs locally after surgery alone; postoperative radiation therapy and fluorouracil are recommended. Fluorouracil is the mainstay of treatment for metastatic colon or rectal cancer, with a response rate of 20%. The addition of leucovorin results in higher response rates and possibly longer survival than fluorouracil alone. In all patients undergoing surgical resection of colon or rectal cancer, a preoperative carcinoembryonic antigen (CEA) level should be measured. A persistently elevated or increasing level may be indicative of residual or recurrent tumor.

4. **Anal cancer.** Chemotherapy with concurrent radiation therapy appears to result in a higher cure rate than surgical resection and usually preserves the anal sphincter and fecal continence (*Am. J. Med.* 78:211, 1985). Surgical resection should be used only as salvage therapy.

C. **Genitourinary malignancies**

1. **Bladder cancer** in the United States is usually transitional cell carcinoma. A variety of chemical carcinogens including those in cigarette smoke are implicated. Unifocal tumors confined to the mucosa should be managed with cystoscopy and transurethral resection or fulguration, repeated at approximately 3-month intervals; multifocal mucosal disease is treated with intravesicular BCG, thiotepa, or mitomycin C. Locally invasive cancers should be resected. Adjuvant chemotherapy improves survival when regional lymph node involvement is documented in the cystectomy specimen. In metastatic or recurrent disease, the highest response rates are seen with cisplatin-containing regimens.

2. **Prostate cancer.** Local control of the primary lesion may be achieved with either prostatectomy or radiation therapy; the risk of impotence may be lower with radiation therapy. Although not useful as a routine screening test, prostate-specific antigen may be used as a marker for recurrence, bulk of disease, and response to therapy; when available, it has supplanted acid phosphatase. In patients with metastatic disease, bilateral orchiectomy, luteinizing hormone releasing hormone (LHRH) analogs, or diethylstilbesterol (DES) relieve bone pain in about 85% of cases for a median of 18–24 months. Disease that has relapsed after hormonal therapy seldom responds to further hormonal therapy. The role of chemotherapy has yet to be established. Anemia and bone pain dominate the advanced phases of this disease and are best relieved with transfusions and palliative radiation therapy.

3. **Renal cell cancer** is treated by surgical resection, which may be curative in localized disease; there is no effective adjuvant therapy. In metastatic disease, progestational agents (e.g., medroxyprogesterone) produce tumor regression in less than 15% of patients. Chemotherapy, alpha-interferon, and interleukin-2 have reported response rates of 15–30%.

4. **Cancer of the testis** is one of the malignancies most curable with chemotherapy. The patient suspected of having cancer of the testis should only have tissue obtained through an inguinal orchiectomy because a transscrotal

incision facilitates tumor spread to the inguinal lymph nodes. The initial evaluation should include a serum alpha-fetoprotein (AFP) and beta subunit of human chorionic gonadotropin (β-HCG), a CT scan of the abdomen and pelvis, and possibly a lymphangiogram. Most cases of seminoma should be treated with radiation therapy.

In a nonseminomatous germ cell cancer, a retroperitoneal lymph node dissection is performed as further staging except in the instance of bulky abdominal disease or pulmonary metastasis. If microscopic disease is identified at surgery, two alternatives are acceptable: (1) two cycles of postoperative chemotherapy or (2) observation until relapse followed by institution of chemotherapy. In the setting of gross metastatic disease, cisplatin-based chemotherapy is curative in the majority of germ cell cancers. If tumor markers normalize after chemotherapy but a radiographic mass persists, exploratory surgery should be performed; the lesion will prove to be residual cancer in about one-third of the cases. Patients with residual cancer should receive additional chemotherapy (*J. Clin. Oncol.* 8:1777, 1990).

D. Gynecologic malignancies

1. **Cervical cancer.** The recognized risk factors are multiparity, multiple sexual partners, and human papillomavirus. Carcinoma in situ and superficial disease may be treated by endocervical cone biopsy. Microinvasive disease is treated with an abdominal hysterectomy. Advanced local disease, either by invasion of the cervix or local extension, is treated with radiation therapy and surgery. Inoperable cancer may be controlled with radiation therapy. Metastatic disease is treated with cisplatin-based chemotherapy.

2. **Ovarian cancer** is primarily a disease of postmenopausal women. Because symptoms are uncommon with localized disease, most patients present with advanced local disease, malignant ascites, or peritoneal metastases. Surgical staging and treatment include an abdominal hysterectomy, bilateral oophorectomy, lymph node sampling, omentectomy, and peritoneal cytology as well as removal of all gross tumor. If the tumor is localized to the ovary, the surgery may be curative and further treatment is not routinely recommended. However, if microscopic foci of cancer are identified, chemotherapy is administered postoperatively. The serum marker **CA-125**, though not specific, is elevated in more than 80% of women with epithelial ovarian cancer and is a sensitive indicator of response. After a response is achieved, a "second-look laparotomy" is performed to restage and to debulk. About one-third of the patients who are in pathologic complete remission after a second-look laparotomy are cured. Those who have residual cancer should receive additional chemotherapy.

E. Head and neck cancer is usually squamous cell cancer, may arise in a variety of sites, and each has a different natural history. Early lesions may be cured with surgery, radiation therapy, or both. Despite aggressive surgical and radiation therapy, approximately 65% of patients with head and neck cancer have uncontrolled local disease. Chemotherapy is used for the treatment of disseminated disease and produces high response rates with a modest improvement in survival.

F. Lung cancer is the most common cause of cancer death in the United States. Because of its relationship to cigarette smoking, it is also the most preventable. Treatment is based on the histology and stage of the disease. Small-cell lung cancer is defined as either limited (confined to one hemithorax and ipsilateral regional lymph nodes) or extensive. Non–small-cell lung cancer includes several histologic subtypes that all behave in a similar fashion. Whenever possible, surgical resection should be attempted for non–small-cell lung cancer because this affords the best chance of cure.

1. **Small-cell lung cancer** is responsible for a number of paraneoplastic syndromes (see Complications of Cancer, sec. **II**). In limited disease, combination chemotherapy results in an 85–90% response rate, a median survival of 12–18 months, and a cure in 5–15%; in extensive disease, the median survival is 8–9 months, but cures are rare. For patients achieving a complete

remission with chemotherapy, **prophylactic whole-brain radiation** therapy should be administered to decrease the risk of CNS relapse. The role of radiation therapy to the chest as consolidation therapy remains controversial and is not routinely recommended.

2. **Non–small-cell lung cancer** survival rates after resection are not improved with adjuvant chemotherapy or radiation therapy. Radiation therapy is the conventional treatment for unresectable disease that is confined to the lung and regional lymph nodes. The role of chemotherapy before or concurrent with radiation therapy is not established. In patients with metastatic disease, cisplatin-based combination chemotherapy may modestly improve survival.

G. **Malignant melanoma** should be considered in any changing or enlarging nevus, and suspicious lesions should undergo excisional biopsy. Subsequently, a wide local excision is performed to remove possible vertical as well as radial spread of tumor. The depth of invasion is inversely related to the prognosis. Neither adjuvant radiation therapy nor chemotherapy improves the results of surgery alone. Systemic disease may respond to dacarbazine (DTIC), alpha-interferon, or interleukin-2 in 10–30% of patients.

H. **Sarcomas** are tumors that arise from mesenchymal tissue and occur most commonly in soft tissue or bone. Initial evaluation should include a CT scan of the chest, since hematogenous spread to the lungs is very common.

1. **The prognosis for soft tissue sarcoma** is primarily determined by the grade and not the cell of origin. Surgical resection should be performed when feasible and may be curative. In low-grade tumors, local and regional recurrence is most common and adjuvant radiation therapy may be of benefit. High-grade tumors frequently recur systemically, but no advantage to the routine use of adjuvant chemotherapy has been consistently demonstrated. In metastatic disease, doxorubicin, ifosfamide, and DTIC produce responses in 40–55%.

2. **Osteogenic sarcomas** are treated with surgical resection followed by adjuvant chemotherapy for 1 year. Treatment of isolated pulmonary metastasis by surgical resection is associated with long-term survival.

3. **Kaposi's sarcoma** in an immunocompetent patient is generally a low-grade lesion of the lower extremities that is readily treated with local radiation therapy or vinblastine. When Kaposi's sarcoma complicates organ transplantation or AIDS, it is more aggressive and may arise in visceral sites. Cutaneous disease may be observed or treated with alpha-interferon or low-dose vinca alkaloid. Advanced cutaneous disease or visceral disease, especially pulmonary, should be treated with a vinca alkaloid, bleomycin, or etoposide (*Am. J. Med.* 87:57, 1989).

I. **Cancer with an unknown primary site.** Approximately 5% of cancer patients present with symptoms of metastatic disease, but no primary tumor site is identifiable on physical examination, routine bloodwork, and chest x-ray. A search for the primary lesion should be directed by the histopathologic cell type and the site of the metastasis. Immunohistochemical stains may identify specific tissue antigens that help to define the origin of the tumor and guide subsequent therapy. **In general, systemic therapy is only helpful if the primary site is identified;** "broad-spectrum" chemotherapeutic regimens do not improve survival when compared to palliative therapy. Two potentially curative circumstances deserve separate mention:

1. **Cervical adenopathy** suggests cancer of the lung, breast, head and neck, or lymphoma. In this case, initial evaluation usually includes panendoscopy (nasendoscopy, laryngopharyngoscopy, bronchoscopy, and esophagoscopy) and biopsy of any suspicious lesion prior to excision of the lymph node. If squamous cell carcinoma is identified, the patient is presumed to have primary head and neck cancer and radiation therapy may be curative.

2. **Midline mass in mediastinum or retroperitoneum.** In both sexes, a midline mass in the mediastinum or retroperitoneum may be an extragonadal germ cell cancer. Elevations in AFP or β-HCG further suggest this diagnosis. This neoplasm is potentially curable (see sec. **II.C.4**).

III. Therapy of hematologic tumors

A. Lymphoma is usually diagnosed by biopsy of an enlarged lymph node.

1. The staging for both Hodgkin's disease and non-Hodgkin's lymphoma is as follows:

a. Stage I—disease localized to a single lymph node or group.

b. Stage II—more than one lymph node group affected but confined to one side of the diaphragm.

c. Stage III—disease in the lymph nodes or the spleen and occurring on both sides of the diaphragm.

d. Stage IV—liver or bone marrow involvement.

e. B symptoms. Fever above 38.5°C, night sweats requiring a change in clothes, and a 10% weight loss over 6 months are B symptoms, which suggest bulky disease and worsen the prognosis.

2. Hodgkin's disease usually presents with cervical adenopathy and spreads in a predictable manner along lymph node groups. Treatment is based on the presenting stage of the disease; the cell type is relatively unimportant in the natural history and prognosis. Initial evaluation includes a CT scan of the abdomen and pelvis, bilateral bone marrow biopsies, and lymphangiogram to determine the clinical stage of the disease. Exploratory laparotomy with splenectomy and liver biopsy is performed if the findings will change the stage of disease and therefore the treatment. **Stage IA and IIA** disease are treated with radiation therapy unless a mediastinal mass exceeding one-third of the chest width is present, in which case chemotherapy is included. **Stage IIIA** disease may be treated by either radiation therapy or chemotherapy, while all **stage IV** patients should receive combination chemotherapy. When B symptoms are present, chemotherapy is recommended regardless of the stage.

3. Non-Hodgkin's lymphoma is currently classified as low-, intermediate-, or high-grade based on the histologic type. Staging workup is the same as for Hodgkin's, but non-Hodgkin's lymphoma has a less predictable pattern of spread. Advanced stage disease (stage III or IV) is usually apparent, and exploratory laparotomy and lymphangiogram are rarely necessary.

a. Low-grade lymphoma often involves the bone marrow at diagnosis, but the disease has an indolent course. Since this tumor is rarely eradicated, immediate treatment has no impact on survival. Radiation therapy or an alkylating agent (e.g., cyclophosphamide) are used to ameliorate symptoms. Radiation therapy may produce a long-term complete remission in stage I or II disease.

b. Intermediate-grade lymphoma has a more aggressive course, seldom involves the bone marrow at diagnosis, and may be cured with chemotherapy. Complete response rates currently exceed 80%. Bulky disease, defined by a tumor mass greater than 10 cm in diameter or a serum lactate dehydrogenase (LDH) above 500 IU/liter, is less likely to be cured.

c. High-grade lymphoma, including **Burkitt's, lymphoblastic, and immunoblastic lymphomas,** are the most aggressive subtypes and have a high frequency of CNS and bone marrow involvement. Cerebrospinal fluid (CSF) cytology should be included as part of the initial evaluation. Combination chemotherapy is the mainstay of treatment and should include CNS prophylaxis if the CSF is cytologically free of tumor. If tumor cells are seen in the CSF, additional therapy may be indicated (see Complications of Cancer, sec. **I.B**). Prophylaxis to prevent **tumor lysis syndrome** (see Complications of Treatment, sec. **I.F**) should be performed prior to induction chemotherapy.

B. Leukemia presents with cytopenias, lymphadenopathy, splenomegaly, or leukostasis. The peripheral blood smear usually distinguishes between acute and chronic leukemia, but a bone marrow aspirate should be performed to confirm the diagnosis and further classify the disease by immunophenotype and cytogenetics.

1. Acute nonlymphocytic leukemia (ANL) constitutes about 80% of acute leukemia in adults. Cytosine arabinoside is the cornerstone of induction therapy and is usually administered with daunorubicin to induce remission. After achieving a complete remission, at least one additional cycle of chemotherapy is given as consolidation. Alternatively, allogeneic bone marrow transplantation may be used for consolidation.

2. **Acute lymphocytic leukemia (ALL)** in adults is significantly more difficult to cure than in children. CNS prophylaxis is necessary. After achieving a complete remission, consolidation chemotherapy is followed by maintenance chemotherapy for at least 1 year.

3. **Chronic lymphocytic leukemia (CLL)** usually presents with lymphocytosis, but lymphadenopathy, splenomegaly, anemia, and thrombocytopenia may occur during the course of the disease. Treatment is similar to that for **low-grade lymphoma** (see sec. **III.A.3.a**) and should be given for control of symptoms. Lymphocytosis alone is not an indication for therapy. Immune hemolytic anemia or immune thrombocytopenia may develop as a complication of CLL and is treated with glucocorticoids (e.g., prednisone, 1 mg/kg PO qd). CLL does not evolve into acute leukemia, but transformation to an **intermediate- or high-grade lymphoma** may occur (Richter's syndrome).

4. **Chronic myelogenous leukemia (CML)** is diagnosed when the Philadelphia chromosome t(9;22) is identified. Leukocytosis and thrombocytosis may be controlled with hydroxyurea for several years before transformation into a **blast crisis** that mimics acute leukemia. Myeloblast transformation responds poorly to therapy, but in lymphoblastic crisis, treatment with vincristine and prednisone is warranted. In either case, the blast phase of CML is seldom cured with chemotherapy. Allogeneic bone marrow transplantation for CML in the chronic phase has been associated with prolonged remissions.

5. **Hairy-cell leukemia** should be considered in patients with splenomegaly and pancytopenia.

C. **Multiple myeloma** is a malignant plasma cell disorder that may present with hypercalcemia, bone pain, or acute renal failure. The initial evaluation should include a radiographic bone survey, bone marrow aspirate, serum and urine protein electrophoresis, beta-2 microglobulin, sedimentation rate, and quantitative immunoglobulins. Since the bone lesions are predominately osteolytic, radionuclide bone scans are rarely helpful. Treatment generally includes a combination of an oral alkylating agent, vincristine, and a glucocorticoid. Local radiation therapy should be used to relieve painful bone lesions.

Complications of Cancer

I. **Complications related to tumor mass**
   A. **Brain metastasis.** Patients with parenchymal brain metastasis may present with headache, mental status changes, weakness, or focal neurologic deficits. Papilledema is observed in only 25% of patients. In patients with malignancy, a CT scan of the head showing one or more round, contrast-enhancing lesions surrounded by edema is usually sufficient for the diagnosis. If cancer has not previously been diagnosed, tissue should be obtained from the brain lesion or a more accessible site prior to initiating radiation therapy. Initial therapy with dexamethasone, 10 mg IV or PO, is intended to decrease cerebral edema and should be continued at a dosage of 4–6 mg PO q6h throughout the course of radiation therapy or longer, if symptoms related to edema persist. Subsequent therapy depends on the number and location of the brain lesions, as well as the prognosis of the underlying cancer. Patients with a chemotherapy-responsive neoplasm and a solitary, accessible lesion should be considered for surgical resection. All patients who have not received prior radiation therapy should receive whole-brain radiation therapy.

   B. **Meningeal carcinomatosis** should be suspected in a cancer patient with headache or cranial neuropathies. This pattern of spread is most often seen with lung or breast cancer, melanoma, or lymphoma; the diagnosis is confirmed by cytology of the CSF. In general, a CT scan of the head is performed to rule out parenchymal metastases or hydrocephalus prior to performing a lumbar puncture. Local radiation therapy or intrathecal chemotherapy may provide temporary relief of symptoms (see Chemotherapy, sec. **II.C**). Meningeal lymphoma may respond to intravenous cytosine arabinoside.

C. Spinal cord compression is most commonly caused by hematogenous spread of cancer to the vertebral bodies followed by expansion into the spinal canal or ischemia of the spinal cord. Back pain is the first symptom and may precede neurologic deficits by weeks to months. Weakness generally antedates sensory loss and autonomic dysfunction of the bowel or bladder. The most common malignancies that cause spinal cord compression are breast, lung, and prostate cancer, but the diagnosis should be considered in any patient with cancer complaining of back pain. Initial evaluation should include radiographs of the painful area. Further evaluation and therapy are discussed in Chap. 25.

D. Superior vena cava (SVC) obstruction is most commonly caused by cancers that arise in or spread to the mediastinum, such as lymphoma or lung cancer. The compressed SVC leads to swelling of the face or trunk, chest pain, cough, or shortness of breath. Dilated superficial veins of the chest, neck, or sublingual area suggest an engorged collateral circulation. The presence of a mass by chest radiograph or CT scan usually confirms the diagnosis. Formerly, SVC obstruction was felt to put the cerebral venous circulation in jeopardy and was considered an oncologic emergency. However, collateral veins develop rapidly so that serious complications in this setting are usually limited to the mediastinal mass compromising the airway. If the histologic origin of the obstruction is unknown, tissue may be obtained for diagnosis via bronchoscopy or mediastinoscopy. Therapy is directed at the underlying disease. Chemotherapy should be administered through a vein not obstructed by the lesion. Neoplasms not responsive to chemotherapy are treated with radiation therapy (*J. Clin. Oncol.* 2:961, 1984).

E. Malignant effusions

1. **Malignant pericardial effusion** commonly results from cancer of the breast or lung. In some patients, the initial presentation is acute cardiovascular collapse from **cardiac tamponade,** requiring emergent pericardiocentesis. After cardiovascular stabilization, some patients may improve with treatment if the tumor is chemotherapy-sensitive. When the pericardial effusion is a complication of uncontrolled disease, palliation may be achieved by pericardiocentesis; the effusion should be completely drained followed by instillation of 30 or 60 mg of bleomycin through the drainage catheter, which is subsequently clamped for 10 minutes and then withdrawn (*Int. J. Cardiol.* 16:155, 1987). Subxiphoid pericardiostomy may be performed in patients who fail to respond to other treatment (*J.A.M.A.* 257:1088, 1987).

2. **Malignant pleural effusion** develops as a result of pleural invasion by tumor or obstruction of lymphatic drainage. When systemic control is not feasible and reaccumulation of fluid occurs rapidly after drainage, removal of the fluid followed by instillation of a sclerosing agent into the pleural space is recommended. Resistant effusions may be controlled with pleurectomy (see Chap. 10).

3. **Malignant ascites** is most commonly caused by peritoneal carcinomatosis and is best controlled through systemic chemotherapy. Therapeutic paracenteses can provide symptomatic relief. Intraperitoneal instillation of chemotherapy has been used but is not routinely recommended.

II. Paraneoplastic syndromes are complications of malignancy that are not directly caused by a tumor mass effect. They may be the presenting symptom. The effects are presumed to be mediated by either secreted tumor products or the development of autoantibodies. Paraneoplastic syndromes have been described that affect virtually every organ system, and in most cases, successful treatment of the underlying malignancy will eliminate these effects.

A. Metabolic complications

1. **Hypercalcemia** is the most common metabolic complication in malignancy

and can cause mental status changes, gastrointestinal discomfort, and constipation. Acute and chronic management of hypercalcemia is discussed in Chap. 23.

2. **Syndrome of inappropriate antidiuretic hormone (SIADH)** should be considered in a euvolemic cancer patient with unexplained hyponatremia (see Chap. 3). Although a variety of neoplasms have been described in association with SIADH, small-cell lung cancer is most frequently responsible. If chemotherapy is ineffective, radiation therapy may decrease the tumor mass and relieve symptoms (see Chap. 3 for management).

3. **Cancer cachexia** refers to the clinical syndrome of anorexia, distortion of taste perception, and loss of muscle mass. The asthenic appearance of patients is more often related to tumor type than to tumor burden. Megestrol acetate, 160 mg PO qd, has been used as an appetite stimulant, resulting in weight gain in some patients (*Semin. Oncol.* 14:37, 1986).

B. Neuromuscular complications

1. **Polymyositis (PM) and dermatomyositis (DM)** (see Chap. 24). DM more often than PM has been associated with a variety of malignancies, including non–small-cell lung, colon, ovarian, and prostate cancer. In some patients, successful treatment of their malignancy has resulted in resolution of the symptoms. An exhaustive search for an underlying malignancy is not recommended because a primary malignancy will be found in less than 20% of patients (*N. Engl. J. Med.* 326:363, 1992).

2. **Lambert-Eaton myasthenic syndrome** is characterized by proximal muscle weakness, decreased or absent deep tendon reflexes, and autonomic dysfunction. EMG using high-frequency nerve stimulation may show post-tetanic potentiation. Small-cell lung cancer is most frequently associated with this syndrome, and effective chemotherapy may result in improvement. If cancer therapy is ineffective, diaminopyridine, 10–25 mg PO qid, may be of benefit. Worsening symptoms have been reported with the use of calcium channel antagonists; these agents are contraindicated in this syndrome (*N. Engl. J. Med.* 321:1567, 1989).

C. Hematologic complications include anemia, neutropenia, and thrombocytopenia, which may be associated with the malignancy or its treatment (see Complications of Treatment, sec. **I.B**).

1. **Erythrocytosis** is a rare complication of hepatoma, renal cell cancer, and benign tumors of the kidney, uterus, and cerebellum. Debulking the tumor with surgery or radiation therapy generally results in resolution of the erythrocytosis. Occasionally, therapeutic phlebotomy is indicated (see Chap. 18).

2. **Granulocytosis (leukemoid reaction)**, in the absence of infection, occurs in cancer arising in the stomach, lung, pancreas, and brain and in lymphoma. Since the neutrophils are mature and seldom exceed 100,000/μl, complications are rare and intervention is unnecessary.

3. **Thrombocytosis** in patients with cancer may be due to splenectomy, iron deficiency, acute hemorrhage, or inflammation; treatment is not usually necessary. **Thrombocytopenia** may occur following chemotherapy, with splenomegaly, with malignant infiltration of the bone marrow, or by an immune mechanism (see Chap. 17).

4. **Thromboembolic complications.** Mucin-secreting adenocarcinomas of the gastrointestinal tract and lung cancer have been associated with a "hypercoagulable state" resulting in recurrent venous and arterial thromboembolism. Nonbacterial thrombotic (marantic) endocarditis, usually involving the mitral valve, may also occur. Heparin should be instituted, and treatment of the underlying cancer should begin. Heparin, IV or SQ, to maintain the partial thromboplastin time (PTT) at 1.5–2.0 times normal, appears to be more effective than warfarin in the prevention of subsequent thrombi (*Blood* 62:14, 1983). In many patients, biochemical evidence of disseminated intravascular coagulation coexists with thromboemboli (see Chap. 17).

D. Glomerular injury resulting in renal failure has been observed as a paraneoplastic syndrome. Minimal change disease is often associated with lymphoma, especially Hodgkin's disease; membranous glomerulonephritis is more often seen with solid tumors. The process may be reversed with treatment of the underlying cancer.

E. **Clubbing** of the fingers and **hypertrophic osteoarthropathy** (polyarthritis and periostitis of long bones) are most often observed in non–small-cell lung cancer but are also seen with lesions metastatic to the mediastinum. Some improvement in the osteoarthropathy may be achieved with nonsteroidal anti-inflammatory agents, but definitive therapy requires treatment of the underlying malignancy.

F. **Fever** may accompany lymphoma and renal cell cancer and may also occur with hepatic metastasis. Once an infectious etiology for the fever has been excluded, nonsteroidal anti-inflammatory agents (e.g., ibuprofen, 400 mg PO qid, or indomethacin, 25–50 mg PO tid) may provide symptomatic relief.

G. **Bone metastases** are a common pattern of tumor spread and may be identified on x-rays or radionuclide bone scan. Radiation therapy is used for palliation of painful lesions and to prevent fracture in weight-bearing bones.

Chemotherapy

I. **Administration of chemotherapeutic drugs.** The dosage of chemotherapy is usually based on body surface area (Table 19-1); for some agents, dosage is determined by body weight. Chemotherapy dosage should be adjusted when changes in body weight occur. One to two weeks following the first dose of chemotherapy, a complete blood count should be obtained to determine the degree of myelosuppression. Dosage usually must be adjusted for the following conditions: (1) neutropenia, (2) thrombocytopenia, (3) stomatitis, (4) diarrhea, or (5) limited metabolic capacity for the drug. **The advice of an oncologist and precise adherence to a treatment plan is mandatory because of the low therapeutic index of chemotherapeutic agents.**

II. **Route of administration**

A. **Oral drug administration** may be accompanied by nausea and vomiting, necessitating antiemetic therapy. For some agents, oral absorption is erratic and parenteral administration is preferred.

B. **Intravenous drug administration** should be performed by experienced personnel. Care should be taken to ensure free flow of fluid to the vein, and adequate blood return should be verified prior to instillation of chemotherapy. In general, infusions should be through a large-caliber, upper extremity vein. When possible, veins of the antecubital fossa, wrist, dorsum of the hand, and arm ipsilateral to an axillary lymph node dissection should be avoided. In patients with poor peripheral venous access or those requiring many doses of chemotherapy, **indwelling venous catheter devices** should be considered (*J.A.M.A.* 253:1590, 1985).

C. **Intrathecal (IT) chemotherapy** is given for the treatment of meningeal carcinomatosis or as CNS prophylaxis. Side effects include acute arachnoiditis, subacute motor dysfunction, and progressive neurologic deterioration (leukoencephalopathy). Decreased cognitive function has been documented in children. Impaired cognitive function and leukoencephalopathy occur more often when IT chemotherapy is given with whole-brain radiation. **Methotrexate,** 10–12 mg, is diluted in 5 ml of preservative-free, nonbacteriostatic, isotonic solution. Prior to administration, 5–10 ml of CSF should be allowed to drain; methotrexate is then injected into the spinal canal over 5–10 minutes. To decrease the risk of arachnoiditis, patients should remain supine for 15 minutes after the infusion is completed. To avoid systemic side effects from methotrexate, leucovorin, 5–10 mg PO q6h, should be administered for 8 doses beginning 12–24 hours after intrathecal treatment. **Cytosine arabinoside (ara-C),** 50–100 mg in 5–10 ml of diluent, may be administered in a similar manner.

D. **Intracavitary instillation** of chemotherapy may be useful in some circumstances. Thiotepa, 30–60 mg, is commonly instilled in the bladder for the treatment of

Table 19-1. Doses and common toxicities of antineoplastic agents

	Dose range/schedule	N&V	Mucositis	Diarrhea	Days to nadir	Skin	Lung	Neurologic	Dose modification for
Antimetabolites									
Cytosine arabinoside	20 mg/m² IV infusion/day × 14–21 days	0	0	+	10–14 +++	0	0	0	
	100–200 mg/m² IV/day × 5–7 days	++	+	++	10–14 +++	Alopecia	0	0	
Fluorouracil	3–6 g/m² IV qd × 3–6 days	+++	+	++	10–14 ++	Phlebitis	0	Cerebellar	
	350–450 mg/m² IV × 5 days	0–+	+++	+	7–14 ++	Phlebitis	0	Cerebellar	
	200–100 mg/m² infusion × 5 days	0–+		+++	7–14 +	Hand-foot*	0	Cerebellar	
Methotrexate	20 mg/m² IV qd × 28–56 days With leucovorin	0	+	+++	None	Hand-foot*	0	0	
	10–60 mg/m² IV q1–3wk	+	++	++	7–14 ++	Dermatitis	+	0	Effusions, renal failure
	>1.5 g IV qd × 1 with leucovorin	+++	+++	+++	7–14 +++	Dermatitis	+	0	Effusions, renal failure
Pentostatin	5 mg/m² IV qd × 2	+	0	0	?	?	0	Lethargy, coma	
6-Mercaptopurine	75–100 mg/m² PO qd	+	0	0	7–14 ++	Rash	0	0	Allopurinol, renal, hepatic
Thioguanine	100 mg/m² PO qd × 1–4	+	+	0	10–30 ++	0	0	0	Renal
Alkylating agents									
Busulfan	2–4 mg/m² PO qd × 4	0	+	0	14–28 ++	Hyperpigment	0	0	
Chlorambucil	6–14 mg/m² PO qd × 4 each month, or daily	0	0	0	10–14 ++	0	+	0	Barbiturates
Cyclophosphamide	60–150 mg/m² PO qd × 14 each month, or daily	+	0	0	10–12 ++	0	+	0	
	500–1500 mg/m² IV q21d	++	++	+++	7–14 ++	Alopecia	+	0	
	120–200 mg/kg IV with BMR	+++	+++		7–14 +++	Alopecia	+	0	
Dacarbazine (DTIC)	300–1500 mg/m² IV q21–28d	+++	0	0	None	Vesicant	0	0	
Ifosfamide	800–1500 mg/m² IV q21–28d	+++	+	0	7–10 +++	Alopecia, rash	0	Encephalopathy	
Mechlorethamine	8 mg/m² IV q28d	+++	+	+	7–14 ++	Alopecia, rash, vesicant	0	0	

Drug	Dose							
Melphalan	4–8 mg/m² PO qd × 4	0	0	0	10–14++	0	0	0
Nitrosoureas								
Carmustine (BCNU)	60–100 mg/m² IV qd × 3	+++	0	0	28–35++	0	0	0
CCNU	100–300 mg/m² PO q6wk	+++	0	0	21–42++	0	+	0
Streptozocin	500–1500 mg/m² IV qd × 5d	++	0	0	None	0	0	0
Thiotepa	Up to 1.125 g/m² IV with BMR	++	+++	+++	7–14+++	Alopecia, rash	0	Encephalopathy
Tumor antibiotics								
Bleomycin	10–20 mg/m² SQ	0	0	0	None	Erythema	+	Renal
Dactinomycin	0.4–1.0 mg/m² IV	++	++	0	14–21++	Alopecia, rash	0	0
Daunorubicin	45–60 mg/m² IV qd × 3	++	+	+	7–14+++	Alopecia, vesicant	0	Renal, hepatic
Doxorubicin	10–60 mg/m² IV q7–28d	++	+	+	7–14+++	Alopecia, vesicant	0	Renal, hepatic
Mitoxantrone	10–30 mg/m² IV q21–28d	+	+	+	7–14++	Alopecia, vesicant	0	0
Mitomycin C	10–15 mg/m² IV q4–6wk	+	+	0	21–28++	Vesicant	+	0
Plant alkaloids								
Etoposide	50–200 mg/m² PO/IV qd × 5d	0	0	0	10–14++	Vesicant	0	0
Vinblastine	5–10 mg/m² IV q1–4wk	+	+	+	4–10++	Alopecia, vesicant	+	Liver
Vincristine	1–2 mg IV q1–4wk	0	0	0	None	Vesicant	+	Hepatic
Other								
Carboplatin	200–360 mg/m² IV q21–28d	++	0	0	14–28++	0	0	0
Cisplatin	20–120 mg/m² IV × 1–5d	+++	0	0	None	0	+	Renal
Hydroxyurea	500–2,000 mg PO q30d or daily	0	0	0	7–10++	Skin atrophy	0	0
L-Asparaginase	1,000–10,000 IU SQ qd × 3	0	0	0	None	0	0	Encephalopathy
Procarbazine	100–200 mg/m² PO qd × 7–14	+	0	0	7–10++	Rash	0	Encephalopathy

Key: 0 = none; + = mild; ++ = moderate; +++ = severe; N&V = nausea and vomiting; BMR = bone marrow rescue.
* See sec. III.A.2.

bladder carcinoma. Doxorubicin and cisplatin have been given through an implanted peritoneal catheter for the treatment of peritoneal metastasis.

 E. Intraarterial chemotherapy is advocated as a method of achieving high drug concentrations at specific tumor sites. Although of theoretic advantage, there are no absolute indications for chemotherapy administered by this route.

III. Chemotherapeutic agents. A summary of commonly used chemotherapeutic agents, dosage, and toxicities is given in Table 19-1. Class-specific or unique side effects are described below.

 A. Antimetabolites exert antitumor activity by acting as pseudosubstrates for essential enzymatic reactions. In general, their greatest toxicity occurs in tissues that are actively replicating (e.g., gastrointestinal mucosa, hematopoietic).

  1. Cytosine arabinoside (ara-C) is an analog of deoxycytidine that is most useful in hematologic neoplasms. In standard doses, myelosuppression and gastrointestinal toxicity are dose-limiting. In high doses, conjunctivitis is common, and prophylaxis with dexamethasone eyedrops, 2 drops OU tid, should be administered. Cerebellar ataxia, pancreatitis, and hepatitis may also develop. If cerebellar dysfunction occurs during treatment, the cytosine arabinoside must be discontinued.

  2. Fluorouracil (FU) is a pyrimidine analog that is administered as an injection or as a continuous infusion. When administered as a bolus injection, myelosuppression is dose-limiting; with a 4- to 5-day infusion, stomatitis and diarrhea are dose-limiting. Cerebellar ataxia has been reported with both schedules and requires discontinuation of the drug. Chest pain ascribed to coronary artery vasospasm may occur with infusions and, if suspected, should be treated with a calcium channel antagonist (e.g., nifedipine) or by discontinuing the chemotherapy (*Cancer* 61:36, 1988). Fluorouracil may be administered over 6–8 weeks and is limited by the development of a palmar-plantar erythrodysesthesia (hand-foot syndrome). Leucovorin may be coadministered with fluorouracil to potentiate the cytotoxicity of the fluorouracil; diarrhea is dose-limiting (*J. Clin. Oncol.* 7:1419, 1989).

  3. Methotrexate is an inhibitor of dihydrofolate reductase and causes numerous specific toxicities. Mucositis is dose-limiting.

   a. Prolonged reabsorption. Methotrexate accumulates in effusions and slowly diffuses into the circulation, producing substantial toxicity. Patients with effusions requiring methotrexate should either have the fluid drained prior to receiving this drug or have the dosage drastically reduced.

   b. Interstitial pneumonitis, unrelated to the cumulative dose and associated with a peripheral eosinophilia, may occur. It should be treated with glucocorticoids (e.g., prednisone, 1 mg/kg PO qd or equivalent) and precludes additional use of methotrexate.

   c. Hepatitis may occur with long-term oral administration but also may occur after a single high dose (see Chap. 24).

   d. High-dose methotrexate may be associated with crystalline nephropathy and renal failure. Urine alkalinization with sodium bicarbonate should be maintained to minimize this risk. Leucovorin is used to "rescue" normal tissue after high-dose methotrexate. The **leucovorin dose** depends on the amount of methotrexate used, but the usual dosage is 5–25 mg IV or PO q6h for 8–12 doses or until the serum methotrexate concentration is less than 50 nM.

  4. 6-Mercaptopurine (6-MP) is a purine analog that is partially metabolized by xanthine oxidase; to avoid increased toxicity, patients on allopurinol should receive a 25% dose of 6-MP. Hepatic cholestasis has been observed.

 B. Alkylating agents are useful in a wide variety of malignancies. These drugs cause DNA cross-linking and strand breaks. Most alkylating agents are cytotoxic to resting and dividing cells. Patients should be counseled that sterility, which is often irreversible, may develop after treatment with alkylating agents. Chlorambucil, cyclophosphamide, melphalan, and mechlorethamine have been implicated in the development of acute nonlymphocytic leukemia and myelodysplasia 3–10 years after treatment.

1. **Busulfan (Myleran)** is well absorbed orally and is usually administered on an intermittent schedule. Interstitial pneumonitis, gynecomastia, and a reversible syndrome resembling Addison's disease may develop with chronic daily oral administration.
2. **Chlorambucil (Leukeran)** is a well-tolerated orally administered drug. Myelosuppression is dose-limiting and usually readily reversible.
3. **Cyclophosphamide (Cytoxan)** may cause hemorrhagic cystitis (see Complications of Treatment, sec. **I.E**). Adequate hydration to maintain urine output should be achieved while administering the drug. Oral cyclophosphamide should be given early in the day to ensure adequate hydration. High-dose cyclophosphamide is used as a preparative agent prior to bone marrow transplantation; at these doses a hemorrhagic myocarditis may occur.
4. **Dacarbazine (DTIC)** can produce a flu-like syndrome consisting of fever, myalgias, facial flushing, malaise, and marked elevations of hepatic enzymes.
5. **Ifosfamide** is chemically similar to cyclophosphamide, but the incidence of hemorrhagic cystitis is much higher (occurring in 20–30% of treated patients). Administration of 2-mercaptoethane sulfonate (MESNA) (usually infused with ifosfamide at a dosage of at least 0.6 mg of MESNA to 1 mg of ifosfamide) is recommended to lower the incidence (see Complications of Treatment, sec. **I.E**).
6. **Mechlorethamine (nitrogen mustard)** is a skin irritant; protective gloves and eyewear must be used during drug preparation and administration. Development of a drug rash does not prevent the further use of this agent.
7. **Melphalan (Alkeran)** is only available as an oral agent. An idiosyncratic interstitial pneumonitis may occur, and although usually reversible, it precludes further use of the drug.
8. **Nitrosoureas (Carmustine [BCNU]** and **Lomustine [CCNU])** are lipid soluble and thus penetrate the blood-brain barrier. BCNU is usually administered in an ethanol solution, and toxicity from the vehicle, including giddiness, flushing, and phlebitis, may occur. Since delayed myelosuppression occurs 6–8 weeks after treatment and may be cumulative, these agents are commonly given at 8-week intervals.
9. **Thiotepa** may be administered intravenously with bone marrow rescue. When used intravesically, 60–90 mg is administered in 60–100 ml of water and instilled over 2 hours.

C. **Antitumor antibiotics** intercalate adjacent DNA nucleotides, interrupting replication and transcription and causing strand breaks; they are cell-cycle nonspecific.
   1. **Anthracycline antibiotics** are associated with a cardiomyopathy consisting of **intractable congestive heart failure** and dysrhythmias. **Using doxorubicin,** this complication is seen in about 2% of patients receiving 550 mg/m^2, but the incidence increases dramatically at higher cumulative doses. Concomitant cyclophosphamide or previous chest irradiation may potentiate this toxicity. As the cumulative dose approaches 450–550 mg/m^2, serial radionuclide ventriculograms should be performed and the anthracycline should be discontinued if left ventricular function is compromised. Myocardial damage is related to peak serum concentrations and to cumulative dose; longer (96-hour) infusions have allowed for higher cumulative dosages. These agents may also produce a radiation recall effect consisting of acute toxicity to previous radiation fields, usually to the heart, gastrointestinal region, or lungs.
      a. **Daunorubicin** is used in the treatment of acute leukemia, and bone marrow suppression is expected; the dose-limiting toxicity is usually mucositis. Red urine may be caused by the drug and its metabolites.
      b. **Doxorubicin (Adriamycin)** toxicity is very similar to daunorubicin, although this drug has a broader spectrum of activity.
      c. **Mitoxantrone** is structurally similar to doxorubicin and daunorubicin but is associated with less cardiac toxicity. Mucositis and myelosuppression are dose-limiting; a bluish discoloration of the urine and sclera may occur.
   2. **Bleomycin** is useful in combination chemotherapy because it is rarely

myelosuppressive. **A test dose,** 1–2 mg SQ, should be administered prior to instituting full doses (especially in patients with lymphoma), since severe allergic reactions with hypotension may occur. Interstitial pneumonitis (which occasionally results in irreversible pulmonary fibrosis) is more common in patients with underlying pulmonary disease, previous lung irradiation, or in patients receiving a cumulative dose of 200 mg/m^2. Pulmonary symptoms and chest radiographs should be monitored.

   3. **Mitomycin C** is associated with delayed myelosuppression that worsens with repeated use of the drug. Interstitial pneumonitis has been observed. The **hemolytic-uremic syndrome** has been reported, is exacerbated by red blood cell transfusions, and should be suspected in patients with sudden onset of a microangiopathic hemolytic anemia and renal failure.

D. **Plant alkaloids.** Vincristine and vinblastine inhibit the assembly of microtubules and disrupt mitosis. Rapid intravenous injection of any plant alkaloid may produce hypotension.

   1. **Vincristine** often causes a dose-limiting neuropathy. Paresthesias followed by loss of deep tendon reflexes usually occur. Neuritic pain, jaw pain, diplopia, constipation, abdominal pain, and an adynamic ileus are less likely. Other adverse effects include the syndrome of inappropriate antidiuretic hormone (SIADH) and Raynaud's phenomenon.

   2. **Vinblastine** is less neurotoxic than vincristine and is usually limited by myelosuppression. In high doses, myalgias, obstipation, and transient hepatitis may occur.

   3. **Etoposide (VP-16).** The predominate dose-limiting toxicity is myelosuppression.

E. **Platinum-containing agents** act as intercalators, causing single- and double-strand breaks in DNA.

   1. **Cisplatin** is one of the most potent agents in producing nausea and vomiting; aggressive antiemetic therapy is mandatory (Table 19-2). The patient should be vigorously hydrated with isotonic saline. One liter of saline should be administered over 4–6 hours before and after chemotherapy. The dosage of cisplatin should be reduced for renal insufficiency and should be withheld if the serum creatinine is greater than 3 mg/dl. Other toxicities include hypomagnesemia and ototoxicity.

   2. **Carboplatin** is a recently released cisplatin analog with less neurotoxicity, ototoxicity, and nephrotoxicity than cisplatin; myelosuppression is the dose-limiting toxicity.

F. **Other agents**

   1. **Hydroxyurea,** an oral agent that inhibits ribonucleotide reductase, is used in the management of the chronic phase of CML and other myeloproliferative diseases. The dosage is adjusted to the peripheral blood neutrophil and platelet count.

   2. **L-Asparaginase** hydrolyzes asparagine, depleting cells of an essential substrate in protein synthesis. Allergic or anaphylactic reactions may occur. Other toxicities include hemorrhagic pancreatitis, hepatic failure with depression of clotting factors, and encephalopathy.

   3. **Procarbazine** is an oral agent that inhibits DNA, RNA, and protein synthesis. It is a monoamine oxidase inhibitor, and therefore tricyclic antidepressants, sympathomimetic agents, and tyramine-containing foods must be used with caution. Procarbazine has a disulfiram-like effect, so ethanol should not be ingested while taking this medication.

G. **Hormonal agents** lack direct cytotoxicity. In general, they have few serious adverse effects. In disseminated disease, eventual resistance to hormonal agents should be anticipated.

   1. **Diethylstilbesterol** is an estradiol analog used in the treatment of breast and prostate cancer. The usual dosage is 5 mg PO tid in women and 1–3 mg PO qd in men. Adverse effects include nausea, gynecomastia, fluid retention, hypertension, and thrombophlebitis. Thromboembolic and cardiovascular complications limit its usefulness in prostate cancer.

Table 19-2. Recommendations for antiemetic therapy

See Nausea and Vomiting, Table 19-1:

0	None necessary
+	Phenothiazine ± butyrophenones ± antihistamine
+ +	Phenothiazine ± butyrophenones ± antihistamine ± anxiolytic ± steroids
+ + +	Ondansetron or phenothiazine ± butyrophenones ± antihistamine ± anxiolytic ± steroids ± high-dose metoclopramide

Phenothiazines*
    Prochlorperazine, 10 mg PO or IV q4–6h
    Prochlorperazine, 25 mg PR q4–6h
    Chlorpromazine, 10 mg PO q4–6h
    Trimethobenzamide, 100 mg PO or IM q4–6h
Ondansetron, 0.15 mg/kg IV 30 min prechemotherapy and q4h × 2
Butyrophenones*
    Droperidol, 5 mg IV q4–6h
Metoclopramide,* 1–3 mg/kg IV prior to chemotherapy and q2h × 3
Antihistamines
    Diphenhydramine, 50 mg PO or IV q4–6h
Anxiolytics
    Lorazepam, 1–2 mg PO or IV tid–qid
Steroids
    Dexamethasone, 10–30 mg IV prior to chemotherapy

* May cause extrapyramidal side effects, which may be treated with either diphenhydramine, 50 mg PO or IV q4–6h, or benztropine mesylate, 1–2 mg IV or PO q4–6h.

2. **Gonadotropin agonists.** Two LHRH agonists are used in the treatment of metastatic prostate cancer. Leuprolide acetate is associated with an initial flare in tumor symptoms, bone pain, fluid retention, hot flashes, sweats, and impotence. A long-acting analog, goseralin acetate, is also available.
3. **Progestational agents.** Megestrol acetate, 40 mg PO qid, and medroxyprogesterone, 10 mg PO qd, have been used in the treatment of a variety of neoplasms. Principal toxicities include weight gain, fluid retention, hot flashes, and vaginal bleeding with discontinuation of therapy. Both agents have been used in the treatment of cachexia associated with cancer and AIDS (see Complications of Cancer, sec. II.A.3).
4. **Tamoxifen** is an estrogen antagonist. The usual dosage is 10 mg PO bid. After 7–14 days of treatment, a **hormone flare** (increasing bone pain, erythema, and hypercalcemia) occurs in approximately 5% of women with estrogen receptor–positive breast cancer and bone metastases. The symptoms abate over 7–10 days, and 75% of these patients respond to tamoxifen. Palliation of pain, control of hypercalcemia, and continuation of the drug are recommended. The long-term administration of tamoxifen is not associated with a systemic anti-estrogen effect (vaginal atrophy, osteoporosis, or increased risk of heart disease).
H. **Immunotherapy.** In general, the use of immunotherapeutic agents such as interleukin-2, monoclonal antibodies, and gamma-interferon must be regarded as investigational. BCG vaccine, methane extracted residue (MER), and *Corynebacterium parvum* have not proved effective as immunoadjuvants.
    1. **Levamisole** is administered with fluorouracil as adjuvant therapy in colon cancer (see Approach to the Cancer Patient, sec. II.B.3). The dosage of 50 mg PO tid for 3 days q2wk is well tolerated and does not appear to add to the toxicity of fluorouracil.
    2. **Alpha-interferon** is currently used for hairy-cell leukemia and the chronic phase of CML. Toxicity includes nausea and vomiting, flu-like symptoms, and

headaches. The acute toxicity may respond to acetaminophen; with continued administration these symptoms subside.

I. **Retinoids** have been used as therapeutic and chemopreventive agents. 13-Cis-retinoic acid, 50–100 mg/m^2 PO qd for 12 months, has been shown to lower the incidence of second primary tumors in patients previously treated for head and neck cancer (*N. Engl. J. Med.* 323:795, 1990). All-trans-retinoic acid, 45–100 mg/m^2 PO qd, has resulted in resolution of disseminated intravascular coagulation and remissions in acute promyelocytic leukemia. Common toxicities include dry skin, headaches, nausea and vomiting, and elevation of transaminases (*Blood* 76:1704, 1990).

Complications of Treatment

I. **Chemotherapy** frequently causes serious or life-threatening toxicity. The most common and predictable toxicities are to rapidly proliferating cells of hematopoietic and mucosal tissue. Since repair of these tissues cannot be accelerated, palliation during the healing process is the primary goal.

A. **Extravasation** of certain chemotherapeutic agents from venous infusion sites may lead to severe local tissue injury. Offending agents are identified as vesicants in Table 19-1. Initial symptoms of pain or erythema may appear within hours or be delayed for up to 1–2 weeks. When extravasation occurs, the following steps should be taken:

1. **Stop the chemotherapy infusion.** While the venous catheter is still in place, approximately 5 ml of blood should be aspirated to remove any residual drug.

2. **Certain drugs require hot or cold** compresses and are neutralized by instillation of agents locally through the catheter and subcutaneously into the nearby tissue:

Drug	Compresses	Antidote
Dacarbazine	Hot	Isotonic thiosulfate IV and SQ
Daunorubicin	Cold	DMSO applied topically to the vein
Doxorubicin	Cold	DMSO applied topically to the vein
Mechlorethamine		Isotonic thiosulfate IV and SQ
Mitomycin C		Isotonic thiosulfate IV and SQ
Vinblastine	Hot	Hyaluronidase, 150 U/ml; 1–6 ml SQ × 1
Vincristine	Hot	Hyaluronidase, 150 U/ml; 1–6 ml SQ × 1
VP-16	Hot	Isotonic thiosulfate IV and SQ

3. **Follow the area closely** for signs of tissue breakdown; surgical intervention for debridement or skin grafting may be necessary. Extravasation injuries usually result in severe pain, so adequate analgesia should be supplied (*J. Clin. Oncol.* 5:1116, 1987).

B. **Myelosuppression** from most agents reaches its peak 7–14 days following treatment (see Table 19-1). Prophylactic measures to reduce bleeding are mandatory; however, empiric antibiotics or antifungal agents are not generally recommended.

1. **Risk of infection** increases dramatically when the neutrophil count is less than 500/μl and is directly related to the duration of the neutropenia. In the absence of neutrophils, signs of infection or inflammation may be muted. A febrile neutropenic patient should be presumed to be infected and must be evaluated and treated quickly. Physical examination must be performed to localize any sites of infection, with particular attention to indwelling catheter sites, sinuses, and the oral and rectal areas. **Cultures** of blood, urine, stool, sputum, and other foci suspected of bacterial infection are collected, and a chest radiograph is obtained. **Empiric antibiotic treatment** should be initiated immediately after cultures are obtained. In the absence of any obvious source, the antibiotics should provide broad coverage of gram-negative bacilli and

gram-positive cocci. In choosing a regimen, local susceptibility patterns should also be considered. Empiric therapy may consist of an aminoglycoside and semisynthetic penicillin, a double beta-lactam combination, or a single agent such as cefoperazone, 1–2 g IV bid; ceftazidime, 1–2 g IV q8h; or imipenem, 500–1,000 mg IV qid. **Modification of the antibiotic regimen** according to the culture data or clinical picture may become necessary. Additional agents to treat *Staphylococcus epidermidis, Clostridium difficile,* or anaerobic infections are commonly necessary. Persistent fever, in the absence of other data, usually does not warrant an empiric change in the antibacterial therapy. Amphotericin B (0.5–1.0 mg/kg qd) should be added empirically if the fever continues longer than 72 hours (see Chap. 12). Antibiotics are continued until the neutrophil count is greater than 500/µl.

2. **Thrombocytopenia** below 20,000/µl that is the result of chemotherapy should be treated with platelet transfusions to minimize the risk of spontaneous hemorrhage (see Chap. 18). When prolonged thrombocytopenia is anticipated, histocompatibility testing should be performed prior to therapy so that HLA-matched single-donor platelets may be provided when alloimmunization makes the patient refractory to random donor platelets.

3. **Red blood cell transfusions** are indicated for patients who have (1) symptoms of anemia, (2) active bleeding, or (3) a hemoglobin concentration below 7–8 g/dl (see Chap. 18). Because of anecdotal reports of graft-versus-host disease associated with transfusions, radiation of all blood products is generally recommended for immunosuppressed marrow transplant patients.

C. **Gastrointestinal toxicity**
1. **Stomatitis** is an unpleasant consequence of many chemotherapeutic agents (see Table 19-1) and is commonly the dose-limiting toxicity of methotrexate and fluorouracil. With simultaneous administration of radiation therapy, the toxicity is more severe. Healing generally occurs within 7–10 days of the development of symptoms. The severity of stomatitis ranges from mild (oral discomfort) to severe (ulceration, impaired oral intake, and hemorrhage). In mild cases, oral rinses (chlorhexidine, 15–30 ml swish and spit tid or the combination of equal parts diphenhydramine elixir, saline, and 3% hydrogen peroxide) may provide relief. In severe cases, intravenous morphine is appropriate. **IV fluids** should be used to supplement oral intake as needed. Patients with moderate or severe stomatitis may develop aspiration; precautions should include elevation of the head of the bed and availability of a hand-held suction apparatus. In severe or prolonged episodes, superinfection with *Candida* or *Herpes simplex* may be present and requires appropriate diagnosis and antimicrobial intervention.

2. **Diarrhea** is the result of cytotoxicity to the rapidly proliferating cells of the intestinal mucosa. In some cases, IV fluids are necessary to avoid dehydration. The use of oral opioid agents as antidiarrheals is commonly limited by abdominal cramping. The severe diarrhea associated with fluorouracil and leucovorin has been reported to respond to octreotide, 150–500 µg SQ tid.

3. **Nausea and vomiting** may develop in varying degrees and frequency. Suggestions for antiemetic agent(s) are listed in Table 19-2 according to the severity of nausea and vomiting outlined in Table 19-1.

D. **Interstitial pneumonitis** may develop as a dose-related, cumulative toxicity or as an idiosyncratic reaction. The implicated agent should be discontinued, and institution of glucocorticoids (e.g., prednisone, 1 mg/kg PO qd or equivalent) may be of some benefit. The long-term outcome is unpredictable.

E. **Hemorrhagic cystitis** may develop with either cyclophosphamide or ifosamide. Continuous bladder irrigation with isotonic saline should continue until the hematuria resolves.

F. **Tumor lysis syndrome** occurs in patients with rapidly proliferating neoplasms that are highly sensitive to chemotherapy. Rapid tumor kill releases intracellular contents and causes hyperkalemia, hyperphosphatemia, and hyperuricemia. Although reported in the treatment of a variety of malignancies, it is usually associated with **high-grade non-Hodgkin's lymphoma** and **acute**

leukemia. During induction chemotherapy, prophylactic measures should include allopurinol, 300–600 mg PO or IV qd, and aggressive intravenous hydration (e.g., 3,000 ml/m^2 daily). The addition of sodium bicarbonate, 50 mEq/1,000 ml of hydration fluid, to alkalinize the urine above pH 7 may prevent uric acid nephropathy and acute renal failure. When hyperphosphatemia accompanies hyperuricemia, urine alkalinization should be avoided because calcium phosphate precipitation may result in renal failure. Despite these preventive measures, hemodialysis may be needed for hyperkalemia, hyperphosphatemia, acute renal failure, or fluid overload.

II. **Radiation therapy** toxicity is related to the location of the therapy, total dose delivered, and the rate of delivery. Larger fractions per dose are associated with more acute normal tissue toxicity than a more protracted delivery.

    A. **Acute toxicity** develops within the first 3 months of therapy and is characterized by an inflammatory reaction. Such toxicity may respond to anti-inflammatory agents such as glucocorticoids. Local irritations or burns in the treatment field will generally resolve with time. Close observation and treatment of any infections as well as palliation of symptoms such as pain, dysphagia, dysuria, or diarrhea (depending on the site of treatment) are the mainstay of supportive care until healing has occurred.

    B. **Subacute toxicities** between 3 and 6 months of therapy and **chronic toxicity,** after 6 months, are less amenable to therapy, as fibrosis and scarring are present.

20

Diabetes Mellitus

Matthew J. Orland

Diabetes Mellitus

Diabetes mellitus (DM) refers to a group of disorders manifested by hyperglycemia. Although the pathogeneses of these disorders are diverse, patients with DM ultimately demonstrate an inability to produce insulin in amounts necessary to meet their metabolic needs.

I. **Classification**

   A. **Diabetes mellitus** includes three diagnostic types.

      1. **Insulin-dependent (type I) diabetes mellitus** most commonly occurs in children and young adults but may occur at any age. Among individuals with a genetic predisposition, the immune-mediated destruction of insulin-producing cells leads to a progressive, nearly total loss of endogenous insulin. Exogenous insulin is essential to achieve glycemic control, to prevent diabetic ketoacidosis (DKA), and to sustain life.

      2. **Non–insulin-dependent (type II) diabetes mellitus** usually occurs after age 30. A strong genetic predisposition is evident, but the pathogenesis is different from that of type I DM. Most individuals are obese, and resistance to insulin action is present in many cases. Endogenous insulin production is usually adequate to avoid ketoacidosis, but DKA may occur with intense stress. Exogenous insulin can be used to treat hyperglycemia but is not required for survival.

      3. **Other (secondary) diabetes mellitus** associates hyperglycemia to another established cause, including pancreatic disease, pancreatectomy, drugs or chemical agents, Cushing's syndrome, acromegaly, and a number of uncommon genetic disorders.

   B. **Impaired glucose tolerance** is a classification appropriate for those who manifest abnormal plasma glucose levels but who do not meet the defined diagnostic criteria for DM (see sec. **II**).

   C. **Gestational diabetes mellitus** refers to patients in whom hyperglycemia develops during pregnancy. These individuals usually revert to normal glucose tolerance following delivery but have an increased risk for development of DM later in life.

II. **Diagnosis of diabetes mellitus** can be established when classic symptoms accompany unequivocal hyperglycemia, and also when specific diagnostic criteria are met in asymptomatic individuals. Screening is appropriate in patients with a strong family history of DM; with significant obesity; with recurrent skin, genital, or urinary tract infections; or with a pregnancy history complicated by gestational diabetes, prematurity, or birth weight greater than 9 pounds. In these patients a random plasma glucose (PG) greater than 160 mg/dl or fasting PG greater than 115 mg/dl is an indication for diagnostic testing and close follow-up. Reversible conditions that promote hyperglycemia (Table 20-1) should be sought and corrected, if possible, before the diagnosis of DM is established.

   A. **Symptomatic patients** with polyuria, polydipsia, and weight loss can be diagnosed when a random plasma glucose is greater than 200 mg/dl, and no further testing is needed. When glucose is less than 200 mg/dl, testing as for asymptomatic patients (see sec. **II.B**) is usually warranted.

   B. **Asymptomatic patients.** Diagnostic testing should be performed when an

Table 20-1. Conditions that promote hyperglycemia in patients with diabetes mellitus[a]

I. Increased dietary intake (particularly of carbohydrate)
II. Limitation of physical activity
III. Reduction of hypoglycemic therapy
IV. Limitation of endogenous insulin production
    A. Pancreatic diseases (or pancreatectomy)[b]
    B. Drug treatment[b]
        1. Destruction of insulin-producing cells
            a. Streptozocin
            b. Pentamidine isethionate
        2. Reversible inhibition of insulin secretion
            a. Diazoxide
            b. Thiazide diuretics
            c. Phenytoin
    C. Electrolyte disorders
        1. Hypokalemia
        2. Hypomagnesemia
V. Development of insulin resistance[b]
    A. Infection
    B. Inflammation
    C. Myocardial or other tissue ischemia, or infarction
    D. Trauma
    E. Surgery
    F. Emotional stress
    G. Pregnancy
    H. Drug treatment
        1. Glucocorticoids
        2. Estrogens (including oral contraceptives)
        3. Sympathomimetic agents
        4. Nicotinic acid
    I. Antibodies to insulin
    J. Antibodies to insulin receptors

[a] These conditions (particularly IV and V) should also be investigated in patients with diabetic ketoacidosis or nonketotic hyperosmolar syndrome.
[b] These conditions may also promote transient hyperglycemia among patients without established DM.

abnormal screening result is obtained or when a strong clinical suspicion of DM (see sec. II) is present. These **tests should be repeated** and abnormal results should be demonstrated on more than one occasion before a diagnosis is made.
1. **Fasting plasma glucose,** after an overnight fast, should be greater than 140 mg/dl.
2. **Oral glucose tolerance testing** can be performed when fasting plasma glucose does not establish a diagnosis. Results are valid only when patients are not stressed, when physical activity is unrestricted, and when daily carbohydrate intake is greater than 150 g. Nonpregnant adults should be given 75 g of glucose in the morning after an overnight fast. Plasma glucose should be measured initially, and at half-hour intervals for 2 hours after glucose administration. A normal test shows (1) a fasting PG less than 115 mg/dl, (2) a 2-hour PG less than 140 mg/dl, and (3) no values greater than 200 mg/dl. A diagnosis of DM can be made if the PG is 200 mg/dl or greater (1) at 2 hours and (2) on at least one of the earlier samples. Intermediate values define impaired glucose tolerance.
  C. **Modified criteria are defined for pregnant patients.**
III. **Management of diabetes mellitus.** Objectives of diabetes therapy should be (1) to avoid the immediate consequences of insulin insufficiency, including symptomatic

hyperglycemia (i.e., polyuria, polydipsia, and weight loss), DKA, and nonketotic hyperosmolar syndrome (NKHS); and (2) to ameliorate the complications of long-standing disease. There is evidence that the chronic complications of DM result from metabolic abnormalities, and that control of hyperglycemia may reduce their incidence (*Ann. Intern. Med.* 105:254, 1986). For each patient, the physician should attempt to formulate a treatment plan that yields the best glycemic control possible without producing frequent or severe hypoglycemia. Clinical practice recommendations are established by the American Diabetes Association (*Diabetes Care* 14 (suppl 2):1, 1991).

A. Monitoring of therapy. The objectives of management demand careful attention to the status of glucose control and of any acute or chronic complications.

 1. **Patient assessment** should include a careful investigation for symptomatic hyperglycemia, including occurrence of nocturia, polyuria, or polydipsia, as well as more subtle symptoms such as fatigue or blurred vision. Physical examination should focus on manifestations of complications of DM affecting the eyes, cardiovascular system, kidneys, nerves, and skin (see sec. **III.I**). Symptoms of hypoglycemia should also be assessed in patients using pharmacologic therapy (see Hypoglycemia).

 2. **Glucose measurements** are necessary to document efficacy and to guide modification of therapy.

    a. **Plasma glucose measurement** is appropriate for screening and diagnosis (see sec. **II**) and is the traditional therapeutic parameter. Falsely low PG values may occur as a result of glycolysis in the collection tube; this can be minimized by routine use of glycolytic inhibitors and rapid processing of samples.

    b. **Capillary blood glucose measurement** allows a rapid measurement of glucose in whole blood. The widespread use of blood glucose monitoring with glucose oxidase reagent strips and portable reflectance meters allows a convenient and cost-effective alternative to frequent PG determinations. Errors may occur when a blood sample is inadequate or when the timing of the reaction is not measured correctly (*Arch. Intern. Med.* 144:2029, 1984). Most meters require routine cleaning and calibration.

       (1) **Self-monitoring of blood glucose (SMBG)** using these methods is the preferred means of following glucose control. SMBG is appropriate for all patients with DM. Frequency of monitoring may vary based on goals for glycemic control and stability of glucose levels. Considerations for frequency of monitoring should include a routine schedule and an intensified program appropriate when therapy is changed or illness occurs (see sec. **III.F**). Measurements should be recorded in an organized fashion by the patient, so that they can be reviewed during regular assessment of therapy.

       (2) **Reliability of measurements** depends on proper instruction and should be periodically reassessed by the physician and by a diabetes nurse–educator.

    c. **Urine glucose determinations** monitor blood glucose levels above a variable renal glucose threshold (i.e., 150–350 mg/dl). Glucose oxidase strips or tape provide a semiquantitative measurement of urine glucose, influenced by both glucose and water excretion; therefore, results correlate poorly with blood glucose levels. Urine assays cannot detect hypoglycemia. Urine glucose measurements can be used when blood glucose monitoring is impractical.

 3. **Glycosylated hemoglobin measurements** are important tools for periodic assessment of glycemic control. These assays quantify nonenzymatic, covalent glycosylation of hemoglobin that develops during the life span of circulating red blood cells and is linearly correlated with mean blood glucose levels over 2–3 months preceding measurement. A percentage of stably glycosylated hemoglobin (hemoglobin A_{1C}) in blood serves to validate patient SMBG data (*Diabetes Care* 7:602, 1984). Hemoglobinopathies may affect hemoglobin A_{1C} levels, and underestimation of chronic hyperglycemia may

occur in conditions in which red blood cell survival is reduced (e.g., uremia, hemolytic anemia).

4. **Ketone assays** employ the nitroprusside reaction to measure ketones in blood and urine. Ketone overproduction may occur with DKA, prolonged fasting, or alcohol intoxication.

   a. **Serum ketone measurements** are important to document DKA (see Insulin-Dependent [Type I] Diabetes Mellitus). Titration may allow a semiquantitative determination of ketone concentrations, but this is seldom useful.

   b. **Urine ketone determinations** are a sensitive means of monitoring ketones in blood and should be performed by patients prone to DKA when persistent hyperglycemia is noted or when illness or stress is present.

B. **Patient education.** Optimum treatment of DM requires an informed patient. Management is facilitated when the properly educated patient can make appropriate decisions in daily care.

1. **Early education** should emphasize the practical aspects of management, including diet planning and techniques for the monitoring of glucose and ketones. The relationships of diet, physical activity, and medications should be conveyed. Specific instructions should be given regarding care in emergencies or for complicating illnesses, including careful monitoring (see secs. **III.A.2.b.(1)**, **III.F**, **III.G**, and **III.H**). When insulin or an oral hypoglycemic drug is prescribed, patients must know how to prevent, recognize, and manage hypoglycemia. Basic instructions should also be given to family members and roommates. Useful publications from the American Diabetes Association are available to help patients develop an understanding of their disease and their treatment plan.

2. **Team support.** Instruction by the physician, by a diabetes nurse–educator, and by a dietitian is important.

C. **Dietary modification** is important in all types of DM and may also be beneficial to patients with impaired glucose tolerance. The objectives of dietary management differ according to (1) the diagnostic type of diabetes, (2) the degree of obesity, (3) the coexistence of lipid abnormalities, (4) the presence of diabetic complications, and (5) the concurrent medical therapy. The meal plan should be prepared with consideration of patient preferences, resources, and needs.

1. **Caloric goals** should be those required to achieve and to maintain ideal body weight (see Chap. 2). Reduction of caloric intake is desirable only in overweight patients.

2. **Consistency** in composition and timing of meals is important, particularly for patients using fixed insulin regimens or oral hypoglycemic drugs. Exchange lists allow a motivated patient to construct a consistent diet and yet maintain some freedom in choice of foods.

3. **Food composition.** The optimum nutrient composition in DM is uncertain (*Diabetes Care* 6:197, 1986). Considerations include not only effects of the diet on blood glucose levels but also the impact dietary modification might make toward a reduction of atherosclerosis and other chronic complications.

   a. **Carbohydrate** (55–60%) is essential to maintain caloric intake. Foods with a high refined sugar content should be limited but can be included as part of a balanced meal. Complex carbohydrates are a preferred calorie source. Carbohydrate-containing foods can be classified by a glycemic index (*Diabetes Care* 11:149, 1988) related to effects on postprandial blood glucose.

   b. **Protein** (10–20%) should be sufficient to maintain nitrogen balance and to promote growth (see Chap. 2). Limitation of protein intake may be appropriate for patients with diabetic nephropathy (see Chap. 11).

   c. **Fat** (25–30%) should be restricted. Cholesterol intake should be less than 300 mg/day, and saturated fat intake should be replaced by polyunsaturated fat when possible.

   d. **Fiber** (25 g/1000 kcal) in the diet can retard the absorption of sugars and can ameliorate postprandial blood glucose elevation. Fiber-containing foods that aid glucose control include beans, legumes, and guar gum; bran and guar fiber may also help to lower total and low-density lipoprotein (LDL) cholesterol (*Diabetes Care* 11:160, 1988).

  e. Artificial sweeteners are available as a substitute for sucrose in soft drinks and many foods. Aspartame and saccharin are helpful in reducing sucrose intake while maintaining a palatable diet.

4. Alcohol use should be limited. Alcohol inhibits hepatic gluconeogenesis and may promote hypoglycemia in patients using insulin or oral hypoglycemic drugs. Sugar-containing alcoholic beverages may also cause hyperglycemia. Alcohol contributes to acute and chronic hypertriglyceridemia (see Chap. 22) and perturbs sulfonylurea metabolism (see sec. **IV**). A limited consumption of alcohol among patients with DM is acceptable, with meals, and should be defined as fat in a meal plan (see sec. **III.C.3.c**). Patients with neuropathy should avoid alcohol, as worsening impairment may occur.

D. Physical activity offers both benefits and risks for patients with DM. In normal individuals, increased glucose utilization of exercising muscle is balanced by hepatic glucose production; this balance is regulated by insulin and is often disturbed in diabetes. During exercise marked hyperglycemia and ketosis can occur when DM is poorly controlled, and hypoglycemia may be promoted by abundant exogenous insulin or by the endogenous insulin stimulated by oral hypoglycemic drugs. Careful planning of meals and dosing are required when insulin-treated patients increase activity or attempt strenuous exercise. Snacks can be used during a period of intense physical activity to balance the effects of fixed exogenous insulin or oral hypoglycemic drug treatment. Exercise may also be detrimental to patients with chronic complications of DM; cardiovascular disease, neuropathy, and retinopathy may yield a functional impairment. Preventive management, including cardiovascular evaluation, proper footwear, and ophthalmic care, is appropriate, and patient education is essential.

E. Pharmacologic therapy includes treatment with insulin or with oral hypoglycemic drugs (see secs. **IV** and **V**).

  1. Decisions in drug treatment should be based primarily on the type of DM and on the need for control of blood glucose.

  2. Modification of therapy should be guided by the goals set for each patient to control blood glucose. Changes in drugs or dosing should be accompanied by patient education and by an intensification of glucose monitoring.

F. Hyperglycemic exacerbations. Therapy of DM must address not only the control of glucose in the stable patient but also the management of situations in which routine treatment is inadequate. The stress of illness or trauma increases metabolic demands for insulin, and special attention to diabetes care is required. As treatment is adjusted, the physician should consider (1) the nature of the precipitating stress, (2) the diagnostic type of diabetes, (3) the therapeutic goals established for the patient, (4) the compliance to the usual treatment regimen, and (5) the complications that might result from an adjustment.

  1. Intensification of monitoring should be prompted by changes from the usual glucose profile and should be continued until stability returns and further changes are not anticipated.

  2. Identification of precipitating factors. Correction of an illness or other condition promoting hyperglycemia (see Table 20-1) is the most important aspect of successful treatment. A diagnostic evaluation is warranted when causes of worsening hyperglycemia are not apparent. When possible, a time course of the precipitating stress should be anticipated; resolution usually reverses the increase in insulin demands.

  3. Modification of therapy is required when symptomatic hyperglycemia is evident or when DKA might occur (see Insulin-Dependent [Type I] Diabetes Mellitus). Dietary modifications are not routinely indicated but may be necessary when a precipitating event has perturbed dietary intake (see sec. **III.G**) The initiation of insulin or oral hypoglycemic drugs must be accompanied by appropriate patient education (see sec. **III.B**), even when needs are expected to be temporary.

G. **Inability to maintain dietary intake** may occur secondary to gastrointestinal illness, surgery, trauma, or depression. If insulin or an oral hypoglycemic drug is used, management must include meticulous monitoring. Drug dosage reductions and use of oral, sugar-containing fluids or intravenous dextrose are appropriate measures to prevent hypoglycemia (see Hypoglycemia).

H. **Infection** occurs frequently in diabetic patients, and the coexistence of infection and diabetes affects management of both. Patients with uncontrolled DM are often immunologically compromised, with impaired granulocyte function; improvement in resistance to infection can follow control of blood glucose.

   1. **Urinary tract infection** occurs commonly in women with DM. Pathogens include enteric gram-negative bacteria, as well as staphylococci, enterococci, and fungi. Antibiotic therapy is appropriate. Antibiotic prophylaxis may be helpful to patients with recurrent infections or neurogenic bladder (see Chronic Complications of Diabetes Mellitus).

   2. **Cellulitis** is common in patients with DM. Streptococci and *Staphylococcus aureus* are frequent pathogens; gram-negative and anaerobic infections may also occur when an open ulcer or necrotizing inflammation is present. Cellulitis is often more difficult to treat in extremities compromised by neuropathy or vascular insufficiency.

   3. **Skin abscesses** are usually caused by *Staph. aureus*. Large abscesses require drainage; all warrant antibiotic therapy.

   4. **Vulvovaginitis** is commonly due to *Candida albicans,* and topical antifungal therapy is appropriate (see Chap. 13).

I. **Assessment for chronic complications of diabetes** is important in the routine management of patients with type I DM beginning at 5 years' duration, for all patients with type II or other DM, and during diabetic pregnancy. The routine outpatient evaluation should include ophthalmoscopy, cardiac and vascular assessment, neurologic examination, and examination of the feet. Urinalysis should include an assessment for protein. Plasma creatinine and electrolytes should be measured periodically. Monitoring of serum lipid levels is recommended. A yearly ECG is advised, and surveillance for retinopathy requires at least yearly examinations by an ophthalmologist (see Chronic Complications of Diabetes Mellitus).

J. **Preventive care.** The severity of some diabetic complications may be reduced by specific prophylactic management.

   1. **Identification.** Patients with DM should carry information about the type of diabetes, complications, and treatment regimens that can be used when emergency care is necessary.

   2. **Vaccinations.** Pneumococcal vaccine should be considered for all patients. Yearly influenza vaccination is prudent.

   3. **Attention to other risk factors for cardiovascular disease.** Detection and management of hypertension and hyperlipidemia (see Chaps. 4 and 22) and abstinence from cigarette smoking are particularly important health maintenance objectives.

   4. **Foot care** is essential for patients with neuropathy (see Chronic Complications of Diabetes Mellitus, sec. **VII**).

K. **Drug therapy for other conditions** should be chosen with consideration of side effects that may compromise management of hyperglycemia (see Table 20-1) or worsen diabetic complications. In general, therapy should not be withheld if indications for use are sound. Patient education and intensification of glucose monitoring, including SMBG in outpatients, should accompany initial use, changes in dosage, and discontinuation of any drug.

IV. **Oral hypoglycemic drugs.** The sulfonylureas lower blood glucose in patients capable of endogenous insulin production. These drugs affect glucose metabolism by stimulation of insulin secretion, and perhaps by reduction of insulin resistance. They are indicated for nonpregnant adults with type II and most secondary DM.

A. **Preparations.** Sulfonylureas differ in potency, in duration of action (Table 20-2), and in certain peculiar side effects.

B. **Contraindications.** Sulfonylureas should not be used in type I DM, in children,

Table 20-2. Characteristics of the oral hypoglycemic drugs (sulfonylureas)[a]

Generic name	Initial dosage[b]	Maximum dosage	Duration of activity (hr)[c]
Glyburide	1.25–5.0 mg PO qd	10 mg PO bid	24–60
Glipizide	2.5–5.0 mg PO qd	20 mg PO bid	12–24
Chlorpropamide	100–250 mg PO qd	250 mg PO bid	48–90
Tolazamide	100–250 mg PO qd	500 mg PO bid	10–24
Acetohexamide	250–500 mg PO qd	750 mg PO bid	12–24
Tolbutamide	250–500 mg PO bid	1000 mg PO tid	6–12

[a] Drugs are listed in order of decreasing potency. Maximum efficacy is similar for all of the drugs at the maximum dosage listed.
[b] The lower dosages are appropriate when initiating treatment in elderly patients, in patients with uncertain meal schedules, or in patients with mild hyperglycemia.
[c] Activity of the sulfonylureas is prolonged in both hepatic and renal failure.

or during pregnancy or lactation. Use should be avoided in patients with severe hepatic or renal failure.

   C. Complications of sulfonylurea therapy can occur with any of these drugs. The augmented hypoglycemic potency of glyburide and glipizide may permit their effective usage with fewer drug interactions and dose-related toxic reactions.

     1. Hypoglycemia from sulfonylureas can be severe and prolonged, often warranting observation and therapy well beyond the expected duration of action of the offending drug (see Table 20-2). Alcohol, chloramphenicol, clofibrate, methyldopa, miconazole, monoamine oxidase inhibitors, phenylbutazone, probenecid, salicylates, sulfonamides, and warfarin may potentiate the hypoglycemic effects of sulfonylureas, and concurrent use of these drugs requires an intensification of glucose monitoring and dosage adjustment (see Hypoglycemia).

     2. Toxic reactions include skin rash, blood dyscrasias, and cholestatic jaundice. Flushing, tachycardia, nausea, and headache may occur following the consumption of alcohol.

     3. An increased risk of cardiovascular mortality has been shown (*Diabetes* 19 (suppl 2):747, 1970) with use of sulfonylureas. This risk must be weighed against their therapeutic benefit in treatment of patients with type II or other DM.

     4. Chlorpropamide may cause hyponatremia and fluid retention.

V. Insulin. Exogenous insulin lowers blood glucose in all types of DM. Optimal insulin treatment, however, should approximate physiologic insulin delivery, which at best is difficult with subcutaneous injections, or even with continuous insulin infusion. A variety of formulations are available to help match release of subcutaneously injected insulin to the estimated basal needs, observed between meals and during sleep, and to the diet and activity schedules.

   A. Insulin formulations differ (1) in type, which is designed to influence the rate of absorption after subcutaneous injection (Table 20-3); (2) in composition, according to animal or human species; and (3) in concentration.

     1. Rapid-acting insulins include regular and semilente types. Only regular insulin is appropriate for intravenous use; both can be given subcutaneously.

       a. Intravenous regular insulin can be given as a bolus or as a continuous infusion. An intravenous insulin bolus produces its maximum effect at 10–30 minutes and may last for 1–2 hours. For most clinical uses an insulin infusion can be prepared by adding 100 units of insulin to 500 ml of 0.45% saline (i.e., 0.2 units/ml, 1 unit/5 ml). Like many peptides, insulin adheres to containers and to plastic infusion lines; administration should be preceded by flushing lines with roughly 50 ml of the solution to saturate binding sites. Effects of insulin infusions also last for roughly 1–2 hours after cessation, with lower doses waning more rapidly.

Table 20-3. Pharmacokinetics of insulin after subcutaneous injection*

Insulin type	Onset of action (hr)	Peak effect (hr)	Duration of activity (hr)
Rapid-acting			
Regular	0.25–1.0	2–6	4–12
Semilente	0.5–1.0	3–10	8–18
Intermediate-acting			
NPH	1.5–4.0	6–16	14–28
Lente	1.0–4.0	6–16	14–28
Long-acting			
PZI	3.0–8.0	14–26	24–40
Ultralente	3.0–8.0	8–28	24–40

Key: NPH = neutral protamine Hagedorn; PZI = protamine zinc insulin.
* Variations in pharmacokinetics are related to patient differences, species composition, and insulin dose. Human insulins may produce a faster peak effect and a shorter duration of activity than bovine or beef–pork insulins. Larger doses may have a more marked peak effect and a more prolonged duration of activity. Activity may be prolonged in renal failure.

    b. Intramuscular regular insulin produces its maximum effect at 30–60 minutes after injection in patients with normal circulation and lasts for 2–4 hours. The activity is variable and often delayed in hypotensive patients.

    c. Subcutaneous regular insulin is prescribed most commonly. Maximum activity occurs 2–6 hours after injection with an insulin syringe (see sec. **V.C**), with activity lasting for 4–12 hours (see Table 20-3). When the dose of insulin is increased, absorption kinetics are affected; a more marked peak effect and a more prolonged duration of activity can be anticipated with larger doses (see sec. **V.C**).

  2. Intermediate-acting insulins include neutral protamine Hagedorn (NPH) and lente insulins (see Table 20-3), which release insulin from a subcutaneous site during most of the day after morning injection. This release is not constant; insulin activity reaches a peak 6–16 hours after injection, followed by a slower decline in level and in activity. As with regular insulin, pharmacokinetics are dose dependent.

  3. Long-acting insulins include ultralente insulin and protamine zinc insulin (PZI), which are absorbed more slowly than the intermediate-acting insulins. They can be administered to provide a nearly constant level of circulating insulin when given in daily or bid injections.

  4. Species composition. Insulins from bovine, porcine, and human sources differ in amino acid composition. Human and porcine insulins are less immunogenic than bovine insulin (see sec. **V.D**). Pharmacokinetics may also differ; human insulins are often absorbed more rapidly, showing earlier peak effects and shorter durations of activity than the similarly formulated insulins of porcine or bovine composition. The differences may be important in certain treatment situations; a faster-acting regular insulin of human composition may be the best to manage an ensuing meal, while a slower-acting ultralente insulin of bovine (or beef–pork) composition may be the best to provide basal doses in multiple daily insulin injection (MDII) regimens (see Insulin-Dependent [Type I] Diabetes Mellitus). Because of the pharmacokinetic variabilities, care should be taken when a change in species composition is prescribed; dosage adjustments may be necessary.

  5. Concentration. Almost all insulins used in adults are prepared as 100 units/ml, or U-100. Lower concentrations (e.g., U-40) are often used in children and in subcutaneous infusion pumps. A U-500 insulin is available for patients with severe insulin resistance.

B. **Mixed insulin therapy** using different insulin types is employed to meet needs for variable insulin delivery while providing a convenient dosing regimen. Most commonly used is a combination of rapid-acting and intermediate-acting insulins, mixed in a syringe immediately before administration. When two different insulin types are drawn from the same syringe, care should be taken to avoid cross-contamination of the bottles; when regular insulin is used, it should be drawn first. Insulin mixtures may change pharmacokinetics of component types and yield unexpected results. A delay in the peak activity of regular insulin may be observed when it is mixed with lente or ultralente insulins, but when regular insulin is mixed with NPH insulin the respective activities are not changed. Commercially prepared mixtures of regular and NPH insulins are available, and they may provide a convenient option for patients whose needs match the available formulations. PZI insulin should not be mixed with other types.

C. **Subcutaneous insulin administration.** Methods and timing of insulin administration are at least as important as the insulin dosage for effective treatment of hyperglycemia. The strategy of insulin delivery is guided by the type of DM and the individualized goals for blood glucose control (*Diabetes Care* 13:955, 1990).

1. **Syringe injection.** Disposable syringes with fine (27–29 gauge) hypodermic needles are the preferred tools for insulin administration. Doses must be measured with precision. Bottles of NPH and ultralente insulins should be agitated gently (avoiding formation of bubbles) before an aliquot is removed for injection. Most insulin syringes are calibrated in 1- to 2-unit increments that may be difficult for a visually impaired patient to see. Nondisposable, cartridge-loaded syringe injectors, using replaceable needles, provide an alternative to syringes and are particularly attractive for patients who use MDII.

2. **Jet injection.** Jet injector devices present an alternative to hypodermic needles. Because of dissimilar absorption kinetics, effective doses of insulins may be different from those defined by syringe injection; jet injectors produce a roughly 10–20% augmented and 30-minute earlier peak activity for most insulin types. This may present an advantage with regular insulin taken before meals but a disadvantage with intermediate-acting and long-acting insulins prescribed to provide stable levels during the day.

3. **Sites of injection.** Subcutaneous tissue of the anterior abdominal wall, anterior thighs, buttocks, and posterior arms can be used for injection. Sites should be clean, and areas of infection, inflammation, scarring, or lipodystrophy should be avoided. The site of injection may affect the kinetics of insulin absorption; absorption is generally fastest from the abdomen and slower from the extremities. It is prudent to alternate (rotate) subcutaneous injection sites, but rotation may not be desirable when marked variations in absorption are suspected (*Practical Diabetology* 9:1, 1990). Exercise or massage of injection sites may accelerate insulin absorption. Peripheral vasoconstriction may retard absorption.

4. **Portable infusion pumps** can deliver continuous, programmable infusions of insulin, allowing an alternative to injections. Abdominal sites are most suitable for placement of a subcutaneous infusion catheter; these sites should be rotated and must be inspected regularly for signs of infection.

D. **Complications of insulin therapy**

1. **Hypoglycemia** is the most frequent and serious complication of insulin treatment (see Hypoglycemia). Severity and duration of hypoglycemia can be estimated from the dosage, the methods of injection (e.g., SQ, IM, IV), and the pharmacokinetics of the types of insulin administered (see Table 20-3).

2. **Insulin allergy** may occur, particularly when insulin therapy is intermittent. Reactions are usually related to species composition, but allergy can develop with any preparation. Protamine, a component of NPH and PZI formulations, rarely promotes an allergic response. Most reactions are local, characterized by erythema, induration, and pruritus at a recent injection site. Serious manifestations can include urticaria and anaphylaxis. Skin tests may aid

diagnosis. Uninterrupted treatment with purified insulins of human (or porcine) composition is beneficial during treatment and for subsequent prevention.

  a. Treatment of local reactions is often unnecessary. Pruritus or urticaria may respond to antihistamines (see Chap. 1).

  b. Treatment of systemic reactions should be guided by the severity of manifestations. Generalized urticaria may respond to antihistamines (see sec. **V.D.2.a**); however, these patients should be observed for more serious reactions. Standard measures for the management of anaphylaxis are appropriate (see Chap. 26), including the administration of epinephrine and glucocorticoids.

  c. Desensitization regimens can be used for patients with significant insulin allergy requiring insulin therapy (*Med. Clin. North Am.* 62:663, 1978).

  3. Antibody-mediated insulin resistance may occur at any time but is most common within the first 6 months of initiation or reinstitution of insulin therapy. Low titers of insulin antibodies are common; however, levels sufficient to raise daily insulin requirements are rare. Hyperglycemia that does not respond to a usual insulin dosage is the primary manifestation; other causes of hyperglycemic exacerbations must be excluded (see Table 20-1). Change to human insulins is appropriate. When patients require high doses of insulin, U-500 preparations can be prescribed.

  4. Lipodystrophy may occur at sites of insulin injection. **Lipoatrophy** has been related to impure insulin preparations and can be treated with repeated injections of small doses of purified insulin into the periphery of the affected sites. **Lipohypertrophy** occurs when insulin is injected frequently at a single site; if the site is avoided, further treatment is usually unnecessary.

Insulin-Dependent (Type I) Diabetes Mellitus

The absence of endogenous insulin in insulin-dependent diabetes demands perpetual treatment with exogenous insulin. Analogous to the needs of normal individuals, estimated at 0.6–1.2 units/kg/day (35–50 units/day in adults), daily insulin needs of patients with type I DM can be divided into a **basal requirement** (40–50%), which is needed to maintain glycemic control between meals and during sleep, and a **dietary requirement** (50–60%), which is devoted to the control of nutrient intake. The basal requirement should be supplied in an uninterrupted fashion to avoid DKA and death. Successful management respects the basal requirement without compromise and adjusts the dietary requirement as needed to accommodate meal and activity schedules. This can be achieved with twice-daily (conventional) insulin treatment but often warrants more frequent insulin dosing. Among those motivated to perform frequent SMBG, and to make careful decisions in an effort to avert hypoglycemia, an intensive insulin regimen may allow better glycemic control and perhaps a means to reduce chronic complications.

I. Management of hyperglycemia requires an individualized treatment plan. The plan must consider basal needs, dietary intake, physical activity, and preferences in insulin dosing schedules.

  A. Dietary objectives. Basic considerations in dietary therapy apply (see Diabetes Mellitus, sec. **III.C**).

  1. Caloric goals should be defined to achieve normal growth and development among children and adolescents and to maintain ideal body weight in adults.

  2. Consistency must be maintained among patients using fixed daily insulin regimens. A plan that does not allow some flexibility, however, is usually not conducive to long-term compliance. For patients using two daily (bid) insulin injections (see sec. **I.B**), the safest plan includes breakfast, lunch, dinner, and a snack at bedtime. Snacks between meals are also appropriate in some patients to balance activities of injected insulins or effects of physical activity.

B. **Conventional methods of insulin therapy.** Effective management in type I DM warrants more than one daily insulin injection and usually more than one insulin type to address both the basal and the dietary insulin requirements. Conventional therapy employs rapid-acting and intermediate-acting insulins, injected twice daily. Basal and dietary requirements are not met separately, but basal insulin needs are accommodated while the peak effects of the insulins are adjusted to conform to the daily meal plan and activity schedule.

1. **Initiation of insulin therapy.** Although a daily insulin requirement of 35–50 units/day can be defined in most adults, a partial insulin lack is common at the time of diagnosis of type I DM, and lower doses (e.g., 20–40 units/day) often are more appropriate in initial treatment. An empiric algorithm divides the estimated daily insulin requirement into thirds, with two thirds given before breakfast and one third before the evening meal. The morning dose is split into two-thirds intermediate-acting insulin and one-third rapid-acting insulin, and the evening dose is split evenly between the intermediate-acting and rapid-acting insulins. Therapy should be carefully monitored in the hospital, and frequent SMBG should be followed closely after discharge.

2. **Timing of insulin administration** must be set with respect to meals and activity. Before insulin is injected, attention must be given to the plan for the following hours; once the dose is given, the plan must be followed to avoid treatment complications. Practical considerations include diagnostic tests and meal distribution procedures in the hospital, and fixed work and meal schedules in outpatients.

3. **Dosage adjustments.** The initial insulin regimen is seldom satisfactory; frequent modification is usually necessary to accommodate changes in diet and activity. Effects of these changes cannot be predicted in the hospital; thus, it is appropriate to provide a conservative regimen that maintains blood glucose in the range of 100–250 mg/dl and is not likely to produce hypoglycemia at home. Guided by SMBG, outpatient insulin doses may later be modified to meet individual goals. Soon after initiation of treatment many patients with type I DM experience a "honeymoon period" with a marked decrease in insulin requirements. This may allow glycemic control with modest amounts of insulin for several months.

   a. **Frequent blood glucose measurement** is the most satisfactory means to assess therapy. Four measurements daily, preceding meals and at bedtime (qid), usually give ample data for safe and effective insulin adjustment.

   b. **Persistent hyperglycemia should be documented** before the insulin dosage is adjusted. When hyperglycemia occurs daily during one preprandial period, the timing and distribution of insulin activity can be modified without a substantial change in the total daily insulin dose (see secs. **I.B.3.d** and **e**). When all glucose values are higher than treatment goals, an increase in the total daily dose is appropriate, and the distribution of insulins should be maintained until a new profile is established.

   c. **Hypoglycemia should be avoided** by conservative changes in insulin dosing. When glucose values are within 100–250 mg/dl in a stable patient, dose changes of more than 10% are seldom needed, and frequent adjustments should be avoided unless motivated by changes in diet or physical activity. Ample communication between the physician and the patient is essential (see Hypoglycemia).

   d. **Adjustments of intermediate-acting insulin** are usually made to control blood glucose (1) before breakfast, with the evening dose, or (2) before supper, with the morning dose. Increases in the evening dose should be made with caution, as nocturnal hypoglycemia may result. Optimum management may warrant the administration of the evening dose at bedtime, maintaining rapid-acting insulin before supper, resulting in a three-injection regimen.

   e. **Adjustments of rapid-acting insulin** are usually made to control blood glucose (1) before lunch, with the morning dose, or (2) before bedtime, with the evening dose. The administration of regular insulin at bedtime should be avoided in routine management.

    f. **Patient variability in insulin absorption** should be considered in adjustments of individual insulin doses (see Diabetes Mellitus, sec. **V.A**, and Table 20-3).

    g. **Changes in diet and activity** should be followed carefully with a modification of insulin dosing. When oral intake is restricted, the basal insulin requirement may be met by bid injections of intermediate-acting insulin, totaling one half (40–50%) of the usual total daily insulin dose.

C. **Multiple daily insulin injections (MDII)** are an alternative to the conventional, twice-daily, insulin treatment in type I DM. Principles of therapy with MDII are based on an emulation of insulin delivery by the normal pancreas, with administration specifically devoted to the basal and the dietary insulin requirements. The basal insulin is provided by daily or twice-daily injections of long-acting or intermediate-acting insulins (or both), and the dietary needs are met by doses of regular insulin given before each meal. Initially reserved for intensive insulin therapy aimed at the near-normalization of hemoglobin A_{1C} levels, MDII regimens may also be preferred in the management of patients with varied meal schedules (e.g., travelers, shift workers). Ultimately, many patients prefer MDII regimens because of the freedom gained in meal selection and in timing of meals, which is not so critical as when fixed insulin schedules are prescribed. MDII should be recommended only for motivated and careful patients, and close physician contact is mandatory until educational goals are met.

    1. **Initiation of MDII therapy** should follow an interval of conventional treatment, during which the patient should show competence in dietary management and both an ability and a willingness to perform frequent SMBG. Initially, 40% of the daily insulin dose should be given as one or two injections of long-acting insulin; one injection may be sufficient when bovine or beef–pork insulin is used and the dose is less than 30 units, but bid dosing is preferable with higher doses or with human insulin (see Diabetes Mellitus, sec. **V.A.4**). The remainder (i.e., 60%) should be divided among meals, and doses can be varied as indicated by size and composition of each meal; thus, doses are usually different for breakfast, lunch, dinner, and snacks, accommodating different meal sizes and carbohydrate contents. The total daily insulin dose with MDII may be less than that seen with conventional treatment, because of an improved distribution of insulin activity.

    2. **Timing of insulin administration.** When long-acting insulin is used, any consistent qd or bid schedule may achieve basal insulin requirements. Regular insulin doses should be given approximately 30 minutes before meals, allowing time for the absorption of injected insulin to match nutrient delivery from the intestine; meals can be eaten earlier, however, if the preprandial blood glucose is low. Because the activity of subcutaneous regular insulin may persist for longer than postprandial nutrient delivery, care must be taken in the management of physical activity after meals.

    3. **Dosage adjustments** should be guided by at least qid blood glucose monitoring; intensive management may warrant eight measurements daily. Although individual guidelines must be set, an objective of (1) a preprandial glucose of 80–100 mg/dl and (2) a 2-hour postprandial glucose of less than 200 mg/dl is achievable in a closely monitored patient with type I DM. Although this goal can be met, it confers a risk of complicating hypoglycemia and demands multiple management decisions each day.

    a. **Adjustments of long-acting insulin** should be made on the basis of trends occurring in (1) morning preprandial blood glucose (see sec. **I.C.3.c**), (2) blood glucose at night (i.e., 3:00 AM), or (3) late postprandial glucoses not responsive to adjustments of preprandial insulin doses. When change from a stable glucose profile is encountered, recommendations for the treatment of hyperglycemic exacerbations apply (see Diabetes Mellitus, sec. **III.F**). Several days should be allowed between dosage adjustments to verify a consistent response.

    b. Adjustments of regular insulin should consider (1) the size and composition of the ensuing meal, (2) the level of any anticipated physical activity, and (3) the preprandial blood glucose. Although selection of proper preprandial insulin doses is initially difficult, therapy is ultimately facilitated by education and experience.

    c. Increased morning insulin requirements may be observed in patients using MDII, manifested by hyperglycemia in the morning, increasing from normal at 3:00 AM to relative hyperglycemia at 6:00 AM, despite an otherwise optimum glycemic profile. Management of this "dawn phenomenon" can be achieved with a small dose of intermediate-acting insulin (e.g., 2–3 units) at bedtime, or by a change to alternative methods of insulin delivery (see sec. **I.D**).

   4. Complications. The aim of achieving near-normal glucose with any insulin regimen increases the risk of hypoglycemia. MDII should be discontinued or goals for glucose control should be revised if frequent or severe hypoglycemia occurs.

  D. Continuous subcutaneous insulin infusion (CSII) represents an alternative to insulin injections and provides a method of achieving glucose control analogous to MDII. Principles of treatment with CSII are also modeled after the normal pancreas; the basal insulin requirement is met by a continuous infusion of insulin, and the dietary requirement is addressed by boluses of insulin administered before meals. Sophistication in delivery of basal insulin allows adjustment for regular physical activity schedules and management of the dawn phenomenon. Like MDII, CSII is best reserved for motivated patients who are in close communication with an experienced physician.

   1. Initiation of CSII is best suited to patients experienced in diabetes care and preferably capable of management with MDII. Thus, dosage can be based on previous requirements, similar to those established by an MDII regimen (see sec. **I.C**).

    a. Catheter placement and care should be reviewed. The sites should be kept meticulously clean (see Diabetes Mellitus, sec. **V.C.3**) and must be examined regularly.

    b. Patients should examine pumps before use and should become adept in their operation to avoid complications.

   2. Timing of insulin administration and dosage adjustments are managed similarly to those of MDII regimens (see secs. **I.C.2 and 3**), and must be followed by frequent blood glucose monitoring.

   3. Complications. Hypoglycemia can occur (see sec. **I.C.4**). Subcutaneous infections, often with *Staph. aureus,* may develop at infusion sites. Severe hyperglycemia or DKA may result from an obstruction or dislodgment of catheters not noticed by the patient, or by pump failure. If CSII is discontinued, an MDII regimen can be substituted using similar basal and preprandial dosing; careful monitoring is needed.

  E. Hemoglobin A$_{1C}$ should be measured at 2- to 3-month intervals in patients with type I DM to support the blood glucose data used for management of therapy. Optimum hemoglobin A$_{1C}$ levels are slightly above the normal range; normal levels are attainable, but often at the expense of frequent hypoglycemia.

II. Diabetic ketoacidosis occurs as a result of severe insulin insufficiency (usually with a compromise of the basal requirement) and with an excess of counterregulatory hormones (e.g., glucagon). The predisposition to DKA is characteristic of type I DM and may be a presenting manifestation. However, DKA may occur in any patient with diabetes who is sufficiently provoked. The occurrence of DKA requires an explanation, such as an interruption of insulin therapy or a precipitating stress (see Table 20-1), which increases basal insulin needs. The therapy of DKA should include (1) restoration of volume, (2) appropriate electrolyte management, (3) reversal of acidosis and severe ketosis, and (4) control of blood glucose.

  A. Diagnosis. DKA often presents with weight loss, polyuria, and polydipsia. Common symptoms include vomiting and abdominal pain that is typically vague and without localizing signs. A severe acidosis promotes hyperventilation.

Shock or coma may occur. **Laboratory evaluation** reveals metabolic acidosis with an elevated anion gap, and the presence of serum ketones (see sec. **II.D**). Plasma glucose is almost always elevated. Other laboratory features may include hyponatremia, hyperkalemia, increased serum urea nitrogen and creatinine, hyperosmolarity, and an elevated level of serum amylase unrelated to abdominal pathology.

B. **Precipitating factors.** Common conditions leading to DKA include insufficient or interrupted insulin therapy and infection or other stress (see Table 20-1). Because an infection is often occult, cultures of blood and urine, careful examination of the skin and feet, and a chest radiograph are indicated. Myocardial infarction (MI) may precipitate DKA; an ECG is useful both for cardiac assessment and for the evaluation of hyperkalemia (see Chap. 3). Pregnancy may also precipitate DKA.

C. **Supportive measures.** Stabilization of patients in shock (see Chap. 26) and management of coma (see Chap. 25) should proceed without delay, as should initiation of specific therapy.

D. **Monitoring of therapy.** Frequent measurements of glucose and electrolytes are essential to assess response to therapy in DKA. A safe approach is to measure blood glucose with glucose oxidase reagent strips q30–60min and to measure plasma electrolytes q1–2h. Arterial blood gases should be repeated to assess the response of pH when bicarbonate therapy is used or when plasma bicarbonate does not respond to 4–6 hours of insulin treatment. Serial measurements of serum ketones are not helpful, because the most prevalent ketone body in DKA is beta-hydroxybutyrate, which is not detected by the nitroprusside reaction; the anion gap is a more reliable parameter of ketoacidosis unless lactic acidosis is also present (see sec. **II.M.1**). Ketonuria can persist following the correction of acidosis, and urine ketones are of only limited utility in following therapy. Pertinent clinical and laboratory data should be recorded in an organized fashion on a flow sheet; this facilitates evaluation of therapy.

E. **Fluid management.** Restoration of intravascular volume should be prompt, guided by ongoing considerations of cardiac and renal function. Initial fluids should include isotonic (0.9%) saline or lactated Ringer's solution, without additives. Patients with normal cardiac function should receive the first liter of fluid within one hour. Shock may warrant more rapid infusion. Volume replacement can then proceed at 1 liter/hour (or more) until the intravascular deficit has been restored.

1. **Monitoring of volume.** Frequent assessment of the heart rate, blood pressure, and urine output is important to guide fluid replacement. Bladder catheterization should be avoided as a routine procedure but can be used to assess urine output in hypotensive or comatose patients, or when neurogenic bladder is present. Suspected heart failure, myocardial infarction, or renal failure may warrant the monitoring of central venous pressure (CVP) or pulmonary artery occlusive pressure (PAOP) (see Chap. 6).

2. **Correction of free water deficit.** A hypotonic solution, such as 0.45% saline, can be used as an alternative to isotonic saline to restore intravascular volume when the serum sodium is greater than 155 mEq/liter.

3. **Maintenance fluids.** When the intravascular volume has been restored, a maintenance infusion of 0.45% saline (see secs. **II.G** and **I**) is appropriate in all patients. A rate of 150–250 ml/hour is proper among patients with normal heart and renal function. Fluid input and output should be followed. Sodium bicarbonate can also be used in maintenance fluids (e.g., 44 mEq in a liter of 0.45% saline) regardless of any specific indications for bicarbonate therapy initially. This measure may reduce the transient hyperchloremia that often results from sodium chloride administration.

F. **Bicarbonate therapy** should be considered initially when (1) DKA is accompanied by shock or coma, (2) arterial pH is less than 7.1, or (3) severe hyperkalemia is present (see Chap. 3). Bolus infusion of bicarbonate should be avoided except as an emergency resuscitation measure. A solution of sodium bicarbonate, 88 mEq (two ampules) in a liter of 0.45% saline, can be infused as a substitute for isotonic saline (see sec. **II.E**) until indications for bicarbonate are no longer present.

G. **Potassium replacement** is a fundamental part of the therapy of DKA. Although hyperkalemia may be observed initially due to metabolic acidosis, patients with DKA are usually deficient in potassium, and life-threatening hypokalemia can develop during insulin treatment. Administration of potassium should begin when the ECG shows no evidence of hyperkalemia; when ample urine output is demonstrated, this should occur within the first 2 hours of treatment, at an initial rate of 10 mEq/hour. When plasma potassium is less than 4 mEq/liter at presentation, or when hypokalemia occurs, the infusion of potassium chloride may approach 15–20 mEq/hour (see Chap. 3). Measurements of plasma potassium can be used to guide potassium administration, but delays from the clinical laboratory should not obstruct therapy. In patients with oliguria or renal failure, potassium levels must be monitored meticulously, and continuous ECG monitoring may be warranted. Potassium should be administered only in **peripheral** intravenous solutions.

H. **Insulin treatment** in DKA reverses ketogenesis and restores normal nutrient utilization. Although insulin acts to lower the blood glucose in DKA, the resolution of acidosis and ketone production is the therapeutic objective, and a dextrose infusion is needed (see sec. **II.I**) to avoid hypoglycemia during treatment.

   1. **Initial dose.** In adults, initial therapy should include regular insulin, 10–20 units IV, given as a bolus.

   2. **Continuous intravenous insulin infusion** is the treatment of choice in DKA. Administration at 10 units/hour (see Diabetes Mellitus, sec. **V.A.1.a**) is appropriate initially.

   3. **Intramuscular insulin injections** provide an alternative to IV infusion. The IM route should be avoided in hypotensive patients, as absorption is unpredictable. An initial dosage of 10 units IM q1h should be given.

   4. **Adjustments of insulin dosage** should be guided initially by blood glucose. After the first hour of treatment, the glucose levels should fall by at least 50 mg/dl/hour; a slower response may be indicative of insulin resistance, inadequate fluid administration, or improper insulin delivery. When dextrose is given (see sec. **II.I**), the plasma bicarbonate and anion gap are more appropriate measures of insulin effect. If insulin resistance is suspected, the dosage of IV insulin should be increased by 50–100% in hourly increments; it may be prudent to advance IM insulin more slowly. Insulin can be tapered, with care to maintain the basal requirements (e.g., 1–2 units/hour), when plasma bicarbonate rises to more than 15 mEq/liter and the anion gap resolves. Subsequently, when oral intake is resumed, subcutaneous insulin can be given and the IV or IM insulin discontinued (see secs. **II.K** and **L**).

I. **Dextrose administration.** Because the fall in blood glucose caused by insulin treatment is usually more prompt than is the resolution of ketoacidosis, administration of dextrose is needed during therapy. Normalization of blood glucose is not advised in the initial therapy of DKA because of a risk for serious hypoglycemia complicating the administration of high doses of rapid-acting insulin. A reasonable goal is to maintain glucose at 200–300 mg/dl; fluids should contain 5–10% dextrose when the blood glucose falls to within this range. When the initial blood glucose is less than 400 mg/dl, dextrose-containing fluids are appropriate as part of the starting regimen.

J. **Phosphate administration.** Insulin treatment promotes cellular uptake of phosphate with a reduction of plasma phosphate levels. Complications of hypophosphatemia in DKA are rare. The use of potassium phosphate in maintenance IV fluids (total dose ≤20 mEq K^+) is usually sufficient to mitigate hypophosphatemia until stores can be repleted with oral supplements. When patients are incapable of oral intake for prolonged periods, additional intravenous phosphate can be given with care to avoid potential complications of treatment, including hypocalcemia and renal failure (see Chap. 23).

K. **Initiation of oral intake.** Nausea, vomiting, and abdominal pain usually resolve during the first few hours of treatment. Patients can eat when they can tolerate food, but ketoacidosis should be corrected before a full diet is resumed.

L. Prevention of recurrent DKA should be guaranteed by correction of precipitating factors and by maintenance of uninterrupted insulin therapy with respect for the basal insulin requirement. Delay in the subcutaneous administration of insulin following IV or IM therapy in DKA should be avoided, and care should be taken to maintain the administration of insulin in doses sufficient to meet metabolic requirements. Rapid-acting insulin should be given SQ, alone or in a mixed injection, before the IV insulin is discontinued or concurrently with the last IM injection, so that continuous insulin activity is maintained and the basal needs are met. Measurements of electrolytes should continue at q4h intervals until stability is clearly demonstrated.

M. Complications of DKA. Management of shock (see Chap. 26) and coma (see Chap. 25) should accompany specific therapy.

1. **Lactic acidosis** may accompany ketoacidosis, particularly when shock, sepsis, or necrotizing inflammation is also present. Lactic acidosis should be suspected when the pH and anion gap do not respond to insulin therapy. Lactic acidosis may respond to volume replacement, but infusion of bicarbonate may be required until the cause is corrected.

2. **Cerebral edema** may occur during therapy of DKA (especially in children), and is manifested by headache, altered mental status, and papilledema. Computed tomography can establish the diagnosis. Prompt therapy is warranted for this often fatal complication (see Chap. 25).

3. **Arterial thrombosis** has been recognized as a complication of DKA and may present as stroke, myocardial or other organ infarction, or limb ischemia. Management is specific to the affected area of the body. Thrombectomy and anticoagulation (see Chap. 17) may be appropriate.

Non–Insulin-Dependent (Type II) and Other Diabetes Mellitus

Treatment of non–insulin-dependent and secondary DM is variable, depending most on the extent of endogenous insulin insufficiency observed in each patient. This insufficiency may be related to impaired insulin production, insulin resistance, or both. The absolute deficiency of insulin is usually not severe enough to compromise basal insulin requirements (except in diabetes secondary to severe pancreatic disease or near-total pancreatectomy); thus, patients are resistant to ketoacidosis unless a severe stress is present. Fasting plasma glucose is a rough indicator of the extent of insulin insufficiency. Patients with type II and other DM are vulnerable to chronic complications that are related to both the duration and the severity of their hyperglycemia; thus, management goals reflect a premise that glycemic control is beneficial.

I. Management of hyperglycemia. Both short-term and long-term goals should be considered in individual treatment, particularly among obese patients with type II DM. Weight reduction can reduce insulin requirements and improve glucose tolerance; an optimal plan is one that attempts to achieve and maintain ideal body weight.

A. Dietary objectives. General principles of dietary management apply (see Diabetes Mellitus, sec. III.C).

1. **Caloric reduction** is important for overweight patients with type II DM. Benefits to glucose control may be apparent after only modest weight reduction. Crash dieting for rapid weight loss is seldom beneficial in long-term management, but a hypocaloric diet may be worthwhile in combination with a program of behavior modification to revise long-term eating habits. A goal to reduce weight by roughly 1 pound/week is appropriate and can be achieved in most cases when caloric intake is reduced by 500 kcal/day. Input from a dietitian is desirable to help construct an individualized meal plan and

to encourage dietary compliance among outpatients. Caloric reduction is not desirable for those patients already at or near their ideal body weight.

   2. Adequate nutrition should be established, particularly in patients requiring caloric reduction. Vitamin supplements are indicated when daily intake is less than 1200 kcal.

B. Physical activity. A program of regular physical activity is an important adjunct in achieving weight control and also may improve glucose management by enhancing sensitivity to insulin. A graded exercise program should be used in untrained patients only after medical evaluation; in patients over age 40 the evaluation should include a resting ECG and stress test. Patient education and monitoring may help to avert potential complications (see Diabetes Mellitus, sec. **III.D**).

C. Oral hypoglycemic drugs can be used in conjunction with dietary modification when indicated (see Diabetes Mellitus, sec. **IV**).

   1. Efficacy. Sulfonylureas are effective in patients with mild to moderate fasting hyperglycemia. Roughly 70% of patients with type II DM initially achieve an appropriate reduction of fasting blood glucose (i.e., to less than 110 mg/dl) with these drugs. Response may be better among type II patients with (1) onset of diabetes after age 40, (2) hyperglycemia of less than 5 years' duration, and (3) no previous history of insulin therapy. Among the patients using sulfonylureas who initially achieve adequate blood glucose control, secondary failures may occur, suggesting a need for insulin therapy. Efficacy of sulfonylureas may also be reduced by concurrent administration of drugs that potentiate hyperglycemia (see Table 20-1).

   2. Indications. Hyperglycemia unresponsive to diet and physical activity warrants treatment with sulfonylureas or insulin. Decisions between these two modalities are usually based on clinical criteria and on patient acceptance of the treatment alternatives. The oral drugs can be used in the treatment of mild hyperglycemic exacerbations due to a self-limited or treatable illness; patients who are severely stressed often are not responsive. Frequent glucose monitoring is essential to avert complications (see Diabetes Mellitus, sec. **III.F**).

   3. Administration. Sulfonylurea therapy should be initiated with the lowest effective drug dosage (see Table 20-2). The dosage should be increased until treatment goals are achieved or a maximum dose is given. Particular care in initial dose selection and adjustment is appropriate in elderly patients. When blood glucose, monitored frequently (i.e., 2–4 times/day), falls to less than 200 mg/dl, changes in dosage should be gradual (e.g., weekly) to avoid hypoglycemia.

D. Insulin therapy. Patients with type II and other DM often need exogenous insulin to manage hyperglycemia. In some, insulin can be considered as an alternative to oral drug therapy; in others, insulin represents the only effective treatment. Insulin is not a substitute for proper dietary modification.

   1. Efficacy. Insulin therapy should allow glycemic control in all patients. Resistance to insulin action may be severe in some individuals, with exogenous insulin requirements greater than 100 units daily, implying a total insulin requirement (met by both endogenous and exogenous sources) that is far greater, and not well estimated by the 0.6–1.2 units/kg/day requirement of normal individuals. An increase in appetite may be perceived and a weight gain may be observed after initiation of insulin treatment; this does not limit efficacy of insulin in lowering blood glucose but underscores a need for dietary modification and strict weight control measures.

   2. Indications. Although appropriate in chronic management, insulin may be essential to control hyperglycemia during periods of acute stress, such as with surgery, infection, or pregnancy (see Diabetes Mellitus, secs. **III.F** and **V**).

   3. Initiation of insulin therapy. The dosage of insulin required to reduce blood glucose in type II and other DM is highly variable. Initially, 10–20 units of an intermediate-acting insulin can be given subcutaneously before breakfast; degree of obesity and severity of hyperglycemia aid in selection of a dose within this range. A lower dose (e.g., 10 units) is appropriate in elderly patients and when switching treatment to insulin from oral hypoglycemic drugs.

4. **Dosage adjustments** should be based on results of blood glucose monitoring. It is prudent to measure blood glucose before meals and at bedtime (qid) when adjusting therapy. Measurements before breakfast and dinner are often the most useful when treatment is limited to a single injection of intermediate-acting insulin given in the morning; the value before dinner usually corresponds to the peak activity of the NPH or lente insulin. When the lowest of the qid glucose measurements is within the desired range, the insulin activity should be distributed by adding other insulin types (see Table 20-3), additional injections, or both, according to the glucose profile. Gradual adjustments of insulin dosage (i.e., q2–3d) are prudent when measurements are near the therapeutic goals, as fluctuations may also be related to diet, physical activity, injection site, and changes in insulin sensitivity occurring during treatment. Only persistent hyperglycemia, recurring at one or more times a day, should prompt an increase in daily dosage.

   a. **Fasting hyperglycemia** with an otherwise acceptable glucose profile is an indication for (1) distributing 10–25% of the total daily insulin dose to a second injection of intermediate-acting insulin given before bedtime, (2) distributing 30–40% of the total daily insulin dose to a second injection of intermediate-acting insulin given before supper, or (3) considering the use of long-acting insulin.

   b. **Late-morning or evening hyperglycemia** can be treated with injections of rapid-acting insulin given before breakfast or supper, respectively. When mixed insulins are given in twice-daily injections, management becomes similar to conventional therapy of type I DM (see Insulin-Dependent [Type I] Diabetes Mellitus, sec. **I.B**).

E. **Therapy with both insulin and oral hypoglycemic drugs** has been suggested as an option in the management of type II DM by the results of several research protocols. Combined therapy may be beneficial in some isolated cases, but general application is not recommended (*Clinical Diabetes* 5:73, 1987).

F. **Hemoglobin A_{1C}** measurements should be used to assess chronic therapy. Measurement at 2- to 6-month intervals is appropriate. Normal hemoglobin A_{1C} levels in patients with type II DM are an acceptable treatment objective and can be achieved without frequent or severe hypoglycemia in patients using pharmacologic therapy, guided by SMBG.

II. **Nonketotic hyperosmolar syndrome (NKHS)** occurs predominantly in patients with type II and other DM, in whom dehydration and severe hyperglycemia may occur without development of ketoacidosis. NKHS may occur as a sequel to severe stress (see Table 20-1) and may follow stroke or an excessive carbohydrate intake. The pathogenesis of NKHS usually includes impaired renal excretion of glucose; thus, antecedent renal insufficiency or prerenal azotemia is common. As the basal insulin requirement is usually not compromised, excessive ketone production does not occur. Therapy of NKHS should include (1) the restoration of volume and osmolarity and (2) the management of hyperglycemia. Methods of treatment resemble those for DKA (see Insulin-Dependent [Type I] Diabetes Mellitus, sec. **II**).

A. **Diagnosis.** Patients often present with obtundation or coma, severe dehydration, and an underlying illness. Laboratory evaluation should reveal (1) hyperglycemia, often greater than 600 mg/dl; (2) absence of significant ketonemia; and (3) plasma osmolarity of greater than 320 mOsm/liter. Associated findings may include severe azotemia and lactic acidosis.

B. **Recognition of precipitating factors.** Considerations are similar to those for DKA. Insufficiency of insulin is often aggravated by glucocorticoids, and diuretic medications may augment volume depletion. An evaluation for infection and myocardial infarction is indicated. Repeated neurologic examination is important, as focal deficits or seizures may become apparent during therapy.

C. **Supportive measures** should include management specific to shock (see Chap. 26) and coma (see Chap. 25). Patients taking glucocorticoids should be given doses appropriate for severe stress (see Chap. 21).

D. Monitoring of therapy. It is appropriate initially to measure electrolytes hourly and to assess blood glucose at half-hour intervals. Monitoring may be less frequent when improvement is evident, but care should be taken to avoid hypoglycemia.

E. Fluid replacement. Initial therapy should correct the volume deficit, and isotonic (0.9%) saline is appropriate. Initial fluids should be given without additives, and a rapid rate of administration is appropriate (e.g., 1 liter/hr or more) until the intravascular volume is restored. When serum sodium or osmolarity measurements become available to guide therapy, 0.45% saline can be given to correct a relative free water deficit. Caution is indicated in the elderly and in those with MI, heart failure, or renal insufficiency. Frequent clinical assessment is imperative; bladder catheterization and monitoring of CVP or PAOP may be warranted (see Chap. 6). **After volume is restored** and hyperglycemia has responded to insulin therapy, a 5% dextrose in water (D/W) solution can be given to patients with persistent hyperosmolarity and hypernatremia. Maintenance fluids should be given at 100–250 ml/hour. Prolonged infusion of hypotonic solutions may be needed, particularly among elderly patients with sustained hyperosmolarity (see Chap. 3).

F. Electrolyte management. Potassium deficit should be anticipated during insulin treatment and may be severe in patients taking thiazide or loop diuretics. A lactic acidosis often responds to volume replacement, but bicarbonate administration may be needed (e.g., for pH <7.2), particularly when secondary to necrotizing inflammation or sepsis. Considerations for proper electrolyte replacement and the use of bicarbonate in maintenance fluids are similar to those for DKA. Phosphate should be monitored.

G. Insulin treatment in NKHS serves to restore normal glucose homeostasis; thus, blood glucose is the principal determinant of therapy. Regular insulin, 20 units IV, should be given initially when plasma glucose is greater than 600 mg/dl at presentation; smaller doses can be given when hyperglycemia is less marked. Insulin should then be given by infusion (or IM injection) to lower blood glucose gradually, roughly to 200 mg/dl, before initiation of subcutaneous insulin treatment.

Diabetes Mellitus in Pregnancy

Maintenance of normal blood glucose levels is particularly important in pregnancy. Patients with preexisting DM who become pregnant are particularly vulnerable to fetal complications, and maternal health can be compromised when diabetic complications occur. The outcome of a diabetic pregnancy can be improved by proper management; ideal care includes the initiation of an intensive insulin regimen before conception, monitored by meticulous SMBG (i.e., 4–8 times/day) and documented with near-normal hemoglobin A_{1C} levels. The stress of pregnancy also may provoke gestational DM; these patients deserve prompt diagnosis and specialized prenatal management.

I. **Diagnosis of gestational diabetes mellitus** may be suggested from symptoms or glycosuria or from a screening glucose tolerance test revealing a PG of greater than 150 mg/dl 1 hour after a 50-g oral glucose load, recommended at 24–28 weeks in all pregnant women. Normal fasting plasma glucose in pregnancy is 60–80 mg/dl; DM can be diagnosed when a fasting PG of greater than 105 mg/dl is shown on more than one occasion. When the fasting PG is equivocal, or when a screening test is positive, gestational DM can be established by a 100-g, 3-hour glucose tolerance test using specific criteria.

II. **Management of hyperglycemia** is facilitated by dietary modification and insulin treatment. Careful monitoring of blood glucose is an essential guide to therapy, as demands for insulin and the renal glucose threshold both change during pregnancy. Preprandial blood glucose values of less than 100 mg/dl are an achievable treatment objective, taking care to avert hypoglycemia.

A. Dietary modification. Caloric requirements in pregnancy are roughly 5 kcal/kg more than those in nonpregnant adults (see Diabetes Mellitus, sec. **III.C**). Caloric reduction should not be used for glucose control, and some weight gain during pregnancy should be allowed. A limitation of refined carbohydrate is appropriate. Artificial sweeteners should be restricted, as safety in pregnancy has not been established. Protein intake should be sufficient (i.e., 1.5 g/kg). A consistent diet is usually prescribed, including three meals and a bedtime snack.

B. Insulin treatment is usually required among pregnant patients with preexisting DM and should be used in gestational DM when dietary modification is inadequate. Insulin requirements vary during pregnancy. In general, requirements are lower in the first trimester, increase after 24 weeks, and drop suddenly in the immediate postpartum period, mandating close monitoring.

    1. Patients with preexisting diabetes usually require two daily insulin injections, and most can benefit from MDII or CSII regimens (see Insulin-Dependent [Type I] Diabetes Mellitus). Human insulin should be used. Labile glycemic response may warrant hospitalization and the use of continuous intravenous insulin therapy, particularly in the peripartum period (see Therapy of Diabetes Mellitus in Surgical Patients, sec. **I.D**).

    2. Patients with gestational diabetes often do well with less intensive treatment, reflecting the anticipated degree of insulin insufficiency. In most patients, management emulates that for type II DM (see Non–Insulin-Dependent [Type II] and Other Diabetes Mellitus), but **sulfonylureas should be avoided.**

III. Diabetic ketoacidosis may occur in pregnant patients and may be damaging, if not fatal, to the fetus. Management is the same as for nonpregnant adults (see Insulin-Dependent [Type I] Diabetes Mellitus). Urine ketone assays are useful in screening.

IV. Assessment for chronic complications of diabetes is important in pregnant patients, particularly among those with preexisting DM. Retinopathy and nephropathy may progress rapidly during pregnancy, potentially affecting both maternal and fetal health. Microvascular and macrovascular disease may limit placental circulation and must be considered during the high-risk obstetric assessment.

V. Lactation is associated with an elevated caloric requirement, roughly 500 kcal/day more than that needed before pregnancy. During the postpartum period patients often consider weight loss, and with varying individual needs the management of patients with DM is facilitated by careful SMBG.

Therapy of Diabetes Mellitus in Surgical Patients

Surgery poses a significant stress to diabetic patients and often perturbs dietary management. Careful attention to blood glucose control is necessary to (1) avoid symptomatic hyperglycemia and acute complications (e.g., DKA, hypoglycemia) and (2) allow a normal inflammatory response and wound healing. It is prudent to maintain a blood glucose of 100–250 mg/dl in nonpregnant adults. Elective procedures should be postponed until control is achieved. When possible, minor surgery should be scheduled for early morning to minimize interruption of the usual treatment schedule.

I. Modification of chronic therapy should be guided by the patient's usual treatment and by the nature of the surgery. Blood glucose monitoring should be used to guide adjustments. Recommendations for the treatment of hyperglycemic exacerbations apply (see Diabetes Mellitus, sec. **III.F**). It is important to recognize the nutritional needs of surgical patients, and administration of 5% dextrose in IV solutions, enteral tube feedings, or parenteral nutrition should not be withheld because of hyperglycemia (see Chap. 2).

    A. Patients managed with diet alone usually require no additional measures.

Purified human (or porcine) insulin should be used to manage fasting or preprandial glucose greater than 250 mg/dl.

B. **Patients using oral hypoglycemic drugs** should discontinue them on the day preceding surgery. Insulin should be used (see sec. **I.A**) when control of hyperglycemia is needed.

C. **Insulin-treated patients** require dosage adjustments. Decisions in therapy should be related to the diagnostic type of diabetes and the nature of the surgical stress. When insulin is used, a dextrose infusion should be available to avert hypoglycemia, and careful monitoring is imperative in the perioperative period.

   1. **In insulin-dependent diabetes** maintenance of uninterrupted insulin administration is essential to prevent DKA. Care must be taken that the basal insulin requirement is not compromised. In general, at least half of the usual daily insulin dose must be administered on the day of surgery and subsequently. All or a part of the usual dietary insulin requirement may also be met if a diet is prescribed, or when intravenous dextrose is administered. The administration of 5% dextrose in maintenance IV fluids is appropriate to limit lipolysis and ketogenesis in patients with restricted oral intake. Glucose monitoring is mandatory, and the periodic measurement of plasma electrolytes and urinary ketones is also advised, as DKA can occur in a stressed, postoperative patient even when blood glucose is not markedly elevated.

      a. **Among patients using conventional therapy,** a dose of intermediate-acting insulin can be given in the morning before minor surgery, and then bid. Hyperglycemia can be managed with supplements of regular insulin, given q4–6h, continued until oral intake is resumed. Mixed insulin can then be given, adjusted to dietary intake and blood glucose measurements.

      b. **Among patients using MDII or CSII,** the preoperative basal insulin doses should be continued without interruption in the perioperative period. When oral intake is restricted, regular insulin can be given as above (see sec. **I.C.1.a**). When a diet is ordered, the MDII or CSII regimen can be resumed, with adjustments of regular insulin doses to accommodate changes from the usual dietary regimen.

   2. **In non–insulin-dependent and other DM,** management should reflect the anticipated extent of insulin insufficiency. It may be appropriate to hold insulin in patients scheduled for minor procedures during morning hours and to give modified therapy based on blood glucose and an anticipated diet after surgery. Patients with large exogenous insulin requirements (i.e., >50 units/day) and those undergoing major surgery should be given insulin preoperatively, and in the immediate postoperative period, guided by blood glucose (see sec. **I.C.1.a**). An appropriate prescription is one half to two thirds of the usual daily insulin dose as intermediate-acting insulin in anticipation of surgery, then short-acting insulin as needed to control blood glucose postoperatively.

D. **Intravenous insulin infusion therapy** is a desirable alternative to subcutaneous insulin in the management of patients undergoing very stressful procedures (e.g., coronary artery bypass, renal transplant). An IV insulin infusion (see Diabetes Mellitus, sec. **V.A.1**) can be started preoperatively and continued through the procedure until hemodynamic stability and knowledge of the postoperative insulin requirements permit treatment with subcutaneous insulin (or oral hypoglycemic drugs). The infusion can be started using half of the patient's usual daily insulin dose, prescribed in units/hour; 0.5–1.0 unit/hour is appropriate initially for patients not previously using insulin. Blood glucose should be measured hourly. Among insulin-dependent patients care must be taken when IV infusions are discontinued (see Insulin-Dependent [Type I] Diabetes Mellitus, sec. **II.L**).

II. **Emergency surgery** may be needed despite severe hyperglycemia, DKA, or NKHS. Intensive monitoring is indicated, and use of an IV insulin infusion (see sec. **I.D**) is preferred in perioperative management. When possible, the restoration of intravascular volume should precede surgery.

III. **Assessment for chronic complications of diabetes** is important in the perioperative period. Patients with cardiovascular disease and neuropathy are susceptible to asymptomatic myocardial infarction. Patients with neuropathy are also particularly prone to development of decubitus ulcers, often of the heel, during periods of prolonged immobilization; prophylactic care is warranted. Enteropathy may alter the gastrointestinal responses to surgery and anesthesia.

Chronic Complications of Diabetes Mellitus

I. **Ophthalmic complications** of DM include diabetic retinopathy and diseases of the anterior chamber that affect vision. Prophylactic care includes yearly examination by an ophthalmologist as a minimum requirement for detection of retinopathy, recommended beginning at 5 years after onset in type I DM and at the time of diagnosis in type II DM (which often is after onset of the disease). Ophthalmology consultation is also needed for management of visual disturbance.

   A. **Diabetic retinopathy** includes (1) background retinopathy, which is limited to the retina (i.e., microaneurysms, intraretinal blot hemorrhages, retinal infarcts, hard exudates), and (2) proliferative retinopathy (i.e., neovascularization), which extends anterior to the retina and obscures visualization of the underlying retinal details. Patients with proliferative diabetic retinopathy are especially prone to acute visual loss. **Retinal laser photocoagulation** can reduce the incidence and retard the progression of visual impairment if it is employed before irreversible damage occurs. Vitrectomy may be beneficial to patients experiencing acute vitreous hemorrhage or a traction retinal detachment.

   B. **Visual disturbance** may complicate retinopathy or may follow cataract formation, glaucoma, ischemic optic neuropathy, or paresis of the extraocular muscles. Acute monocular visual loss can be due to hemorrhage, retinal detachment, or embolic retinal infarction. Bilateral visual loss suggests stroke but may also result from a dominant monocular visual loss when vision in the nondominant eye is insidiously impaired. Blurring of vision may occur as a result of lens alterations that follow a change in mean plasma glucose; often, this can take several weeks to resolve. Diplopia may indicate a cranial nerve palsy (i.e., nerves III, IV, VI). "Floaters," "spots," or "webs" may be the presenting descriptions of preretinal or vitreous hemorrhage and mandate prompt ophthalmologic evaluation.

II. **Diabetic neuropathy** may present with sensory symptoms or deficits, motor abnormalities, or autonomic dysfunction.

   A. **Pain** from mononeuropathy may occur in the distribution of a peripheral nerve, often with hyperesthesia. The differential diagnosis includes nerve entrapment and radiculopathy, which warrant specific management. There is no effective, specific therapy for painful diabetic neuropathy, but lowering of blood glucose may help in patients with marked hyperglycemia. Success in treatment of chronic pain has been documented with the use of amitriptyline, 10–150 mg PO qhs (*Neurology* 37:589, 1987). Side effects of amitriptyline may include constipation, postural hypotension, and urinary retention; caution should be used when any of these problems already exist as a manifestation of diabetic autonomic neuropathy (see sec. **II.D**). Potent analgesic drugs may be needed for severe pain (see Chap. 1).

   B. **Sensory deficit** has no specific treatment. Patients must be educated to avoid complications in neuropathic extremities, including trauma, burns, bone injury, and ulcers (see sec. **VII**).

   C. **Motor deficit** may result in muscle weakness and atrophy. Physical therapy may be helpful to patients with disability.

   D. **Autonomic neuropathy** may cause postural hypotension, persistent tachycardia, or neurogenic bladder and may contribute to gastrointestinal complications and impotence. Impaired visceral pain sensation often can obscure symptoms of angina pectoris or myocardial infarction.

      1. **Postural hypotension** should be treated symptomatically. Supportive mea-

sures include rising slowly from the supine or sitting position, particularly from bed in the morning, and limiting supine posturing by elevating the head of the bed at home. Some patients may respond to fludrocortisone, 0.1–0.3 mg PO qd, or sodium chloride, 1–4 g PO qid, or both. Care must be taken to limit supine hypertension, hypokalemia, and volume overload complicating this therapy. Postural changes in blood pressure may interfere with the effective treatment of hypertension; management should avert disabling symptoms.

2. **Neurogenic bladder** should be suspected in patients with recurrent urinary tract infection and requires specific therapy. Urinary retention is often not noticed by patients with DM and should be a consideration in routine management. Manual pressure or intermittent catheterization (i.e., q3–4h during the day) may be required to promote urination.

3. **Incontinence** of urine or feces may occur. Fecal incontinence must be distinguished from diarrhea; the latter may be more amenable to treatment (see sec. **VI.A**).

III. **Diabetic nephropathy** may cause proteinuria, hypertension, and a decline in glomerular filtration rate (GFR), leading ultimately to renal failure.

A. **Management of renal failure** includes dietary modification (see Chap. 11) and treatment of volume overload, if present.

B. **Hypertension** is a manifestation of diabetic nephropathy, and, if untreated, may accelerate renal, retinal, and cardiovascular impairment. Treatment should be prescribed using individualized criteria (*Diabetes Care* 10:764, 1987), but blood pressure should be made normal when possible (see sec. **II.D.1**). Angiotensin-converting enzyme inhibitors may be beneficial in patients with proteinuric renal disease (see sec. **III.E** and Chap. 11).

C. **Iodinated intravenous contrast agents** impair GFR with increased frequency in patients with DM. When possible, diagnostic tests should be chosen to avoid use of these chemicals. If an IV contrast agent is necessary, liberal hydration both before and after administration should be provided, and urine output and serum creatinine should be monitored.

D. **Urinary tract infections** should be treated aggressively (see Diabetes Mellitus, sec. **III.H.1** and Chap. 13).

E. **Hyperkalemia** may result from renal failure, hyporeninemic hypoaldosteronism, or, in some patients, lack of insulin. Potassium-sparing diuretics, angiotensin-converting enzyme inhibitors, and, rarely, beta-adrenergic antagonists may promote hyperkalemia; alternative drugs should be chosen when necessary. Acute treatment measures may be needed (see Chap. 3). When hyperkalemia accompanies a hyperchloremic acidosis, patients may respond to fludrocortisone, 0.05–0.1 mg PO qd. Others may respond to insulin therapy.

IV. **Macrovascular disease** is accelerated in diabetic patients. Severe peripheral vascular disease causes ischemia and predisposes to bacterial infections that are refractory to antibiotic treatment. Surgical management is often needed to treat symptomatic peripheral vascular disease; pentoxifylline, 400 mg PO tid, may be helpful when surgery is not appropriate. Macrovascular disease also leads to stroke and myocardial infarction. Hyperlipidemia and hypertension should be treated as indicated (see Chaps. 22 and 4). **Cigarette smoking should be discouraged.**

V. **Coronary artery disease and myocardial infarction** occur with increased frequency in DM. Heart disease must be considered when dyspnea or unexplained hyperglycemia occurs, even when other symptoms of angina pectoris are atypical or absent. Young age should not preclude the diagnosis of coronary heart disease (see Chap. 5). A yearly ECG should be obtained as part of routine care (see Diabetes Mellitus, sec. **III.I**), and periodic evaluation with a stress test may be appropriate (see Non–Insulin-Dependent (Type II) and Other Diabetes Mellitus, sec. **I.B**).

VI. **Diabetic enteropathy** is a manifestation of autonomic neuropathy, affecting gastrointestinal motility.

A. **Diarrhea** in patients with DM warrants diagnostic evaluation (see Chap. 15); symptomatic therapy is appropriate when a correctable cause is not found. Bacterial overgrowth may respond to tetracycline, 250 mg PO qid.

B. **Impaired gastric emptying** may lead to recurrent nausea and vomiting. Some patients respond to metoclopramide, 10–20 mg PO 30–60 minutes ac and qhs. Goals for glycemic control and methods of therapy for hyperglycemia should be reassessed when timing of nutrient delivery is unpredictable.

VII. **The diabetic foot** is a manifestation of chronic neuropathy, aggravated in many cases by vascular insufficiency and infection. Sensory loss allows tolerance of repeated trauma from tight shoes and improper weight bearing, which leads to skin breakdown, skin ulceration, tissue necrosis, and fracture. Specialized treatment is needed to prevent and to manage foot disease.

A. **Prophylactic foot care** includes properly fitting shoes, daily examination for injury, and care in the management of calluses and in nail cutting and cleaning.

B. **Patients with foot ulcers** must totally avoid local pressure to allow healing; hospitalization is often required to facilitate management with absence of weight bearing. Infection is common, and osteomyelitis can complicate deep ulcers. The most common pathogens are streptococci and *Staph. aureus,* but gram-negative and anaerobic bacteria (e.g., *Bacteroides fragilis*) also infect these wounds. Debridement and broad-spectrum antibiotics or combination antibiotic regimens are appropriate in the initial therapy of infected ulcers (see Chap. 13). Surgical treatment of peripheral vascular disease may be warranted to allow healing. Amputation may be necessary to prevent recurrent septicemia and death, but a conservative approach to chronic management usually is preferred.

Hypoglycemia

Hypoglycemia complicates therapy with oral hypoglycemic agents and with insulin. Less commonly, hypoglycemia occurs in nondiabetic patients. Management in both cases includes prompt treatment and the correction of underlying causes.

I. **Hypoglycemia in patients with diabetes** usually results from (1) a change in content or timing of meals, (2) an increase in physical activity, or (3) a medication overdosage. Severity is the most important determinant of treatment. Management should consider the peak effects and durations of action of insulin or oral hypoglycemic drugs used (see Tables 20-3 and 20-2). Patients manifesting severe or recurrent hypoglycemia may have an impaired counterregulatory response of glucagon and epinephrine (*Diabetes* 30:260, 1981). Goals for management of DM should be reassessed when frequent or severe hypoglycemia complicates therapy.

A. **Diagnosis.** Mild hypoglycemic reactions are characterized by irritability, tremulousness, diaphoresis, tachycardia, and confusion. These symptoms result in part from the secretion of epinephrine, a mediator of the counterregulatory response to falling glucose. Insufficient hypoglycemic counterregulation or medication overdose may allow more serious manifestations, such as seizure, stupor, coma, or focal neurologic findings. Plasma or blood glucose measurements, when available, should be used to validate symptomatic hypoglycemia.

B. **Treatment of hypoglycemic episodes** should be guided by (1) the mental status of the patient, (2) the level of blood glucose, and (3) the anticipated clinical course. Prolonged observation is warranted in sulfonylurea overdose.

1. **Oral carbohydrate** is sufficient for alert patients when drug overdose is not apparent. Oral glucose, sucrose, or sugar-containing fluids often produce hyperglycemia; 1–2 cups of milk, 4 oz of orange juice without additives, a piece of fruit, a granola bar, or cheese and soda crackers are usually adequate for the treatment of mild hypoglycemia detected by glucose monitoring or mild, adrenergic symptoms (see sec. **I.A**). More potent, sugar-containing fluids can be used when initial response is not sufficient, when gastroparesis is suspected, or when ability to maintain oral intake is impaired due to gastrointestinal illness. Frequent monitoring (e.g., q30–60min) should verify efficacy.

2. **Intravenous dextrose** should be given when mental function is impaired, when medication overdosage is suspected, or when prolonged hypoglycemia is anticipated. Initially, 50% dextrose, 25–50 ml, should be given, followed by infusion of 5–10% D/W. Blood glucose should be kept greater than 150 mg/dl, as verified by frequent, serial measurements.

3. **Glucagon,** 1 mg IM (or SQ), can be given to treat severe hypoglycemia in outpatients, or when intravenous access is difficult. Injection of glucagon may cause vomiting, and care should be taken to prevent aspiration of gastric contents. Patients prone to severe hypoglycemia should have glucagon for home use; a family member or roommate must be instructed in preparation and injection technique.

C. **Adjustments of drug therapy** should be aimed at prevention of recurrence. Reduction of sulfonylurea dosage is appropriate. A change in the distribution and timing of insulin injections is indicated when hypoglycemia recurs at a particular time of day, but a total dose reduction is indicated when hypoglycemia is severe, prolonged, or unpredictable.

D. **Adjustments of diet and physical activity** may be an alternative to changing drug dosage. Consistency should be ascertained when appropriate. Carbohydrate intake may be increased or activity reduced at times when recurrent low blood glucose is defined.

E. **Hypoglycemia unawareness** is a potential cause and a complication of frequent insulin-induced hypoglycemia. Often with impaired hypoglycemic counterregulation mechanisms, patients afflicted with hypoglycemia unawareness do not develop the normal, epinephrine-mediated symptoms of falling glucose (see sec. **I.A**) and are predisposed to insidious development of stupor or coma, heralded by diaphoresis in some cases. Goals for glycemic control among patients with hypoglycemia unawareness must be considered carefully; intensive regimens are not advised when frequent or severe hypoglycemia is threatened. SMBG is an essential management tool among these patients. **Beta-adrenergic antagonists may contribute to hypoglycemia unawareness;** alternative treatments should be chosen when severe or recurrent hypoglycemia occurs in patients taking these drugs.

II. **Spontaneous hypoglycemia** in patients not using insulin or oral hypoglycemic drugs can be classified as fasting or reactive.

A. **Fasting hypoglycemia** occurs when hepatic glucose production does not match cellular glucose uptake. Normal adults can maintain blood glucose with 72 hours of fasting. Hypoglycemia may result from an insulinoma, severe liver disease, alcohol intoxication, adrenocortical insufficiency, hypothyroidism, growth hormone deficiency, or malnutrition among patients with renal failure. Presenting symptoms may include dementia, seizure, or bizarre behavior. Therapy should be directed at the cause. **Diazoxide,** 50–100 mg PO tid, can be used to limit insulin secretion in patients with an insulinoma, anticipating surgical resection; prolonged use promotes volume overload, warranting diuretic treatment. Thiazide diuretics potentiate hyperglycemic effects of diazoxide.

B. **Reactive hypoglycemia** occurs in the postprandial state from the action of insulin secreted in response to meals. Symptoms are similar to those of mild insulin-induced hypoglycemia (see sec. **I**). Reactive hypoglycemia occurs often as a sequel to partial gastrectomy; symptoms appear 1–2 hours after meals. Functional symptoms also occur in patients without antecedent surgery, and are often later (e.g., 3–5 hours) in the postprandial period. These patients can respond to a modification of eating habits; frequent, small feedings are appropriate. Often patients with reactive hypoglycemia also manifest impaired glucose tolerance, and dietary management appropriate for diabetes mellitus may be helpful (see Diabetes Mellitus, secs. **I.B and III.C**). Patients unresponsive to dietary modification may perceive a symptomatic benefit from the anticholinergic agent propantheline, 15 mg PO 15–30 minutes ac, which delays gastric emptying.

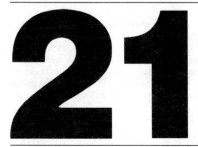

Endocrine Diseases

Clay F. Semenkovich

Hypothyroidism

The lack of thyroid hormone affects every organ system in the body. Hypothyroidism often presents gradually, with symptoms that are extremely prevalent in the general population. Therefore, physicians should maintain a relatively low threshold for screening for hypothyroidism. Primary hypothyroidism (disease of the thyroid gland itself) occurs after prior radioactive iodine (RAI) therapy for hyperthyroidism, thyroidectomy, therapeutic neck irradiation (e.g., for Hodgkin's disease), and iodine–containing drug treatment. The most common cause of primary hypothyroidism in the United States is chronic lymphocytic (Hashimoto's) thyroiditis, which is more common in women than in men. Patients generally have a small goiter that is slightly firm but usually not nodular. Histologic confirmation of the diagnosis is not required; detection of circulating antithyroglobulin and antimicrosomal antibodies can be used to confirm the diagnosis but seldom alters management. Primary hypothyroidism from Hashimoto's thyroiditis may be associated with autoimmune adrenocortical destruction (as part of an autoimmune polyglandular syndrome). Secondary hypothyroidism (due to pituitary disease) may be caused by pituitary surgery or by tumors (see Disorders of the Anterior Pituitary Gland). Secondary hypothyroidism may be associated with deficiencies of other pituitary hormones (e.g., ACTH). **Clinical features** include tiredness, cold intolerance, constipation, weight gain, menorrhagia, bradycardia, edema (particularly of the hands and face), thick dry skin, and prolongation of tendon reflex contraction and relaxation. Creatine kinase (CK) levels are frequently elevated. Serum cholesterol is increased due to decreased clearance of low-density lipoprotein (LDL) cholesterol. Anemia may be due to hypothyroidism, but other types of anemia occur with increased frequency in patients with hypothyroidism, including (1) folate-deficient anemia (due to impaired absorption of folic acid), (2) pernicious anemia occurring in association with Hashimoto's thyroiditis, and (3) iron-deficiency anemia (due to menorrhagia).

I. **Diagnostic evaluation.** If hypothyroidism is suspected, serum T_4 and thyroid-stimulating hormone (TSH) should be measured. An elevated serum TSH in the setting of a low or low-normal T_4 indicates primary hypothyroidism. If the serum TSH is normal or low and clinical suspicion for hypothyroidism is high, attention should be focused on the possibility of hypothalamic or pituitary disease (see Disorders of the Anterior Pituitary Gland). Subclinical hypothyroidism is defined as a normal serum T_4 and an elevated serum TSH and minimal or no symptoms of hypothyroidism. These patients should receive thyroid replacement.

II. **Therapy. Full thyroid hormone replacement may precipitate adrenal crisis** if patients with hypothyroidism and autoimmune polyglandular syndrome or deficiencies of other pituitary hormones are not first treated with cortisol.
   A. **Hypothyroidism in the medically stable patient.** Since hypothyroidism is likely to have been of gradual onset, rapid repletion is rarely necessary. Precipitation of angina or cardiac arrhythmias is a potentially serious complication of treatment, especially in elderly patients or those with underlying heart disease.
      1. **Levothyroxine** is the drug of choice. In most patients therapy may be started with the average replacement dose of 1.6 µg/kg PO qd (usually 100–125

μg PO qd) (*N. Engl. J. Med.* 316:764, 1987). In elderly patients the initial dose should be 25–50 μg PO qd because subclinical coronary disease may be present. The dose should be increased in 25- to 50-μg increments at approximately 4-week intervals until full replacement is achieved. Therapy should be assessed by response of T_4 and serum TSH and improvement in clinical features. TSH may normalize slowly, especially in long-standing hypothyroidism; thus, if adequate clinical improvement has been achieved and T_4 levels are in the normal range, the dose should not be increased simply to normalize TSH in the months following initiation of therapy. Restoration of euthyroidism in a hypothyroid patient promotes metabolic clearance of thyroxine; T_4 levels may decrease and TSH levels increase, requiring an increase in thyroxine dose.

2. **Therapeutic adjustment.** Once patients are receiving a stable dose of thyroid replacement, they should be evaluated yearly with clinical assessment and a serum TSH (*Ann. Intern. Med.* 113:450, 1990). Thyroid hormone requirements decrease with aging, and appropriate decreases in the replacement dose should be made as indicated by the TSH. A suppressed or low TSH reflects overreplacement of thyroid hormone. Despite the fact that patients may feel better on a higher dose of thyroid hormone, even modest overreplacement should be avoided because of potentially adverse effects on the heart and liver (*Mayo Clin. Proc.* 63:1223, 1988) as well as a tendency to diminish bone mass in such patients (*J.A.M.A.* 259:3137, 1988; *Ann. Intern. Med.* 113:265, 1990). Because of the long half-life of T_4, measurements of TSH should be made at intervals of 4 weeks or longer after dosage changes. Once patients are receiving a particular thyroid hormone preparation, it is appropriate to continue to specify that preparation when writing prescriptions.

B. **Hypothyroidism in the patient with known cardiac disease.** Although concern over exacerbating angina or precipitating myocardial infarction is appropriate, concurrent thyroid and cardiac disease can and should be treated optimally. Therapy should be initiated with levothyroxine, 12.5 μg PO qd, with dosage increments of 12.5 to 25.0 μg every 4 weeks until full replacement dosage is achieved. Simultaneously, management of the cardiac condition should be intensified (see Chaps. 5 and 6). If angina increases despite anti-anginal therapy, cardiac catheterization and coronary revascularization may be indicated and can be done safely despite minimal or no thyroid replacement preoperatively; thyroxine therapy may be optimized after successful revascularization. Hypothyroid patients may be difficult to wean from a ventilator after anesthesia (see Chap. 9) but otherwise usually tolerate surgery well.

C. **Hypothyroidism requiring rapid replacement**

1. **Trauma, emergency surgery, and severe infection** may be poorly tolerated by the hypothyroid patient and may lead to myxedema coma. In such circumstances, hypothyroidism should be corrected as rapidly as is safely possible. This is usually accomplished by administration of levothyroxine, 200–500 μg IV, followed by levothyroxine, 100 μg IV qd. To prevent precipitation of relative adrenal insufficiency, hydrocortisone, 100 mg IV q8h, is recommended concurrently. This type of thyroid hormone replacement is necessary only when hypothyroid patients are extremely ill. If the patient has a mild infection, if trauma is not extensive, and if the patient is capable of enteral intake, standard oral replacement therapy is appropriate. Surgery in hypothyroid patients is not necessarily associated with higher permanent morbidity or mortality (*Am. J. Med.* 77:261, 1984) and can be considered in patients in whom presurgery hormone replacement is not feasible. Elective surgery should be delayed until hypothyroidism is corrected.

2. **Myxedema coma** is a rare disorder characterized by hypoventilation, hypotension, hypothermia, hyponatremia, and hypoglycemia. These are nonspecific findings, and low serum T_4 levels are often found in euthyroid patients with severe illness. Many patients with suspected myxedema coma will have other explanations for their illness. If myxedema coma is strongly

suspected, a serum sample should be sent for measurement of T_4, TSH, and free T_4 (by equilibrium dialysis), followed by rapid replacement with IV levothyroxine and hydrocortisone (see sec. **II.C.1**). If clinically indicated, empiric replacement therapy can be given while one awaits the results of thyroid function tests.

Hyperthyroidism

Thyrotoxicosis is a clinical state caused by excessive circulating thyroid hormone. Clinical features include nervousness, diarrhea, heat intolerance, weight loss despite a good appetite, hair loss, palpitations, and amenorrhea or a marked decrease in menstrual flow (in women). Elderly patients may present with wasting and none of the classic signs or symptoms of hyperthyroidism ("apathetic" hyperthyroidism). Physical examination often reveals tachycardia, a widened pulse pressure, lid lag on downward gaze, and a fine tremor of the hands. Other cardiovascular findings (see Chap. 7), particularly atrial fibrillation resistant to conventional therapy, may also occur. **Thyrotoxicosis** may be caused by hyperthyroidism (i.e., overactivity of the thyroid gland) or exogenous hormone ingestion. In hyperthyroidism, a goiter may be present but is often minimal. **As with hypothyroidism, there are no thyroid function tests that provide an unequivocal diagnosis of hyperthyroidism.** A combination of careful clinical assessment and proper interpretation of thyroid function tests is mandatory.

I. **Diagnosis of thyrotoxicosis.** In suspected thyrotoxicosis, serum T_4 and TSH should be measured.
   A. **Thyroid hormones.** An elevated T_4 alone is not diagnostic of thyrotoxicosis. Thyroxine is almost entirely protein bound. The major T_4 binding protein is thyroxine-binding globulin (TBG), which is increased by estrogen administration (e.g., oral contraceptives), pregnancy, and liver disease, and on a genetic basis. In these conditions, the serum T_4 will be moderately elevated, but the TSH will be normal and signs of hyperthyroidism will be absent. However, T_4 elevations of greater than 20 µg/dl usually indicate true thyrotoxicosis and not TBG excess.
   B. **Thyroid-stimulating hormone.** A suppressed TSH alone is not diagnostic of thyrotoxicosis; it may be found in euthyroid individuals with autonomous thyroid nodules, with pituitary disease, pituitary surgery, or irradiation; in euthyroid patients with Graves' ophthalmopathy; and in some euthyroid individuals without any demonstrable thyroid disorder.

II. **Differential diagnosis**
   A. **Graves' disease** is an autoimmune disorder that is the most common cause of hyperthyroidism. About 40% of patients with Graves' disease also manifest ophthalmopathy (*Am. J. Med.* 87:70, 1989), which may include periorbital edema, conjunctivitis, proptosis, and extraocular muscle abnormalities. Graves' disease is frequently familial, is more common in women than in men, and occurs relatively often in the elderly. The best clinical marker for the disease is the presence of ophthalmopathy in the patient or in the family.
   B. **Toxic adenomas,** single and multiple (i.e., toxic multinodular goiter), produce thyrotoxicosis by secreting thyroid hormone autonomously. They do not remit spontaneously and should be treated with RAI or surgery.
   C. **Iodine-induced thyrotoxicosis** occurs after the administration of potassium iodide (saturated solution of potassium iodide [SSKI] and expectorants) and organic iodides (radiographic contrast dyes and amiodarone). Patients with multinodular goiters, endemic goiters, and a history of Graves' disease are susceptible to this complication. A low or absent radioactive iodine uptake (RAIU) is seen with this disorder. Thyrotoxicosis induced by iodine administration is usually mild and self-limited, requiring only symptomatic therapy with beta-adrenergic antagonists. In severe cases of iodine-induced thyrotoxicosis, antithyroid drug therapy may be required.
   D. **Thyroiditis** can produce thyrotoxicosis by causing release of thyroid hormone

from an injured gland. Patients may have a tender thyroid gland on physical examination. This disorder is presumably the result of viral infection and is usually self-limited, requiring only symptomatic treatment with beta-adrenergic antagonists and analgesics.

   E. Choriocarcinoma and hydatidiform mole cause thyrotoxicosis by producing human chorionic gonadotropin, which has some TSH activity. Functioning thyroid cancer, TSH-secreting pituitary adenomas, self-administration of excessive amounts of thyroid hormone (thyrotoxicosis factitia), and ectopic thyroid tissue (e.g., struma ovarii) are rare causes of thyrotoxicosis.

III. Therapy of thyrotoxicosis is either immediate or definitive.

   A. The purpose of immediate therapy is to alleviate symptoms and rapidly reduce thyroid hormone levels.

   1. Propranolol reduces many manifestations of thyrotoxicosis, especially tachycardia and tremor; it also inhibits peripheral conversion of T_4 to T_3, the active form of thyroid hormone. Propranolol is used to control symptoms while awaiting RAI therapy, surgery, or the effects of antithyroid medications. Therapy is initiated at a dosage of 10–20 mg PO q6h and gradually increased until symptoms are alleviated. A reasonable goal is alleviation of resting tachycardia. In most cases, a daily dose of 80–320 mg is sufficient.

   2. Diltiazem, a calcium channel antagonist, may be useful in controlling thyrotoxicosis-associated tachycardia in patients in whom therapy with propranolol may be contraindicated (*Arch. Intern. Med.* 148:1919, 1988). Therapy is initiated at a dosage of 30 mg PO q6h and is gradually increased until symptoms are controlled (which usually requires 180–360 mg/day). Diltiazem should not be used concurrently with propranolol.

   3. Iodide can rapidly decrease the serum T_4 concentration and produce symptomatic improvement of the thyrotoxic state, largely by inhibition of thyroid hormone release. Iodide is not effective for long-term treatment of hyperthyroidism. It interferes with the subsequent administration of RAI and can prolong the time required to achieve euthyroidism with antithyroid drugs. It should be used only to (1) treat thyroid storm, (2) prepare patients for thyroid surgery, (3) prepare hyperthyroid patients for emergency nonthyroidal surgery, or (4) treat patients with severe underlying cardiac disease who require rapid lowering of thyroid hormone levels. SSKI contains 750 mg/ml iodide. The usual dosage is 1–2 drops (approximately 75 mg) PO bid. Side effects include skin rash and sialadenitis.

   B. Definitive therapy. In patients with Graves' disease, the choice of definitive therapy is between RAI therapy, antithyroid medications, and surgery. For most patients, RAI therapy represents the best choice, although several factors, including patient preference, should be considered. In the older patient with greater surgical risk, RAI is the therapy of choice. Most clinicians are reluctant to use RAI therapy in children because of possible long-term risks of radiation exposure, but it is not absolutely contraindicated; surgery is often preferred. Surgery should be considered for patients when compliance with medications or follow-up after RAI is not expected.

   1. Radioactive iodine (I-131). Radioactive iodine delivers a high dose of radiation to the thyroid gland, resulting in tissue ablation. It is concentrated in the thyroid gland, limiting exposure of other tissues to radiation. There is no evidence that such therapy increases risk of cancer, leukemia, or genetic abnormalities, and the subsequent risk of thyroid cancer is probably decreased. The gonadal dose of radiation associated with RAI therapy is equivalent to the exposure associated with approximately two barium enemas or intravenous pyelograms (IVPs) and is considered benign. Radioactive iodine is contraindicated in pregnancy and during lactation.

   a. Dosage and administration. Almost all patients treated with RAI will eventually become hypothyroid. There is no evidence that an intermediate dose of I-131 will prevent this. It is prudent to request, therefore, to attempt thyroid ablation at the time of treatment; most patients will become hypothyroid within months and can then be treated with replacement doses of thyroid hormones. Patients first receive a low dose of RAI (the uptake dose). Twenty-four hours later, RAI uptake is determined and the therapy dose is administered as an oral solution. I-131 not taken up by the thyroid will be eliminated in the urine, sweat, saliva, and feces; close physical contact (especially with infants and young children) and contact with bodily fluids should be restricted for 3 days after receiving a therapy dose of I-131. Radioactive iodine therapy diminishes the synthetic capacity of the thyroid gland but usually does not affect the stored hormone present in the gland. Thus, the effect of RAI on thyroid hormone levels is often not apparent for 2–3 months. During this time, propranolol and, if appropriate, antithyroid medication are continued and the patient is evaluated at monthly intervals with clinical assessment and measurement of serum T_4 levels. If no response is seen after 6 months, RAI treatment should be repeated.

   b. Radiation thyroiditis is rare but may occur within 2 weeks of administration of RAI. This transient exacerbation of thyrotoxicosis is a result of leakage of thyroid hormone. It is seldom clinically significant but can precipitate thyroid storm or cardiac decompensation in patients with severe hyperthyroidism or underlying cardiac disease (*Am. J. Med.* 75:353, 1983). Such patients should be treated with antithyroid medication until clinically and chemically euthyroid before RAI therapy. The medication is stopped 3 days before RAI therapy and may be restarted 3–7 days after the RAI dose is received. This precaution is necessary in only a small number of hyperthyroid patients.

2. **Antithyroid drugs** interfere with organification of iodide to form iodotyrosines, the precursors of thyroid hormone. Propylthiouracil also inhibits the peripheral conversion of T_4 to T_3. The rationale for long-term therapy with these drugs is to render the patient euthyroid while awaiting spontaneous remission of the disease.

   a. Propylthiouracil (PTU) and **methimazole** (Tapazole) are available only in oral form. The usual starting dosage of PTU is 100 mg PO tid in most patients with Graves' disease. Many clinicians use 150–200 mg PO tid in patients with severely symptomatic hyperthyroidism. Up to 1000 mg per day divided into four doses may be required in some cases. The usual starting dose of methimazole is 30 mg PO qd, with dosages of up to 90 mg per day occasionally required (methimazole is contraindicated in pregnancy). In patients with more severe hyperthyroidism, PTU may be preferred because of its ability to decrease the conversion of T_4 to T_3.

   b. Follow-up and duration of therapy. Clinical response usually takes weeks to months since antithyroid drugs prevent hormone synthesis but do not affect release of stored hormone. Maintenance doses are usually lower than those necessary to achieve an initial response, and it is usually appropriate to decrease the dose of antithyroid medication after 4–8 weeks of treatment. Patients usually require concomitant therapy with propranolol and should be evaluated at regular (4–6 week) intervals with clinical examinations and measurement of serum T_4 and TSH levels. Thyrotropin may remain suppressed for several months after the patient is euthyroid. Thyrotropin may also become elevated while the patient is euthyroid during the process of recovering from hyperthyroidism; thus, management should not be altered on the basis of any single measurement of thyroid function. Medication should be continued for about 6 months, then gradually withdrawn and the clinical response assessed.

   c. Efficacy. A long-term remission occurs in approximately one third of cases. Presenting features suggesting that a long-term remission may occur include (1) absence of a goiter and (2) mild hyperthyroidism of relatively recent onset. The majority of relapses occur within 3–6 months of cessation of therapy, at which time alternative treatment is recommended.

   d. Complications of antithyroid drug therapy are usually mild. In perhaps

5% of patients, a rash or urticaria will develop, which can be managed with antihistamines or a change to the alternative antithyroid drug. Transient leukopenia is common and does not usually require any change in therapy. Severe arthralgias or hepatitis can occur and should prompt a discontinuation of drug therapy. Agranulocytosis is the most serious complication of therapy and occurs in about 0.5% of patients. It may be more likely to occur in patients over the age of 40 (*Ann. Intern. Med.* 98:26, 1983). WBC counts obtained at 2-week intervals for the first 3 months of therapy may detect agranulocytosis before the onset of clinically evident infection (*Arch. Intern. Med.* 150:621, 1990). All patients started on antithyroid medication must be told to stop their medication and seek medical attention if fever, pharyngitis, or other manifestations of infection develop.

3. **Surgery.** Subtotal thyroidectomy is very effective in the treatment of hyperthyroidism. The incidence of recurrence with long-term follow-up is approximately 10%. Surgery produces permanent hypothyroidism less frequently than does RAI (*N. Engl. J. Med.* 311:426, 1984). It is appropriate for patients with hyperthyroidism who will not consider RAI therapy and cannot be treated with antithyroid drugs because of adverse reactions, and for pregnant patients with severe thyrotoxicosis or recurrence.

   a. **Perioperative management.** In preparation for surgery, the patient should be made euthyroid with antithyroid drugs. Once euthyroidism is achieved, iodine (SSKI, 1–2 drops PO tid) is given concurrently for up to 2 weeks before surgery to decrease the vascularity of the thyroid gland. In patients who cannot tolerate antithyroid drugs, propranolol alone can be used to prepare them.

   b. **Complications.** In the hands of a skilled surgeon, recurrent laryngeal nerve damage and permanent hypoparathyroidism are rare. Voice fatigue when speaking for prolonged periods may be due to subtle nerve damage. Transient hypocalcemia may occur but usually does not require therapy.

IV. **Severe thyrotoxicosis** may occasionally present a threat to life (**thyroid storm**). Such cases are usually associated with a precipitating event, including surgery, infection, or childbirth. The metabolic abnormalities are so severe that fever, cardiovascular compromise (usually manifested as high-output heart failure or severe arrhythmias), or mental status changes may occur, requiring aggressive treatment.

A. **Supportive measures.** Fluids, electrolytes, and vasopressor agents should be used as indicated. Glucose should be given intravenously to prevent or correct hypoglycemia. Acetaminophen and a cooling blanket can be used to treat fever. In refractory cases, chlorpromazine, 25–50 mg PO or IM q6h, may be helpful.

B. **Specific therapy.** Inhibition of synthesis and release of thyroid hormone are accomplished with antithyroid drugs and iodide.

   1. **Propylthiouracil,** 300–400 mg PO (or by nasogastric tube), should be given initially, followed by 200 mg PO q4h.

   2. **SSKI,** 5 drops PO (or by nasogastric tube) q8h, or **sodium iodide,** 1 g/24h by continuous IV infusion, should be started approximately 1 hour after the patient has received the initial dose of PTU. Iodide has immediate effects on thyroid hormone release.

   3. **Dexamethasone,** 2 mg IV or PO q6h, should be given. Dexamethasone inhibits both release of thyroid hormones and peripheral conversion of T_4 to T_3.

   4. **Propranolol,** 40–80 mg q6h, should be given orally (or by nasogastric tube) when possible. Propranolol can also be administered at a dose of 1 mg/min IV to a maximum dosage of 0.15 mg/kg q6h, with cardiac monitoring (see Chap. 7).

   5. Once clinical improvement is apparent, iodide and dexamethasone are gradually discontinued and arrangements are made for definitive therapy.

V. **Graves' ophthalmopathy** is usually mild and associated with excessive lacrimation and a foreign body sensation. Treatment is supportive, with the use of sunglasses, artificial tears, and methylcellulose ointment at bedtime. Sleeping with the head of the bed elevated may relieve periorbital edema. There is no evidence that any particular therapy for hyperthyroidism exacerbates Graves' ophthalmopathy (*Am. J. Med.* 87:70, 1989). The eye disease frequently follows a course completely independent of thyroid abnormalities. Exophthalmos in Graves' disease can be associated with optic neuropathy, characterized by decreased visual acuity, decreased color sensitivity (especially to the color red), visual field defects, and pallor of the optic disk. These patients require immediate treatment with systemic corticosteroids (e.g., prednisone, 100 mg PO qd) and emergency referral to an ophthalmologist for consideration of orbital decompression.

Multinodular Goiter and Thyroid Nodules

Palpation of the thyroid gland frequently reveals nodules. The clinician should determine whether the entire gland feels nodular; if so, it is likely that the patient has multinodular goiter, a common disorder of uncertain etiology.

I. **Multinodular goiter.** Patients with multinodular goiter are almost always euthyroid and are not at significantly increased risk for thyroid cancer. Nodules in these patients should not be evaluated unless they are symptomatic, or unless a nodule shows sudden change in size or is clearly dominant or different from the remainder of the gland. Thyroid hormone therapy is not recommended and may be deleterious. If a multinodular goiter grows rapidly; causes hoarseness, dysphagia, or respiratory compromise; or is cosmetically unacceptable, it can be surgically removed.

II. **Solitary nodules**

A. **A palpable solitary nodule of the thyroid gland** should be evaluated. For most patients thyroid scanning will not alter management. The detection of a cystic component on sonography does not increase the likelihood that the nodule is not malignant (*Arch. Intern. Med.* 150:1422, 1990). Referral for surgical excision is recommended if any of the following clinical features are present:

1. The presence of **apparent distant metastases** to lung or bone of uncertain etiology.
2. The presence of **cervical lymphadenopathy.**
3. **Rapid growth** of the nodule.
4. The presence of **a very firm nodule that is fixed to the surrounding tissues.**
5. **Vocal cord paralysis.**
6. **A history of thyroid cancer.**
7. **A family history of medullary carcinoma of the thyroid or of multiple endocrine neoplasia type IIa or IIb.**
8. **A history of head or neck irradiation.** This can be difficult to elicit and patients should be specifically asked about prior therapy for acne, tonsillar enlargement, an enlarged thymus, or fungal infections of the skin.

B. **Fine-needle aspiration cytology (FNAC).** Patients without any of the above clinical features have a 10–20% chance of harboring a thyroid cancer within a solitary nodule and should be offered FNAC. The aspiration technique is easy to learn and rarely more traumatic than drawing blood but does require the skills of an experienced cytologist.

1. **Benign nodules.** If benign cytology is clearly shown by FNAC, additional short-term intervention is not necessary. A dose of levothyroxine sufficient to suppress the TSH level is usually given, but it is unclear if such therapy is more effective than placebo in causing regression of thyroid nodules (*N. Engl. J. Med.* 317:70, 1987). Patients with benign nodules should be followed clinically, and if enlargement occurs, FNAC should be repeated or the patient should be referred directly to a surgeon. Patients who have had a benign thyroid tumor resected, especially those with a history of head or neck irradiation, may benefit from treatment with thyroid hormone. However, this treatment does not decrease the risk of cancer in these patients (*N. Engl. J. Med.* 320:835, 1989), and they should be followed carefully.

2. **Nodules with indeterminate or malignant cytology** should be referred for surgical therapy.
3. **Follow-up of patients with resected thyroid cancer** should be done in consultation with an endocrinologist. Therapy may include use of I-131 as adjunctive therapy.

Effects of Nonthyroidal Illness and Drugs on Thyroid Function

Abnormalities in thyroid function tests may erroneously suggest a diagnosis of hypo- or hyperthyroidism in patients who are ill, or in conjunction with certain drug use (*Ann. Intern. Med.* 98:946, 1983).

I. **Euthyroid hypothyroxinemia** is characterized by low levels of T_4. These patients are usually extremely ill and most have a normal serum TSH. The free T_4 by equilibrium dialysis, a better guide for therapy than the TSH in these patients, is usually normal or elevated in nonthyroidal illness. In an extremely ill patient with low levels of T_4 and clinical features of hypothyroidism (unexplained hypercholesterolemia, elevated serum CK, or unexplained effusions), it is reasonable to attempt cautious replacement therapy with thyroid hormone, with reassessment following clinical improvement. This course of therapy does not improve survival in patients with severe nonthyroidal illness (*J. Clin. Endocrinol. Metab.* 63:1, 1986), but it does not appear to be harmful.

II. **Euthyroid hyperthyroxinemia** must be distinguished from true hyperthyroidism. In patients with liver disease (in whom an elevated T_4 is caused by increased TBG), and acute nonthyroidal illness such as trauma, myocardial infarction, or pneumonia, T_4 can be elevated but the TSH is usually normal and the patient is euthyroid. In some patients with acute psychiatric illness, the T_4 is elevated but the TSH is suppressed. With appropriate psychiatric care these laboratory abnormalities resolve.

III. **Drugs.** A variety of commonly used preparations may alter thyroid function tests.
   A. **Phenytoin** consistently lowers serum T_4. The serum TSH is usually normal, and clinical abnormalities of thyroid function do not occur.
   B. **Amiodarone** is iodine rich and fat soluble, features that cause prolonged changes in both thyroid tests and thyroid function. The drug increases serum T_4 and decreases serum T_3. It may increase the level of TSH even in patients receiving thyroxine replacement for hypothyroidism (*Ann. Intern. Med.* 113:553, 1990). True thyrotoxicosis or true hypothyroidism may occur with amiodarone therapy. Therapy of amiodarone-induced thyrotoxicosis can be difficult; thyroidectomy may be appropriate in some patients (*J.A.M.A.* 263:1526, 1990).
   C. **Radiographic contrast dyes,** such as **iopanoic acid** and **ipodate,** produce effects similar to those of amiodarone. Some patients develop true thyrotoxicosis or transient hypothyroidism after receiving these agents.
   D. **Propranolol** in large doses may produce an elevated T_4 with a normal T_3. The TSH in these patients is normal and they are euthyroid.
   E. **Glucocorticoids** in large doses may decrease T_4 (slightly), T_3, and TSH. Patients treated with high-dose glucocorticoids are usually euthyroid.
   F. **Dopamine,** after prolonged infusion, decreases T_4, T_3, and TSH in some patients. These individuals are usually euthyroid.
   G. **Lithium carbonate** directly inhibits thyroid hormone secretion and may produce goiter and true hypothyroidism. Thyroid function and symptoms should be monitored before and during therapy.
   H. **Salicylates** in high doses (4–12 g/day) may decrease T_4 and T_3 by displacing these hormones from protein-binding sites. The TSH in these patients is normal and they are euthyroid.
   I. **Estrogens** and tamoxifen cause an elevation of T_4 with a normal TSH; patients are euthyroid.

Thyroid Disease and Pregnancy

I. **Hypothyroidism.** Some patients with hypothyroidism may require increased replacement doses of levothyroxine during pregnancy (*N. Engl. J. Med.* 323:91, 1990); the thyroxine replacement dose should be adjusted to maintain TSH levels in the normal range.

II. **Hyperthyroidism.** Elevations of T_4 are expected in pregnancy due to increases in TBG induced by estrogen, so the diagnosis of hyperthyroidism must be based on clinical findings, combined with an elevated free T_4 and suppressed TSH. Graves' disease is the most common cause of hyperthyroidism in pregnancy. Propylthiouracil is the treatment of choice (see Hyperthyroidism, sec **III.B.2.a**), but PTU crosses the placenta and can cause fetal goiter and hypothyroidism. Propylthiouracil is started at 100 mg PO tid and the serum T_4, TSH, and clinical response are followed at frequent intervals. Within 3–4 weeks, the dosage can usually be decreased to 50 mg PO tid based on clinical response and a serum T_4 in the mildly thyrotoxic range. It is frequently possible to decrease the dose to 50 mg PO qd or to discontinue the medication completely in the third trimester. **Methimazole is contraindicated** because it may cause fetal scalp defects. Propranolol should be avoided except for the temporary amelioration of severe thyrotoxic symptoms. Iodide should not be used. Subtotal thyroidectomy is an acceptable option for patients in the second trimester who require large doses of PTU (>450 mg per day) or experience significant drug toxicity; patients should be prepared for surgery with PTU alone if possible. **Radioactive iodine is contraindicated in pregnancy.** Careful monitoring of fetal heart rate and intrauterine development is essential in pregnant patients with hyperthyroidism.

III. **Postpartum thyroiditis** occurs in about 5% of all pregnancies (*Arch. Intern. Med.* 150:1397, 1990). Women have typical signs and symptoms of mild hyperthyroidism (that may be overlooked) and may have a small, painless goiter. The disorder usually presents within 4–6 weeks of delivery, resolves within weeks to months, and is frequently associated with a late hypothyroid phase. Up to 25% of patients experience a recurrence with the next pregnancy. Patients should be followed with measurement of TSH levels and have symptoms treated with propranolol during the hyperthyroid phase of the disorder. This therapy should be avoided in women who are breastfeeding since propranolol is excreted in breast milk. Patients who experience a hypothyroid phase can be treated transiently with levothyroxine, but therapy should be discontinued within 2–3 months and the TSH measured 1 month later to verify a return to normal thyroid function.

Disorders of the Anterior Pituitary Gland

The anterior pituitary synthesizes at least 6 hormones: prolactin, adrenocorticotropic hormone (ACTH), growth hormone (GH), follicle-stimulating hormone (FSH), luteinizing hormone (LH), and thyroid-stimulating hormone or thyrotropin (TSH). All are important in normal physiology, but only ACTH and TSH are critical for survival. As with other endocrine glands, the pituitary can be involved in hypo- and hyperfunction and can develop tumors.

I. **Microadenomas** (<10 mm in diameter) are present at autopsy in 10–20% of adults (*Ann. Intern. Med.* 112:925, 1990). These tumors may be detected incidentally during radiologic examinations. Microadenomas do not cause pituitary hypofunction but may cause pituitary hyperfunction. Once hyperprolactinemia is excluded, patients should be evaluated for overproduction of GH, which can result in acromegaly, and overproduction of ACTH, which results in Cushing's disease. Thyrotropin- and gonadotropin-secreting tumors are extremely rare.

II. **Macroadenomas** (>10 mm in diameter) may present with symptoms due to excess hormone production or with symptoms related to tumor size. Macroadenomas may compress or invade adjacent structures and cause visual field defects, cranial nerve defects, or a nasopharyngeal mass. Formal visual field testing and MRI or CT imaging of the pituitary is recommended (see Hyperprolactinemia).

III. **Specific disorders**

A. **Acromegaly** is usually caused by a GH-secreting pituitary tumor and rarely by ectopic secretion of GH or overproduction of growth hormone–releasing hormone. Onset is gradual, with coarsening of facial features, soft-tissue swelling, and extremity enlargement (e.g., increasing ring or shoe size). Headaches, excessive sweating, hypertension, joint pain, paresthesias from peripheral neuropathy, glucose intolerance or diabetes mellitus, macroglossia, and skin tags may also occur.

1. **Diagnostic evaluation.** Most of the growth-promoting effects of GH are mediated by insulin-like growth factor I (also called IGF-I or somatomedin C). Because GH secretion is episodic and its serum half-life is short, measurement of serum IGF-I is the screening test of choice for acromegaly. If the IGF-I level is elevated, MRI of the pituitary using gadolinium is appropriate. The diagnosis may be confirmed by measuring serum GH after administration of 75 g of oral glucose. Sampling should be obtained every 30 minutes for 2 hours; suppression of GH to less than 2 ng/ml occurs in normal subjects.

2. **Therapy.** Transsphenoidal surgery is usually indicated. Most patients achieve satisfactory short-term results, but long-term efficacy of surgery is uncertain. Successful surgery should result in normal IGF-I and GH levels, including normal suppression after glucose. Additional therapy with bromocriptine (see Hyperprolactinemia, sec. **IV.2**) or the long-acting somatostatin analogue octreotide is required for patients who have persistent elevation of IGF-I or GH. Bromocriptine should be used first. It seldom normalizes GH levels, but most patients improve clinically. Octreotide at a dose of 100 μg SQ tid (*Ann. Intern. Med.* 112:173, 1990) is more effective than bromocriptine but is expensive and must be administered subcutaneously. Side effects include mild gastrointestinal discomfort and flatulence. Cholelithiasis develops in a significant percentage of patients treated long-term with octreotide. Radiation therapy may be warranted in acromegaly that is resistant to other forms of therapy.

B. **Cushing's disease** (see Glucocorticoid Excess [Cushing's Syndrome]).

C. **Hypopituitarism.** The most common etiologies are pituitary or hypothalamic tumors, trauma, and prior surgery or irradiation. Postpartum necrosis (Sheehan's syndrome) is rare. Gonadotropin deficiency is the most common disorder, presenting as amenorrhea in women and androgen deficiency and infertility in men. Lack of TSH produces secondary hypothyroidism (see Hypothyroidism). Lack of ACTH produces secondary adrenal insufficiency with nausea, vomiting, and orthostatic hypotension due to glucocorticoid deficiency. Since aldosterone secretion is intact, volume depletion and hyperkalemia are absent. Other clues to hypopituitarism include improved glycemic control in patients with diabetes mellitus, inability to tan after sun exposure, fine wrinkling at the corners of the eyes, and loss of axillary and pubic hair.

1. **Screening** can be performed by measurement of serum thyroxine (T_4) and testosterone (in men) or estradiol (in women) and by performance of a rapid ACTH stimulation test (see Adrenal Insufficiency).

2. **Therapy** includes replacement of deficient hormones and treatment of the underlying cause if needed. If present, adrenal insufficiency should be corrected first. Before committing patients to lifelong replacement therapy, subspecialty consultation is appropriate.

Hyperprolactinemia

Prolactin (PRL) is an anterior pituitary hormone involved in lactation; it also influences pituitary gonadotropin secretion. Prolactin is tonically inhibited by hypothalamic dopamine; thus, interference with dopaminergic activity can elevate prolactin levels. Prolactin secretion is pulsatile and variable; elevations should be confirmed by independent measurements on different days, and early morning sampling should be avoided since elevations can occur normally during sleep.

I. **Clinical manifestations**

    A. In women, hyperprolactinemia may present as amenorrhea, galactorrhea, or, occasionally, infertility with regular menses. Many of these patients have recently started or stopped taking oral contraceptive agents. However, more than 80% of patients with galactorrhea and normal menses have normal PRL levels (*N. Engl. J. Med.* 296:589, 1977).

    B. In men, elevations of prolactin can present as decreased libido, infertility, or impotence (*J. Urol.* 142:992, 1989). Hyperprolactinemia is confirmed when prolactin levels are persistently greater than 20 ng/ml.

    C. Hyperprolactinemia and amenorrhea in women are associated with a decrease in bone mass, which may predispose to osteoporosis. In men, hyperprolactinemic hypogonadism is also associated with decreased bone mass, as well as elevations in serum lipids, which may increase the subsequent risk of atherosclerosis (*Ann. Intern. Med.* 110:526, 1989, and 111:288, 1989).

II. **Causes.** Pregnancy and lactation cause physiologic elevation of plasma prolactin. The most common causes of pathologic elevations are medications and prolactinomas. Pituitary and hypothalamic diseases (e.g., pituitary tumors, tuberculosis, sarcoidosis, metastatic cancer) disrupt normal connections between the pituitary gland and hypothalamus and may cause mild elevations of prolactin. Cranial irradiation also causes prolactin elevation (*J. Clin. Oncol.* 5:1841, 1987).

    A. Prolactinomas. Prolactin-secreting tumors of the pituitary are classified as **microadenomas** (<10 mm in diameter) or **macroadenomas** (>10 mm in diameter). Prolactin levels greater than 200 ng/ml suggest the presence of a macroadenoma. Microadenomas tend to be identified in women of reproductive age; macroadenomas often occur in older men.

    B. Medications. Prolactin elevations secondary to medications are generally less than 100 ng/ml. Withdrawal of oral contraceptive drugs is a common cause of transient hyperprolactinemia, usually lasting less than 6 months. Phenothiazines and related drugs, antihypertensives such as methyldopa and reserpine, antiemetics such as metoclopramide, morphine and related drugs, and cimetidine reduce dopaminergic activity; estrogens, verapamil, and some antidepressant agents increase PRL levels through other mechanisms. Withdrawal of the offending drug is usually sufficient to restore normal prolactin levels. Chronic cocaine abuse followed by abstinence is associated with hyperprolactinemia; observation is sufficient in management (*Am. J. Psychiatry* 145:1094, 1988).

    C. Systemic illness, such as chronic renal failure, liver disease, and psychogenic and physiologic stresses, can elevate PRL levels. Direct nipple stimulation and thoracic nerve stimulation by trauma or herpes zoster can be causative. Nonpuerperal mastitis is commonly associated with hyperprolactinemia (*J.A.M.A.* 261:1618, 1989). **Ectopic production** of PRL is rare but may occur in patients with ovarian teratomas (*Obstet. Gynecol.* 75:540, 1990; *J.A.M.A.* 263:2472, 1990) or acute myeloid leukemia (*Leukemia Res.* 14:57, 1990). Hypothyroidism, the polycystic ovary syndrome, and, rarely, adrenal insufficiency can cause hyperprolactinemia.

III. **Diagnostic evaluation.** A detailed history and physical examination, including a complete drug history, should be performed. A serum creatinine level and thyroid function testing should be obtained; women should have a pregnancy test.

    A. Microadenomas cause mild to moderate PRL elevations. Magnetic resonance imaging using gadolinium or CT of the pituitary gland is appropriate if no other cause of hyperprolactinemia is found.

    B. Macroadenomas usually present with prolactin levels greater than 200 ng/ml. Imaging of the pituitary gland is appropriate. Since **visual loss** is a major potential complication of macroadenomas, MRI is usually the imaging technique of choice for the pituitary. However, in selected patients with invasive macroadenomas, high-resolution CT scanning may be preferred to delineate the degree of bone involvement. If a macroadenoma is detected, patients should undergo formal visual field testing and evaluation of essential pituitary function (see Disorders of the Anterior Pituitary Gland).

IV. Therapy

A. Withdrawal of offending medications

B. Management of prolactinomas

1. **Observation.** Mild to moderate hyperprolactinemia due to a microadenoma (or with normal pituitary imaging) can be managed with clinical observation if fertility is not desired and symptoms are not significant. In the absence of treatment, clinically significant progression is unlikely. In one study, 35% of subjects with untreated hyperprolactinemia showed clinical improvement (*J. Clin. Endocrinol. Metab.* 68:412, 1989). If observation is chosen, PRL levels and pituitary imaging should be obtained yearly for 2 to 3 years, then less frequently if the patient's condition is clinically stable.

2. **Medical therapy. Bromocriptine,** a dopaminergic agonist, normalizes PRL levels in most patients with microadenomas and may cause shrinkage of macroadenomas. The initial dose is 1.25–2.50 mg PO with food at bedtime. An additional dose of 2.5 mg PO with a meal is added at 1-week intervals until a schedule of 2.5 mg tid with food is reached, at which time PRL should be measured. The dose is adjusted to achieve a normal serum prolactin. Prolactin levels are unlikely to be lowered further by doses greater than 20 mg per day. Short-term side effects consist mostly of nausea and orthostatic hypotension, which improve or resolve even with continued therapy. Long-term side effects include nasal congestion and constipation. Many patients achieve normal PRL levels with bid or even qhs administration. Long-term therapy is often required, since stopping the medication usually results in increased PRL levels and reexpansion of prolactinomas. Those who achieve a good response to bromocriptine should have pituitary imaging performed and a prolactin level measured at one year, and then yearly thereafter. Patients with microadenomas who achieve normal PRL levels on bromocriptine can have the medication discontinued for 2 to 3 weeks each year. In this setting PRL levels should be measured to determine if continued therapy is necessary (*Endocrinol. Metab. Clin. North Am.* 18:259, 1989). If symptoms such as headache or visual acuity changes appear, pituitary imaging should be performed regardless of the PRL level (see sec. III.B). Some patients with macroadenomas do not respond to bromocriptine and may require surgery with or without radiation therapy.

3. **Surgery**
   a. **Microadenomas.** Bromocriptine consistently lowers PRL to normal and restores fertility in the great majority of patients. Therefore, surgery is usually necessary only for patients who desire fertility but cannot tolerate or do not respond to bromocriptine.
   b. **Macroadenomas.** Most PRL-secreting macroadenomas shrink with medical therapy. Thus, a trial of bromocriptine is reasonable, even if visual field defects are present. Surgical resection should be performed in patients who do not respond to bromocriptine and in patients who cannot tolerate long-term medical therapy.

4. **Radiation therapy** is reserved for patients with invasive pituitary tumors or those who do not achieve a satisfactory clinical response to medical or surgical therapy. Patients must be followed indefinitely; deficiencies of anterior pituitary hormones may develop many years after pituitary irradiation.

C. Prolactinomas and pregnancy.

Patients with microadenomas who wish to become pregnant should receive bromocriptine in consultation with an endocrinologist. Barrier contraception is recommended until regular menses occur since early pregnancy on therapy may be difficult to detect, and exposure of the fetus to bromocriptine should be avoided. Patients with prolactin-secreting macroadenomas who desire fertility should usually be treated with radiation or surgery in addition to bromocriptine before becoming pregnant. Since both radiation and surgery may interfere with anterior pituitary function and impair fertility, subspecialty consultation is appropriate. Postpartum therapy in a woman who required bromocriptine during pregnancy is determined by symptoms and the results of postpartum CT scanning of the pituitary. Most prolactinomas regress in the postpartum period.

Hirsutism

Hirsutism is the excessive growth of androgen-dependent hair in a woman. Most of the body is covered with androgen-independent, or vellus, hairs. Under the influence of androgens, vellus hairs are converted to dark, terminal hairs in certain regions, including the upper lip, chin, sternum, midline region of the abdomen (especially the region between the umbilicus and the pubis), and upper back. **A careful drug history** should be obtained. Many patients with hirsutism are already taking cosmetic steps to remove hair. In such patients, the upper back and the skin over the sacrum (regions not easily reached by the patient) should be examined to determine the untreated extent of the disorder. Evidence of virilization (frontal balding, acne, deepening of the voice, clitoromegaly, or an increase in shoulder girdle musculature) suggests that a severe hyperandrogenic state, such as that associated with an adrenal or ovarian tumor, may be present.

I. **Diagnosis.** There are numerous causes of hirsutism but the most common are a familial tendency to grow androgen-dependent hair and the polycystic ovary syndrome.

   A. **The polycystic ovary syndrome** (*Ann. Intern. Med.* 110:386, 1989) is a heterogeneous group of disorders characterized by androgen excess. The diagnosis is made clinically in a hirsute woman with obesity, menstrual abnormalities that frequently date from menarche, infertility, insulin resistance, an LH to FSH ratio of greater than 3:1, acne, chronic endometrial stimulation, or hyperprolactinemia. Half of women with the syndrome are not obese. Patients with the polycystic ovary syndrome frequently have an elevated free testosterone, but this finding is not specific for the syndrome.

   B. **Some medications,** including cyclosporine, phenytoin, minoxidil, and diazoxide, can stimulate vellus hair growth. Danazol and other androgenic agents, including those commonly abused by athletes, and some progestins such as norgestrel stimulate terminal hair growth and cause true hirsutism. Withdrawal of the offending drug is appropriate.

   C. **Endocrine disorders** such as Cushing's syndrome, acromegaly, and, rarely, hypothyroidism may be associated with hirsutism. In selected populations, hirsutism is associated with subtle defects in adrenal steroidogenesis (i.e., late-onset or nonclassic congenital adrenal hyperplasia) (*N. Engl. J. Med.* 323:849, 1990, and 323:855, 1990).

   D. **Androgen-producing ovarian or adrenal tumors** can produce hirsutism. Androgen-producing adrenal tumors are usually large, but ovarian neoplasms causing hirsutism can be small and difficult to detect.

   E. **Initial laboratory evaluation.** In patients with mild hirsutism, the initial laboratory evaluation includes total and free testosterone levels and measurement of dehydroepiandrosterone sulfate (DHEA-S). In patients with moderate or severe hirsutism, measurement of total testosterone, free testosterone, DHEA-S, and prolactin, and an overnight dexamethasone suppression test are appropriate. If the total testosterone is greater than 200 ng/dl, or if the DHEA-S is greater than 800 μg/dl, imaging of the adrenal gland (by CT or MRI scanning) or the ovaries (by ultrasonography) is indicated to assess the possibility of an androgen-producing tumor. However, the majority of patients with testosterone levels greater than 200 ng/dl do not have detectable adrenal or ovarian tumors (*Am. J. Obstet. Gynecol.* 153:44, 1985).

II. **Therapy**

   A. **Hypothyroidism** should be treated with thyroid hormone replacement (see Hypothyroidism, sec. **II**), and hyperprolactinemia should be treated with bromocriptine (see Hyperprolactinemia, sec. **IV**).

B. **Many patients with hirsutism** will only have elevated levels of free testosterone. In the setting of obesity, weight loss should be recommended. If fertility is not desired, patients can be started on an oral contraceptive containing low-dose estrogen and a progestin with few androgenic side effects (such as ethynodiol diacetate). Unless undesirable side effects develop (e.g., abnormalities of liver function tests, thrombotic events, hypertension), therapy should be continued for a year before a determination of its clinical effectiveness is made. Therapy is associated with a reduction in free testosterone long before clinical effects are seen; demonstration of normal free testosterone levels is important to document efficacy of therapy. Spironolactone, 50–100 mg PO bid, which has antiandrogenic properties, can be used in patients who cannot tolerate oral contraceptives. Spironolactone should not be used in patients with renal dysfunction; serum potassium levels should be closely monitored to avert hyperkalemia. If this agent is given alone, contraception should be used because of the possibility of adverse fetal effects of spironolactone.

Hypogonadism

Hypogonadism in women occurs as a normal part of the aging process but may also occur in young women as the result of surgery, autoimmune disease of the ovary, or pituitary or hypothalamic disease.

I. **Menopause** is heralded by the onset of irregular menses; atrophy of the urogenital epithelium, which can cause dyspareunia and dysuria; and hot flashes, which characteristically occur at night. Emotional changes may be secondary to disruption of sleep caused by vasomotor symptoms. Menopause is associated with an increased risk of osteoporosis and atherosclerosis.

II. **Evaluation of amenorrhea in young women**

A. **Diagnostic evaluation** should begin with a pregnancy test and measurement of serum prolactin. If these are unrevealing, patients should receive medroxyprogesterone, 10 mg PO qd, for 5–10 days. If menses occur after this therapy, the ovaries are producing sufficient estrogen to cause endometrial proliferation, and there is no anatomic obstruction to menstrual flow; most of these patients are anovulatory because of intense physical activity, weight loss, prior therapy with oral contraceptive agents, or psychological stress that interferes with normal hypothalamic function. Subspecialty consultation may be appropriate. If bleeding does not occur after the administration of medroxyprogesterone, estrogen deficiency is present and serum levels of LH and FSH should be measured. Elevated levels of LH or FSH in this setting indicate ovarian failure. This is usually autoimmune in nature, accounts for more than 10% of cases of secondary amenorrhea (*Am. J. Obstet. Gynecol.* 155:531, 1986), and may be associated with autoimmune thyroiditis and autoimmune adrenal failure. Normal or low levels of LH and FSH indicate a hypothalamic or pituitary disorder or an anatomic obstruction to menstrual flow. The latter is evaluated in consultation with a gynecologist. Patients with ovarian failure and normal or low LH and FSH levels should be tested for hypopituitarism (see Disorders of the Anterior Pituitary Gland) and undergo imaging of the hypothalamus and pituitary gland by MRI or CT scanning. If no tumor is detected, some of these patients may benefit from pulsatile administration of gonadotropin-releasing hormone.

B. **Treatment** of ovarian failure regardless of the patient's age consists of estrogen and progesterone replacement therapy. Unless a specific contraindication exists, such as history of an estrogen-responsive tumor, a history of thrombotic events, vascular headaches clearly related to estrogen therapy, severe liver dysfunction, or hypertension clearly related to estrogen therapy, all postmenopausal women are candidates for hormonal replacement (*Arch. Intern. Med.* 151:75, 1991). The benefits of such therapy include protective effects against osteoporosis and possibly cardiovascular disease and diminution in the symptoms of menopause. Menopausal women and patients with premature ovarian failure should be started on conjugated estrogen, 0.625 mg PO qd, for days 1–25 of each month.

Medroxyprogesterone, 10 mg PO qd, should be added on days 16–25 of each month. Side effects include nausea, weight gain, and breast tenderness that may decrease with continued therapy or can be managed by decreasing the dose of estrogen. Women who have not undergone a hysterectomy often experience withdrawal bleeding with this regimen. Women who have undergone a hysterectomy can be treated with conjugated estrogen, 0.625 mg PO qd, without medroxyprogesterone.

III. **Hypogonadism in men** may present with infertility, loss of libido, impotence, a decrease in muscle mass, or a decrease in androgen-dependent hair.

   A. **Diagnostic evaluation** should include a clinical assessment of body habitus (e.g., a eunuchoid body habitus characterized by long arms and legs); facial, pubic, and axillary hair; the presence of gynecomastia; and testicular size and consistency. Normal testes are approximately 4.5 cm in greatest dimension and should be firm, not soft, with palpation. Laboratory evaluation should include measurement of prolactin, testosterone, LH, and FSH. Semen analysis is helpful only in evaluating suspected infertility in a man with normal hormone levels.

   1. **A low testosterone level with an elevated LH or FSH** indicates a testicular disorder and is referred to as hypergonadotropic hypogonadism. The most common cause is Klinefelter's syndrome, characterized by an XXY genotype and occurring in about 1 of every 500 men. Gynecomastia, disproportionately long legs, and small, firm testes are seen in this syndrome, and patients may be impotent and infertile. These patients may be at increased risk for hypothyroidism, breast cancer, and chronic obstructive pulmonary disease. Primary hypogonadism may also occur as part of an autoimmune polyendocrine disorder (see sec. **II.A**).

   2. **A low testosterone level with normal or low values for LH and FSH** indicates a hypothalamic disorder and should prompt a radiologic evaluation of the hypothalamus and pituitary gland for a tumor as well as evaluation for hypopituitarism (see Disorders of the Anterior Pituitary Gland). Patients with hypogonadotropic hypogonadism who desire fertility may benefit from therapy with a combination of HCG (a source of LH) and human menopausal gonadotropin (HMG, a source of FSH) or pulsatile administration of gonadotropin-releasing hormone.

   3. **Patients who abuse synthetic androgens** (e.g., athletes, body builders) also may have a low serum testosterone level and low or normal LH and FSH. These patients do not have symptoms of hypogonadism, but many have atrophic testes and infertility due to suppression of gonadotropins.

   4. **Hyperthyroidism** may masquerade as hypogonadism since such patients frequently have gynecomastia, decreased libido, and decreased muscle mass. These patients have a high testosterone level due to increased sex hormone–binding globulin.

   B. **Therapy of hypogonadism** consists of testosterone replacement. The usual replacement regimens are testosterone enanthate or testosterone cypionate, IM, at a dose of 100 mg each week, 200 mg every 2 weeks, or 300 mg every 3 weeks. Family members can be taught to administer the therapy. Older men or those with symptoms suggestive of prostatic enlargement should begin therapy with testosterone propionate, 50 mg IM q3–4 days (which has a relatively short half-life and may be helpful if prostatism is exacerbated by androgen therapy). Side effects of replacement therapy are usually minimal and include fluid retention, exacerbation of hypertension, gynecomastia, and acne. Testosterone replacement is contraindicated in patients with prostate cancer. Orally active testosterone derivatives should be avoided.

Adrenal Insufficiency

Adrenal insufficiency may result from inadequate pituitary secretion of ACTH (secondary adrenal insufficiency, see Disorders of the Anterior Pituitary Gland) or from disease of the adrenal gland itself (primary adrenal insufficiency or Addison's disease). The most common etiology of primary adrenal insufficiency is autoimmune destruction of the adrenal gland. This is usually a presumptive diagnosis made when there is no evidence of infection (e.g., no evidence of tuberculosis in other organs or evidence of human immunodeficiency virus [HIV] infection). Patients with presumed autoimmune adrenal failure are at risk for other autoimmune endocrinopathies, including Graves' disease, Hashimoto's thyroiditis, diabetes mellitus, pernicious anemia, and gonadal failure; coexistence of these disorders should be considered in management. Patients with a history of childhood mucocutaneous candidiasis or idiopathic hypoparathyroidism are at high risk for development of adrenal insufficiency and are classified as having autoimmune polyglandular disease type I, or autoimmune polyendocrinopathy–candidiasis–ectodermal dystrophy. This disorder tends to be familial and may present in adulthood (*N. Engl. J. Med.* 322:1829, 1990). Adrenal hemorrhage in the setting of anticoagulant or thrombolytic therapy may cause adrenal insufficiency. Patients with HIV infection are at increased risk for adrenal failure. Adrenal disease in these patients may be due to frank necrosis, Kaposi's sarcoma, or infection with cytomegalovirus, *M. tuberculosis,* atypical mycobacteria, or *Cryptococcus.*

I. **Diagnosis.** Patients with both primary and secondary adrenal insufficiency may manifest anorexia, lethargy, weight loss, nausea and vomiting, and abdominal, muscle, and joint pain as a result of cortisol deficiency. Patients with primary adrenal failure may also have complications due to aldosterone deficiency, including volume depletion, hyponatremia, hyperkalemia, and mild metabolic acidosis. Patients with primary adrenal failure may be hyperpigmented (especially in the palmar creases and regions of the skin exposed to pressure or trauma). Individuals with secondary adrenal insufficiency do not have aldosterone deficiency and do not become hyperpigmented.

A. **The rapid ACTH stimulation test** (cortrosyn stimulation test) screens for both primary and secondary adrenal insufficiency (*Lancet* 1:1208, 1988). The patient must not be taking glucocorticoids and must not have had recent pituitary surgery. The test is performed by obtaining a baseline cortisol and administering 0.25 mg synthetic ACTH 1–24 IV as a bolus, followed by measurement of plasma cortisol 30 minutes after the injection. If either of the cortisol values is 20 µg/dl or greater, the patient does not have clinically important defects in ACTH or cortisol production. Rarely, patients with secondary adrenal insufficiency may have a normal response to the rapid ACTH stimulation test but an abnormal response of cortisol to insulin-induced hypoglycemia. Thus, more extensive testing is appropriate if the results of the rapid ACTH stimulation test are not consistent with the patient's clinical presentation.

B. **Prolonged ACTH infusion.** If the rapid ACTH stimulation test is abnormal and intrinsic adrenal disease is suspected, a prolonged ACTH infusion should be performed. Synthetic ACTH 1–24, 0.25 mg/24 hours as a continuous IV infusion, is administered and plasma cortisol is measured at 0, 12, and 24 hours. The normal plasma cortisol at 24 hours is 40 µg/dl or greater. Patients with secondary adrenal insufficiency may have an intermediate response.

C. **Insulin tolerance testing.** If pituitary disease is suspected, an insulin tolerance test should be performed, usually in consultation with an endocrinologist. The test should not be performed in the elderly or in a clinically unstable patient but otherwise can be safely performed in the physician's office. With the physician present and after an overnight fast, regular insulin, 0.1–0.15 units/kg, is administered by IV bolus to effect a reduction in blood glucose to less than 40 mg/dl. This usually occurs within 30 minutes. Blood glucose and plasma cortisol levels are obtained at 15-minute intervals for one hour. Symptomatic hypoglycemia is necessary for an adequate cortisol response, which is defined as a peak level of 18 µg/dl or greater. Rarely, severe symptoms secondary to hypoglycemia may occur, and a 50-ml ampule of 50% dextrose for IV administration should be available during the test (see Chap. 20).

II. **Management**

A. **Primary adrenal insufficiency (Addison's disease).** In patients without significant concurrent stress, management involves replacement of glucocorticoid and mineralocorticoid function.

1. **Glucocorticoid replacement** is accomplished with prednisone, 5 mg PO qam and 2.5 mg PO qpm. Adequate replacement can only be assessed by symptoms, however, and in some patients signs of cortisol excess may develop on this dose. In these patients replacement should be with prednisone, 5 mg PO qam. During mild intercurrent illness, glucocorticoid doses should be doubled for 3 days; then the replacement dosage should be resumed without tapering. If for any reason the patient becomes unable to take fluids or medications orally, medical attention should be sought; patients should have a syringe and vial of sterile dexamethasone, 4 mg, to be administered intramuscularly in emergencies if immediate medical attention is unavailable.

2. **Mineralocorticoid replacement** is accomplished with fludrocortisone, 0.05–0.2 mg PO qd. The dosage should be titrated to (1) avert supine or postural hypotension, (2) normalize plasma potassium levels, and (3) avoid edema. Patients should be encouraged to maintain a liberal salt intake.

3. **Patient education** should include (1) directions for obtaining a medical alert bracelet imprinted with the words "adrenal insufficiency," (2) instruction on self-administration of IM dexamethasone, (3) counseling on how to adjust glucocorticoid dosage during intercurrent illness, and (4) dietary instruction for periods of mild intercurrent illness (such as gastroenteritis), including adequate salt and fluid intake.

B. **Secondary adrenal insufficiency** in unstressed patients is managed like Addison's disease, except that since mineralocorticoid secretion is intact, therapy with fludrocortisone is not necessary.

C. **Management of adrenal insufficiency perioperatively and during acute illness.** Patients with known or suspected adrenal insufficiency, including patients receiving current or recent glucocorticoid therapy, require glucocorticoid supplementation in the perioperative period and during other periods of severe physiologic stress. Hydrocortisone sodium succinate, 100 mg IV, should be administered on call to the operating room and continued through the day of surgery at 100 mg IV q8h. The dosage should be decreased by 50% each day and either discontinued or reduced to the patient's maintenance dosage by the third postoperative day, assuming that the patient's course is otherwise uncomplicated. During acute illness in the hospital, a similar regimen can be followed, with the goal of reducing glucocorticoid supplementation to replacement or maintenance doses within 3–5 days of the initiating event.

D. **Adrenal crisis** should be considered in any severely ill patient with hypotension. Clinical clues that might suggest a diagnosis of acute adrenal insufficiency include hyperpigmentation, persistent tachycardia after apparent correction of fluid deficits, or hypotension resistant to vasopressor drugs. A plasma cortisol value should be obtained; then hydrocortisone sodium succinate, 100 mg IV, should be given immediately and continued q8h. Concomitant volume repletion should be instituted immediately with IV isotonic saline containing 5% dextrose. The extracellular fluid deficit is frequently large (e.g., 2–3 liters). If the plasma cortisol value obtained before treatment is high, therapy is discontinued. If the value is low, replacement can be changed to dexamethasone (which is not detected by cortisol assays), 4 mg IV q12h, and a prolonged ACTH stimulation test should be performed. If acute adrenal failure is present, the response to therapy is usually rapid. In the setting of therapy with isotonic saline, mineralocorticoid replacement is not necessary. Glucocorticoid therapy should be tapered to replacement doses within 3–5 days, and fludrocortisone should be given (see sec. II.A.2) when IV fluids are discontinued.

E. **Withdrawal of glucocorticoid therapy.** Many medical illnesses are treated with supraphysiologic doses of glucocorticoids. Withdrawal of this therapy consists of tapering the dose of glucocorticoids, with rapidity of the taper determined by disease activity. Monitoring of the hypothalamic/pituitary/adrenal axis is usually not necessary in these patients. If symptoms consistent with adrenal insufficiency develop (see sec. I), they can be treated by decreasing the rate of tapering, or by empirically reinitiating glucocorticoid replacement. Any patient who has received more than 10 mg prednisone or its equivalent for longer than one week should be considered to have a suppressed hypothalamic/pituitary/adrenal axis. This suppression may last for months and perhaps up to a year. These patients should receive glucocorticoid supplementation during periods of severe stress (such as severe infection or surgery).

Glucocorticoid Excess (Cushing's Syndrome)

Cushing's syndrome is most commonly a manifestation of exogenous glucocorticoid administration. Primary or secondary adrenal hyperfunction may also occur. The presenting features include truncal obesity, proximal muscle weakness, hypertension, glucose intolerance or diabetes mellitus, hirsutism, osteoporosis, menstrual irregularities, and thin skin. If hyperpigmentation, hypokalemia, and relative absence of obesity exists, the cortisol excess is likely due to ACTH secretion by a malignant tumor.

I. **Screening and diagnosis.** A screening test for cortisol excess should be performed to distinguish true hypercortisolism from other disorders with similar features. In the presence of psychotic depression or alcoholism, screening tests may be unreliable. Measurement of an 0800 plasma cortisol alone is not a valid screening test for hypercortisolism. Two reasonable screening tests are available.
   A. **A 24-hour urinary free cortisol measurement** is the screening test of choice. Urinary creatinine should also be measured to verify that an adequate collection is obtained (see Chap. 11). Urinary free cortisols that are consistently greater than 100 μg/24 hour are abnormal.
   B. **The single-dose overnight dexamethasone suppression test** is another reliable screening test for Cushing's syndrome. Dexamethasone, 1 mg PO, is administered between 2300 and 2400 hours. An 0800 plasma cortisol level of 5 μg/dl or less the following morning excludes hypercortisolism. False-positive results may occur in patients taking phenytoin or other drugs that enhance the metabolism of dexamethasone, in obese patients, or in those who are stressed due to intercurrent illness.
   C. **Diagnostic evaluation.** If results of either of the screening tests are abnormal, a plasma ACTH should be obtained and more definitive testing performed, usually in consultation with an endocrinologist.

II. **Therapy.** Depending on the site of dysfunction, patients with adrenocortical hyperfunction may be candidates for adrenalectomy or pituitary resection. In most cases treatment will result in primary or secondary adrenal insufficiency, and management is required (see Adrenal Insufficiency).

Adrenal Tumors

Adrenal tumors occur commonly in the general population. Incidental adrenal adenomas are often detected during CT or MRI studies obtained for different reasons. An adrenal mass may be malignant and may produce excessive amounts of cortisol, androgens, aldosterone, or catecholamines. If a hormone excess syndrome is suspected, a biochemical diagnosis should be made first, followed by the appropriate imaging procedure.

I. **Diagnosis of adrenal tumors.** If an adrenal mass is identified incidentally, screening for endocrine hyperfunction should be performed in the proper clinical setting. In the presence of any of the clinical features of Cushing's syndrome, a 24-hour urinary free cortisol should be obtained (see Glucocorticoid Excess [Cushing's Syndrome], sec. **I.A**). In the presence of hirsutism or virilization, serum testosterone and DHEA-S should be measured (see Hirsutism, sec. **I.E**). If the patient is hypertensive, the possibility of aldosterone excess or a pheochromocytoma should be considered.

A. Diagnosis of aldosterone excess. A plasma potassium should be obtained when the patient has been off diuretics for a month. If the patient is hypokalemic, a sample is sent for determination of plasma renin activity. If the plasma renin activity is low, primary aldosteronism can be confirmed by measurement of 24-hour urinary aldosterone. If this value is elevated, consultation with an endocrinologist is appropriate to help identify a lesion that can be corrected by surgery.

B. Pheochromocytoma. A substantial portion of these patients have sustained hypertension. Many but not all patients experience hypertensive paroxysms. Most experience headaches, palpitations, or diaphoresis. Patients with neurofibromatosis, retinal cerebellar hemangioblastomatosis (von Hippel–Lindau disease), or one of the multiple endocrine neoplasia syndromes, may have early pheochromocytomas without symptoms or hypertension.

1. A **24-hour urine collection** for free catecholamines, metanephrines, and creatinine should be obtained. Ideally, this sample should be obtained while the patient is taking no antihypertensive medications. If this is impractical, clonidine is the drug of choice for hypertensive control while this screening test is being performed. A positive test suggests an adrenal pheochromocytoma. Radiographic imaging (CT or MRI) of the abdomen is also appropriate.

2. **Plasma catecholamines** can be helpful in the evaluation of such patients. Marked elevations of norepinephrine are necessary to effect an elevation of blood pressure. Elevations of norepinephrine greater than 2000 pg/ml are consistent with the presence of a pheochromocytoma.

3. **Phenoxybenzamine,** 10 mg PO q12h, is used preoperatively to treat hypertension. Dosage is adjusted to control blood pressure while avoiding symptomatic postural hypotension.

C. Anatomic evaluation. If an adrenal adenoma is not shown to be hyperfunctioning and is less than 4–5 cm in greatest diameter, the issue becomes whether an early adrenal carcinoma is present. Most such masses are benign, and unless invasive characteristics are noted by imaging, these tumors should be initially followed by CT scanning or MRI at 6-month intervals to assess the possibility of enlargement. Evidence suggests that MRI may be capable of identifying adrenal masses that are unlikely to be carcinomas (*A.J.R.* 153:771, 1989). An adrenal mass greater than 5 cm in diameter should be surgically removed.

II. **Adrenal masses and the staging of lung cancer.** The adrenal gland is a fairly common site of metastasis in patients with bronchogenic carcinoma, and adrenal masses are noted frequently during the staging of patients with a lung mass. There is evidence that such adrenal masses are more likely to be incidental adenomas than metastases (*Radiology* 153:217, 1984). These masses can be biopsied with a fine needle under CT guidance before thoracotomy, although some experts believe that MRI characteristics may identify an adenoma and obviate the need for biopsy.

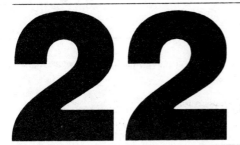

Lipid Disorders

Anne Carol Goldberg

General Considerations

The relationship between the risk of atherosclerotic heart disease and serum lipoproteins is well established. Elevated levels of total cholesterol and low-density lipoprotein cholesterol (LDL-C), and low levels of high-density lipoprotein cholesterol (HDL-C), are associated with increased risk. In some situations, such as familial combined hyperlipoproteinemia (FCHL), dysbetalipoproteinemia, and diabetes mellitus, elevated triglycerides are also a marker of increased risk of cardiovascular disease. Evidence of the beneficial effects of reduction of serum cholesterol and LDL-C has led to the development of guidelines from the National Cholesterol Education Program for detection, evaluation, and treatment of high blood cholesterol levels in adults (*Arch. Intern. Med.* 148:36, 1988). The approach to hyperlipidemia presented in this chapter generally follows these guidelines.

Detection and Evaluation

I. **Serum cholesterol** is used for purposes of case-finding and initial classification of risk. Cholesterol levels should be obtained in everyone over age 20; this may be a nonfasting specimen. Three levels of risk are defined. The presence of nonlipid cardiac risk factors should also be ascertained.
   A. **Desirable blood cholesterol** is less than 200 mg/dl. Individuals in this group should be educated about general dietary and cardiac risk factor modification. Serum cholesterol should be remeasured in 5 years because cholesterol levels may change over time.
   B. **Borderline–high blood cholesterol** is from 200–239 mg/dl. Further management depends on the presence of coronary heart disease (CHD) or two or more cardiac risk factors (Table 22-1).
      1. **In the absence of CHD or at least two risk factors,** the patient should be given information on diet. Serum cholesterol and risk factor assessment should be repeated annually.
      2. **The presence of CHD or two risk factors** requires that lipoprotein analysis be performed. Further decisions are based on the **LDL cholesterol.**
   C. **High blood cholesterol** is greater than or equal to 240 mg/dl. Lipoprotein analysis should be obtained and used for therapeutic decisions.
II. **Lipoprotein analysis** is performed on serum obtained after a **12-hour fast.** Total cholesterol, triglycerides, and HDL-C are measured and LDL-C is calculated using the following formula:

LDL-C = total cholesterol − HDL-C − (triglyceride/5)

where triglyceride/5 represents the cholesterol contained in very low density lipoprotein (VLDL). Because of biologic variability as well as potential measurement error, two or three measurements should be obtained 1–8 weeks apart while the patient is on his or her usual diet. In patients who are losing weight, are pregnant, have had major surgery, or are seriously ill (e.g., myocardial infarction),

Table 22-1. Cardiac risk factors

Male sex
Family history of CHD (myocardial infarction or sudden death before age 55 in
  parent or sibling)
Cigarette smoking
Hypertension
HDL-C concentration below 35 mg/dl (on more than one measurement)
Diabetes mellitus
Presence of cerebrovascular or peripheral vascular disease
Severe obesity (>30% overweight)

cholesterol levels may not be representative, and analysis should be deferred for at
least 6 weeks.

III. **The LDL cholesterol level** is the basis for decisions concerning dietary or drug
therapy.
   A. **Desirable LDL-C** is less than 130 mg/dl. Patients in this group should be given
   general dietary and risk factor information, and total cholesterol can be
   remeasured in 5 years.
   B. **Borderline high-risk LDL-C** is 130–159 mg/dl. The presence or absence of CHD
   or two risk factors determines further management.
      1. **Absence of CHD or two risk factors** requires that the patient be given diet
      counseling. Total cholesterol should be measured annually, and dietary
      counseling should be reinforced.
      2. **Patients with CHD or two risk factors** are treated similarly to those with
      high-risk LDL cholesterol.
   C. **High-risk LDL cholesterol** is greater than 160 mg/dl. Patients should have a
   clinical evaluation including history, physical examination, and laboratory tests
   to identify secondary causes of hyperlipidemia and familial disorders.
      1. **Secondary causes of hyperlipidemia** include diet, hypothyroidism, diabetes
      mellitus, nephrotic syndrome, uremia, and dysproteinemia. Certain **drugs**
      can have effects on lipids. Thiazide diuretics, beta-adrenergic antagonists
      (particularly less selective ones), glucocorticoids, estrogens, progestins, retin-
      oids, anabolic steroids, and alcohol have variable effects on cholesterol,
      triglycerides, and HDL cholesterol.
      2. **Familial hyperlipoproteinemias** are associated with severe elevations of
      serum lipids and often require drug therapy in addition to diet.
      3. **Treatment** begins with diet therapy and may progress to drug therapy. Diet
      therapy continues even if drug therapy is used.
      4. **Age, sex, state of health, and number of cardiac risk factors** of each patient
      must be considered in making decisions about treatment.
IV. **Serum triglyceride** levels may be found to be elevated in the course of cholesterol
evaluation. The Consensus Development Conference on Treatment of Hypertriglyceridemia defined levels of triglycerides to be considered for treatment (*J.A.M.A.*
251:1196, 1984).
   A. **Normal triglycerides** are less than 250 mg/dl.
   B. **Borderline hypertriglyceridemia** levels are between 250 and 500 mg/dl. Diet is
   the initial form of therapy in these patients. Drug therapy may be indicated in
   patients who do not respond adequately to diet and who have coronary artery
   disease, a positive family history, or the presence of other CHD risk factors.
   C. **Definite hypertriglyceridemia** is defined as triglyceride levels above 500 mg/dl.
   Diet is initial therapy, but drug therapy should be considered after an adequate
   trial of dietary therapy in patients who fail to lower their levels to less than 500
   mg/dl, because of the risk of pancreatitis.

Diagnosis of Specific Disorders

I. **Hypercholesterolemia** may be due to a primary disorder.
  A. **Familial hypercholesterolemia (FH)** is an autosomal dominant disorder involving the LDL receptor.
    1. **Heterozygotes** for FH have 50% of the normal number of LDL receptors, elevated LDL-C levels, and cholesterol levels of 350–550 mg/dl. The incidence is approximately 1 in 500 persons. Affected patients often have premature vascular disease and may have tendinous xanthomas. Treatment usually requires drug as well as diet therapy.
    2. **Homozygotes** for FH have few or no LDL receptors and thus have markedly elevated LDL-C levels and blood cholesterol levels of 650–1000 mg/dl. The incidence is 1 in 1 million. Heart disease often begins in early childhood, and many patients die of heart disease in their twenties and thirties. Affected children may have planar and tuberous as well as tendinous xanthomas. They respond poorly to both diet and drug therapy and may require plasmapheresis or liver transplantation.
  B. **Familial combined hyperlipidemia (FCHL)** is associated with an increased risk of vascular disease. The molecular basis of this disorder is unknown, but some patients have been found to be obligate heterozygotes for lipoprotein lipase deficiency. FCHL occurs in 1–2% of the population. The diagnosis is made by the presence of multiple lipoprotein phenotypes within one family. Family members may have elevated VLDL (type IV), elevated LDL-C (type IIa), or increased levels of both VLDL and LDL-C (type IIb). Diet therapy, weight loss, and exercise are useful initial therapies, but many patients will require drug therapy aimed at correcting specific lipoprotein abnormalities.
  C. **Polygenic hypercholesterolemia** is found among the 10% of the adult population whose serum cholesterol levels are above 300 mg/dl and who do not clearly demonstrate a monogenic inheritance of hypercholesterolemia. Some of these patients will be resistant to diet therapy alone and will require medication.

II. **Hypertriglyceridemia** may be secondary to diet, obesity, excess alcohol intake, diabetes mellitus, hypothyroidism, uremia, dysproteinemias, beta-adrenergic antagonists, estrogen, oral contraceptive drugs, and retinoids. Triglyceride levels greater than 500 mg/dl are often associated with an underlying primary disorder. Primary hypertriglyceridemia can be due to FCHL or familial hypertriglyceridemia.

III. **Dysbetalipoproteinemia** (type III hyperlipoproteinemia) is a rare (approximately 1 in 5000) disorder caused by an abnormality of apoprotein E, a protein on the surface of VLDL and other lipoproteins, which is important in the uptake of remnant particles by cell surface receptors. Cholesterol-enriched VLDL (beta-VLDL), an atherogenic particle, accumulates. Both cholesterol and triglycerides are elevated. Diagnosis is made by a combination of ultracentrifugation and isoelectric focusing, which shows an abnormal apoprotein E pattern. Patients may have palmar or tuberous xanthomas, and there is increased risk of vascular disease.

IV. **Hyperchylomicronemia** is diagnosed by the presence of a chylomicron layer when plasma is centrifuged or when chylomicrons float to the top of plasma that has been refrigerated overnight. Chylomicrons can be seen when triglyceride levels are in excess of 1000 mg/dl. The patient may have rare syndromes involving absence of lipoprotein lipase activity or absent apoprotein CII (a cofactor of lipoprotein lipase). Chylomicrons alone may be increased, as in lipoprotein lipase deficiency (type I), or both VLDL and chylomicrons may be elevated (type V). In type V hyperlipidemia, total cholesterol levels are often markedly elevated because of the presence of large numbers of VLDL particles that contain cholesterol as well as triglycerides. In patients with primary hypertriglyceridemia, FCHL, or type III hyperlipidemia, hyperchylomicronemia may develop in the presence of excessive dietary fat intake, uncontrolled diabetes, alcohol excess, obesity, or other secondary causes of hyperlipidemia. The chylomicronemia syndrome may include abdominal pain, hepatome-

galy, splenomegaly, eruptive xanthomas, lipemia retinalis, and pancreatitis. Memory loss, paresthesias, and peripheral neuropathy can also occur.
V. **Low HDL-C levels** (<35 mg/dl) may be due to a genetic disorder or to secondary causes.
   A. **Primary disorders** include familial hypoalphalipoproteinemia, primary hypertriglyceridemias, and rare disorders such as fish-eye disease, Tangier disease, and lecithin–cholesterol–acyl transferase (LCAT) deficiency.
   B. **Secondary causes** of low HDL-C levels include cigarette smoking, obesity, lack of exercise, androgens, progestational agents, anabolic steroids, beta-adrenergic antagonists, and hypertriglyceridemia.
VI. **Family members** of patients with hyperlipidemia should be screened to facilitate diagnosis of primary hyperlipidemias as well as to identify other patients in need of treatment.

Therapy

I. **The rationale for therapy** of hyperlipidemia is to reduce the risk of atherosclerotic cardiovascular disease. In patients with severe hypertriglyceridemia, the aim is to prevent pancreatitis.
   A. **Reduction of cholesterol and LDL cholesterol levels** is associated with a reduction of risk of cardiovascular disease. This has been demonstrated by a number of clinical trials involving both primary and secondary prevention (*J.A.M.A.* 251:351, 1984; *J. Am. Coll. Cardiol.* 8:1245, 1986).
   B. **Hypertriglyceridemia** is less clearly associated with cardiovascular disease, but risk is believed to be increased in FCHL, in patients with triglyceride levels greater than 500 mg/dl, or when other risk factors are present. Triglyceride levels above 1000 mg/dl should be treated to prevent hyperchylomicronemia and pancreatitis.
II. **Diet is the initial therapy** for hyperlipidemia and in most cases should be tried for several months before drug therapy is considered.
   A. **Goals** of therapy of hypercholesterolemia should be set. These are minimal goals, and lower levels of LDL should be attained whenever possible.
      1. **In the absence of CHD or risk factors,** a target goal LDL-C is less than 160 mg/dl.
      2. **The presence of CHD or two or more risk factors** calls for a target goal LDL-C of less than 130 mg/dl. More aggressive therapy may be indicated in patients with CHD.
   B. **Monitoring** can be performed using total cholesterol levels rather than the more expensive lipoprotein analysis. Total cholesterol levels of 240 mg/dl (in patients without CHD or risk factors) and 200 mg/dl (in patients with CHD or two or more risk factors) can be used as surrogate goals.
   C. **Diet therapy** can be done in a stepped fashion.
      1. **Step one diet** involves reduction of dietary fat to less than 30% of total calories, decrease of saturated fat intake to less than 10% of calories, and decrease of cholesterol intake to less than 300 mg/day.
         a. **Saturated fat** intake is reduced by cutting portion sizes of beef, pork, chicken, and fish to 3 oz, and limiting total meat consumption to 6 oz per day. Lean cuts of beef and pork should be well trimmed, skin should be removed from chicken and turkey, and fried foods should be avoided. Vegetable oils that are highly saturated, such as coconut oil and palm oil, should be avoided. Low-fat dairy products can be substituted for whole-milk products. Soft margarine, liquid vegetable oils, and low-fat cheese should replace butter, solid vegetable shortening, and high-fat cheese.
         b. **Polyunsaturated fats** can be obtained from vegetable oils and margarine. Intake of polyunsaturated fat should not exceed 10% of total calories. Very high proportions of polyunsaturated fat in the diet lower HDL-C as well as LDL-C.

   c. **Monounsaturated fat** should be 10–15% of total calories. These fats are found in vegetable oils, especially olive and canola oil. They also make up some of the fat in meats.
   d. **Cholesterol intake** can be reduced by restricting egg yolks and organ meats such as liver, kidney, brains, and sweetbreads. A maximum of four egg yolks per week (including those used in prepared foods) can be used.
   e. **Fresh fruits, vegetables, and whole-grain products** should be used to increase variety and provide nutrients and fiber. Carbohydrates, especially complex carbohydrate, should make up 55–60% of total calories.
   2. **If goal cholesterol is not met** after 6–12 weeks, referral to a **registered dietitian** for reinforcement of step one diet or instruction in the step two diet may be helpful.
   3. **Step two diet** involves further decreases of saturated fat to 7% of calories and of cholesterol intake to less than 200 mg per day.
   4. **Duration of diet therapy** should be at least 6 months in most cases. Cholesterol levels should be monitored at 6- to 8-week intervals to provide incentive for change. Gradual initiation of diet changes often works better than drastic alterations.
   5. **Adjustments in dietary therapy** need to be made for the elderly, who may have poor nutritional intake, and in pregnant women, who have increased requirements for a number of nutrients. Severely restrictive diets should not be used in young children with the exception of those with primary lipoprotein lipase deficiency in whom dietary fat restriction is necessary to prevent hyperchylomicronemia.
   6. **A shorter trial** of diet therapy may be suitable for patients with severe hyperlipidemias, especially in the presence of preexisting CHD or multiple cardiac risk factors.
   7. **Improved compliance may be achieved** by setting realistic goals with an emphasis on gradual change; involving the patient, food preparers, and family in making and implementing decisions; and referring patients to registered dietitians who can offer endorsement and encouragement of diet as a major therapy.
   D. **Hypertriglyceridemic patients** usually respond to restriction of dietary fat and may also require decreased intake of simple sugars and alcohol.
   E. **The chylomicronemia syndrome** requires a diet very low in total fat (10–20% of total calories as fat). Primary lipoprotein lipase deficiency is treated with fat restriction and does not respond to drug therapy.
III. **Weight loss** is beneficial if the patient is overweight. Total calories should be adjusted for **gradual** weight loss. Elevated triglycerides often respond well. HDL cholesterol may increase with weight loss.
IV. **Exercise** is often helpful in lowering triglyceride and cholesterol levels and in raising HDL-C. It can also contribute to weight loss.
V. **Discontinuation of thiazide diuretics and beta-adrenergic antagonists,** if possible, sometimes leads to reduction of triglycerides, cholesterol, and LDL-C, and to increased HDL-C. Substitution of a selective beta-adrenergic antagonist for an unselective one may be helpful.
VI. **Secondary causes of hyperlipidemia** should be treated. Control of hyperglycemia is critical if diabetic dyslipidemia is to be adequately managed.
VII. **Drug therapy** is considered if maximal diet, weight reduction, and exercise efforts do not reduce serum lipids to goal levels after an adequate trial.
   A. **Initiation of drug therapy** of hypercholesterolemia should be considered if LDL-C remains greater than 190 mg/dl in patients without CHD or two or more cardiac risk factors. In patients with CHD or two or more risk factors, the cut-off point is LDL-C greater than 160 mg/dl.
   B. **Goals of therapy** are the reduction of LDL-C to less than 130 mg/dl in patients with CHD or two or more risk factors and to less than 160 mg/dl in patients without CHD or two or more risk factors.
   C. **Diet therapy** is continued even if drug therapy is used.

D. First-choice drugs for hypercholesterolemia are the bile acid sequestrant resins, cholestyramine and colestipol, and nicotinic acid. These drugs have been shown to have both safety and efficacy in reduction of cholesterol and risk of CHD. **Lovastatin,** an HMG CoA reductase inhibitor, is effective in lowering LDL-C. However, its long-term safety has not been established.

E. Second-choice drugs include gemfibrozil, probucol, and clofibrate.

F. Hypertriglyceridemia requiring drug therapy can be treated with nicotinic acid or gemfibrozil.

G. Dysbetalipoproteinemia responds well to diet and weight loss. When drugs are needed, nicotinic acid, gemfibrozil, or clofibrate can be used.

H. In patients with a low level of HDL-C and high LDL-C, cholesterol-lowering drugs that also raise HDL-C, such as nicotinic acid, should be given priority (*Arch. Intern. Med.* 149:505, 1989).

I. Drug combinations may be useful in certain situations.

    1. In severe hypercholesterolemia it is often necessary to use a combination of diet and two drugs to reduce LDL-C to desired levels. Useful combinations include a resin plus nicotinic acid and a resin plus lovastatin.

    2. Combined LDL-C and triglyceride elevations may respond to the combination of a bile acid sequestrant resin with the addition of nicotinic acid or gemfibrozil.

    3. Low doses of two drugs can be combined if higher doses of a single agent are not tolerated by the patient.

J. Response to therapy should be monitored by checking cholesterol and triglyceride levels after 4–6 weeks of therapy. If there is no response to a drug after 2–3 months in spite of dosage adjustments, or if there are unacceptable side effects, the drug should be discontinued. If the initial drug produces only a partial response at tolerated dosage, addition of a second drug with a different mechanism of action may be useful.

VIII. Plasmapheresis and liver transplantation have been used to treat patients with the homozygous form of familial hypercholesterolemia since these patients respond poorly to drug therapy. Plasmapheresis has also been used for some patients with severe heterozygous FH.

Drugs

I. Bile acid sequestrant resins (cholestyramine and colestipol) are insoluble, nonabsorbable, anion-exchange resins that bind bile acids within the intestine, preventing their reabsorption. Since more cholesterol must be used to synthesize bile acids, there is an increase in cell surface receptors for LDL, producing a fall in circulating LDL-C levels. Reduction of LDL-C is dose dependent; up to 35% reduction can be seen. HDL-C may increase, and VLDL will sometimes increase, usually transiently. The use of resins as single-drug therapy is contraindicated in the presence of markedly elevated triglyceride levels.

A. Compliance is enhanced and side effects minimized by starting therapy with low dosages and carefully educating the patient about these drugs. The resins are powders that must be mixed with a liquid. The initial dosage of cholestyramine is 4 g (one scoop or packet) PO bid with meals, gradually increasing to 8–16 g PO bid. A chewable bar form of cholestyramine is also available; the unit dose is one bar (4 g), which is chewed and followed by at least 8 oz of a liquid. The initial dosage of colestipol is one scoop or packet (5 g) PO bid, increasing to a maximum of 15 g PO bid. Lower dosages may be effective in some patients. Increasing the dose gradually and starting at even lower dosages such as one half or one packet per day can be helpful. The drug can be mixed in almost any liquid or semiliquid food. Timing close to meals is important. It should be taken within one hour of a meal, especially the evening meal if once-a-day dosing is used.

B. Side effects include constipation, abdominal pain, nausea, vomiting, bloating, heartburn, belching, and flatulence. These effects will often diminish with continued use of the drug. The resins may interfere with absorption of thiazides, digoxin, warfarin, thyroxine, and cyclosporine; medications should be given at least 1 hour before or 4 hours after the resins.

II. **Nicotinic acid** is a water-soluble vitamin that lowers levels of VLDL up to 40%, can lower LDL-C by 15–30%, and can raise HDL-C by 10–30%.

   A. **Dosage** should be low initially with a gradual increase. Initial dosage is 100 mg PO one to three times per day with meals, increasing slowly (e.g., by 300 mg/day each week), to 2–4 g/day. Few patients can tolerate more than 4 g/day.

   B. **Side effects** limit the use of high dosages. Cutaneous flushing occurs in most patients but tolerance usually develops. Aspirin, 325 mg PO 30 minutes before each dose, can decrease flushing. Other side effects include pruritus, rash, nausea, dyspepsia, anorexia, dizziness, and hypotension. Hyperuricemia, liver function abnormalities, and worsening of glucose intolerance may occur. Baseline liver profiles and uric acid and fasting blood glucose levels should be obtained, and these should be monitored monthly while the dosage is being increased to 1–4 g/day and thereafter every 3–4 months. Use of nicotinic acid is contraindicated in patients with gout, peptic ulcer disease, inflammatory bowel disease, and significant arrhythmias. Diabetes mellitus is not an absolute contraindication, especially in patients receiving insulin, but blood sugar levels must be monitored carefully. Use of some generic sustained-release preparations may be associated with increased toxicity, including severe hepatotoxicity (*Ann. Intern. Med.* 111:253, 1989). Use of such preparations should be avoided. **Niacinamide has no significant effect** on lipid levels.

III. **The HMG CoA reductase inhibitors** are a new class of drugs that inhibit the rate-limiting step in cholesterol biosynthesis. **Lovastatin** is the first drug of this class to be released in the United States. Other drugs in the class are pravastatin and simvastatin, which are similar to lovastatin in structure, effect, and side effects. Inhibition of enzyme activity leads to a decrease in intracellular cholesterol pools and consequently an increase in LDL receptors; plasma levels of LDL-C are reduced by up to 40% (*N. Engl. J. Med.* 318:81, 1988). HDL-C increases slightly, and triglyceride levels may also decrease. **Use of lovastatin should be reserved for hypercholesterolemic patients who do not respond adequately to or cannot tolerate other first-line drugs and who are at high risk for CHD.**

   A. **Initial dosage** of lovastatin is 20 mg PO with the evening meal. The dosage can be increased to 20 mg PO bid and, if necessary, to 40 mg PO bid.

   B. **Side effects** are usually mild and transient, and include bloating, flatulence, dyspepsia, diarrhea, constipation, nausea, abdominal pain, and insomnia. Liver function tests should be followed, preferably at 6-week intervals for the first 12 months. Mild elevations of transaminases may occur after starting therapy; these usually decrease with continued therapy. In 1–2% of patients, transaminase elevations to more than 3 times the upper limit of normal have occurred up to 15 months after starting therapy. In such cases, the drug should be discontinued.

   Lovastatin should be avoided in the presence of active liver disease. Myalgias, myositis, and elevated levels of creatine phosphokinase (CK) have occurred in 2% of patients taking lovastatin. Levels of CK should be checked if patients have muscular complaints, and lovastatin should be discontinued if CK is elevated. The combination of lovastatin with cyclosporine, gemfibrozil, erythromycin, or niacin carries an increased risk of myopathy. Rhabdomyolysis has been reported.

IV. **Gemfibrozil** is a fibric acid derivative that lowers levels of VLDL and raises HDL-C. It produces 0–15% reduction of LDL-C in patients with type IIa or IIb hyperlipidemia. LDL may increase in patients with type IV hyperlipidemia. It is useful in patients with hypertriglyceridemia and in combination with resins for combined hyperlipidemia. A primary prevention trial (*N. Engl. J. Med.* 317:1237, 1987) showed decreased risk of cardiac disease in hypercholesterolemic and hypertriglyceridemic men treated with gemfibrozil over a 5-year period.

   A. **Dosage** is 600 mg PO bid before meals.

   B. **Side effects** include bloating, abdominal pain, diarrhea, nausea, headaches, and occasional rashes. Liver enzymes should be monitored 2 months after starting the drug. Gemfibrozil potentiates the effects of warfarin and may be lithogenic.

V. Probucol reduces levels of LDL-C by 8–15% but also reduces HDL-C by up to 25%. Triglyceride levels are not affected. It may be useful for hypercholesterolemic patients who do not tolerate other drugs. It has also been used with bile acid sequestrant resins for combination therapy of severely hypercholesterolemic patients.

A. Dosage is 500 mg PO bid with meals.

B. Side effects are uncommon; they include diarrhea, flatulence, nausea, and abdominal pain. Prolongation of the QT interval can occur. Probucol accumulates in adipose tissue and has a long half-life; it can remain in the body for months after discontinuation.

VI. Clofibrate is a fibric acid derivative. It is now used infrequently because of questions of long-term safety. It is used mostly for severe hypertriglyceridemia and in some patients with dysbetalipoproteinemia.

A. Dosage is 1 g PO bid.

B. Side effects include nausea, diarrhea, liver dysfunction, and rashes. Clofibrate has been reported to cause a myopathic syndrome, especially in patients with renal failure. The incidence of gallstones is increased. The drug also potentiates the effects of phenytoin, tolbutamide, and warfarin.

VII. Neomycin and D-thyroxine have a high potential for serious side effects and are not recommended for general use.

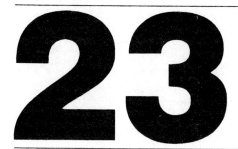

Mineral and Metabolic Bone Disease

William E. Clutter

Mineral Disorders

I. **Calcium** is essential for bone formation and neuromuscular function. Approximately 99% of body calcium is in bone; most of the other 1% is in the extracellular fluid (ECF). About 50% of serum calcium is ionized (free) and the remainder is complexed, primarily to albumin. The normal range of serum total calcium is 8.9–10.3 mg/dl (1 mg/dl = 0.25 mM/liter). Changes in serum albumin, especially hypoalbuminemia, alter total calcium concentration without affecting the clinically relevant ionized calcium level. Total calcium concentration can be "corrected" for hypoalbuminemia by adding 0.8 mg/dl for every 1 g/dl that the serum albumin falls below 4.0 g/dl. However, this correction is imprecise, and if serum albumin is abnormal, clinical decisions should be based on ionized calcium levels, which must lie within a narrow range (4.6–5.1 mg/dl) for normal neuromuscular function. Calcium metabolism is regulated by **parathyroid hormone (PTH)** and metabolites of **vitamin D. Parathyroid hormone increases serum calcium** by stimulating bone resorption, increasing renal calcium reabsorption, and promoting renal conversion of vitamin D to its active metabolite calcitriol (1,25-dihydroxyvitamin D $[1,25(OH)_2D]$). Parathyroid hormone also increases renal phosphate excretion. Serum calcium regulates PTH secretion by a negative feedback mechanism; hypocalcemia stimulates and hypercalcemia suppresses PTH release. Secreted PTH is rapidly metabolized, and inactive carboxyterminal fragments constitute most of circulating PTH immunoactivity. **Vitamin D** is absorbed from food and synthesized in skin exposed to sunlight. The liver converts it to 25-hydroxyvitamin D $[25(OH)D]$, which in turn is converted by the kidney to $1,25(OH)_2D$. The latter metabolite increases serum calcium by promoting intestinal calcium absorption and plays a role in bone formation and resorption. It also enhances phosphate absorption by the intestine. Synthesis of $1,25(OH)_2D$ is stimulated by PTH and hypophosphatemia and inhibited by increased serum phosphorus.

A. **Hypercalcemia** (Table 23-1) (*Endocrinol. Metab. Clin. North Am.* 18:389, 1989). Hypercalcemia is almost always caused by both increased entry of calcium into the ECF (from bone resorption or intestinal absorption) and decreased renal calcium clearance. More than 90% of cases are due to primary hyperparathyroidism or malignancy.

Primary hyperparathyroidism causes most cases of hypercalcemia in ambulatory patients. It is a common disorder, especially in elderly women, in whom the annual incidence is about 2 per 1000. About 85% of cases are due to an adenoma of a single gland, 15% to hyperplasia of all four glands, and 1% to parathyroid carcinoma. The majority of patients have asymptomatic hypercalcemia found incidentally. Patients may have symptoms of hypercalcemia (see sec. **I.A.1**), nephrolithiasis, osteopenia affecting primarily cortical bone (*Am. J. Med.* 89:327, 1990), or, rarely, a specific bone disorder, osteitis fibrosa.

Malignancy is responsible for most hypercalcemia in hospitalized patients, acting via two major mechanisms. In **local osteolytic hypercalcemia,** tumor cell products, such as cytokines, act locally to stimulate osteoclastic bone resorption. This form of malignant hypercalcemia occurs only with extensive bone involvement by tumor, most often due to breast carcinoma, myeloma, and lymphoma. In **humoral hypercalcemia of malignancy (HHM),** tumor products act systemically

Table 23-1. Causes of hypercalcemia

Common
   Primary hyperparathyroidism
   Malignancy
Uncommon
   Sarcoidosis, other granulomatous diseases
   Vitamin D toxicity
   Hyperthyroidism
   Thiazides
   Lithium
   Milk-alkali syndrome
   Immobilization
   Familial hypocalciuric hypercalcemia
   Associated with renal failure

to stimulate bone resorption and, in many cases, to decrease calcium excretion. PTH–related peptide, which acts via PTH receptors but is not detected by PTH immunoassays, is an important mediator of this syndrome (*N. Engl. J. Med.* 322:1106, 1990). Tumor-derived growth factors may also play a role, but PTH itself does not. HHM is most often caused by squamous carcinoma of the lung, head and neck, or esophagus, or by renal, bladder, or ovarian carcinoma. Patients with malignant hypercalcemia of either type almost always have advanced, clinically obvious disease.

Other causes of hypercalcemia (see Table 23-1) are uncommon and are almost always clinically evident. Thiazide diuretics cause persistent hypercalcemia only in patients with increased bone turnover—for example, due to mild primary hyperparathyroidism.

1. **Clinical manifestations.** Most symptoms of hypercalcemia are present only if serum calcium is above 12 mg/dl and tend to be more severe if hypercalcemia develops rapidly. **Renal** manifestations include polyuria and nephrolithiasis. **Gastrointestinal** symptoms include anorexia, nausea, vomiting, and constipation. **Neurologic** findings include weakness, fatigue, confusion, stupor, and coma. **ECG manifestations** include a shortened QT interval. Patients with hypercalcemia are more susceptible to digoxin toxicity. If serum calcium is above 13 mg/dl, renal failure and ectopic soft tissue calcification may develop. Polyuria combined with nausea and vomiting may cause marked dehydration, which impairs calcium excretion and may cause rapidly worsening hypercalcemia.

2. **Diagnosis.** Increases in serum albumin can raise the total calcium level slightly, without affecting the clinically relevant ionized calcium concentration. Mildly elevated serum calcium levels should be repeated and the **serum ionized calcium** should be measured to determine whether hypercalcemia is actually present. The differential diagnosis of hypercalcemia requires distinction of primary hyperparathyroidism from malignancy.

   a. **The history and physical examination** should focus on (1) the **duration of hypercalcemia** (if present for more than 6 months without obvious cause, primary hyperparathyroidism is almost certain), (2) history of **renal stones** (which are not seen in hypercalcemia of malignancy), (3) clinical evidence for any of the unusual causes of hypercalcemia, and (4) **symptoms and signs of malignancy** (which almost always precede malignant hypercalcemia).

   b. **The serum PTH level** should be measured (*Endocrinol. Metab. Clin. North Am.* 18:611, 1989). Most current immunoassays (termed midmolecule or C-terminal assays) recognize the carboxyterminal fragment of PTH and discriminate well between primary hyperparathyroidism and other causes of hypercalcemia. However, in renal failure, carboxyterminal fragments accumulate in serum and PTH levels may be falsely elevated with these assays. In this situation, newer two-site immunometric assays for intact PTH are more specific.

c. Other tests should include a complete blood count, serum electrolytes, and multichannel chemistry screening. Any evidence of malignancy or other causes of hypercalcemia should be carefully evaluated. Bone scans or x-rays should be done only if clinical findings suggest bone involvement.

d. Hypercalcemia due to malignancy or the uncommon causes listed in Table 23-1 is almost always evident from the history, physical examination, and routine laboratory tests; serum PTH levels are not elevated in these disorders (unless renal failure is present). In a patient with hypercalcemia, an elevated serum PTH, and no clinical evidence of malignancy, the diagnosis of primary hyperparathyroidism is secure. Chronic asymptomatic hypercalcemia is almost always due to primary hyperparathyroidism.

3. Therapy of hypercalcemia (*Endocrinol. Metab. Clin. North Am.* 18:807, 1989) includes measures that increase calcium excretion and decrease resorption of calcium from bone.

a. Extracellular fluid volume restoration. Severely hypercalcemic patients are almost always dehydrated, and the first step in therapy is ECF volume repletion with 0.9% saline to restore the glomerular filtration rate (GFR) and promote calcium excretion. The initial infusion rate should be 300–500 ml/hour and should be reduced after the ECF volume deficit has been partially corrected. At least 3–4 liters should be given in the first 24 hours.

b. Saline diuresis. After ECF volume is restored, infusion of 0.9% saline, 3–6 liters/day (125–250 ml/hr), promotes calcium excretion. Therapy should be monitored with careful records of fluid intake and output, daily weight, and frequent evaluation for evidence of heart failure. **Serum electrolytes,** calcium, and magnesium should be measured q6–12h. Adequate replacement of potassium and magnesium is essential (see sec. **III.B.3** and Chap. 3). **Furosemide,** 20–40 mg IV bid-qid, can be given if clinical evidence of heart failure develops but must not be used before ECF volume is restored and is seldom necessary if cardiac and renal function are normal. **Thiazide diuretics must be avoided,** since they impair calcium excretion.

c. Bisphosphonates inhibit bone resorption. **Etidronate,** 7.5 mg/kg in 250 ml 0.9% saline, is infused IV over 2 hours daily, until serum calcium is normal, or for a maximum of 7 days. **Pamidronate** appears to be more effective. A single dose of 60–90 mg in one liter of 0.9% saline or 5% D/W is infused over 24 hours (*Med. Lett.* 34:1, 1992); for severe hypercalcemia (>13.5 mg/dl), 90 mg should be used. Serum calcium and creatinine should be measured q12–24h. Hypercalcemia abates gradually over several days and may remain suppressed for 1–2 weeks. Repeated courses of therapy can be given when hypercalcemia recurs. Bisphosphonates lower serum calcium in most patients, with few side effects. Pamidronate may cause a transient fever. The serum creatinine level may rise, especially if other nephrotoxic drugs are used. Etidronate should be avoided if serum creatinine is greater than 2.5 mg/dl.

d. Plicamycin (mithramycin) inhibits bone resorption and reliably lowers serum calcium. Because of its toxicity, it is used only in malignant hypercalcemia. A single dose of 25 µg/kg in 500 ml 5% dextrose in water (D/W) is infused IV over 4–6 hours. Serum calcium gradually falls, reaching a nadir in 2–4 days; the duration of effect varies from 5–15 days. Treatment can be repeated when hypercalcemia recurs. Monitoring should include complete blood count, prothrombin time, serum creatinine, and liver enzymes q2–3 days. Side effects include nausea, vomiting, thrombocytopenia, platelet dysfunction, coagulation factor deficiency, renal failure, and hepatic dysfunction. Severe toxicity is uncommon with the initial dose but more likely with repeated doses. Plicamycin is contraindicated in patients with a bleeding diathesis and should be used only with

caution in renal failure, hepatic dysfunction, or during myelotoxic chemotherapy.

e. **Calcitonin** is a peptide hormone that inhibits bone resorption and increases renal calcium excretion. The dose of salmon calcitonin is 4–8
IU/kg IM or SQ q6–12h. Serum calcium may fall by 1–3 mg/dl within
hours. The hypocalcemic effect usually wanes after several days but may
be prolonged by concomitant glucocorticoid therapy. Side effects include
flushing, nausea, and, rarely, allergic reactions. Calcitonin is less consistently effective than other inhibitors of bone resorption but has no serious
toxicity and is safe in renal failure. It can be used early in the therapy of
severe hypercalcemia to achieve a rapid response but is not useful for
long-term therapy.

f. **Glucocorticoids** lower serum calcium by inhibiting cytokine release, by
direct cytolytic effects on some tumor cells, and by inhibiting intestinal
calcium absorption. They are effective in hypercalcemia due to myeloma,
other hematologic malignancies, sarcoidosis, and vitamin D intoxication.
Other tumors, such as breast carcinoma, rarely respond. The initial dose
is prednisone, 20–50 mg PO bid, or its equivalent. It may take 5–10 days
for serum calcium to fall. After serum calcium stabilizes, the dose should
be gradually reduced to the minimum needed to control symptoms of
hypercalcemia. Toxicity, discussed in Chap. 24, limits the usefulness of
glucocorticoids for long-term therapy.

g. **Oral phosphate** inhibits calcium absorption and promotes calcium deposition in bone and soft tissue. It should be used only if the serum
phosphorus is less than 3 mg/dl and renal function is normal (to minimize
the risk of soft tissue calcification). Doses of 0.5–1.0 g elemental phosphorus PO tid (see sec. **II.B.3**) modestly lower serum calcium in some patients.
Serum calcium, phosphorus, and creatinine should be monitored frequently, and the dose should be reduced if serum phosphorus exceeds 4.5
mg/dl or the product of serum calcium and phosphorus (measured in
mg/dl) exceeds 60. Side effects include diarrhea, nausea, and soft tissue
calcification. Intravenous phosphate should never be used to treat hypercalcemia.

h. **Gallium nitrate** inhibits bone resorption and was approved for therapy of
malignant hypercalcemia in 1991. A regimen of 200 mg/m^2 in 1 liter 5%
D/W or 0.9% saline infused IV over 24 hours, and repeated daily for 5 days,
lowered serum calcium to normal in 18 of 24 patients (*Ann. Intern. Med.*
108:669, 1988). A saline diuresis of at least 2 liters/day should be
maintained during treatment. Side effects include hypophosphatemia and
a transient increase in serum creatinine; in a few patients receiving
higher doses, optic neuritis has developed. The place of gallium nitrate in
treatment of malignant hypercalcemia is not yet established.

i. **Cis-platinum** has been reported to ameliorate malignant hypercalcemia
independent of its antitumor effect (*Arch. Intern. Med.* 147:329, 1987). Its
place in treatment of malignant hypercalcemia is not yet established.

4. **Acute management** is warranted if severe symptoms are present or serum
calcium is greater than 12 mg/dl. The goal is to alleviate symptoms; it is not
necessary to achieve a normal serum calcium. These measures allow time to
complete diagnostic studies and begin treatment of the underlying disease.
Mild, asymptomatic hypercalcemia requires only treatment of its cause.
The first step is **replacement of ECF volume** with 0.9% saline. Intake should
exceed output by at least 2 liters in the first 24 hours, and **saline diuresis**
with 0.9% saline, 3–6 liters/day, should then be continued. A drug that
inhibits bone resorption should be given early. **Pamidronate** is the therapy of
choice for most patients. **Plicamycin** is also effective, but more toxic; it can be
used in malignant hypercalcemia if bisphosphonates are ineffective. **Calcitonin** can be used in patients with renal failure or added to another drug to
rapidly control severe hypercalcemia but is seldom active for more than a few

days. In oliguric renal failure that cannot be treated with IV saline, **hemodialysis** with a calcium-free dialysate will lower serum calcium temporarily.

5. **Chronic management of hypercalcemia**

   a. The only effective therapy for **primary hyperparathyroidism** is parathyroidectomy. However, in the asymptomatic majority of patients, the issue is whether surgery is indicated (*J. Clin. Endocrinol. Metab.* 70:1489, 1990). The natural history of asymptomatic hyperparathyroidism is not fully known, but in many patients the disorder has a benign course, with little change in clinical findings or serum calcium for years. The major concern is the possibility of progressive loss of bone mass and increased risk of fracture; deterioration of renal function is also possible but unlikely in the absence of nephrolithiasis. Currently, it is impossible to predict which patients will develop problems. **Indications for surgery** include (1) symptoms due to hypercalcemia, (2) nephrolithiasis, (3) reduced bone mass (more than 2 standard deviations below mean for age), (4) serum calcium more than 11.5 or 12 mg/dl, (5) age less than 50, and (6) infeasibility of long-term follow-up. Surgery is a reasonable choice in healthy patients even if they do not meet these criteria, since it has a high success rate with low morbidity and mortality. However, asymptomatic patients can be followed by assessing clinical status, serum calcium and creatinine levels, and bone mass (with single-photon absorptiometry of the forearm) at 6- to 12-month intervals. Surgery should be recommended if any of the above criteria develop or if there is progressive decline in bone mass or renal function.
   Parathyroidectomy by a surgeon experienced in the procedure has a success rate of 90–95%. After surgery, Chvostek's and Trousseau's signs and serum calcium should be monitored daily for several days. There is often a brief (1–2 days) period of mild, asymptomatic hypocalcemia. In the rare patients with overt bone disease, hypocalcemia may be severe and prolonged (the hungry bone syndrome), requiring therapy (see sec. **I.B.3**). Other complications include permanent hypoparathyroidism and injury to the recurrent laryngeal nerve. Reexploration has a lower success rate and a greater risk of complications and should be performed at a referral center. Localization procedures (*Ann. Intern. Med.* 107:64, 1987) are not indicated before initial neck exploration but may be helpful before reexploration.
   Medical therapy has not been shown to be beneficial. However, in postmenopausal women with primary hyperparathyroidism, ethinyl estradiol, 30 μg PO qd, lowers serum calcium slightly and may help to preserve bone mass (*Endocrinol. Metab. Clin. North Am.* 18:715, 1989). In patients with symptomatic hypercalcemia who refuse or cannot tolerate surgery, physical activity should be encouraged, along with a diet containing at least 2–3 liters of fluid and 8–10 g of salt per day. Dietary calcium restriction is not appropriate and thiazide diuretics must be avoided. Oral phosphate therapy (see sec. **I.A.3.g**) may lower serum calcium but also raises serum PTH levels; its benefits do not clearly outweigh risks, and it should be used only if symptomatic hypercalcemia cannot be surgically corrected (*J. Clin. Endocrinol. Metab.* 56:953, 1983).

   b. Therapy of **malignant hypercalcemia** may control symptoms while antineoplastic therapy takes effect but rarely succeeds for long unless the cancer responds to treatment. Since patients usually have extensive, unresectable disease, with median survival less than 3 months, the initial decision should be whether therapy is warranted. This judgment depends on the prospect for effective treatment of the cancer and the expected quality of life. Treatment of hypercalcemia may palliate symptoms such as anorexia, nausea, and malaise that could be attributed to cancer (*Ann. Intern. Med.* 112:499, 1990). However, in comatose patients with advanced cancer for which no further antineoplastic therapy is planned, hypercalcemia should generally not be treated.

After acute management of hypercalcemia, physical activity and a diet containing at least 2–3 liters of fluid and 8–10 g of salt should be encouraged, and nausea should be treated. Restriction of dietary calcium is not helpful. Repeated doses of IV **pamidronate** or **plicamycin** can be given when hypercalcemia recurs. Pamidronate is preferred if myelosuppressive chemotherapy is being given. **Prednisone**, 20–50 mg PO bid, usually controls hypercalcemia in multiple myeloma and other hematologic malignancies. Oral **phosphate** can be tried if serum phosphorus is low and renal function is normal.

c. **Hypercalcemia due to other disorders.** Vitamin D toxicity should be treated with prednisone and a low-calcium diet (<400 mg/day). The effects of vitamin D itself may take 2 months to abate, but the toxicity of its metabolites is more short-lived. Hypercalcemia due to sarcoidosis responds to prednisone, and a dose of 10–20 mg/day may be sufficient for long-term control.

B. **Hypocalcemia.** The most common cause of low total serum calcium is **hypoalbuminemia.** If serum free calcium is normal, then no disorder of calcium metabolism is present. **Causes of low serum free calcium** include renal failure, hypoparathyroidism (either idiopathic or postsurgical), severe hypomagnesemia, hypermagnesemia, acute pancreatitis, rhabdomyolysis, tumor lysis syndrome, vitamin D deficiency, pseudohypoparathyroidism (PTH resistance), and, rarely, multiple citrated blood transfusions. Low free calcium is common in critically ill patients, sometimes without evident cause.

1. **Clinical manifestations** vary with the degree and rate of onset; chronic hypocalcemia may be asymptomatic. Alkalosis augments calcium binding to albumin and increases the severity of symptoms. Increased excitability of nerves and muscles causes paresthesias and **tetany,** including carpopedal spasms. **Trousseau's sign** is development of carpal spasm when a blood pressure cuff is inflated above systolic pressure for 3 minutes. **Chvostek's sign** is twitching of facial muscles when the facial nerve is tapped anterior to the ear. The presence of these signs is known as **latent tetany.** Severe hypocalcemia may cause lethargy, confusion, and, rarely, laryngospasm, seizures, or reversible heart failure. The ECG may show a prolonged QT interval. Chronic hypocalcemia may cause cataracts and calcification of the basal ganglia.

2. **Diagnosis.** The **history and physical examination** should focus on (1) previous neck surgery (hypoparathyroidism may develop immediately or gradually over years), (2) disorders associated with idiopathic hypoparathyroidism (e.g., hypothyroidism, adrenal failure, candidiasis, vitiligo), (3) family history of hypocalcemia (which may be positive in hypoparathyroidism or pseudohypoparathyroidism), (4) drugs that cause hypomagnesemia (see sec. **III.B**), (5) conditions that cause vitamin D deficiency (see Metabolic Bone Disease, sec. **II**), and (6) findings of pseudohypoparathyroidism (short stature, short metacarpals). **Laboratory studies** should include serum free calcium, phosphorus, magnesium, creatinine, and PTH. Serum phosphorus is elevated in most causes of hypocalcemia except vitamin D deficiency, in which it is low. Serum PTH is elevated in disorders other than hypoparathyroidism and magnesium deficiency.

3. **Acute management.** Symptomatic hypocalcemia should be treated as an emergency with 10% **calcium gluconate** (90 mg elemental calcium/10 ml), 2 ampules (20 ml) IV over 10 minutes, followed by infusion of 60 ml in 500 ml 5% D/W (1 mg/ml) at 0.5–2.0 mg/kg/hr. Serum calcium should be measured q4–6h. The infusion rate should be adjusted to avoid recurrent symptomatic hypocalcemia and to maintain the serum calcium between 8 and 9 mg/dl. The underlying cause should be treated, or long-term therapy started, and the IV infusion then gradually tapered. **Hypomagnesemia,** if present, must be treated to correct hypocalcemia (see sec. **III.B.3**). In patients taking digoxin,

the ECG should be monitored since calcium potentiates digitalis toxicity. **Calcium and bicarbonate are not compatible IV admixtures.**

4. **Long-term management** of hypoparathyroidism and pseudohypoparathyroidism requires calcium supplements and vitamin D or its active metabolite to increase intestinal calcium absorption. Since PTH cannot limit urinary calcium excretion in these diseases, hypercalciuria and nephrolithiasis are potential side effects. **The objective is to maintain serum calcium slightly below the normal range (between 8.0 and 9.0 mg/dl)**, which usually prevents manifestations of hypocalcemia and minimizes hypercalciuria. While the dose of vitamin D is being titrated, serum calcium should be measured twice a week. When a maintenance dose is achieved, serum and 24-hour urine calcium should be monitored every 3–6 months, since unexpected fluctuations may occur. If urine calcium exceeds 250 mg/24 hr, the dose of vitamin D should be reduced. **If hypercalcemia develops,** vitamin D and calcium should be stopped until serum calcium falls to normal, then both should be restarted at lower doses. Hypercalcemia due to calcitriol usually resolves within 1 week, and serum calcium should be monitored q24–48h. Hypercalcemia due to vitamin D itself may take over 2 months to resolve; if symptomatic, it should be treated with prednisone (see sec. **I.A.3.f**). In mild vitamin D toxicity, serum calcium can be monitored at weekly intervals until it returns to normal. Therapy of vitamin D deficiency and malabsorption are discussed in Metabolic Bone Disease, sec. **II.**

   a. **Oral calcium supplements. Calcium carbonate** (Oscal, 250 or 500 mg elemental calcium/tablet; Tums Extra-Strength, 400 mg elemental calcium/5 ml; or various generics) is the least expensive compound. The initial dosage is 1–2 g elemental calcium PO tid during the transition from IV to oral therapy. For long-term therapy, the typical dosage is 0.5–1.0 g PO tid, with meals. Calcium carbonate is only soluble at an acid pH but is well absorbed when taken with food, even in subjects with achlorhydria. Side effects include dyspepsia and constipation.

   b. **Vitamin D.** Dietary deficiency can be corrected by 400–1000 IU/day, but treatment of other hypocalcemic disorders requires much larger doses of vitamin D or use of an active metabolite. **Calcitriol** or $1,25(OH)_2D$ (Rocaltrol, 0.25 or 0.5 µg/capsule) has a rapid onset of action. The initial dose is 0.25 µg PO qd, and most patients are maintained on 0.5–2.0 µg PO qd. The dose can be increased at 2- to 4-week intervals. **Vitamin D** (50,000 IU or 1.25 mg/capsule) requires weeks to achieve full effect. The initial dose is 50,000 IU PO qd, and usual maintenance doses are 50,000–100,000 IU PO qd. The dose can be increased at 4- to 6-week intervals. Calcitriol is much more expensive than vitamin D, but its lower risk of toxicity makes it the best choice for most patients.

   c. **Other measures.** In patients with severe hyperphosphatemia, serum phosphorus should be lowered to less than 6.5 mg/dl with oral phosphate binders (see sec. **II.A.2.b**) before vitamin D is started. If hypercalciuria develops at serum calcium levels less than 8.5 mg/dl, hydrochlorothiazide, 50 mg PO qd, can be used to reduce urinary calcium excretion.

II. **Phosphorus** is critical for bone formation and cellular energy metabolism. About 85% of body phosphorus is in bone and most of the remainder is within cells; only 1% is in the ECF. Thus, serum phosphorus levels may not reflect total body phosphorus stores. Phosphorus exists in the body as phosphate, but serum concentration is expressed as mass of phosphorus (1 mg/dl phosphorus = 0.32 mM/liter phosphate). The normal range is 3.0–4.5 mg/dl, with somewhat higher values in children and postmenopausal women. Serum phosphorus is best measured in the fasting state, since there is diurnal variation with a morning nadir, and since carbohydrate ingestion and glucose infusion lower serum phosphorus, while a high phosphate meal raises it. Major regulatory factors include **PTH,** which lowers serum phosphorus by increasing renal excretion; **$1,25(OH)_2D$,** which increases serum phosphorus by enhancing intestinal phosphate absorption; **insulin,** which lowers serum levels by shifting phosphate into cells; dietary phosphate intake; and renal function.

Table 23-2. Causes of severe hypophosphatemia (<1 mg/dl)

Alcohol abuse and withdrawal
Respiratory alkalosis
Malabsorption
Oral phosphate binders
Refeeding after malnutrition
Hyperalimentation
Severe burns
Therapy of diabetic ketoacidosis

A. **Hyperphosphatemia** is most often due to **renal failure** but also occurs in hypoparathyroidism, pseudohypoparathyroidism, rhabdomyolysis, tumor lysis syndrome, and metabolic and respiratory acidosis, and after excess phosphate administration.
   1. **Clinical manifestations** are due to hypocalcemia (see sec. **I.B.1**) and ectopic calcification of soft tissues, including blood vessels, cornea, skin, kidney, and periarticular tissue. Chronic hyperphosphatemia contributes to renal osteodystrophy.
   2. **Management** (*N. Engl. J. Med.* 320:1140, 1989) includes:
      a. **Restriction of dietary phosphate** to 0.6–0.9 g/day.
      b. **Oral phosphate binders.** In patients with renal failure, **calcium carbonate** (see sec. **I.B.4.a**) is given at an initial dosage of 0.5–1.0 g elemental calcium PO tid with meals. The dosage can be increased at intervals of 2–4 weeks to a maximum of 3 g tid. The goal of therapy is to maintain serum phosphorus between 4.5 and 6 mg/dl. Serum calcium and phosphorus should be measured frequently and the dose adjusted to keep the serum calcium less than 11.0 mg/dl and the calcium–phosphorus product less than 60, to minimize the risk of ectopic calcification. If hyperphosphatemia persists despite doses of calcium that cause hypercalcemia, small doses of aluminum (Al) gels can be added—for example, **Al hydroxide** (600 mg/tablet or 320 mg/5 ml) or **Al carbonate** (600 mg/tablet or 400 mg/5 ml), 5–10 ml or 1–2 tablets PO tid with meals. Side effects of Al gels include nausea and constipation; prolonged use in renal failure may cause Al toxicity (see Chap. 11).
      c. **Saline diuresis** (see sec. **I.A.3.b**) will reduce acute hyperphosphatemia in patients without renal failure.
      d. **Dialysis** is required to treat hyperphosphatemia in severe renal failure.
B. **Hypophosphatemia** may be caused by impaired intestinal absorption, increased renal excretion, or redistribution of phosphate into cells. **Severe hypophosphatemia** (<1 mg/dl, Table 23-2) usually indicates total body phosphate depletion. However, during therapy of diabetic ketoacidosis, hypophosphatemia seldom reflects severe phosphate depletion and very rarely causes clinical manifestations. **Moderate hypophosphatemia** (1.0–2.5 mg/dl) is common in hospitalized patients and may not indicate total body phosphate depletion. In addition to the conditions listed in Table 23-2, moderate hypophosphatemia may be caused by (1) infusion of glucose, (2) dietary vitamin D deficiency or malabsorption, and (3) increased renal phosphate loss due to hyperparathyroidism, the diuretic phase of acute tubular necrosis, renal transplantation, familial X-linked hypophosphatemia, Fanconi's syndrome, oncogenic osteomalacia, and ECF volume expansion.
   1. **Clinical manifestations** typically occur only if there is total body phosphate depletion and serum phosphorus is less than 1 mg/dl. Muscular abnormalities include weakness, rhabdomyolysis, impaired diaphragmatic function, respiratory failure, and congestive heart failure. Neurologic abnormalities include paresthesias, dysarthria, confusion, stupor, seizures, and coma. Hemolysis, platelet dysfunction, and metabolic acidosis rarely occur. Chronic hypophos-

phatemia causes rickets in children and osteomalacia in adults (see Metabolic Bone Disease, sec. II).

2. **Diagnosis.** The cause is usually apparent, but if not, urine phosphorus helps to define the mechanism. Excretion of more than 100 mg/day during hypophosphatemia indicates excessive renal loss. Family history, serum calcium and PTH, and urine amino acids help to distinguish among renal causes, and low serum 25(OH)D suggests dietary vitamin D deficiency or malabsorption.

3. **Management**

   a. **Moderate hypophosphatemia** (1.0–2.5 mg/dl) is usually asymptomatic and requires no therapy except correct of the cause. Persistent hypophosphatemia should be treated with oral phosphate supplements, 0.5–1.0 g of elemental phosphorus PO bid-tid. Preparations include Neutra-Phos (250 mg elemental phosphorus and 7 mEq each of sodium and potassium per capsule) and Neutra-Phos K (250 mg elemental phosphorus and 14 mEq potassium per capsule). The contents of capsules should be dissolved in water. Fleet Phospho-Soda (815 mg phosphorus and 33 mEq sodium per 5 ml) can also be used. For patients who require long-term therapy, bulk powder is more economical; a 64-g bottle of Neutra-Phos dissolved in 1 gallon of water provides 250 mg elemental phosphorus/75 ml. Serum phosphorus, calcium, and creatinine should be measured daily as the dose is adjusted. Side effects include diarrhea, which often limits the dose, and nausea. Hypocalcemia and ectopic calcification are rare unless hyperphosphatemia occurs.

   b. **Severe hypophosphatemia** (<1 mg/dl) may require IV phosphate therapy when associated with serious clinical manifestations. However, IV phosphate does not improve the outcome of therapy in diabetic ketoacidosis; unless there is evidence of preexisting phosphate depletion from another cause, the risks of IV phosphate outweigh the benefits in this disorder (*N. Engl. J. Med.* 313:447, 1985).

   Intravenous preparations include potassium phosphate (1.5 mEq potassium/mM phosphate) and sodium phosphate (1.3 mEq sodium/mM phosphate). An infusion of 0.08–0.16 mM phosphate/kg (2.5–5.0 mg elemental phosphorus/kg) in 500 ml 0.45% saline is given IV over 6 hours. Further doses should be based on symptoms, and the serum calcium, phosphorus, and potassium, which should be measured every 6 hours. Intravenous infusion should be stopped when serum phosphorus is greater than 1.5 mg/dl or when oral therapy is possible. Because of the need to replenish intracellular stores, 24–36 hours of infusion may be required. **Extreme care must be used to avoid hyperphosphatemia,** which may cause hypocalcemia, ectopic soft tissue calcification, renal failure, hypotension, and death. In renal failure, IV phosphate should be given only if absolutely necessary. Hypophosphatemic patients are frequently hypokalemic and hypomagnesemic, and these disorders must be corrected as well. (Conversion equations for phosphate therapy are: 1 mM phosphate = 31 mg phosphorus, and 1 mg phosphorus = 0.032 mM.)

III. **Magnesium** (*D.M.* 34:161, 1988) plays an important role in neuromuscular function. About 60% of body magnesium is in bone and most of the remainder is within cells. Only 1% is in the ECF, and, thus, serum magnesium levels may not reflect total body magnesium content. Normal serum concentrations are 1.3–2.2 mEq/liter.

   A. **Hypermagnesemia** occurs in **renal failure,** usually after therapy with magnesium-containing antacids or laxatives, and during treatment of preeclampsia with IV magnesium.

      1. **Clinical manifestations** are usually seen only if serum magnesium is greater than 4 mEq/liter. Neuromuscular abnormalities include areflexia, lethargy, weakness, paralysis, and respiratory failure. Cardiac findings include hypotension; bradycardia; prolonged PR, QRS, and QT intervals; complete heart block; and asystole. Hypocalcemia may occur.

2. **Therapy.** Hypermagnesemia can be prevented by avoiding magnesium preparations in renal failure. Asymptomatic hypermagnesemia requires only withdrawal of this therapy. Severe, symptomatic hypermagnesemia should be treated with **10% calcium gluconate**, 10–20 ml IV over 10 minutes to temporarily antagonize the effects of magnesium. Prompt supportive therapy is critical, including mechanical ventilation for respiratory failure and a temporary pacemaker for bradyarrhythmias. In severe renal failure, **hemodialysis** is required for definitive therapy. In patients without severe renal failure, 0.9% saline with 20 ml of 10% calcium gluconate/liter can be given at 150–200 ml/hour to promote magnesium excretion.

B. **Hypomagnesemia** may be caused by (1) decreased intestinal absorption due to malnutrition, malabsorption, prolonged diarrhea, or nasogastric aspiration, or (2) increased renal excretion caused by hypercalcemia, osmotic diuresis, and several drugs: **loop diuretics, aminoglycosides, amphotericin B, cis-platinum,** and **cyclosporine.** Hypomagnesemia often complicates **alcoholism** and **alcohol withdrawal.**

1. **Clinical manifestations.** Hypomagnesemia often causes **hypokalemia** and **hypocalcemia,** which contribute to the clinical picture. Neurologic abnormalities include lethargy, confusion, tremor, fasciculations, ataxia, nystagmus, tetany, and seizures. ECG abnormalities include prolonged PR and QT intervals. Atrial and ventricular arrhythmias may occur, especially in patients treated with digoxin.

2. **Diagnosis.** The cause is usually evident, but if not, urine magnesium helps to define the mechanism. Excretion of more than 2 mEq/day during hypomagnesemia indicates excessive renal loss.

3. **Treatment** must be given with extreme care in renal failure because of the risk of hypermagnesemia.

   a. **Mild or chronic hypomagnesemia** can be treated with 240 mg elemental magnesium PO qd–bid. Magnesium oxide preparations include Mag-Ox 400 (240 mg elemental magnesium/400-mg tablet) and Uro-mag (84 mg elemental magnesium/140-mg tablet). The major side effect is diarrhea.

   b. **Severe, symptomatic hypomagnesemia** can be treated with 50% magnesium sulfate (4 mEq/ml), 2–4 ml IV over 15 minutes, followed by an infusion of 48 mEq in 1 or more liters of IV fluid over 24 hours. Because of the need to replenish intracellular stores, the infusion should be continued for 3–7 days. Serum magnesium should be measured q12–24h and the infusion rate adjusted to keep serum magnesium less than 2.5 mEq/liter. Tendon reflexes should be tested frequently, since hyporeflexia suggests hypermagnesemia. Reduced doses must be used in even mild renal failure. Magnesium sulfate can be given intramuscularly but is painful. (Conversion equations for magnesium therapy are: 1 mM = 2 mEq = 24 mg elemental magnesium.)

Metabolic Bone Disease

Metabolic bone diseases decrease the mass and strength of the skeleton, predisposing to fracture. Bone mass increases until about age 30, then gradually declines. In women, after menopause or premature ovarian failure, estrogen deficiency leads to a period of accelerated bone loss lasting 5–10 years. **Osteopenia** (Table 23-3) is a general term for abnormally low bone mass. Its clinical importance is due to the morbidity and mortality of fractures, which may occur with minimal trauma. The most common cause of osteopenia is **osteoporosis;** other causes include **osteomalacia** and the bone disease of **hyperparathyroidism.**

I. **Osteoporosis** (Table 23-3) is defined as low bone mass with a normal ratio of mineral to osteoid (the organic matrix of bone). Primary osteoporosis is the most common form and is classified into two major types (*J. Clin. Endocrinol. Metab.* 70:1229, 1990). **Postmenopausal or type I osteoporosis** becomes clinically manifest about 10 years after menopause, with a peak incidence in the 60s and early 70s.

Table 23-3. Causes of osteopenia

Osteoporosis
  Primary
    Postmenopausal (type I)
    Senile (type II)
    Idiopathic (in younger men and women)
  Secondary
    Cushing's syndrome (including glucocorticoid therapy)
    Hyperthyroidism
    Hypogonadism in men
    Immobilization
    Chronic heparin administration
    Osteogenesis imperfecta and related disorders
Primary hyperparathyroidism
Osteomalacia
Myeloma
Mastocytosis
Renal osteodystrophy

Predominantly trabecular bone is lost, leading to vertebral crush fractures and Colles' fractures of the distal forearm. Other symptoms include acute or chronic back pain, kyphosis, and loss of height. **Senile or type II osteoporosis** presents after about age 70 in both sexes. Both cortical and trabecular bone is lost, leading to increased risk of hip and vertebral fractures. The most important **risk markers for osteoporosis** are female sex, white or Oriental race, early menopause (spontaneous or due to oophorectomy), and therapy with glucocorticoids. Lean body habitus, positive family history of osteoporosis, low calcium intake, lack of exercise, smoking, alcohol abuse, therapy with phenytoin, subtotal gastrectomy, chronic obstructive pulmonary disease, and chronic liver disease may also indicate increased risk. Therapy with thiazide diuretics appears to reduce risk.

A. Diagnosis. Osteoporosis may be detected because of fractures that occur with minimal trauma, as an incidental finding on an x-ray, or by measurement of bone density. Diagnosis of primary osteoporosis requires exclusion of secondary forms of osteoporosis and other causes of osteopenia (Table 23-3). The history, physical examination, and a few basic laboratory tests usually suffice. Testing should include a complete blood count, multichannel chemistry screening, serum thyroid-stimulating hormone (TSH), urinalysis, and serum protein electrophoresis. Serum calcium and phosphorus are normal in osteoporosis, and alkaline phosphatase is normal except for brief elevations after a fracture; abnormal values suggest a cause other than primary osteoporosis. If osteomalacia (see sec. II) is suspected because of a history of gastrointestinal disease or abnormal serum chemistry values, serum 25(OH)D should be measured. Bone biopsy is not necessary in patients with typical osteoporosis. However, in premenopausal women or men younger than 65, it may help to diagnose other causes of osteopenia.

Bone mass measurements are the most sensitive and specific tests for osteopenia and predict the risk of fracture. Several methods are in current use. Single-photon absorptiometry measures bone mass in the distal forearm with high precision. It is widely available and relatively inexpensive. Quantitative computed tomography measures lumbar trabecular bone mass with somewhat lower precision and is more expensive. Dual-energy x-ray absorptiometry measures total bone mass of the lumbar spine and proximal femur with high precision.

Indications for bone mass measurement are not clearly established (*N. Engl. J. Med.* 324:1105, 1991). Nonselective screening is not recommended. However, in perimenopausal women, measurement of bone mass is useful if it will influence the decision to start long-term estrogen replacement. Another indication is evidence of osteoporosis on conventional x-rays. Since apparent osteopenia and minimal vertebral deformities are not specific, bone mass measurement can determine whether evaluation and therapy of osteopenia are warranted.

B. **Prevention** is preferable to treatment of established osteoporosis, since no therapy can substantially increase bone mass. In perimenopausal women, **risk factors** for osteoporosis (see sec. I) should be assessed. If multiple risk factors are present, or if an estimate of fracture risk will help determine whether to prescribe preventive therapy, **bone mass** should be measured. If bone mass is low compared with norms for age and sex, then preventive measures, usually estrogen replacement, should be recommended. Estrogen replacement is indicated for all women with **premature menopause** and no contraindications (see sec. I.B.2). The ratio of benefit to risk is also very favorable for women who have had a **hysterectomy** because of benign disease.

1. **Calcium.** Many women avoid dairy products and have deficient dietary calcium. In postmenopausal women with low calcium intake, calcium supplementation slows loss of bone mass (*N. Engl. J. Med.* 323:878, 1990). The recommended intake for premenopausal women and men is 1000 mg/day, and for postmenopausal women, 1500 mg/day. Most women require calcium supplements, 500–1000 mg/day, to achieve this level of intake. Calcium carbonate (see Mineral Disorders, sec. **I.B.4.a**) is the least expensive preparation. Side effects include dyspepsia, constipation, and hypercalciuria.

2. **Estrogen replacement** after menopause inhibits bone resorption, slows the loss of bone mass, and reduces the risk of fractures. A **cyclic regimen** including estrogen and a progestin should be used, giving estrogen on days 1–25 of each month. Appropriate doses include (1) conjugated estrogens (Premarin), 0.625 mg PO qd; (2) ethinyl estradiol, 20 µg PO qd; or (3) estradiol, 1 mg PO qd (*Mayo Clin. Proc.* 63:453, 1988). Transdermal estradiol, 0.05 mg patch twice a week, is also effective (*Lancet* 336:265, 1990). In women who have side effects at these doses, conjugated estrogen, 0.3 mg PO qd, is effective when given with 1500 mg calcium/day. **Medroxyprogesterone** (Provera), 5–10 mg PO qd, should be started between days 12 and 15 and continued to day 25 of each month. Progesterone is not needed if the patient has had a hysterectomy. Replacement should begin as soon as possible after the menopause to delay the rapid phase of bone loss; however, therapy may be beneficial as late as age 70. The optimal **duration** of therapy is not established, but there is consensus that it should continue for at least 10 years. Women with premature menopause should be treated at least until the time of normal menopause (about age 50). **Regular evaluation** should include breast examinations, annual mammography, and prompt evaluation of unexpected vaginal bleeding with endometrial biopsy. **Contraindications** include a history of breast or endometrial cancer, recurrent thromboembolic disease, acute liver disease, and unexplained vaginal bleeding. **Relative contraindications** include fibrocystic disease of the breast, uterine myomata, endometriosis, or a family history of breast cancer. **Side effects** include menstrual bleeding, weight gain, nausea, headache, and breast tenderness, which may be alleviated by a reduction in dose. Estrogen therapy increases the risk of endometrial carcinoma, but cyclic therapy with added progestin greatly reduces or eliminates the excess risk. No consistent increase in risk of breast carcinoma has been found. Postmenopausal estrogen replacement does not cause hypertension or increased risk of thromboembolism. In contrast to these risks, considerable epidemiologic evidence indicates that estrogen replacement reduces the risk of myocardial infarction, stroke, cardiovascular death, and death from all causes (*Circulation* 75:1102, 1987; *N. Engl. J. Med.* 325:756, 1991).

3. **Exercise.** Regular walking or other weight-bearing exercise for 1 hour 3 times a week can protect bone mass (*Ann. Intern. Med.* 108:824, 1988).

4. **Prevention of injury** (*N. Engl. J. Med.* 320:1055, 1989). Most hip and wrist fractures are caused by falls. Risk factors for falls, including visual and

balance disorders, postural hypotension, and home environmental hazards should be corrected. Use of sedatives, antihypertensives, and alcohol should be minimized. Since vertebral collapse is precipitated by flexion of the spine, lifting should be minimized.

5. **Excessive thyroid hormone replacement** should be avoided (*Ann. Intern. Med.* 113:265, 1990).

C. **Treatment of established osteoporosis** includes the measures discussed in sec. **I.B.** Estrogen therapy slows bone loss up to age 70 (*Am. J. Obstet. Gynecol.* 156:1511, 1987). Two other drugs can be used in women over 70, women for whom estrogen is contraindicated, and men with osteoporosis. Supplemental calcium, 0.5–1.0 g/day, should be given with each.

1. **Etidronate,** given in 3-month cycles, increases vertebral bone density and decreases the rate of vertebral fracture (*N. Engl. J. Med.* 322:1265, 1990). The regimen is 400 mg PO qd for the first 2 weeks of each 3-month cycle, followed by 2½ months without therapy. The drug should be taken in the middle of a 4-hour fast to assure absorption, and the calcium supplement should not be taken simultaneously. The optimal duration of therapy is not established, but treatment for 3 years increased vertebral bone density by 5%. Side effects include nausea and diarrhea.

2. **Calcitonin** (*Endocrinol. Rev.* 8:377, 1987). In women with osteoporosis, salmon calcitonin in a dosage ranging from 50 IU SQ 3 times a week to 100 IU SQ qd, stabilizes or increases vertebral bone density for periods of 12–24 months. The optimal duration of treatment has not been established. Most patients begin losing bone mass after 12–18 months of treatment, and it is not clear that continuing therapy beyond this time is beneficial. Calcitonin has not been shown to reduce the risk of fracture. Side effects include nausea, flushing, and, rarely, allergic reactions. Other drawbacks include the high cost and need for injections.

II. **Osteomalacia** (Balliere's *Clin. Endocrinol. Metab.* 2:125, 1988) is characterized by defective mineralization of osteoid. Bone biopsy reveals increased thickness of osteoid seams and decreased mineralization rate, assessed by tetracycline labeling. **Causes of osteomalacia** include (1) vitamin D deficiency (rare except in the housebound elderly); (2) **malabsorption** of vitamin D and calcium (the most common cause in the United States) due to gastrectomy, or to intestinal, hepatic, or biliary disease; (3) disorders of vitamin D metabolism (renal disease, vitamin D–dependent rickets); (4) vitamin D resistance; (5) chronic hypophosphatemia (see Mineral Disorders, sec. **II.B**); (6) renal tubular acidosis; (7) hypophosphatasia; and (8) therapy with anticonvulsants, fluoride, etidronate, or aluminum compounds.

A. **Clinical manifestations** include diffuse skeletal pain, proximal muscle weakness, waddling gait, and propensity to fractures. X-ray findings include osteopenia and radiolucent bands perpendicular to bone surfaces (pseudofractures or Looser's zones). Serum phosphorus is typically low and alkaline phosphatase elevated. Serum calcium may be normal but is often low in severe cases.

B. **Diagnosis.** In a patient with osteopenia, elevated serum alkaline phosphatase or low serum phosphorus suggests osteomalacia. **Serum 25(OH)D** levels are low in vitamin D deficiency or malabsorption. In an appropriate clinical setting, these tests are usually sufficient to establish the diagnosis, but in atypical cases, a bone biopsy may be required for definitive diagnosis.

C. **Management**

1. **Dietary vitamin D deficiency** can initially be treated with vitamin D, 50,000 IU PO weekly for several weeks to replete body stores, followed by long-term therapy with 400–1000 IU/day. Preparations include calcium supplements containing vitamin D (Os-Cal + D, 125 IU/250- or 500-mg tablet), many multivitamins (400 IU/tablet), and vitamin D drops (200 IU/drop or 8000 IU/ml).

2. **Malabsorption of vitamin D** may require therapy with high dosages, ranging from 50,000 IU PO per week to 50,000 IU PO qd. The dose should be adjusted to maintain serum 25(OH)D levels within the normal range. Calcium supplements, 1 g PO qd-tid, may also be required. Serum 25(OH)D, serum

calcium, and 24-hour urine calcium should be monitored every 3–6 months (see Mineral Disorders, sec. **I.B.4**). If osteomalacia does not respond to high doses of vitamin D, calcifediol (25(OH)D, 20 or 50 μg/capsule), 20–100 μg PO qd, may be better absorbed. If the underlying disease responds to therapy, the dose of vitamin D must be reduced accordingly.

III. Renal osteodystrophy (*Kidney Int.* 38:193, 1990) refers to the skeletal disorders seen in chronic renal failure (see Chap. 11).

IV. Paget's disease of bone (Balliere's *Clin. Endocrinol. Metab.* 2:267, 1988) is a focal skeletal disorder characterized by rapid, disorganized bone remodeling. It usually occurs after age 40 and most often affects the pelvis, femur, spine, and skull. Clinical manifestations include bone pain and deformity, degenerative arthritis, pathologic fractures, neurologic deficits due to nerve root or cranial nerve compression (including deafness), and, rarely, high-output heart failure and osteogenic sarcoma. Most patients are asymptomatic, with disease discovered incidentally because of elevated serum alkaline phosphatase or an x-ray taken for other reasons.

A. Diagnosis. A bone scan can be used to identify involved areas, which are then evaluated with x-rays. The radiographic appearance is usually diagnostic and biopsy is rarely necessary. Serum alkaline phosphatase is elevated, reflecting the activity and extent of disease. Serum and urine calcium are usually normal but may increase with immobilization, as after a fracture.

B. Management. Most patients require no therapy, or analgesics only. Indications for specific therapy include (1) bone pain not relieved by analgesics, (2) nerve compression syndromes, (3) pathologic fracture, (4) elective skeletal surgery, (5) progressive skeletal deformity, (6) immobilization hypercalcemia, (7) hypercalciuria with nephrolithiasis, and (8) high-output heart failure. Serum alkaline phosphatase should be measured during treatment; a 50% reduction, along with symptomatic improvement, indicates an adequate therapeutic response.

1. Etidronate (Didronel, 200 or 400 mg/tablet) inhibits both bone resorption and formation and is generally the drug of first choice. It is given as a 6-month course, 5 mg/kg PO qd, taken with water at the midpoint of a 4-hour fast. After each course, the drug should be omitted for at least 6 months, to avoid the osteomalacia seen with longer therapy. After a treatment course, symptoms and serum alkaline phosphatase are followed; prolonged remissions may occur. Repeated courses can be given for evidence of recurrence. Side effects include nausea and diarrhea; osteomalacia is rare with this regimen. Etidronate should not be used if lytic disease of weight-bearing bones is present.

2. Calcitonin inhibits bone resorption. The initial dose of **salmon calcitonin** is 100 IU SQ or IM qd. When an adequate response is achieved (usually after several months), the dosage is decreased to 50 IU SQ 3 times a week. If resistance to salmon calcitonin develops, **human calcitonin**, 0.5 mg SQ or IM qd, is often effective. Calcitonin is indicated for treatment of fractures and lytic disease of weight-bearing bones. Side effects include flushing, nausea, and, rarely, allergic reactions. Other drawbacks include the high cost and need for injections.

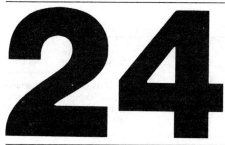

Arthritis and Rheumatologic Diseases

Leslie E. Kahl

Approach to the Patient with a Single Painful Joint

The first step in diagnosis is to **identify the structures involved.** Pain arising in periarticular (e.g., tendon, bursa), muscular, and neurologic structures may be perceived as joint pain. If the pain comes from the joint itself and a **single joint** is involved, the major disorders in the differential diagnosis are **trauma, infection,** and **crystalline arthritis.**

I. **Laboratory studies**
   A. **Radiographs** of the joint may be useful in documenting trauma or preexisting joint disease. The presence of chondrocalcinosis on x-ray suggests pseudogout but is not diagnostic (see Crystal-Induced Synovitis). Radiographs are usually normal in acute infectious or crystalline arthritis.
   B. **Synovial fluid** (Table 24-1). Aspirations of joint fluid should be performed in all patients with monoarticular arthritis who do not have a preexisting diagnosis consistent with the clinical picture. Polyarticular disorders such as rheumatoid arthritis (RA) or systemic lupus erythematosus (SLE) occasionally present initially as monoarthritis, but when a single joint is inflamed out of proportion to the other joints in this setting, **infection must be excluded.**
II. **Management** is based on the results of radiographs and synovial fluid analysis. **Trauma** or **internal derangement** of the joint can be managed by immobilization of the joint and consultation with an orthopedic surgeon. The treatment of **infectious arthritis** and **crystalline disorders** is detailed below. If the synovial fluid appears to be inflammatory (Table 24-1) and crystals are not seen, the patient with monoarthritis should be presumed to have infectious arthritis and treated accordingly.

Joint Aspiration and Injection

I. **Indications.** Joint aspiration should be performed (1) when an effusion is present and its etiology is unclear, (2) for symptomatic relief in a patient with a known arthritis diagnosis, and (3) to monitor the response to therapy in infectious arthritis. Analysis of aspirated synovial fluid should include a cell count, microscopic examination for crystals, Gram's stain, and culture (see Table 24-1). Intra-articular glucocorticoid therapy can be used to suppress inflammation when only one or a few peripheral joints are inflamed and infection has been excluded. The joint should be aspirated to remove as much fluid as possible before steroid injection.
II. **Contraindications. Infection** overlying the site to be injected is an absolute contraindication; significant hemostatic defects and bacteremia are relative contraindications to aspiration and injection.
III. **Complications** following proper joint aspiration and injection are rare. However, the patient should be cautioned to report any increase in pain, swelling, or warmth following arthrocentesis. **Infection** occurs in less than 0.1% of patients when careful sterile technique is employed.

Table 24-1. Classification of synovial fluid

	Normal	Noninflam-matory	Inflammatory	Septic
Color	Colorless	Straw	Yellow	Variable
Clarity	Transparent	Transparent	Translucent	Opaque
WBC/mm^3	<200	200–2000	2000–75,000	>75,000
PMN	<25%	<25%	40–75%	>75%
Culture	—	—	—	May be +
Crystals	—	—	May be +	—
Examples		Osteoarthritis	RA	Bacterial
		Trauma	Gout	infection
		Aseptic	Pseudogout	Tuberculosis
		necrosis	SLE	
		SLE	Seronegative	
			spondyloar-	
			thropathies	

Key: PMN = polymorphonuclear leukocyte.

Postinjection synovitis may occur as a result of phagocytosis of glucocorticoid ester crystals. Such reactions usually resolve within 48–72 hours, and more persistent symptoms suggest the possibility of iatrogenic infection. Localized skin **depigmentation and atrophy** may occur after glucocorticoid injection, particularly when fluorinated steroids such as triamcinolone are used. Accelerated **deterioration of bone and cartilage** may occur when frequent injections are administered over an extended period. Any single joint should therefore be injected no more frequently than every 3–6 months.

IV. Intra-articular medications

A. Glucocorticoids. Available preparations include methylprednisolone acetate, triamcinolone acetonide, and triamcinolone hexacetonide. The dose used is arbitrary, but the following guidelines may be useful:

1. Large joints, such as the knee, ankle, shoulder: 20–40 mg.

2. Wrists and elbows: 10–20 mg of any of the above preparations.

3. Small joints of the hands and feet: 5–15 mg of any of the above preparations.

B. Lidocaine (or its equivalent), up to 1 ml of a 1% solution, can be mixed in a single syringe with the glucocorticoid to promote immediate relief.

V. Technique.

The site of aspiration should be cleansed with povidone/iodine solution. Topical ethylchloride spray can be used as a local anesthetic. Local infiltration with 1% lidocaine can also be used.

A. Knee (Fig. 24-1). The leg should be positioned by gently flexing the knee 10–15 degrees. A rolled towel can be placed in the popliteal fossa to support the knee and allow the quadriceps to relax. The joint is then entered either medially or laterally, immediately beneath the undersurface of the patella.

B. Ankle (Fig. 24-2). Aspiration should be performed with the patient supine and the foot perpendicular to the leg. Medial aspiration is performed immediately medial to the extensor hallucis longus tendon, which can be identified by alternately extending and flexing the great toe. A lateral approach can also be used by introducing the needle just distal to the fibula.

C. Wrist (Fig. 24-3). Aspiration is performed on the dorsum of the wrist with the wrist joint slightly flexed. The point of entry for lateral aspiration is just distal to the end of the radius, immediately on the ulnar side of the extensor tendon of the thumb. Medial aspiration can also be performed between the distal ulna and the carpus.

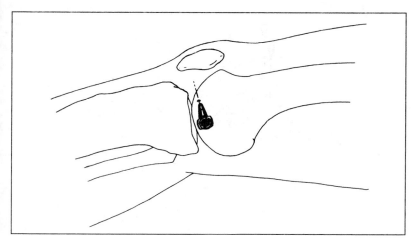

Fig. 24-1. Arthrocentesis of the knee: medial approach. (From J. F. Beary III, C. L. Christian, and N. A. Johanson [eds.]. *Manual of Rheumatology and Outpatient Orthopedic Disorders* [2nd ed.]. Boston: Little, Brown, 1987.)

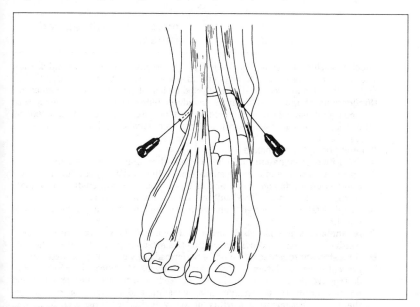

Fig. 24-2. Arthrocentesis of the ankle: medial and lateral approaches. (From J. F. Beary III, C. L. Christian, and N. A. Johanson [eds.]. *Manual of Rheumatology and Outpatient Orthopedic Disorders* [2nd ed.]. Boston: Little, Brown, 1987.)

   D. Joints of the hands and feet. Small joints of the hands and feet are entered
      similarly by introducing the needle from the dorsal surface immediately beneath
      the extensor tendon from either the lateral or medial side. Because these joints
      yield only small amounts of fluid, flushing the aspirate from the syringe with
      saline may increase the yield when attempting analysis for crystals.

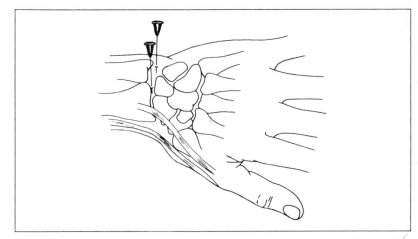

Fig. 24-3. Arthrocentesis of the wrist: medial and lateral approaches. (From J. F. Beary III, C. L. Christian, and N. A. Johanson [eds.]. *Manual of Rheumatology and Outpatient Orthopedic Disorders* [2nd ed.]. Boston: Little, Brown, 1987.)

Infectious Arthritis and Bursitis

Infectious arthritis is generally divided into gonococcal and nongonococcal disease. The usual presentation is with fever and an acute monoarticular arthritis, although multiple joints may occasionally be affected by hematogenously spread pathogens. **Nongonococcal** infectious arthritis in adults tends to occur in patients with previous joint damage or compromised host defenses. In contrast, **gonococcal arthritis** causes one half of all septic arthritis in otherwise healthy, sexually active young adults.

I. **General principles of treatment**
   A. **Joint fluid examination,** including Gram's stain and culture, is mandatory to make a diagnosis and to guide management. In addition, a joint fluid leukocyte count is useful diagnostically and as a baseline for serial studies to evaluate response to treatment. Blood cultures should also be obtained.
   B. **Hospitalization** is indicated to ensure drug compliance and careful monitoring of the clinical response.
   C. **IV antibiotics** provide good serum and synovial fluid drug concentrations. Neither oral nor intra-articular antibiotics are appropriate as initial therapy.
   D. **Repeated arthrocenteses** should be performed daily or as often as necessary to prevent reaccumulation of fluid. Arthrocentesis is indicated to (1) remove destructive inflammatory mediators, (2) reduce intra-articular pressure and promote antibiotic penetration into the joint, and (3) monitor response to therapy by documenting sterility of synovial fluid cultures and decreasing leukocyte counts.
   E. **Surgical drainage** is indicated in the following situations: (1) septic hip, (2) joints in which large amounts of tissue debris or loculation of pus prevent adequate needle drainage (most commonly the shoulder), and (3) joints that do not respond in 5–7 days to appropriate therapy and repeated arthrocentesis.
   F. **General supportive measures.** Splinting of the joint may relieve pain, but prolonged immobilization of the joint can result in stiffness. A nonsteroidal anti-inflammatory drug (NSAID) (see Rheumatoid Arthritis, sec. **I.A**) is often useful to reduce pain and increase joint mobility but should not be used until response to antibiotic therapy has been demonstrated by symptomatic and laboratory improvement.

II. **Nongonococcal septic arthritis** is most often due to *Staphylococcus aureus* (70%) and *Streptococcus* species. Gram-negative organisms are less common, except in the setting of IV drug abuse, neutropenia, coincident joint disease and urinary tract infection, or postoperatively. Initial therapy is based on the clinical situation and a carefully performed Gram's stain. General guidelines are given below (see also Chap. 13). IV antibiotics are usually given for at least 2 weeks, followed by 1 to 2 weeks of oral antibiotics, with the course of therapy tailored to the patient's response.

A. **Gram-positive cocci.** Antistaphylococcal therapy (e.g., nafcillin, 500 mg IVPB q4h, or cefazolin, 1000 mg IVPB q8h) is appropriate. If the Gram's stain reveals typical streptococci, aqueous penicillin G, 1 million units IVPB q4h alone, is adequate.

B. **Gram-negative bacilli.** Empiric therapy must reflect the clinical setting. A third-generation cephalosporin (e.g., ceftriaxone, 2 g IVPB q24h) is appropriate initial coverage. Intravenous drug abusers, neutropenic patients, and postoperative patients should receive agents with antipseudomonal activity (e.g., an antipseudomonal beta-lactam agent such as piperacillin, 2–3 g IV q4–6h, plus an aminoglycoside such as gentamicin, 1 mg/kg IV q8h).

C. **Nondiagnostic Gram's stain**

1. In an **otherwise healthy adult,** empiric coverage should include an antistaphylococcal agent. If the patient is at risk for gonococcal disease, ceftriaxone or penicillin G should be added (see Chap. 13).

2. In the **compromised host,** antibiotic coverage must be individualized but should include agents with activity against staphylococci and gram-negative bacilli.

III. **Gonococcal arthritis,** the articular manifestation of disseminated gonococcal infection (DGI), is the joint infection seen most commonly at urban medical centers. The clinical spectrum of disease often includes migratory or additive polyarthralgias, followed by tenosynovitis and/or arthritis of the wrist, ankle, or knee, and dermatitis. In contrast to nongonococcal septic arthritis, Gram's stain of synovial fluid and cultures of blood or synovial fluid are usually negative. **Throat, cervical, urethral,** and **rectal cultures** should also be obtained. Hospitalization is advised for most patients. Treatment includes penicillin G, 4–10 million units IV/day, or, in areas with penicillin-resistant gonococci, ceftriaxone, 2 g IVPB q12h, along with splinting of the affected joint. Clinical response is usually noted after 2–3 days, at which time treatment can be switched to penicillin V or ampicillin, 500 mg PO qid, for 1–2 weeks of outpatient treatment (see Chap. 13).

IV. **Nonbacterial septic arthritis.** Transient arthralgias and arthritis are common with many viral infections, especially rubella, mumps, infectious mononucleosis, parvovirus, and hepatitis. They are usually self-limited, last for less than 6 weeks, and respond well to a conservative regimen of rest and NSAIDs. A variety of fungi (especially *Sporothrix schenkii*) and mycobacteria can cause septic arthritis and should be considered in patients with a chronic monoarticular arthritis. Treatment is based on culture results.

V. **Septic bursitis,** usually involving the olecranon or prepatellar bursa, can be differentiated from septic arthritis by localized, fluctuant superficial swelling, and by generally painless joint motion (except with full flexion or extension). Most patients have a history of previous trauma to the area or an occupational predisposition (e.g., housemaid's knee, writer's elbow). *Staphylococcus aureus* is the most common pathogen. The principles of management are similar to those for septic arthritis, although outpatient therapy is appropriate for otherwise healthy individuals (e.g., dicloxacillin, 500 mg PO qid for 10 days). Preventive measures (e.g., knee pads) should be used in patients with occupational predispositions.

VI. **Lyme disease** is caused by the tick-borne spirochete *Borrelia burgdorferi*. Arthritis is usually preceded by an erythematous annular rash called erythema chronicum migrans (ECM). Diffuse arthralgia or an oligoarticular arthritis, commonly involving the knees, may be present and may recur. Synovial fluid white blood cell counts average about 25,000 cells/mm^3, with polymorphonuclear leukocytes predominating. Systemic symptoms, meningoencephalitis, and cardiac conduction abnormalities may be associated with this disease. Antibiotic therapy is indicated as discussed in Chap. 13. NSAIDs are a useful adjunct for arthritis.

Crystal-Induced Synovitis

Deposition of microcrystals in joints and periarticular tissues results in **gout, pseudogout, and apatite disease.** A definitive diagnosis of gout or pseudogout is made by identification of polymorphonuclear cells containing phagocytosed crystals in joint fluid examined with compensated polarized light microscopy. Urate crystals, which are diagnostic of gout, are needle-shaped and strongly negatively birefringent; calcium pyrophosphate dihydrate (CPPD) crystals seen in pseudogout are pleomorphic and weakly positively birefringent. Hydroxyapatite complexes, diagnostic of apatite disease, and basic calcium phosphate complexes can be identified only by electron microscopy and mass spectroscopy; in most cases, the arthritides associated with these compounds are clinically suspected but never confirmed.

I. **Primary gouty arthritis** is a metabolic disorder characterized by hyperuricemia, due to either overproduction (10% of cases) or underexcretion (90% of cases) of uric acid. Urate crystals may deposit in the joints, subcutaneous tissues (tophi), and kidneys. Men are much more commonly affected than women; most premenopausal women with gout have a family history of the disease. The clinical phases of gout can be divided into (1) asymptomatic hyperuricemia, (2) acute arthritis, (3) an interval phase, and (4) chronic arthritis.

  A. **Asymptomatic hyperuricemia** (uric acid levels >8 mg/dl in men and >7 mg/dl in women) is present in about 5% of the American male population, of whom 5–10% will develop acute gout. Treatment of asymptomatic hyperuricemia is not routinely recommended because of expense, potential drug toxicity, and the low risk for adverse outcome from the hyperuricemia itself (*Am. J. Med.* 82:421, 1987).

  B. **Acute gouty arthritis** occurs as an excruciating attack of pain, usually in a single joint of the foot or ankle. Occasionally, a polyarticular onset can mimic RA. Attacks are generally separated by pain-free intervals lasting months to years. Attacks may be precipitated by surgery, dehydration, fasting, binge eating, or copious ingestion of alcohol. Although the acute gouty attack will subside spontaneously over several days, prompt medical attention can abort the attack within hours. The serum uric acid level is normal in 30% of patients with acute gout and, if elevated, should not be manipulated until an attack has resolved. If alteration of the uric acid level is planned after the acute attack subsides, maintenance oral colchicine should be used simultaneously to prevent a new attack.

    1. **NSAIDs** are effective in acute gout, although clinical response may require 12–24 hours (see Table 24-2). Initial doses should be high, followed by rapid tapering over 2–8 days. For example, indomethacin is begun at 50 mg PO q6h for 2 days, followed by 50 mg PO q8h for 3 days, and then 25 mg PO q8h for 2–3 more days. The long-acting NSAIDs are generally not recommended for acute gout. The ease of administration and lower toxicity of NSAIDs make them the **drugs of choice** in most settings.

    2. **Colchicine** is most effective if given in the first 12–24 hours of an acute attack and usually brings relief in 6–12 hours. It is available in oral and IV preparations.

      a. **Oral administration** is effective but often associated with severe gastrointestinal toxicity. The dosage is 1.0–1.2 mg given immediately, followed by either 0.5–0.6 mg q1–2h or 1.0–1.2 mg q2h until symptoms abate, gastrointestinal toxicity develops, or the maximum dose of 6 mg in a 24-hour period is reached. The dosage should be reduced in patients with renal or hepatic impairment. No more than 1.8 mg a day should be used thereafter during that attack.

      b. **Intravenous colchicine** results in more rapid relief with fewer gastrointestinal side effects but has the potential for severe myelosuppression, myopathy, and neuropathy. This drug is particularly useful for postoperative gout in patients who are not permitted oral medications. A rapid response to IV colchicine is relatively specific for a crystal-induced

Table 24-2. Nonsteroidal anti-inflammatory drugs

Generic name	Trade name (partial listing)	Tablet size (mg)	Starting dosage (mg)	Maximum daily dose (mg)
Salicylates				
Aspirin[a] (acetylsalicylate)	Aspirin	325	650–1300 q4–6h	b
	Encaprin	500	1000 q6–8h	b
	ZORprin	800	1600 q12h	b
Magnesium salicylate[a]	Mobidin	600	600–1200 tid–qid	b
	Magan	545	545–1090 tid–qid	b
Choline salicylate	Arthropan liquid	1 tsp = 870		b
Choline magnesium trisalicylate[a]	Trilisate	500, 750, 1000 1 tsp = 500	1000–1250 bid	b
Salsalate	Disalcid	500	1000 bid–1500 tid	b
Nonsalicylates				
Diclofenac sodium	Voltaren	25, 50, 75	50–75 bid	200
Diflunisal	Dolobid	250, 500	250 bid	1500
Etodolac	Lodine	200, 300	400 bid–tid	1200
Fenoprofen calcium	Nalfon	200, 300, 600	300–600 qid	3200
Flurbiprofen	Ansaid	50, 100	50–100 tid	300
Ibuprofen	Motrin, Rufen	400, 600, 800	400 qid	3200
Indomethacin	Indocin	25, 50, 75	25 tid–qid	200
	Indocin SR	75	75 qd	200
	Indocin suppositories	50	50 bid	200
Ketoprofen	Orudis	50, 75	75 tid	300
Meclofenamate sodium	Meclomen	50, 100	50 tid–qid	400
Naproxen[a]	Naprosyn	250, 375, 500	250–500 bid	1250
Naproxen sodium	Anaprox	275	275 q6–8h	1375
Phenylbutazone	Butazolidin	100	100 tid	600
Piroxicam	Feldene	10, 20	20 qd	20
Sulindac	Clinoril	150, 200	150–200 bid	400
Tolmetin sodium	Tolectin	200, 400, 600	400 tid	1600

[a] Available as a suspension.
[b] Determined by measurement of serum salicylate level.

arthritis. The drug is diluted in 10–20 ml of sterile water or normal saline and given slowly over 3–5 minutes through a freely flowing IV route to avoid extravasation and tissue necrosis. **Colchicine should not be diluted with or injected into IV tubing containing 5% dextrose** because precipitation will occur. The initial dose is 2 mg, followed by another 1–2 mg in 6 hours if necessary. The total IV dose during a given attack should not exceed 4 mg. The dosage should be reduced in the elderly, if the patient has been receiving chronic oral colchicine, or if the patient has significant renal or hepatic disease (*J. Rheumatol.* 15:495, 1988). No further colchicine should be given orally or intravenously for 7 days.

3. **Glucocorticoids** are indicated for patients in whom colchicine or NSAIDs are contraindicated or for unusual attacks refractory to conventional therapy. Prednisone, 40–60 mg PO qd, should be given until a response appears, then tapered rapidly. Intra-articular glucocorticoids are efficacious, although rarely needed.

C. **Intercritical gout** is defined as the period between attacks. Initially, intercritical periods are long (months to years), asymptomatic, and without abnormal physical findings. With time, acute attacks occur more frequently, intercritical periods are shorter, and chronic joint deformity may appear. In patients with infrequent attacks of gout and normal serum uric acid levels, no intercritical phase medications are necessary. For those with more frequent attacks, prophylactic colchicine (0.5–0.6 mg PO qd or bid) can be used. Patients should be advised to avoid aspirin (uricoretentive), most diuretics, large alcohol intake, prolonged fasts, and foods high in purines (sweetbreads, anchovies, sardines, liver, and kidney). If arthritic attacks are frequent, renal damage is present, or serum or urine uric acid levels are consistently significantly elevated, the serum uric acid level should be lowered. **Maintenance colchicine, 0.5–0.6 mg PO bid, should be instituted a few days before manipulation of the uric acid level to prevent precipitation of an acute attack.** Colchicine is the only drug that is prophylactic for acute gout; NSAIDs are not. If no attacks occur after the uric acid has been maintained in the normal range for 6–8 weeks, colchicine can be discontinued.

1. **Allopurinol,** a xanthine oxidase inhibitor, is an effective therapy for hyperuricemia in most patients.

   a. **Dosage and administration.** The initial dose of allopurinol is usually 300 mg qd. Allopurinol is metabolized by the liver to oxypurinol, a renally excreted active form with a half-life of 30 hours. Therefore, the dose should be reduced in patients with renal or hepatic impairment. Daily dosages can be decreased by 100–200 mg every 2–4 weeks to achieve the minimum maintenance dosage that will keep the uric acid level within the normal range. The concomitant use of a uricosuric agent may hasten the mobilization of tophi but is rarely necessary. If an acute attack occurs while the patient is receiving allopurinol, the drug should be continued at the same dosage while other agents are used to treat the attack.

   b. **Toxicity.** Hypersensitivity reactions are the most common adverse side effect of allopurinol therapy, occurring in up to 5% of patients. Reactions may range from a minor skin rash to a diffuse exfoliative dermatitis with fever, eosinophilia, and renal and hepatic injury. Patients with mild renal insufficiency who are receiving diuretics are at greatest risk. **Severe cases are potentially fatal** and usually require glucocorticoid therapy. Ampicillin rashes may also be more common among patients taking allopurinol. Gastrointestinal intolerance occurs occasionally. Allopurinol may potentiate the effect of oral anticoagulants. Allopurinol blocks metabolism of 6-mercaptopurine and azathioprine, necessitating a 60–75% reduction in dosage of these cytotoxic drugs.

2. **Uricosuric drugs** lower serum uric acid levels by blocking renal tubular reabsorption of uric acid. A 24-hour measurement of creatinine clearance and urine uric acid should be obtained before initiation of therapy. Uricosuric agents are ineffective with glomerular filtration rates of less than 50 ml/min

and are contraindicated in patients who already have high levels of urine uric acid ($\geq$800 mg/24 hr). Enhanced urinary uric acid excretion increases the risk of urate stone formation. This risk can be minimized by maintaining a high fluid intake and alkalinizing the urine. If these drugs are being used when an acute gouty attack begins, they should be continued while other drugs are used to treat the acute attack.

    a. Probenecid is completely absorbed from the gastrointestinal tract, has a half-life of 6–12 hours, and is excreted in the urine. The initial dose is 500 mg PO qd, which can be raised in 500-mg increments every week until serum uric acid levels normalize or urine uric acid level exceeds 800 mg/24 hours. The maximum dose is 3000 mg daily. Most patients require a total of 1.0–1.5 g/day in 2–3 divided doses. Salicylates and probenecid are antagonistic and should not be used together. Probenecid decreases renal excretion of penicillin, indomethacin, and sulfonylureas. Side effects are minimal; hypersensitivity rashes, mild gastrointestinal distress, flushing, and dizziness can occur. Rare complications include hemolytic anemia (in patients with glucose 6-phosphate dehydrogenase deficiency) and peptic ulcerations.

    b. Sulfinpyrazone has similar efficacy and toxicity to probenecid, but sulfinpyrazone also inhibits platelet function. The initial dose is 50 mg twice a day. The dosage can be increased in 100-mg increments weekly until serum uric acid levels normalize, to a maximum dose of 800 mg daily. Most patients require 300–400 mg/day in 3–4 divided doses.

D. Chronic tophaceous gout results from chronic hyperuricemia. Recurrent attacks of arthritis and tophaceous deposits in the joints lead to bone erosions, remodeling of the joint surface, and impaired joint motion. Colchicine, 0.5–0.6 mg PO bid, may prevent new attacks, NSAIDs can decrease existing inflammation, and allopurinol or uricosuric agents will help to mobilize tophi. Rehabilitation includes physical and occupational therapy as well as corrective surgery.

II. Secondary gout, like primary, may be due either to defective renal excretion of uric acid or to overproduction. Intrinsic renal disease, diuretic therapy, low-dose aspirin, nicotinic acid, cyclosporine, and ethanol all interfere with renal excretion of uric acid. Acute articular gout is, however, uncommon in renal failure. Starvation, lactic acidosis, dehydration, preeclampsia, diabetic ketoacidosis, and heavy use of alcohol can also induce hyperuricemia. Overproduction of uric acid occurs in myeloproliferative and lymphoproliferative disorders, hemolytic anemia, polycythemia, and cyanotic congenital heart disease. Management includes treatment of the underlying disorder and allopurinol therapy.

III. Pseudogout results when CPPD crystals deposited in bone and cartilage are released into synovial fluid and induce acute inflammation. **Risk factors** include older age, advanced osteoarthritis, neuropathic joint, gout, hyperparathyroidism, hemochromatosis, diabetes mellitus, hypothyroidism, hypomagnesemia, and hypophosphatasia. Chondrocalcinosis is seen radiographically in 75% of patients, although its presence is not diagnostic. The disease may present as an acute monoarthritis or oligoarthritis mimicking gout, or as a chronic polyarthritis resembling RA or osteoarthritis. The knee is usually affected, although any synovial joint may be involved. Dehydration, acute illness, and surgery (especially parathyroidectomy) are common precipitants of an acute attack of pseudogout. A brief, high-dose course of an NSAID (see Table 24-2) is the therapy of choice for most patients. Colchicine (PO or IV) may also relieve symptoms promptly and is used in the same dosage as for acute gout. Maintenance colchicine may diminish the number of recurrent attacks in some patients. Aspiration of the inflammatory joint fluid often results in prompt improvement, and an intra-articular injection of glucocorticoids may hasten the response.

IV. Apatite disease may present with periarthritis or tendinitis, particularly in patients with chronic renal failure. An episodic oligoarthritis may also occur, and apatite disease should be suspected when no crystals are present in the synovial fluid. Erosive arthritis may be seen, particularly in the shoulder ("Milwaukee shoulder"). The treatment of apatite disease is similar to that of pseudogout.

Rheumatoid Arthritis

Rheumatoid arthritis (RA) is a systemic disease of unknown etiology, characterized by symmetric inflammation of synovial tissues. Serum rheumatoid factor is usually present. Extra-articular manifestations include, in order of decreasing frequency, (1) rheumatoid nodules, (2) pulmonary fibrosis, (3) serositis, and (4) vasculitis. **Felty's syndrome**—the triad of RA, splenomegaly, and granulocytopenia—occurs in a subset of patients who are at risk for recurrent bacterial infections and nonhealing leg ulcers. **Sjögren's syndrome,** characterized by failure of exocrine glands, also occurs in a subset of patients with RA, producing sicca symptoms (dry eyes and mouth), parotid gland enlargement, dental caries, and recurrent tracheobronchitis. The course of the arthritis in RA is variable but tends to be chronic and progressive. Most patients can benefit from a combined program of medical, rehabilitative, and surgical services designed with three distinct goals: (1) suppression of inflammation in the joints and other tissues, (2) maintenance of joint and muscle function and prevention of deformities, and (3) repair of joint damage to relieve pain or improve function. **Patients with RA and a single joint inflamed out of proportion to the remainder of the joints must be evaluated for infectious arthritis.** This complication occurs with increased frequency in RA and carries a 20–30% mortality (*Am. J. Med.* 88:503, 1990).

I. **Medical management.** This is usually provided in a "stepped" approach.

 A. **Nonsteroidal anti-inflammatory drugs** (see Table 24-2), including salicylates, are inhibitors of prostaglandin synthetase. All NSAIDs are antipyretic, analgesic, and anti-inflammatory, and may have efficacy in RA. Individual responses to these agents are variable; if one drug is not effective during a 2- to 3-week trial at full dosage, another should be tried.

 The major side effects of the NSAIDs include dyspepsia, nausea, and, less frequently, headaches, tinnitus, dizziness, and confusion. Localized **gastrointestinal irritation** may be minimized by administration after food or the use of enteric-coated preparations. However, all NSAIDs have a systemic effect on gastric mucosa, resulting in increased membrane permeability to gastric acid. Misoprostol, a synthetic prostaglandin analogue, may decrease the risk of NSAID-induced gastric ulceration (*Lancet* 2:1277, 1988).

 All NSAIDs **inhibit platelet aggregation** reversibly (except aspirin, which is irreversible) and should be used cautiously in patients with bleeding tendencies or those taking warfarin (*Br. J. Rheumatol.* 28:46, 1989). Reversible elevations of **serum transaminases** may occur. Patients known to have **hypersensitivity to aspirin** (asthma, angioedema, urticaria, and nasal polyps) should avoid all NSAIDs except nonaspirin salicylates (see Table 24-2).

 Although serious **renal toxicity**, including acute renal failure, nephrotic syndrome, and acute interstitial nephritis, may occur rarely, prerenal azotemia with increased serum creatinine and hyperkalemia occurs more commonly, particularly in individuals whose renal function is already compromised (*N. Engl. J. Med.* 310:563, 1984). Therefore, periodic monitoring of renal function is recommended, particularly in elderly patients. NSAIDs should not be given to patients with acute renal or hepatic failure and should be used only with caution in patients with chronic renal or hepatic disease. These agents can also cause sodium retention, edema, or worsening of congestive heart failure and may decrease the effectiveness of antihypertensive agents. Other toxicities, including a variety of rashes, blood dyscrasias, and aseptic meningitis, have been reported. Although combinations of NSAIDs are generally not used, the addition of a long-acting drug at bedtime may significantly decrease morning stiffness. Long-acting preparations improve compliance but should be used with caution in elderly patients. None of the NSAIDs is recommended for use during pregnancy or lactation. Specific precautions regarding individual NSAIDs include the following:

 1. **Salicylates** in combination with other drugs (e.g., phenacetin, antihistamines, acetaminophen, caffeine) are no more effective than aspirin alone and

may be more toxic. Serum salicylate levels vary widely among individuals taking identical doses. Maximum therapeutic anti-inflammatory levels are 20–30 mg/dl, and at these levels a small dosage increase may produce a substantial increase in the salicylate level. Serum levels of greater than 40 mg/dl are toxic and may lead to salicylism with mixed acid-base disturbances, tinnitus, noncardiogenic pulmonary edema, fever, coma, and ultimately dehydration, renal failure, and cardiovascular collapse (see Chap. 26). Symptoms of salicylism are easily overlooked in children and older adults, and salicylate levels should be checked periodically. Salicylate levels can also be used to monitor patient compliance or to diagnose subtle salicylism but add little to drug efficacy (*J. Rheumatol.* 11:457, 1984).

Salicylates should be used carefully, if at all, in patients with hyperuricemia; low dosages of salicylates (1.0–2.5 g/day) cause urate retention, whereas high dosages (3–5 g/day) are uricosuric. Salicylates can counteract the effects of probenecid and sulfinpyrazone and should not be given with these drugs. Magnesium salicylate, choline salicylate, choline magnesium trisalicylate, and salsalate are **nonaspirin salicylate derivatives** that are as effective as aspirin but cause less gastrointestinal distress and can be safely used in patients allergic to aspirin (*Br. Med. J.* 1:67, 1975).

2. **Indomethacin,** one of the most potent NSAIDs, produces severe headaches in over 10% of patients. Other CNS side effects are most common in elderly patients and may include dizziness, confusion, hallucinations, and even seizures.

3. **Sulindac** has been reported to cause less interference with renal blood flow than other NSAIDs but should still be used with caution in patients with any impairment in renal function.

4. **Meclofenamate sodium** has been associated with a high incidence of severe diarrhea.

5. **Phenylbutazone**'s toxicities, including severe bone-marrow suppression (e.g., leukopenia, agranulocytosis, thrombocytopenia, aplastic anemia) and severe gastric ulceration, usually preclude long-term use. In addition, phenylbutazone prolongs the prothrombin time in patients on warfarin and may potentiate the hypoglycemic effect of oral hypoglycemic agents.

B. **Glucocorticoids.** Although glucocorticoids are not curative and probably do not alter the natural history of RA, they are among the most potent anti-inflammatory drugs available. Unfortunately, once systemic glucocorticoid therapy has been initiated, few RA patients are able to discontinue it completely without an increase in symptoms.

1. **Indications** for systemic glucocorticoids
   a. Persistent synovitis in multiple joints despite adequate trials of a series of NSAIDs and disease-modifying antirheumatic drugs (see sec. **I.C**).
   b. Severe constitutional symptoms (e.g., fever and weight loss), anemia, or extra-articular disease (vasculitis, episcleritis, or pleurisy).
   c. Occasionally, a patient incapacitated by arthritis can be treated with glucocorticoids for symptomatic relief while awaiting a response to slower-acting, disease-modifying agents (see sec. **I.C**).

2. **Metabolism** (see Systemic Lupus Erythematosus, sec. **II.B**).

3. **Systemic administration.** In non–life-threatening situations, alternate-day glucocorticoid therapy is recommended, since it reduces the incidence of undesirable side effects (except cataracts and osteopenia). A cumulative 2-day dose is given q48h in the morning. Short-acting glucocorticoid preparations must be used to obtain these beneficial effects (Table 24-3). Generally, 10–15 mg prednisone PO qod is quite effective in RA, although some patients do not tolerate the increase in symptoms likely to occur on the off day. For these patients, 5–10 mg prednisone PO qd is usually effective.

4. **Intra-articular administration.** This technique may provide temporary symptomatic relief when only a few joints are inflamed (see Joint Aspiration and Injection for preparations, dosages, and techniques). The beneficial effects of

Table 24-3. Glucocorticoid preparations

Generic name	Approximate equivalent dose (mg)	Usual starting dose (mg/day)	
		Moderate illness	Severe illness
Short-acting			
Hydrocortisone[a] (cortisol)	20.0	80–160	
Cortisone[a]	25.0	100–200	
Prednisone	5.0	20–40	60–100
Prednisolone[a]	5.0	20–40	60–100
Methylprednisolone[a]	4.0	16–32	48–80[b]
Intermediate-acting			
Triamcinolone[a]	4.0	16–32	48–80
Paramethasone	2.0	8–16	24–40
Long-acting			
Dexamethasone[a]	0.75	3–6	9–15
Betamethasone[a]	0.6	2.4–4.8	7.2–12.0

[a] Parenteral forms available. Dosages of oral and parenteral preparations are generally comparable.
[b] High-dose parenteral therapy is often used for severe illness (see Systemic Lupus Erythematosus, secs. **II.C.2** and **II.D.7**).

intra-articular steroids may persist for days to months. This approach may delay or negate the need for systemic glucocorticoid therapy.

5. **Contraindications and side effects** (see Systemic Lupus Erythematosus, sec. **II.D**).

C. **Disease-modifying antirheumatic drugs (DMARDs).** This group of drugs appears to alter the natural history of RA by retarding the progression of bony erosions and cartilage loss, unlike the NSAIDs, which only relieve symptoms. DMARDs are characterized by a delayed onset of action and the potential for serious toxicity and should be prescribed with the guidance of a rheumatologist or other physician experienced in their use.

Indications for DMARD use include: (1) active synovitis not responding to conservative management, including salicylates or other NSAIDs, and (2) rapidly progressive, erosive arthritis.

1. **Methotrexate,** a folic acid antagonist, has recently assumed a prominent position among the DMARDs and is now the initial DMARD prescribed by many rheumatologists. It has also been used successfully in psoriatic arthritis and may improve the leukopenia of Felty's syndrome.

   a. **Metabolism.** Methotrexate is rapidly absorbed from the gastrointestinal tract, in a dose-dependent manner. The drug undergoes hepatic conversion to active metabolites and is eventually excreted in the urine.

   b. **Dosage and administration.** Although methotrexate can be given parenterally (either IV or IM), the initial dose is usually both 7.5 mg PO, taken as a single dose, **once a week.** Toxicity is related to both the total weekly dose and the frequency of administration. Clinical response is usually noted in 4–8 weeks, which is considerably earlier than with other DMARDs. If no response is attained after 6–8 weeks of therapy, the dosage can be increased in 2.5-mg increments every other week to a maximum of 20 mg weekly until improvement is observed. Patients who manifest improvement without toxicity are maintained on methotrexate at the lowest effective dosage indefinitely. Relapse occurs 4–6 weeks after discontinuation of the drug, and remissions are very rare.

c. **Contraindications and side effects. Methotrexate is teratogenic** and should not be used during pregnancy. It should be avoided in patients with significant hepatic or renal impairment. Major side effects include gastrointestinal intolerance, marrow toxicity, liver damage, and hypersensitivity pneumonitis. Blood and platelet counts should be obtained monthly during the first 3–4 months and every 6–8 weeks thereafter. Macrocytosis may herald serious hematologic toxicity (*Arthritis Rheum.* 32:1592, 1989). Although serum transaminase levels should be measured, the exact relationship between abnormalities of liver function tests and progressive liver damage remains unclear. Persistent elevations of serum transaminase levels or reduced serum albumin levels may indicate serious liver toxicity, and liver biopsy or discontinuation of therapy should be considered. Routine liver biopsy should be considered after every 2–4 g methotrexate (*Am. J. Med.* 90:711, 1991). Alcohol consumption dramatically increases the risk of methotrexate hepatotoxicity. Patients with preexisting pulmonary parenchymal disease may be at increased risk of methotrexate pneumonitis and should be instructed to report changes in pulmonary status immediately. A divided-dose regimen (dosage split over 2 or 3 consecutive 12-hour intervals) may reduce gastrointestinal discomfort. Stomatitis, hair loss, headache, and rashes have also been reported. Folic acid supplementation may reduce methotrexate toxicity without interfering with its beneficial effects in RA (*Arthritis Rheum.* 33:9, 1990).

2. **Gold salts** produce significant improvement in approximately half of patients with RA who can tolerate the drug. Gold has also been used successfully in juvenile rheumatoid arthritis, psoriatic arthritis, and Felty's syndrome.

   a. **Metabolism. Parenteral gold** salts are water-soluble, are absorbed rapidly from IM injection sites, and reach maximum plasma concentrations in a few hours. The salts are deposited throughout the body, especially in the reticuloendothelial system (liver and spleen), the renal tubules, and sites of inflammation such as the synovium. Excretion is primarily renal and is very slow, with 60% of each dose retained for at least 1 week. **Oral gold** is only approximately 25% absorbed, with excretion by both renal and fecal routes. At steady state (approximately 3 months), oral gold has a half-life of 8 days.

   b. **Dosage and administration**

      (1) **Parenteral gold salts** are given by deep IM injection. Gold sodium thiomalate (Myochrysine) is an aqueous solution of the drug; aurothioglucose (Solganal) is a suspension in oil that slows absorption. The latter is the preferred drug, with an initial adult dose of 50 mg. Test doses are required with gold sodium thiomalate to prevent nitritoid reactions (see sec. **I.C.2.d.(4)**). If the initial dose is tolerated without adverse effects, 50 mg should be given weekly thereafter.

      (2) **Oral gold** (auranofin) is somewhat less effective than parenteral gold, but also less toxic. The recommended initial dosage is 3 mg PO bid.

   c. **Response to therapy** with either parenteral or oral gold is gradual and continuous; it is usually not seen until after 3–6 months of therapy. An NSAID should be continued for symptomatic treatment of arthritis while gold is introduced and withdrawn slowly only after the gold has produced improvement. **Parenteral** gold is given weekly to a cumulative dose of approximately 1000 mg. If no improvement occurs at that dosage, gold should be discontinued. In patients with improvement after 800–1000 mg total dose of gold, the interval between 50-mg injections can be gradually increased to every 4 weeks. If relapse occurs, the preceding shorter dosage interval should be reinstituted until the relapse remits. If parenteral gold is discontinued, symptoms often worsen within a few months and may be refractory to reinstitution of the drug. Therefore, responders who do not have adverse effects are maintained for prolonged periods (often indefinitely) on monthly gold injections. Some patients who have attained remission with parenteral gold can be switched to oral gold therapy without a loss of efficacy. Synovitis refractory to gold administration occurs in many patients after a few years of good response, and a major change in drug therapy is then required.

Oral gold therapy is continued at a dose of 3 mg PO bid for 6 months. If the response is inadequate, an increase to 3 mg tid can be attempted. If no improvement occurs after a 3-month trial of 9 mg/day, the drug should be discontinued. Good responders are treated indefinitely with either 6 or 9 mg/day auranofin.

d. Contraindications and side effects. Gold is contraindicated in patients with a known gold allergy or history of a severe toxic reaction. Gold should be used cautiously, if at all, in patients with impaired renal or hepatic function. Approximately 30% of patients treated with parenteral gold discontinue the drug because of toxicity, compared to 10% treated with oral gold. Conversely, 10% of patients discontinue parenteral gold because of lack of efficacy, compared to 18% with oral gold (*Arthritis Rheum.* 33:1449, 1990). Adverse reactions can occur at any time during therapy.

  (1) Dermatitis, the most common manifestation of parenteral gold toxicity, is often preceded by pruritus or eosinophilia. Stomatitis may accompany the rash or can occur alone. Injections should be stopped until the skin and mucous membrane lesions resolve. A small test dose can then be given and, if it is tolerated, therapy can be restarted at a lower dose (e.g., 25 mg). If this is tolerated, therapy as previously outlined can be resumed. Rash is rare with oral gold.

  (2) Gold nephropathy is usually manifested by proteinuria and occurs in up to 25% of patients receiving IM gold, but only about 1% with oral gold. A urinalysis should be performed before each gold injection, or at monthly intervals in patients taking oral gold. If proteinuria develops, 24-hour quantification is required. With less than 1.5 g protein/24 hours, gold therapy can be cautiously continued. Proteinuria greater than 1.5 g/24 hours requires cessation of therapy. Proteinuria usually resolves slowly over 12–18 months; advancement to permanent renal failure is rare. Microscopic hematuria is occasionally noted, but only rarely progresses to clinically significant renal disease.

  (3) Hematologic toxicity. The most serious adverse effects of parenteral gold are thrombocytopenia, leukopenia, agranulocytosis, and aplastic anemia. Blood and platelet counts should be done every 1–2 weeks for the first few months of parenteral therapy. If no changes occur after 3–4 months, testing can be done at 2- to 4-week intervals and, ultimately, at 6- to 8-week intervals. Gold therapy should not be restarted in patients who develop cytopenias. Cytopenias are less common with auranofin therapy, and blood counts should be monitored monthly.

  (4) Nitritoid reactions consist of flushing, sweating, dizziness, and syncope occurring within minutes of an injection. These reactions are self-limited and may be avoided by use of oil-based aurothioglucose rather than gold sodium thiomalate.

  (5) Gastrointestinal side effects are common with auranofin (up to 50%) and infrequent with parenteral gold therapy. Diarrhea, abdominal pain, nausea, and vomiting may be treated symptomatically but usually require dosage reduction, discontinuation of therapy, or a change to parenteral gold therapy.

  (6) Rare side effects include reversible cholestatic jaundice, diffuse pulmonary injury, neuropathy, and colitis.

3. Penicillamine is an effective disease-modifying agent in the treatment of RA, with benefit and toxicity profiles very similar to those of parenteral gold. Traditionally, however, it is used after patients fail or cannot tolerate gold therapy.

  a. Metabolism. Penicillamine is rapidly absorbed from the gastrointestinal tract and excreted in the urine.

b. **Dosage and administration.** Penicillamine is administered orally qd or bid, between meals to avoid chelation with dietary metals. Toxicity is related to both the daily dose and the rate of dose increase. Thus, a dosage of 250 mg PO qd for 4–6 weeks is followed by a 125- or 250-mg increase in daily dosage every 4–8 weeks until clinical improvement occurs, or until a daily dose of 1000 mg is reached.

c. **Clinical improvement** is usually seen after 3–6 months. Concomitant NSAID therapy should be continued and tapered only when penicillamine produces a good response. Patients who manifest improvement without toxicity are maintained on penicillamine indefinitely, at the lowest effective dosage. **Gold and penicillamine should not be used together** because of the potential for additive renal and hematologic toxicity.

d. **Contraindications and side effects.** Although some toxicity is seen in more than 50% of patients receiving penicillamine, therapy is discontinued because of toxicity in only 20–30%. Allergy to penicillin does not predict potential reactions to penicillamine; skin testing is not recommended. **Penicillamine is teratogenic** and should not be used during pregnancy.

(1) **Dermatitis** is the most common side effect of treatment. A generalized eruption or stomatitis, or both, occurring in the first few weeks of therapy will usually disappear when the drug is withdrawn and may not recur if the drug is reintroduced at lower doses. Rashes seen after several months of therapy are often pruritic, may resemble pemphigus, and require permanent discontinuation of the drug. When rash occurs with fever, rechallenge should be avoided.

(2) **Hematologic toxicity** includes thrombocytopenia, leukopenia, agranulocytosis, and aplastic anemia. Blood and platelet counts should be obtained every 2 weeks for 3–4 months and at least monthly thereafter. Because counts can drop precipitously despite close monitoring, patients need to be alerted to the signs of these potential complications.

(3) **Proteinuria** due to an immune complex–mediated membranous glomerulonephropathy occurs in up to 15% of patients. Hematuria is less common. Urinalysis should be obtained monthly. Renal complications usually begin after 6–12 months of treatment and may require up to 2 years to resolve after therapy is discontinued. If proteinuria exceeds 2 g/day, the drug should be discontinued. The dosage of penicillamine should never be increased in the presence of proteinuria.

(4) **Other side effects. Autoimmune syndromes** are seen rarely and include myasthenia gravis, diabetes, Goodpasture's syndrome, polymyositis, SLE, and fibrosing alveolitis. Symptoms usually resolve after discontinuation of the drug. Dysgeusia (alteration of taste) is common in the first few months of therapy but usually abates even if therapy is continued. Nausea and dyspepsia occur in up to 15% of patients. Cholestatic jaundice, increased skin friability, and impaired wound healing are occasionally reported.

4. **Hydroxychloroquine** (Plaquenil) is an antimalarial agent with moderate anti-inflammatory and disease-modifying effects in RA. It has also been used successfully in discoid and systemic lupus erythematosus.

a. **Indications.** Hydroxychloroquine is used in patients with RA of mild to moderate severity who fail to respond to therapy with NSAIDs or who are unable to take gold or penicillamine.

b. **Metabolism.** Hydroxychloroquine is well absorbed from the gastrointestinal tract and deposited in many tissues. The drug and its metabolites undergo slow renal excretion.

c. **Dosage and administration.** Therapy is usually initiated at a dosage of 400 mg PO qd. Hydroxychloroquine is taken after meals to minimize dyspepsia and nausea. Clinical improvement is usually seen after 2–6 months. Concomitant NSAID therapy should be continued until hydroxychloroquine produces a good response. Once maximum clinical benefit has been reached and maintained for several months, the dosage can be reduced to the lowest effective level to minimize ocular toxicity.

   d. Contraindications and side effects. Hydroxychloroquine should not be used in patients with porphyria, glucose 6-phosphate dehydrogenase deficiency, or significant hepatic or renal impairment. It should be avoided during pregnancy. The most common side effects are allergic skin eruptions and gastrointestinal disturbances. Serious ocular toxicity occurs but is rare with currently recommended dosages.

   Hydroxychloroquine can be deposited in the cornea, leading to blurred vision or the appearance of halos around lights, an effect that is often reversible if the drug is stopped promptly. Retinal deposition can lead to irreversible damage, although blindness is rare. Because early detectable retinal lesions may precede symptoms, each patient must have a complete ophthalmologic examination at 6-month intervals, including color vision and static visual field testing. At the first sign of visual impairment, particularly reduced sensitivity to red light, the drug should be stopped. Rare complications of hydroxychloroquine therapy include neuropathy, ototoxicity, bone-marrow suppression, emotional changes, bleaching of hair, and cardiomyopathy.

D. Other immunosuppressive agents. Two other immunosuppressive drugs have been used successfully as DMARDs in patients with RA: the purine antagonist azathioprine and the alkylating agent cyclophosphamide. These drugs are indicated only in patients with severe disabling RA (active synovitis or systemic manifestations) who are refractory to or intolerant of standard DMARD therapy. Because of the potential for serious toxicity, these medications should be prescribed with the guidance of a rheumatologist or other physician experienced in their use and given only to well-informed, cooperative patients who are willing to comply with meticulous follow-up.

Drug dosages must be individualized to avoid toxicity, especially myelosuppression. Peripheral blood counts must be monitored closely: 10–14 days after each dosage change and monthly while on a stable dosage. The dosage is usually adjusted to maintain a white blood cell count of 3500–4500 cells/μl, with at least 1000 neutrophils. The lowest dose of medication producing adequate disease control should be used. Objective evidence of improvement may begin after 6–12 weeks of therapy. If there is no response after 16 weeks, the drug should be discontinued. After synovitis has been controlled for several months, these agents should be tapered slowly and maintained at the lowest effective dosage. Potential short-term benefit must be weighed against the possible increased risk of malignancy (lymphoma, leukemia) with long-term use. Chronic or intermittent therapy may be required to control disease activity.

   1. Azathioprine is initiated at approximately 1.5 mg/kg/day PO, given as a single dose or in 2 divided doses. The dosage can be increased to a maximum of 2.5 to 3.0 mg/kg/day to obtain the desired WBC count. The dose of azathioprine should be reduced by 60–75% if it is given concomitantly with allopurinol, which blocks its metabolic pathway.

   2. Cyclophosphamide is initiated at a **daily morning dose** of 1.0–1.5 mg/kg PO. The dosage can be increased to a maximum of 2.5–3.0 mg/kg/day to obtain the desired WBC count. Patients should be encouraged to take the medication with a large amount of fluid, to void frequently, and to void before going to bed to minimize the risk of hemorrhagic cystitis.

   3. Contraindications and side effects (see Chap. 19).

E. Other therapies. Sulfasalazine has shown encouraging results in RA and may be another DMARD (*J. Rheumatol.* 17:764, 1990). The initial dose is usually 500 mg PO qd for 1 week. The dosage is then increased in 500-mg increments weekly until a total daily dose of 2000–3000 mg is reached, with serial monitoring of total blood counts. Clinical improvement may be noted in 6–12 weeks. **Experimental therapies** include total lymphoid irradiation, plasmapheresis, leukopheresis, and cyclosporine. These unproved therapeutic modalities are reserved for the patient who is unresponsive to conventional therapy.

II. **Surgical management.** Corrective surgical procedures including synovectomy, total joint replacement, and joint fusion may be indicated in patients with RA to reduce pain and improve function. Carpal tunnel syndrome, caused by entrapment of the median nerve at the wrist, produces paresthesias in the thumb and first two digits. Surgical repair may be curative if local injection therapy is unsuccessful. **Synovectomy** may be helpful if major involvement is limited to one or two joints and if a 6-month trial of medical therapy has failed. Usually, however, this procedure is only temporarily effective. Prophylactic synovectomy and debridement of the ulnar styloid should be considered in patients with severe wrist disease to prevent rupture of the extensor tendons. Other procedures that may be beneficial include **total joint replacement** of the hip, shoulder, and knee joints and resection of metatarsal heads in patients with bunion deformities and subluxation of the toes. Reconstructive hand surgery may be useful in carefully selected patients. Surgical **fusion of joints** usually results in freedom from pain but also in total loss of motion; this is well tolerated in the wrist and thumb. Cervical fusion of C1 and C2 is indicated for significant subluxation. When cartilage loss or joint deformity is contributing significantly to pain and disability, management by a team including an internist, an orthopedic surgeon, and a rehabilitation expert is desirable.

III. **Adjunctive measures**
A. **Reactive depression** and sleep disorders are frequently encountered in patients with rheumatic diseases. Judicious use of antidepressants and sedatives may greatly improve the functional status of selected patients.
B. **Rehabilitative therapy** should be managed by a team of physicians, physical and occupational therapists, nurses, social workers, and psychologists.
   1. **Acute** care of arthritis involves joint protection and pain relief. Proper joint positioning and splints are important elements in joint protection. Heat is a useful analgesic.
   2. **Subacute** disease therapy should include a gradual increase in passive and active joint movement.
   3. **Chronic** care encompasses instruction in joint protection, work simplification, and performances of activities of daily living. Adaptive equipment, splints, and mobility aids may be useful. Specific exercises designed to promote normal joint mechanics and strengthen affected muscle groups are useful. Overall cardiac conditioning also improves functional status.
C. **Patient education** about the disease process is helpful. Pamphlets and support groups are available in many communities through the Arthritis Foundation and the Lupus Foundation.

Spondyloarthropathies

The spondyloarthropathies are an interrelated group of disorders characterized by one or more of the following features: (1) spondylitis, (2) sacroiliitis, (3) inflammation at sites of tendon insertion (enthesopathy), and (4) asymmetric oligoarthritis. Extra-articular features of this group of disorders may include: (1) inflammatory eye disease, (2) urethritis, and (3) mucocutaneous lesions. The spondyloarthropathies aggregate in families, where they are associated with human leukocyte antigen (HLA)–B27.

I. In **ankylosing spondylitis** (AS), the major clinical problem is inflammation and ossification of the joints and ligaments of the spine and of the sacroiliac joints. Hips and shoulders are the most commonly involved peripheral joints. Because progressive fusion of the apophyseal joints of the spine cannot be either predicted or prevented, the therapeutic goal is to maximize the likelihood that fusion will occur in a straight line, to minimize possible late postural defects and respiratory compromise. Patients should be instructed to sleep supine on a firm bed without a pillow and to practice postural and deep-breathing exercises regularly. Cigarette smoking should be strongly discouraged. Although high-dose salicylate therapy is usually ineffective in controlling pain, other NSAIDs may provide symptomatic relief; indomethacin is the NSAID most commonly used (see Table 24-2). Sulfasalazine also appears to be of benefit in some patients (see Rheumatoid Arthritis, sec. **I.E**) (*Arthritis Rheum.* 31:1111, 1988). Glucocorticoids and immunosuppressive therapy have occasionally been used in patients who do not respond to other agents. Surgical procedures to correct some spine and hip deformities may result in significant rehabilitation in carefully selected patients. Acute anterior uveitis occurs in up to 25% of patients with AS and should be managed by an ophthalmologist. This problem is generally self-limited, although glaucoma and blindness are unusual secondary complications.

II. Arthritis of inflammatory bowel disease. In 10–20 percent of patients with Crohn's disease or ulcerative colitis, an arthritis develops that is very similar to that of ankylosing spondylitis. Clinical features include spondylitis, sacroiliitis, and peripheral arthritis, particularly in the knee and ankle. Although peripheral joint disease may correlate with the activity of the colitis, spinal disease does not. Extra-articular features of the disease including erythema nodosum, stomatitis, uveitis, and pyoderma gangrenosum are also more closely related to peripheral joint disease. Joint aspiration may be useful in this setting to exclude an associated septic arthritis, but antibiotics are not effective in the management of sterile synovitis associated with colitis. As in ankylosing spondylitis, NSAIDs (other than aspirin) are the treatment of choice. Local injection of glucocorticoids and physical therapy are useful adjunctive measures. Enteropathic arthritis may also be associated with intestinal bypass surgery and Whipple's disease.

III. Reiter's syndrome and reactive arthritis. Reiter's syndrome occurs predominantly in young men and may occur with increased frequency in patients infected with human immunodeficiency virus (HIV) (*Ann. Intern. Med.* 106:19, 1987). The clinical syndrome consists of asymmetric oligoarthritis, urethritis, conjunctivitis, and characteristic skin and mucous membrane lesions. The syndrome is usually transient, lasting from one to several months, but recurrences associated with varying degrees of disability are common. A reactive enteropathic arthritis may follow dysentery due to *Shigella flexneri, Salmonella* species, or *Yersinia enterocolitica* infections. Articular manifestations are identical to those of Reiter's syndrome; extra-articular manifestations may occur but tend to be mild.

Conservative therapy is indicated for control of pain and inflammation in these diseases. Spontaneous remissions are common, making evaluation of therapy difficult. High-dose salicylates are usually ineffective, but other NSAIDs (especially indomethacin) are often useful (see Rheumatoid Arthritis, sec. **I.A**). As in AS, sulfasalazine may provide symptomatic relief in some patients. In unusually severe cases, therapy with glucocorticoids or methotrexate may be required to prevent rapid joint destruction. Conjunctivitis is usually transient and benign, but ophthalmologic referral and treatment with topical or systemic glucocorticoids is indicated for iritis.

IV. Psoriatic arthritis. Seven percent of patients with psoriasis have some form of inflammatory arthritis. Four major patterns of joint disease occur: (1) asymmetric oligoarticular arthritis, (2) predominant distal interphalangeal joint (DIP) involvement in association with nail disease, (3) symmetric rheumatoid-like polyarthritis, and (4) spondylitis and sacroiliitis. High-dose salicylates or NSAIDs (see Rheumatoid Arthritis, sec. **I.A**), particularly indomethacin, are used to treat the arthritic manifestations of psoriasis, in conjunction with appropriate measures for the skin disease. Intra-articular glucocorticoids may be useful in the oligoarticular form of disease, but injection through a psoriatic plaque should be avoided. Gold and hydroxychloroquine (see Rheumatoid Arthritis, sec. **I.C**) may have disease-modifying effects in polyarthritis, but the latter has been reported to cause exacerbation of psoriasis in some patients. Severe skin and joint disease generally responds well to low-dose methotrexate (see Rheumatoid Arthritis, sec. **I.C.1**). When reconstructive joint surgery is performed on patients with psoriatic arthritis, the risk of wound infection is increased approximately fivefold due to colonization of psoriatic skin with *Staph. aureus.*

Systemic Lupus Erythematosus

Systemic lupus erythematosus (SLE) is a multisystem disease of unknown etiology that primarily affects women of childbearing age. The course of this disease is highly variable and unpredictable. Disease manifestations are protean, ranging in severity from fatigue, malaise, weight loss, arthritis or arthralgias, fever, photosensitivity, and serositis to potentially life-threatening thrombocytopenia, hemolytic anemia, nephritis, cerebritis, vasculitis, pneumonitis, myositis, and myocarditis. Numerous autoantibodies are found in the serum; antinuclear antibodies are present in more than 95% of patients. Low C3, C4, or CH_{50} levels and high levels of anti-DNA antibodies are associated with disease exacerbations (especially nephritis) in more than half of patients. Treatment of this disorder is problem oriented and directed at the suppression of disease manifestations; no therapy is curative.

I. **Conservative therapy** should be used if the patient's manifestations are mild.
  A. **General supportive measures.** Mild disease exacerbations may subside after a few days of bed rest. Adequate sleep, midafternoon naps, and avoidance of fatigue are strongly recommended. Although skin eruptions in photosensitive patients can be reduced by lotions that contain para-aminobenzoic acid and have a sunscreen rating of 15 or greater, avoidance of sun exposure is recommended. Isolated skin lesions may respond to topical corticosteroids (see Chap. 1).
  B. **NSAIDs** usually control arthritis, arthralgias, fever, and serositis, although they are less effective than glucocorticoids. Fatigue, malaise, and major organ system involvement usually do not respond to NSAIDs. Hepatic and renal toxicities of the NSAIDs appear to be increased in SLE (see Rheumatoid Arthritis, sec. **I.A**), and rare cases of aseptic meningitis have also been reported. NSAIDs should be avoided in patients with active nephritis and used carefully if at all in patients with renal insufficiency.
  C. **Hydroxychloroquine** (see Rheumatoid Arthritis, sec. **I.C.4**) may be effective in the treatment of rash, photosensitivity, arthralgias, arthritis, alopecia, and malaise associated with SLE, and in the treatment of discoid and subacute cutaneous lupus erythematosus. Skin lesions may begin to improve within a few days, but joint symptoms may take 6–10 weeks to subside. The drug is not effective for treating fever or renal, CNS, and hematologic problems.
II. **Glucocorticoid therapy**
  A. **Indications** for the use of systemic glucocorticoids include life-threatening or debilitating manifestations such as glomerulonephritis, CNS involvement, thrombocytopenia, hemolytic anemia, myositis, severe serositis, myocarditis, vasculitis, and other severe systemic involvement unresponsive to conservative regimens.
  B. **Pharmacology.** Glucocorticoids are both anti-inflammatory and immunosuppressive. Oral forms of hydrocortisone and its synthetic analogues are well absorbed by the intestine. The serum half-life of synthetic glucocorticoids varies from a few minutes to several hours, but anti-inflammatory effects and adrenal suppression are not directly related to this half-life.
  C. **Preparations, dosages, and routes of administration** (see Table 24-3). The goal of glucocorticoid therapy is to suppress disease activity with the minimum effective dosage of drug. Prednisone (PO) and methylprednisolone (IV) are generally the preferred drugs because of cost and half-life considerations. Intramuscular absorption is quite variable and is not advised. The route and frequency of administration are determined by the severity of disease manifestations.
    1. **Patients with severe or potentially life-threatening complications** of SLE should be treated with prednisone, 60–100 mg PO qd, which is often given initially in divided doses. After the disease is controlled, therapy should be consolidated to a single daily dose, then slowly tapered, reducing the dosage by no more than 10% every 7–10 days; a more rapid reduction may result in

relapse. The maintenance dosage of prednisone is generally 10–20 mg PO qd or 20–40 mg PO qod.

2. **Intravenous pulse therapy** has been utilized in SLE in such life-threatening situations as rapidly progressive renal failure, active CNS disease, and severe thrombocytopenia. Intravenous infusion of 500 mg methylprednisolone in 0.9% saline or 5% D/W is given over 30 minutes q12h for 3–5 days. Patients who do not show improvement with this regimen are probably unresponsive to steroids, and other therapeutic alternatives must be considered. Prednisone, 50 mg PO bid, is begun after completing pulse therapy and is slowly tapered when clinically feasible.

3. **Alternate-day schedules** (see Rheumatoid Arthritis, sec. **I.B.3**) markedly reduce many of the adverse effects of long-term glucocorticoid therapy, particularly the infectious complications. However, this approach is not indicated in the initial management of patients with severe, active disease.

D. **Side effects.** All glucocorticoid preparations have similar side effects, which are related to both dosage and duration of administration.

1. **Adrenal suppression.** Glucocorticoids suppress the hypothalamic–pituitary–adrenal axis. This effect may persist for months after therapy is stopped, depending on the dose, frequency, and duration of glucocorticoid therapy. Adrenal suppression is minimized by the use of low-dose, short-acting preparations such as prednisone (least expensive) or methylprednisolone, rather than long-acting preparations such as dexamethasone. Whenever possible, a single daily dose should be given in the morning to more closely approximate the normal morning cortisol surge. For alternate-day use, a short-acting steroid is indicated and is also given as a single morning dose. In patients who are receiving chronic glucocorticoid therapy, hypoadrenalism may appear at times of severe stress (e.g., infection, major surgery, serious intercurrent illnesses), presenting as anorexia, weight loss, lethargy, fever, and postural hypotension. Mineralocorticoid activity, however, is preserved, and the hyperkalemia and hyponatremia characteristic of primary adrenal insufficiency are not seen. These patients should wear a medical alert bracelet or carry identification to inform medical personnel that they should receive supplemental glucocorticoids in an emergency situation. Patients who have received more than 10 mg of prednisone (or the equivalent) daily for several weeks may have some degree of axis suppression for up to 1 year following cessation of therapy (see Chap. 21).

2. **Immunosuppression.** Glucocorticoid therapy reduces resistance to infections. Bacterial infections, in particular, are related to dose of glucocorticoid and remain a major cause of morbidity and mortality in SLE. Thus, minor infections may become systemic, quiescent infections may be activated, and organisms that are usually nonpathogenic may cause disease. Local and systemic signs of infection can be partially masked, although fever associated with infection is generally not completely suppressed by glucocorticoids. Immunizations with influenza and pneumococcal vaccines do not appear to activate SLE and are advised as prophylactic measures. A skin test for tuberculosis should be placed before glucocorticoid therapy is instituted when possible.

3. **Changes in physical appearance** may include cushingoid facies, weight gain, redistribution of fat, acne, hirsutism, purple striae, and easy bruisability. These changes can be emotionally disturbing, although most are at least partially reversible as the dosage is reduced.

4. **Changes in mental status** may range from mild nervousness, euphoria, and insomnia to severe depression or psychosis (which can be confused with the CNS manifestations of SLE).

5. **Hyperglycemia** may be induced or severely aggravated by glucocorticoids but is usually not a contraindication to therapy. Insulin therapy may be required, although ketoacidosis is rare.

6. **Fluid and electrolyte abnormalities** include sodium retention and hypokalemia. Patients with congestive heart failure and peripheral edema may have particular difficulty tolerating these drugs.

7. **Hypertension** may be induced or aggravated by glucocorticoids. Pulse IV steroid therapy frequently exacerbates preexisting, poorly controlled hypertension.

8. **Osteopenia** with vertebral compression fractures is common among patients receiving long-term steroid therapy. Supplemental calcium, 1.0–1.5 g/day PO, should be given. Vitamin D and thiazide diuretics may be of benefit (see Chap. 23). Estrogen therapy may be indicated in postmenopausal women at high risk for osteopenia, but its use is controversial in SLE. Calcitonin and diphosphonates can also be considered (see Chap. 23). A judicious exercise program may also be beneficial in stimulating bone formation.

9. **Steroid myopathy** generally involves the hip and shoulder girdle musculature. Muscles are weak but not tender and, in contrast to inflammatory myositis, muscle enzymes and electromyography (EMG) are normal. Biopsy is indicated only in rare cases, to rule out inflammatory myositis. Steroid-induced myopathy should resolve with a reduction in glucocorticoid dosage and an aggressive exercise program, but recovery may take months.

10. **Ocular effects** include increased intraocular pressures (sometimes precipitating glaucoma) and the formation of posterior subcapsular cataracts.

11. **Ischemic bone necrosis** (aseptic necrosis, osteonecrosis, avascular necrosis) may be induced by glucocorticoids. The process is often multifocal, affecting the femoral head, humeral head, and tibial plateau most commonly. Early changes may be demonstrated by bone scan or MRI. Characteristic bone changes on plain radiographs are evidence of long-standing disease. Surgical intervention with core decompression in early ischemic bone necrosis may be beneficial but remains controversial (*Medicine* 59:143, 1980).

12. **Other undesirable effects** of glucocorticoid therapy include hyperlipidemia, menstrual irregularities, increased perspiration with night sweats, and pseudotumor cerebri. Thrombophlebitis, necrotizing arteritis, and pancreatitis, and peptic ulcer disease have been attributed to glucocorticoid therapy, but evidence supporting these associations is weak.

III. **Immunosuppressive agents** used in SLE include azathioprine and cyclophosphamide (see Rheumatoid Arthritis, sec. I.D). These drugs can be used in patients refractory to or intolerant of glucocorticoid therapy, or as steroid-sparing agents. Azathioprine and cyclophosphamide can be administered orally but require 2–4 weeks to exert a beneficial effect. In addition, monthly pulse IV cyclophosphamide (0.5–1.0 g/m^2 IV) for active lupus nephritis may offer a better outcome for renal function than glucocorticoids alone. The blood count should be checked at 10–14 days to determine the degree of bone-marrow suppression (see Chap. 19 for contraindications and side effects). The goal of therapy is to achieve a nadir total WBC count of 3500–4500 cells/μl, with at least 1000 neutrophils. The dosage for the subsequent pulse or oral therapy should be adjusted accordingly.

IV. **Plasmapheresis** has been used on an investigational basis. This therapy may produce a reduction in circulating immune complexes, which sometimes corresponds to clinical improvement. It is most often used in life-threatening situations to control disease until concomitant steroid or immunosuppressive therapy, or both, have taken effect. However, because serologic and clinical manifestations of disease generally rebound on discontinuation of plasmapheresis, concomitant high-dose steroid or cytotoxic therapy is necessary to maintain stability. Plasmapheresis is an impractical long-term therapy for most patients, and its short-term use remains controversial.

V. **Transplantation and chronic hemodialysis** have been utilized in SLE patients with renal failure. Clinical and serologic evidence of nonrenal disease activity often disappear when renal failure ensues. The survival rate in these patients is equivalent to that of patients with other forms of chronic renal disease. Recurrence of nephritis in the allograft occurs rarely.

VI. **Pregnancy in SLE** may be complicated by an increased incidence of spontaneous abortion, fetal death in utero, and prematurity. The correlation between fetal wastage and antibodies to cardiolipin or the lupus anticoagulant is unclear. No controlled study has proved the efficacy of treating pregnant women who have the lupus anticoagulant with glucocorticoids or anticoagulation. Many SLE patients experience an exacerbation in the activity of their disease in the third trimester or peripartum period. Differentiation between active SLE and preeclampsia is frequently difficult. Even in the asymptomatic patient, many rheumatologists advocate a prophylactic increase in the glucocorticoid dosage at the termination of pregnancy.

Scleroderma

Scleroderma (systemic sclerosis [SS]) is a systemic illness of unknown cause characterized by sclerotic skin changes and usually accompanied by multisystem visceral disease. Most of the manifestations of scleroderma have a vascular basis (Raynaud's phenomenon, telangiectasias, nailfold capillary changes, early edematous skin changes, nephrosclerosis), but frank vasculitis is rarely seen. The label scleroderma includes both diffuse scleroderma and the **CREST** (Calcinosis, Raynaud's phenomenon, Esophageal dysmotility, Sclerodactyly, Telangiectasias) syndrome variant. Diffuse scleroderma is characterized by extensive skin disease, the potential for hypertensive "renal crisis," and shortened survival. The CREST variant has limited skin involvement but may be associated with primary pulmonary hypertension or biliary cirrhosis. Anticentromere antibodies are found almost uniquely in CREST. No curative therapy for scleroderma exists; instead, treatment focuses on particular organ involvement in a problem-oriented manner.

I. **Raynaud's phenomenon.** This reversible vasospasm of the digital arteries can result in ischemia of the digits. Patients must be instructed to avoid exposure of the entire body to cold, protect the hands and feet from cold and trauma, and discontinue cigarette smoking. Most pharmacologic approaches have had limited success. Vasodilating drugs, such as **calcium channel antagonists**, prazosin, phenoxybenzamine, reserpine, and guanethidine, are occasionally helpful, but significant side effects, especially orthostatic hypotension, may preclude their use. Sympathetic ganglion blockade with a long-acting anesthetic agent may be useful when a patient has progressive digital ulceration that fails to improve with conservative therapy.

II. **Skin and periarticular changes.** Used early in diffuse scleroderma, penicillamine (see Rheumatoid Arthritis, sec. **I.C.3**) may soften skin and improve joint contractures and may prolong survival. Moisturizing lotions may provide symptomatic relief. Physical therapy is important to retard and reduce joint contractures. Secondary infections at sites of calcinosis or digital ulcers should be treated with appropriate topical (and occasionally systemic) antimicrobials, and debrided if necessary. Although there is no effective therapy for calcinosis, the pruritus and inflammation that sometimes accompany calcinosis may respond to colchicine.

III. **Gastrointestinal involvement.** Reflux esophagitis resulting from lower esophageal abnormalities responds to a vigorous antacid regimen and elevation of the head of the bed during sleep. H_2-receptor antagonists and sucralfate are also useful in some patients. Calcium channel antagonists used for Raynaud's phenomenon may worsen esophageal reflux. Mechanical esophageal dilatation may occasionally be necessary for strictures. Decreased motility of bowel segments can occur, leading to bacterial overgrowth, malabsorption, and weight loss. Treatment with broad-spectrum antimicrobials such as tetracycline or metronidazole often improves the malabsorption (see Chap. 15), and metoclopramide may reduce bloating and distention.

IV. **Renal involvement.** The appearance of hypertension and renal insufficiency, often associated with a microangiopathic hemolytic anemia, signals a poor prognosis. Aggressive blood pressure control with **angiotensin-converting enzyme inhibitors** may delay or prevent the onset of uremia, particularly in patients with a serum creatinine of less than 3.0 mg/dl (*Ann. Intern. Med.* 113:352, 1990). Dialysis and transplantation are appropriate when vigorous medical antihypertensive therapy fails to preserve renal function.

V. **Cardiopulmonary involvement.** Patchy myocardial fibrosis can result in congestive heart failure or arrhythmias. Standard therapies for these conditions are used. Symptomatic pericarditis with an effusion, which can lead to tamponade, is often responsive to glucocorticoids. Coronary artery vasospasm can cause angina pectoris and may respond to calcium channel antagonists. Pulmonary involvement includes pleurisy with effusion, interstitial fibrosis, pulmonary hypertension, and cor pulmonale. Glucocorticoids or NSAIDs can be used to treat pleurisy. Vasodilator therapy may decrease pulmonary artery pressure in pulmonary hypertension but should never be initiated in an unmonitored patient (see Chap. 10).

Necrotizing Vasculitis

Necrotizing vasculitis is characterized by inflammation and necrosis of blood vessels. This entity includes a broad spectrum of disorders having various causes and involving vessels of different types, sizes, and locations. The immunopathogenic process often involves immune complexes, but in most cases the specific antigen and antibody involved have not been identified. Clinical features are diverse and include systemic manifestations such as fever and weight loss, and localized problems including rash, arthritis, myositis, neuropathies, CNS disease, nephritis, pulmonary infiltrates, and gastrointestinal catastrophes. The response to therapy and long-term prognosis of these disorders are highly variable. In the differential diagnosis of most multisystem disorders, vasculitis, infection, and occult emboli (e.g., atrial myxoma, cholesterol emboli) should all be considered.

I. **Specific disorders. Hypersensitivity vasculitis** affects small vessels, presenting with rash and, occasionally, nephritis. It may occur in the setting of infection, connective tissue disease, drug reaction, and malignancy. **Polyarteritis nodosa** (PAN) usually attacks medium-sized vessels in major organs such as kidney, liver, gut, and peripheral nerves. **Wegener's granulomatosis** is typified by involvement of small- to medium-sized vessels in upper and lower airways and kidney disease. **Rheumatoid vasculitis,** which often presents when arthritis is clinically inactive, may produce skin ulcers, nailfold infarcts, scleritis, pericarditis, and peripheral neuropathy. Diagnosis of a specific form of vasculitis usually requires both clinical features and either biopsy specimens or, in PAN, angiography.

II. **Management** should include consultation with a physician experienced in the treatment of these disorders. Treatment should be tailored to the severity of organ system involvement.

A. **Glucocorticoids** are the usual initial therapy and may be beneficial in most vasculitides. Although vasculitis limited to the skin may respond to lower dosages, the initial dosage for visceral involvement should be high (60–100 mg/day prednisone). If life-threatening manifestations are present, a brief course of high-dose pulse therapy with methylprednisolone, 500 mg IV q12h for 3–5 days, should be considered (see Systemic Lupus Erythematosus, sec. **II.C**).

B. **Immunosuppressive agents.** The addition of cyclophosphamide, 1.5–2.0 mg/kg PO qd, to steroid treatment regimens should be considered when major organ system involvement (e.g., lung, kidney, or nerve) is rapidly progressive. **Early addition of cyclophosphamide is appropriate in Wegener's granulomatosis and polyarteritis nodosa.** Patients who are unresponsive to steroid therapy or intolerant of steroid side effects should also be considered for immunosuppressive agents.

C. **Short-term plasmapheresis** to remove presumed pathogenic immune complexes has been advocated for life-threatening vasculitis but should be used in conjunction with an immunosuppressive drug to prevent rebound immune complex production (see Systemic Lupus Erythematosus).

Polymyalgia Rheumatica and Temporal Arteritis

Polymyalgia rheumatica (PMR) presents in elderly patients as proximal limb girdle pain (without weakness or elevated muscle enzymes), morning stiffness, fatigue, weight loss, low-grade fever, anemia, and an erythrocyte sedimentation rate (ESR) of greater than 50 ml/hr. **Temporal arteritis (TA)** is a form of giant cell arteritis also seen primarily in the elderly. Up to 40% of patients with PMR also have TA. Temporal arteritis can present with symptoms of PMR, as well as with headache, scalp tenderness, claudication of jaw muscles, visual disturbances (including blindness), stroke, and an ESR greater than 50 ml/hr. Rarely, major branches of the thoracic and abdominal aorta are affected.

I. **Management of PMR.** If PMR is present without evidence of TA, prednisone, 10–15 mg PO qd, usually produces dramatic clinical improvement within a few days. The ESR should return to normal during initial treatment, but subsequent therapeutic decisions should be based on both ESR and clinical status. Glucocorticoid therapy can be gradually tapered to a maintenance dose of 5–10 mg PO qd. Treatment is required for a minimum of 1 year, and relapses may occur after therapy is discontinued. NSAIDs may facilitate reduction in prednisone dosage.

II. **Management of TA.** Patients suspected of having TA should be treated promptly with prednisone, 60–80 mg PO qd, to prevent irreversible blindness. Alternate-day therapy has no role in the initial management of this disease (*Ann. Intern. Med.* 82:613, 1975). The diagnosis of TA should be confirmed by temporal artery biopsy. Biopsy results will not be altered by 3–5 days of prednisone therapy. High-dose steroid therapy should be continued until symptoms have abated and the ESR has returned to normal. The dosage should then be gradually tapered by not more than 10% per week and should be continued for 1–2 years with close monitoring of the ESR and clinical status. A maintenance dosage of prednisone, 10–20 mg PO qd, may be required for years.

Cryoglobulin Syndromes

Cryoglobulins are serum proteins that reversibly precipitate in the cold. More than half of cryoglobulinemic patients have an underlying disease such as an immunoproliferative process, autoimmune disorder, or underlying infection; the remainder have no obvious underlying disease (essential or idiopathic cryoglobulinemia). Clinical manifestations of cryoglobulins may be mediated by immune complex deposition (arthralgias, purpura, Raynaud's phenomenon, glomerulonephritis, and neuropathy) or by hyperviscosity (headache, lethargy, blurred vision).

I. **Diagnosis** requires the proper collection of serum for the detection of cryoglobulins. Blood should be collected in prewarmed tubes and kept at 37°C while clotting occurs. Serum should be promptly harvested after centrifugation at 37°C and then incubated at 4°C for at least 72 hours. Normal values vary considerably among laboratories, but trace amounts of cryoglobulins may be found in normal persons. Whenever cryoglobulins are identified, immunoelectrophoresis should be performed to identify the proteins as monoclonal (associated with immunoproliferative diseases) or polyclonal.

II. **Therapy** of secondary cryoglobulinemic states is directed at the underlying disease. Essential cryoglobulinemia may respond to prednisone or immunosuppressive agents. Hyperviscosity responds dramatically to plasmapheresis.

Polymyositis and Dermatomyositis

Polymyositis (PM) is an inflammatory myopathy that presents as weakness and, occasionally, tenderness of the hip and shoulder girdle musculature. **Dermatomyositis (DM)** is, by definition, PM with a concomitant rash. PM–DM can occur in three forms: (1) alone, (2) in association with any of the other autoimmune diseases, or (3) with a variety of neoplasms. Men with DM, cutaneous vasculitis, and disease onset after the age of 50 years are at greatest risk of having an associated malignancy (*J. Rheumatol.* 10:85, 1983).

I. **Diagnosis.** Abnormal electromyographic patterns and elevated muscle enzyme levels (creatine kinase, aldolase, SGOT, and lactate dehydrogenase) are usually present. Although the diagnosis is confirmed by muscle biopsy, the disease is patchy, and a biopsy may miss involved areas or show nonspecific changes.

II. **Treatment.** When PM–DM occurs without associated disease, it usually responds well to prednisone, 40–80 mg PO qd. Alternate-day therapy (see Rheumatoid Arthritis, sec. **I.B.3**) can also be successful and should be tried if the patient is not severely ill. Systemic complaints such as fever and malaise respond to therapy first, followed by muscle enzymes and, finally, muscle strength. Once serum enzyme levels normalize, the prednisone dosage should be slowly reduced to maintenance levels of 10–20 mg PO qd or 20–40 mg PO qod. The appearance of steroid-induced myopathy and hypokalemia may complicate therapeutic assessment. PM–DM associated with neoplasia tends to be less responsive to glucocorticoid therapy. In a few patients, removal of an associated malignant tumor has resulted in complete remission of PM–DM. Patients who fail to respond or cannot tolerate the side effects of glucocorticoids may respond to methotrexate or azathioprine (*Ann. Intern. Med.* 111:143, 1989) (see Rheumatoid Arthritis, secs. **I.C** and **I.D**). Complications of severe disease include interstitial lung disease, cardiomyopathy, and respiratory failure due to aspiration pneumonia or diaphragmatic weakness. Because of the pulmonary involvement in myositis, particular care must be used if methotrexate is prescribed. Physical therapy is essential in the management of myositis. Bed rest with active-assisted range of motion is appropriate during very active disease, with more active exercise prescribed to improve strength once inflammation has been controlled.

Osteoarthritis

Osteoarthritis (OA), or degenerative joint disease, is characterized by deterioration of articular cartilage, with subsequent formation of reactive new bone at the articular surface. The disease is more common in the elderly but may occur at any age, especially as a sequel to joint trauma, chronic inflammatory arthritis, or congenital malformation. The joints most commonly affected are the distal and proximal interphalangeal joints of the hands, the hips and knees, and the cervical and lumbar spine. Osteoarthritis of the spine may lead to spinal stenosis (neurogenic claudication), with aching or pain in the legs or buttock on standing or walking.

I. **Medical management.** The objectives of therapy include relief of pain and prevention of disability. NSAIDs and nonnarcotic analgesics usually provide some relief. Intra-articular glucocorticoid injections are sometimes beneficial. Systemic steroids and narcotic analgesics should be avoided.

II. **Adjunctive measures.** Patient education regarding the indolent nature of this disorder, and the preservation of function despite deformity, may relieve unnecessary concerns. When weight-bearing joints are affected, support in the form of a cane, crutches, or walker can be helpful, and weight reduction may be advised. A physical therapy program should provide exercises to prevent or correct muscle atrophy. When serious disability results from severe pain or deformity, surgery may be indicated. Total hip or knee replacement usually relieves pain and increases function in selected patients. Prophylactic correction of childhood abnormalities (e.g., dislocation of the hip) will often prevent the development of OA in later years.

Osteoarthritis of the spine may cause radicular symptoms from pressure on nerve roots and often produces pain and spasm in paraspinal soft tissues. Physical supports (cervical collar, lumbar corset), local heat, and exercises to strengthen cervical, paravertebral, and abdominal muscles may provide relief in some patients. Laminectomy and spinal fusion should be reserved for severe disease with intractable pain or neurologic complications. Lumbar spinal stenosis may require extensive decompressive laminectomy for relief of symptoms.

Fibrositis

Fibrositis (fibromyositis, fibromyalgia) is an extremely common nonarticular musculoskeletal disorder that consists of pain, stiffness, fatigue, and nonrestorative sleep. Commonly associated disorders include tension headache, irritable bowel syndrome, and dysmenorrhea. Pain is poorly localized but spares the joints. The physical examination is notable for characteristic tender points occurring bilaterally over the trapezius ridge, second costochondral junction, posterior cervical musculature, and upper gluteal area and at the anserine and trochanteric bursae. Fibrositis is a diagnosis of exclusion. Fibrositis does not usually respond to NSAIDs or glucocorticoids. **Tricyclic antidepressants** can be given in low doses at bedtime (e.g., amitriptyline, 10–50 mg PO, or cyclobenzaprine, 5–30 mg PO) to correct the disorder of stage 4 sleep characteristic of fibrositis (*Arthritis Rheum.* 29:1371, 1986). **Physical therapy** and **aerobic fitness** programs may also be helpful.

Tendinitis, Tenosynovitis, and Bursitis

Inflammation of periarticular soft tissue structures may result from trauma induced by strain or direct injury and from various rheumatic processes (e.g., RA, Reiter's syndrome, gout). Infection, particularly gonorrhea, must also be considered. Common sites of inflammation include the shoulder (supraspinatus or bicipital head tendinitis), elbow (epicondylitis—tennis elbow or golfer's elbow), thumb (de Quervain's disease), hip (trochanteric bursitis), knee (prepatellar bursitis), and heel (Achilles or calcaneal bursitis). Rest and immobilization provide adequate relief for most patients; joint rest is essential when weight-bearing tendons (patellar, Achilles) are involved. A local injection of 10–40 mg triamcinolone plus 1 ml of 1% lidocaine usually provides immediate relief and may last indefinitely in some patients. NSAIDs are often useful, particularly if multiple areas are involved.

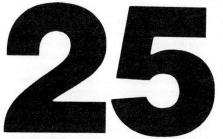

Neurologic Emergencies in Internal Medicine

Barbara Dappert and
Robert G. Kaniecki

Coma

Coma is a sleeplike state of unresponsiveness to external stimulation. A wide variety of metabolic and structural disorders can produce this state. Effective treatment of coma requires correct diagnosis of the underlying cause, which is best accomplished by a systematic approach. (For a complete discussion of coma, see F. Plum and J. B. Posner. *The Diagnosis of Stupor and Coma* [3rd ed.]. Philadelphia: Davis, 1980.)

I. **Pathophysiology.** Stupor and coma result from disease affecting (1) **both cerebral hemispheres** or (2) the **brainstem.** Lesions affecting only a single cerebral hemisphere (e.g., infarction of the middle cerebral artery) rarely cause stupor or coma. However, unilateral cerebral lesions with mass effect (e.g., tumor, hemorrhage, large infarction with secondary edema) can impair consciousness by causing compression of the contralateral hemisphere or the brainstem. Similarly, mass-producing lesions in the cerebellum may impair consciousness by causing brainstem compression. Brainstem lesions impair consciousness by disruption of the reticular formation. Metabolic disorders impair consciousness by diffuse effects on the reticular formation or both cerebral hemispheres.

II. **Assessment**

A. **History** often establishes a diagnosis. The types and temporal course of premonitory symptoms, preexisting medical (e.g., diabetes) or neurologic (e.g., epilepsy) illness, drug use, trauma, and toxin exposure need to be determined. The circumstances in which a comatose patient is found may suggest a diagnosis. People who have had recent contact with the patient, including friends, relatives, police, and ambulance drivers, should be questioned.

B. **General physical examination** may reveal the presence of a systemic illness associated with coma. For example, evidence of cirrhosis suggests hepatic failure, a purpuric rash suggests meningococcemia, and herpetic lesions or oral candidiasis may suggest AIDS.

C. **Neurologic examination** should be repeated at frequent intervals to evaluate the clinical course. Careful examination should localize the anatomic lesion, which in turn should suggest a differential diagnosis. Multifocal signs (i.e., not referable to a single anatomic site) strongly suggest a metabolic cause.

1. **Level of consciousness** is judged by the patient's responses to various stimuli and the amount of stimulation required. Does the patient arouse when called by name, or is shouting, shaking, or painful stimulation needed to elicit a response? Are the responses appropriate?

2. **Pupil size and light reactivity should be noted.**

a. **Midposition (4–6 mm) and fixed pupils** imply a midbrain lesion.

b. **A unilaterally dilated and fixed pupil** implies a third cranial nerve lesion, as might be caused by uncal herniation.

c. **Small but reactive pupils** are seen in metabolic encephalopathy, diencephalic or pontine lesions, and narcotic overdose.

d. **Bilaterally dilated and fixed pupils** are seen with severe anoxic encephalopathy or intoxication with drugs such as scopolamine, glutethimide (Doriden), or methyl alcohol.

3. **Position of the eyes at rest should be noted.**
   a. **Dysconjugate gaze** may suggest a cranial nerve palsy. Deviation of the eye laterally and inferiorly (unopposed VI and IV) suggests a third nerve lesion; deviation of the eye medially suggests a sixth nerve lesion.
   b. **Conjugate eye deviation away** from a hemiparesis suggests a lesion on the side of the gaze preference (above the pons and usually in the frontal lobe). Looking toward the hemiparesis suggests a brainstem lesion contralateral to the hemiparesis (usually in the pons).

4. **Eye movements** are assessed by the oculocephalic and oculovestibular tests. Absence of all eye movements indicates a bilateral pontine lesion or drug-induced ophthalmoplegia (e.g., sedatives, phenytoin, tricyclic antidepressants). Unidirectionally impaired conjugate gaze (i.e., neither eye deviates to one side of midline) usually indicates a lesion in the pons on the side of impaired gaze. An acute hemispheric lesion can also cause a conjugate gaze palsy not overcome by caloric stimulation. Horizontal dysconjugate gaze (i.e., one eye moves less well than the other) suggests a third nerve (defective medial movement) or sixth nerve (defective lateral movement) lesion or a medial longitudinal fasciculus (internuclear ophthalmoplegia) lesion.
   a. **The oculocephalic (doll's eyes) test** is performed by quickly turning the head laterally or vertically while watching the eyes. This test should not be performed if cervical spine injury is suspected. When the brainstem pathways within the pons and midbrain are functioning normally, the eyes move conjugately in the direction opposite to that of head movement.
   b. **The oculovestibular (cold calorics) test** is more potent than the oculocephalic maneuver in producing conjugate eye movements. This test is used if no eye movements can be elicited by the oculocephalic test or if cranial or cervical trauma is suspected. The external auditory canals must be free of obstruction, and the tympanic membranes must be intact. The head is tilted 30 degrees above horizontal while the tympanic membrane is lavaged with 10–50 ml of ice water. In a comatose patient with the brainstem intact from pons to midbrain, the eyes deviate conjugately toward the ear being stimulated. Vertical gaze can be assessed with simultaneous stimulation of both tympanic membranes.

5. **Motor responses,** both spontaneous and induced, should be tested. Spontaneous movement should be observed for symmetry and purpose. Preferential use of the limbs on one side indicates paresis of the unused limbs. Painful stimulation can be used to prompt movement. Stereotyped posturing, rather than purposeful, protective movements, in response to a painful stimulus is not of localizing value and can occur in metabolic coma. Muscle tone should be assessed, particularly for symmetry. The position of the limbs at rest (e.g., external rotation of one leg) and the rate of fall when the limbs are lifted and released are sensitive indicators of hypotonia. Deep tendon reflexes and plantar responses should be assessed, particularly for symmetry.

D. **Ancillary tests** are often needed to establish the cause of coma.
   1. **Serum chemistries** should include glucose, electrolytes, arterial blood gases (ABGs), prothrombin time (PT), partial thromboplastin time (PTT), CBC, calcium, magnesium, BUN, transaminases, and creatinine. Urine and blood should be obtained for toxicologic screening.
   2. **Computed tomography** should be performed when a structural brain lesion is suspected. Aneurysm, arteriovenous malformation, tumor, bilateral subdural hematomas, and subacute infarction may not be visualized by CT unless intravenous iodinated contrast material is used. Normal renal function and absence of contrast allergy should be confirmed prior to administration of dye. MRI is more sensitive for some lesions and does not require dye.
   3. **Skull and cervical spine radiographs** should be obtained if there is a possibility of trauma.
   4. **Other diagnostic tests** include lumbar puncture, EEG, and angiography as dictated by the clinical picture. Treatment efficacy in bacterial meningitis depends on the speed with which antibiotic therapy is instituted. For this

reason, lumbar puncture should be performed early in the evaluation of coma, unless neurologic signs of brain herniation are present (see Increased Intracranial Pressure). **Never postpone treatment of suspected meningitis if there is a delay in obtaining the cerebrospinal fluid (CSF).** (See Chap. 13 for antimicrobial treatment of meningitis).

III. **Treatment.** Certain therapeutic measures should be initiated immediately, in conjunction with assessment.

   A. **Ensure adequate ventilation, circulation, and body temperature.** A plastic nasal or oral airway or endotracheal intubation may be necessary. A large-bore IV catheter should be placed, anticipating the need for rapid administration of fluids or medication.

   B. **Thiamine,** 100 mg IV, is given initially (before dextrose), followed by 100 mg IM qd for 3 days.

   C. **Dextrose,** 50 ml of a 50% solution IV, should be administered if the blood glucose level is low (< 50 mg/dl) or unobtainable.

   D. **Naloxone hydrochloride (Narcan),** 0.4–1.2 mg IV, should be given. Larger doses may be needed for suspected pentazocine or propoxyphene overdoses. With opiate intoxication, a response should be seen within minutes. Repeat doses may be necessary to treat deterioration following initial improvement.

   E. **Flumazenil,** 0.2 mg IV, should be administered over 30 seconds followed by 0.3 mg at 1 minute and then 0.5 mg q1min to a total of 3 mg. If no response has occurred, benzodiazepines are unlikely to be the cause of sedation.

   F. **Treat increased intracranial pressure** (see Increased Intracranial Pressure).

IV. **General care of the immobile patient**

   A. **Protect the airway.**

   B. **Nutrition and vitamin supplementation** must be provided. A duodenal feeding tube should be placed if patients require long-term care.

   C. **Hydration** should be maintained with IV fluids or by duodenal feeding tube. Excessive secretion of antidiuretic hormone is common with neurologic illness and requires close monitoring of fluid and electrolyte balance.

   D. **Cutaneous pressure sores** should be prevented by repositioning the patient every 2 hours. A textured foam (egg-crate) mattress and protective heel pads are beneficial.

   E. **Joint mobility** should be maintained with passive exercise. Fitted boots should be used to prevent contractures of the Achilles tendon.

   F. **Corneal abrasions** can be prevented by taping the eyelids closed after applying methylcellulose drops (1 drop in each eye q4h).

   G. **In-dwelling urinary catheters** are a common source of infection and should be used judiciously. Condom catheters may be more appropriate in male patients, but penile maceration may result from prolonged use.

   H. **Gastric stress ulceration** and attendant hemorrhage may be prevented by frequent administration of antacids via nasogastric tube or intravenous administration of histamine H_2 antagonists (see Chap. 14).

   I. **Heparin, 5,000 units SQ q12h,** should be given to prevent deep venous thrombosis and subsequent pulmonary embolism.

Increased Intracranial Pressure

Management of an acute, life-threatening increase in intracranial pressure (ICP) requires prompt determination of the underlying cause, followed by specific therapeutic measures. The differential diagnosis includes tumor, hematoma, subarachnoid hemorrhage, cerebral edema, abscess, and hydrocephalus.

I. **Presentation**

   A. **Nonspecific signs** include headache, nausea, vomiting, increased blood pressure, bradycardia, papilledema, sixth cranial nerve palsy, transient impairment of vision, and alteration in the level of consciousness.

   B. **Herniation** is due to a pressure gradient that shifts brain tissue. The location of the pressure-producing lesion determines the clinical presentation.

1. **Diencephalic herniation** is caused by a medial supratentorial lesion that forces the diencephalon through the tentorial notch. This process produces (1) Cheyne-Stokes respirations, (2) small but reactive pupils, (3) paresis of upward gaze, and (4) altered mental status.

2. **Uncal herniation** is caused by a lateral supratentorial lesion that forces the medial portion of the temporal lobe (the uncus) through the tentorial notch. The subsequent pressure on midbrain structures results in (1) alteration of consciousness; (2) a dilated, unreactive pupil ipsilateral to the mass, from third nerve compression; and (3) hemiparesis on either side. Eye movements need not be impaired.

3. **Tonsillar herniation** results from pressure that forces the inferior portion of the cerebellum through the foramen magnum, compressing the medulla. This produces (1) altered consciousness and (2) respiratory irregularity or apnea.

II. **Treatment.** Neurosurgical intervention is the definitive treatment for some focal causes of acutely increased ICP, including epidural, subdural, and cerebellar hematomas. Surgery is not helpful for increased ICP following ischemic, anoxic, or metabolic brain necrosis. When increased ICP occurs in a neurosurgical candidate, forced hyperventilation and osmotic agents should be used to delay advancing herniation.

A. **Hyperventilation** using endotracheal intubation produces a fall in arterial PCO_2, thereby reducing cerebral blood flow. Arterial PCO_2 should be maintained at approximately 25 mm Hg. Peak effect occurs within 2–30 minutes.

B. **Osmotic agents,** including mannitol, glycerol, and urea, rely on an intact blood-brain barrier to draw water from the brain tissue compartment into the systemic vascular compartment. Mannitol should be infused IV as a 20% solution (100 g of mannitol in 500 ml of 5% D/W) over 10–20 minutes with a bolus of 1–2 g/kg and maintenance of 50–300 mg/kg IV q6h. A filter should be used to exclude crystals. Therapeutic effect begins within minutes, reaches a peak in about 90 minutes, and decreases over hours. These agents are generally used only in anticipation of more definitive treatment (e.g., evacuation of hematoma). **Complications of osmotic use include a rebound increase in ICP,** acute intravascular volume expansion with pulmonary edema or congestive heart failure, and osmotic diuresis with subsequent dehydration and hypernatremia.

C. **Corticosteroids** are effective in reducing the edema surrounding a tumor and may also be beneficial for trauma and abscess. Dexamethasone, 10 mg IV (or IM), is given initially, followed by 4 mg IV, IM, or PO q6h. Edema due to anoxia and infarction does not respond to steroids. (For a more complete discussion, see R. A. Fishman. *Cerebrospinal Fluid in Diseases of the Nervous System.* Philadelphia: Saunders, 1981.)

Head Injury

Treatment and prognosis of head trauma depend on the extent and pathologic type of brain injury. Clinical assessment must define the cause, type, location, and extent of injury.

I. **Assessment**

A. **History** should document the temporal course of all symptoms, particularly loss of consciousness. Amnesia is related to the severity of the blow and should diminish over time as the patient recovers.

B. **General physical examination** must establish whether the vital signs are stable and if other significant trauma is present.

C. **Neurologic examination** should be repeated at frequent intervals to document any progression of neurologic deficits.

D. **Radiography of the skull** (posteroanterior, Towne's, and lateral views) and cervical spine (open-mouth posteroanterior and lateral views, inclusive of C1–C7) should be obtained.

E. **Computed tomography** of the head should be obtained in patients with focal neurologic deficits, open or penetrating head trauma, depressed or comminuted skull fractures, or mental status abnormalities that are prolonged, progressive, of delayed onset, or suggestive of a focal lesion (e.g., aphasia).

II. **Treatment.** Proper treatment depends on the type of injury.

   A. **Concussion** is a transient abnormality of consciousness (e.g., loss of consciousness, confusion, agitation, amnesia) without focal motor or sensory impairment. Close observation for at least 24 hours, with or without hospitalization, is necessary because onset of intracranial hemorrhage and edema can be delayed.

   B. **Contusion** can be diagnosed by inspection (e.g., penetrating injury), CT scan, and clinical inference from focal neurologic signs. Patients with contusion should be observed in the hospital until stable (at least 24 hours). Prophylactic anticonvulsant therapy is suggested to minimize the risk of early (the first week) posttraumatic seizures, but long-term efficacy depends on individual risk factors (*N. Engl. J. Med.* 323:497, 1990).

   C. **Skull fractures require neurosurgical assessment.** Basilar skull fractures are diagnosed more reliably by the presence of otorrhea, rhinorrhea, hematotympanum, postauricular hematoma, and periorbital hematoma than by radiographs.

   D. **Epidural hematoma** is typically caused by a skull fracture crossing the path of a meningeal artery or vein. Precipitous deterioration often occurs after an initial asymptomatic period. Without immediate surgical evacuation, brain herniation will rapidly ensue.

   E. **Subdural hematoma** results from disruption of the dural venous sinuses or the veins passing from the brain to the dural sinuses. Signs may develop acutely or chronically.

      1. **Acute subdural hematoma** is a neurosurgical emergency.

      2. **Chronic subdural hematoma** is most common in aged, debilitated, and alcoholic patients, and those receiving anticoagulants. Antecedent trauma is often minimal. Symptoms tend to be nonspecific (e.g., headache, confusion, lethargy) and can fluctuate markedly. Small, bilateral subdural hematomas can be difficult to detect with CT scan, unless iodinated contrast material is given IV.

      3. **Spinal fracture and dislocation** are commonly seen with head trauma. In every instance of significant head trauma, the neck must be stabilized in a cervical collar until the integrity of the spine is established.

Spinal Cord Compression

I. **Presentation.** Spinal cord compression often presents with rapid functional deterioration. Difficulty walking, back pain, and incontinence are common presenting symptoms. Signs and symptoms of spinal injury may be secondary to nerve root compression (radicular signs) or spinal cord compression (myelopathic signs).

   A. **Radicular signs** follow the dermatomal and myotomal distributions of the nerve root and are helpful in localizing the lesion.

      1. **Pain** tends to be lancinating, shooting along the dermatome. Valsalva maneuvers and movement will often induce radicular pain.

      2. **Sensory loss** also follows the dermatome but need not be complete. A zone of hypersensitivity and paresthesias may exist between the normal and insensate regions.

      3. **Weakness** is restricted to the muscles supplied by the root. Tone is diminished, as radicular lesions affect the lower motor neuron.

      4. **Reflexes** are diminished at the level of the involved root but are unaffected elsewhere.

      5. **Bowel and bladder function** are impaired only if coccygeal roots are involved.

   B. **Myelopathic signs** (from cord compression) are characterized by the presence of a "level" above which function is preserved and below which function is compromised bilaterally ("para" distribution). The lowest normal dermatomal level indicates the spinal cord level of the lesion. Sensory testing usually affords the most exact clinical determination of lesion location.

1. **Pain** is often diffuse and poorly localized.
2. **Sensory loss** involves all modalities. A zone of hyperpathia and paresthesias, but with normal sensory thresholds, often separates normal from insensate areas.
3. **Weakness** tends to be diffuse and bilateral, involving all muscle groups below the level of the lesion. In slowly progressive lesions, tone is diminished in muscles at the level of the lesion (lower motor neuron sign) but increased in muscles below the level of the lesion (upper motor neuron sign). In acute lesions, tone is diminished throughout (spinal shock).
4. **Reflexes** in slowly progressive lesions are diminished at the level of the lesion but hyperactive below that level. In acute lesions (spinal shock), reflexes are diminished throughout.
5. **Incontinence** of bowel and bladder is a hallmark of spinal cord compression.

II. **Etiology**
   A. **Traumatic spinal injury.** Spinal injuries include fracture dislocations, pure fractures, and pure dislocations. Underlying cervical spondylosis increases the likelihood of cervical cord injury. The portions of the spine with greatest mobility are the levels most subject to trauma and include C1–C2, C4–C6, and T11–L2. **Whenever head injury is present, the neck should be stabilized until physical and radiologic examination have excluded cervical fracture or dislocation.** Treatment of spinal cord injury with methylprednisolone, 30 mg/kg IV bolus, followed by an infusion of 5.3 mg/kg/hour for 23 hours, improves neurologic recovery when administered within 8 hours of injury (*N. Engl. J. Med.* 322:1405, 1990). Immediate neurosurgical consultation should be obtained.
   B. **Spinal cord compression** from epidural metastases is a frequent complication of systemic cancer. The location of epidural metastatic lesions may be thoracic (68%), lumbosacral (16%), or cervical (15%). Breast, lung, and prostate are the most common primary tumor types; others include lymphoma, myeloma, melanoma, kidney, and gastrointestinal malignancies (*Ann. Neurol.* 3:40, 1978).
      1. **History** most commonly includes a complaint of pain (97%), either in the involved vertebra or in a radicular pattern. Weakness is a frequent (76%) complaint and often progresses gradually but may progress rapidly to paralysis. Sensory or autonomic disturbance is sometimes present.
      2. **Physical examination** may reveal vertebral tenderness with percussion or palpation. **Sensory loss** is often present (51%), involves pinprick as often as vibration or position, and usually localizes the lesion within two vertebral levels. Ataxia is occasionally the only clinical sign.
      3. **Ancillary diagnostic tests** should begin with plain x-rays of the spine, which reveal metastatic disease of the vertebral bodies at the level of the lesion in a high percentage of cases. MRI scanning or metrizamide myelography with follow up CT scan is often needed to determine the exact level and extent of the lesion. Neurosurgical consultation should be obtained prior to myelography, as acute decompensation can occur and may require emergency decompressive laminectomy.
      4. **Emergent intervention is imperative,** as neurologic progression may be rapid and irreversible.
         a. **Dexamethasone,** 10 mg IV followed by 4 mg IV q6h, should be started immediately. Higher doses may result in better pain relief but do not affect motor outcome (*Ann. Neurol.* 3:40, 1978; *Neurology* 39:1255, 1989).
         b. **Early radiation therapy** combined with high-dose steroids is usually recommended. Outcome correlates best with the condition of the patient when therapy is initiated; paralysis or autonomic dysfunction is a poor prognostic sign. Radiation therapy should be administered to the area of tumor in a field extending above and below the lesion in all patients who can tolerate the treatment.
         c. **Prompt decompression laminectomy** is indicated in several circumstances: (1) for complete obstruction of CSF if within 24 hours of neurologic deterioration; (2) with radiation-resistant cancer such as renal cell cancer or melanoma; (3) in patients who have already received

maximal radiation therapy to the involved area; (4) in patients without a tissue diagnosis of cancer; and (5) with rapid and relentless deterioration of neurologic function despite medical and radiation therapies.

Cerebrovascular Disease

I. **Ischemia and infarction. Cerebral ischemia** presents with the acute onset of a focal (i.e., within a specific vascular territory) neurologic deficit. **Infarction** occurs when ischemia is prolonged. Accurate localization of the site of ischemic damage is necessary for proper diagnosis and treatment. Systemic hypotension (e.g., due to cardiac arrhythmia or orthostasis) typically presents with syncope and rarely causes focal ischemia or infarction. However, when systemic hypotension is prolonged (e.g., cardiac arrest), infarction may occur in zones between major vascular territories or areas prone to hypoxic-ischemic damage.

A. **Assessment**

1. **History** should establish the pattern of onset and duration of symptoms. The abrupt onset of a focal deficit without a change in level of consciousness is characteristic of ischemia and infarction but may also occur with intracranial hemorrhage, tumor, or migraine. A history should be sought for systemic diseases that can cause stroke, such as cardiac disease predisposing to embolism, connective tissue disease, carcinoma, or IV drug abuse.

2. **General physical examination** should search for cardiac etiologies of cerebral embolism, such as atrial fibrillation, rheumatic valvular disease (particularly mitral stenosis), infective endocarditis, recent anteroseptal myocardial infarction, or ventricular aneurysm. Approximately one-fifth of cerebral infarctions result from cardiogenic embolism (*Arch. Neurol.* 46:727, 1989). Acute systemic illnesses frequently cause focal neurologic signs from a previous stroke to recur, mimicking acute ischemia. Carotid bruits do not accurately predict the side of greatest atherosclerosis or whether atherosclerosis is symptomatic.

3. **Neurologic examination** is the most accurate means of determining lesion location in acute ischemia or infarction.

   a. **Carotid circulation** lesions most commonly cause contralateral hemiparesis, hemisensory loss, or homonymous hemianopsia. Permanent or transient (**amaurosis fugax**) ipsilateral, monocular visual loss resulting from retinal ischemia may occur. **Conjugate eye deviation** away from the side of the hemiparesis indicates a lesion above the pons. **Aphasia** is caused by ischemia or the dominant cerebral hemisphere (i.e., the left hemisphere in right-handed patients and over 75% of left-handed patients); hemineglect results from nondominant hemisphere lesions. Dysarthria may occur with lesions of either hemisphere.

   b. **Vertebral-basilar circulation impairment** produces neurologic deficits referable to the brainstem or the occipital and temporal lobes. Those deficits referable to the brainstem include unilateral or bilateral weakness, sensory loss, diplopia, ataxia, nystagmus, dysarthria, hoarseness, dysphagia, hearing loss, and vertigo. Conjugate eye deviation toward the hemiparetic side occurs with brainstem disease or with active irritative (seizure) foci in the cerebral cortex. Cranial nerve signs contralateral to somatic signs (e.g., left facial weakness and right body weakness) occur with brainstem lesions. **Syncope** or light-headedness is due to a disorder of the cardiovascular system (e.g., postural hypotension, arrhythmia) rather than brainstem ischemia. Vertigo without other brainstem signs is usually due to labyrinthine or eighth nerve disease.

4. **Ancillary diagnostic tests** are often necessary in the evaluation of ischemia and infarction.

   a. **Computed tomography** is performed to exclude structural abnormalities (e.g., tumor, abscess, intracerebral hematoma, subdural hematoma, subarachnoid hemorrhage) that may present with symptoms similar to ischemia. Infarction is usually not evident on a noncontrast CT within the first 36 hours, while acute intracerebral hemorrhage is well seen. Hemorrhage into an infarct can develop 1–7 days after the infarction.

b. **Lumbar puncture** should be performed on all patients suspected of septic embolism from bacterial endocarditis. Meningeal infections with a variety of bacterial, spirochetal, and fungal agents can produce an inflammatory vasculitis that may present as a stroke. A CSF leukocytosis may precede fever, positive blood cultures, and other clinical clues of these diagnoses (*Stroke* 17:332, 1986; *Stroke* 18:544a, 1987).

c. **Laboratory tests** should include CBC, platelet count, clotting studies (PT, PTT), VDRL, and erythrocyte sedimentation rate (ESR) to screen for systemic causes of stroke such as polycythemia, blood dyscrasias, or connective tissue disease. **Serum chemistries,** including glucose and sodium, are mandatory. Metabolic abnormalities present with focal neurologic signs and a relatively intact sensorium.

d. **An electrocardiogram (ECG) and a chest radiograph** should be obtained on all patients. Two-dimensional echocardiography should be obtained if a cardiac source is suspected. In patients over age 50, two-dimensional echocardiography is warranted only if there is evidence of heart disease by history, examination, or ECG. The role of transesophageal echocardiography and contrast echocardiography is not yet defined.

e. **Angiography** may be used to diagnose vasculitis or intracranial atherosclerosis and is essential for the preoperative evaluation of candidates for endarterectomy (see sec. **I.B.2.b**). It is also indicated when the patient is young or poses a diagnostic dilemma. Noninvasive Doppler studies of the carotids are often used as a screen for significant stenosis.

B. **Treatment selection** must weigh several factors, including the likelihood that a cardiogenic embolus was causal, the vascular distribution of the lesion, circulation still at risk, and the general condition of the patient.

1. **Cardiogenic embolus** is an indication for full systemic anticoagulation. The aim of anticoagulant therapy is to prevent subsequent central nervous system (CNS) emboli; the timing for its use in acute stroke remains controversial and depends on the size of the infarct, associated hemorrhage, the presence of systemic hypertension, and the risk of recurrent embolism (*Arch. Neurol.* 46:727, 1989). Therapy should be continued for as long as the embolic source remains (see Chap. 17). Heparin is used acutely to prolong the partial thromboplastin time to 1.5–2.0 times normal. Warfarin is used for chronic anticoagulation (*J. Am. Coll. Cardiol.* 8:41b, 1986). Systemic hypertension is a relative contraindication to long-term anticoagulation, since the risk of intracranial hemorrhage is increased (see Chap. 17). Dipyridamole and warfarin in combination are more effective than warfarin alone in the prevention of embolism from prosthetic cardiac valves (*Mayo Clin. Proc.* 56:265, 1981; *Am. J. Cardiol.* 51:1537, 1983). Mitral valve prolapse (MVP) may be an embolic source, but appropriate treatment has not been defined.

2. **Transient ischemic attacks (TIAs)** are focal, are abrupt in onset, and usually last for 5–20 minutes; they may last as long as 24 hours. Signs of ischemia lasting longer than 24 hours and less than 7 days define reversible ischemic neurologic deficit (**RIND**). Approximately one-third of patients with TIA or RIND will experience cerebral infarction within 5 years. This risk is greatest immediately following the event and diminishes with time. **Treatment of TIA and RIND** is intended to decrease the risk of subsequent stroke. When cardiac disease and other systemic illnesses are not causal, TIA in patients older than 50 years is presumed to result from atherosclerotic disease of the cerebral vasculature and is treated with the following therapeutic measures:

a. **Aspirin** has been shown to reduce the incidence of stroke and death in prospective, randomized studies. Dosages ranged from 300 mg PO tid to 325 mg PO qid. Lower dosages (300 mg qd) have fewer adverse side effects (*Br. Med. J.* 296:316, 1988), but benefit has not been proved. Other antiplatelet agents (e.g., dipyridamole, sulfinpyrazone), alone or in combination with aspirin, are not effective. Ticlopidine (250 mg PO bid) is an alternative to aspirin for stroke prophylaxis (*N. Engl. J. Med.* 321:501, 1989).

b. **Carotid endarterectomy** decreases the risk of stroke and death in patients with recent TIAs or nondisabling strokes and ipsilateral high-grade (70–99%) carotid stenosis (*Stroke* 22:816, 1991; *N. Engl. J. Med.* 325:445, 1991). Benefit has not yet been documented in patients with either moderate symptomatic stenosis or asymptomatic stenosis of any degree. **Cerebral angiography** is the standard method for visualizing extracranial and intracranial vessels prior to surgery. In skilled hands, the combination of extracranial and intracranial Doppler for detecting high-grade stenosis and occlusion may prove useful as a preliminary, low-risk screening assessment.

c. **Anticoagulant therapy** in the treatment of TIA and RIND due to atherosclerosis is controversial. Randomized prospective studies have failed to show prevention of stroke or death. Chronic anticoagulation increases the risk of intracerebral hemorrhage.

d. **Extracranial-intracranial bypass grafting** is not beneficial in the treatment of intracranial atherosclerotic disease.

3. **Progressing stroke** refers to a stepwise progression of neurologic signs due to ischemia or infarction while the patient is under observation. Patients with progressing stroke can deteriorate quickly and require repeated neurologic assessment. Intravenous heparin may be beneficial in the treatment of ischemic, nonhemorrhagic, progressive stroke, but this is controversial (*Stroke* 19:10, 1988).

4. **Completed stroke** is a stable, nonprogressing neurologic deficit. Most progression is complete within the first 96 hours following onset of stroke. No therapy is known that reduces the extent of a completed event. The goal of treatment is the prevention of recurrence and rehabilitation.

a. **Risk factors, especially hypertension,** should be chronically treated. However, in acute stroke, reduction of blood pressure should be avoided, since blood vessel autoregulation is disturbed. Even very high levels of blood pressure should be left untreated, unless evidence of systemic end-organ damage is present such as proteinuria, hematuria, papilledema, or heart failure (see Chap. 4). Blood pressure elevation secondary to brain ischemia usually returns to normal levels within days without treatment.

b. **Aspirin and ticlopidine** reduce the incidence of stroke recurrence in patients with mild completed stroke. Anticoagulants have no role in therapy of stroke in the absence of a cardiogenic source.

c. **Endarterectomy** is indicated in some circumstances (see sec. **I.B.2.b**).

d. **Cerebral edema** following large infarctions is maximal at **24–72 hours** and may cause late deterioration. Medical therapy is usually not effective. Surgical decompression is indicated for cerebellar infarctions when edema causes brainstem compression. Surgical decompression is rarely helpful for infarctions of the cerebral hemispheres.

II. **Intracranial hemorrhages** arise in the intracerebral, subarachnoid, epidural, or subdural spaces. The latter two are discussed in association with head injury.

A. **Intracerebral hemorrhage** usually presents as the sudden onset of a focal neurologic deficit. Signs of sudden increase in intracranial pressure, including alteration in mental status, headache, and vomiting, are present when the hemorrhage is extensive. Focal deficits depend on location and size of the hemorrhage. With massive bleeding, brain herniation may occur (see Increased Intracranial Pressure). Intracerebral hemorrhage often cannot be distinguished clinically from cerebral ischemia without the aid of CT scan.

1. **Chronic systemic hypertension** is the most frequent cause. The locations of hypertensive intracerebral hemorrhage are basal ganglia (70%), pons (10%), cerebellum (10%), and cerebral white matter (10%). Less commonly, intracerebral hemorrhage results from trauma, anticoagulant therapy, saccular aneurysm, arteriovenous malformation, tumor, blood dyscrasia, angiopathy, or vasculitis.

2. **Treatment** consists of supportive care and correction of precipitating factors.
   a. **Systemic blood pressure** should be lowered gradually, over days, with close observation for evidence of cerebral ischemia. Normal vascular autoregulatory mechanisms are unpredictably impaired in chronically hypertensive patients.
   b. **Surgical consultation** should be obtained for patients with cerebellar hematomas, since brainstem compression or obstructive hydrocephalus may develop, requiring immediate surgical treatment. Superficial cerebral hematomas causing significant mass effect can be evacuated, sometimes with clinical improvement. Evacuation of deep cerebral hematomas is rarely beneficial.

B. **Subarachnoid hemorrhage (SAH)** can result from intracerebral hemorrhage, ruptured aneurysm, arteriovenous malformation, blood dyscrasia, head trauma, cocaine or amphetamine abuse, or tumor. Rupture of saccular or **"berry" aneurysms** caused by defects in the arterial media and internal elastic membrane is the most common cause. Other types of aneurysm include the fusiform aneurysm, thought to be secondary to atherosclerosis, and the mycotic aneurysm, from septic embolism. Sudden onset of severe **headache** may be the only symptom of subarachnoid hemorrhage. **Altered mental status** (including coma), fever, vomiting, nuchal rigidity, low back pain, focal neurologic deficits, seizures, and retinal hemorrhages (subhyaloid hemorrhages) also occur. ECG abnormalities are frequent (70%). **Complications** of SAH include rebleeding (20% at 2 weeks), vasospasm with ischemia (days 4–14), hydrocephalus, seizures, and the syndrome of inappropriate antidiuretic hormone (SIADH).

1. **Diagnosis is mandatory** when the history and physical examination suggest SAH.
   a. **Computed tomography** will show blood in the subarachnoid spaces of the sulci and cisternae in 90% of patients within the first 24 hours. Parenchymal and intraventricular hemorrhage can accompany SAH following the rupture of a saccular aneurysm, but suspicion of another etiology should be raised. The source of SAH, especially arteriovenous malformation, may be shown by CT after intravenous administration of iodinated contrast material, but most patients require angiography for definitive diagnosis.
   b. **Lumbar puncture** should be performed when the clinical impression of SAH is not confirmed by CT. When hemorrhagic CSF is obtained, immediate centrifugation should be done to look for a xanthochromatic (yellow) supernatant. Xanthochromia, resulting from RBC lysis, takes several hours to develop and indicates SAH rather than a traumatic lumbar puncture. If doubt still remains, comparison of the first and last specimens of CSF will show a significant decline in RBC count when the blood is from traumatic puncture, but not when it is from true SAH. (A handy approximation: An increase of 1 white blood cell is expected for every 700 red blood cells, and 1,000 red blood cells correspond with an increase of 1 mg/dl of protein.)
   c. **Angiography** is needed preoperatively to determine aneurysm size and location.

2. **Treatment of choice** for saccular aneurysm is surgical repair. Timing is controversial and depends on the clinical condition of the patient. Supportive measures to be used while awaiting surgery include bed rest, sedation, analgesia, and laxatives to prevent sudden increases in intracranial pressure or blood pressure. Only extreme elevations in blood pressure (diastolic > 130 mm Hg) should be treated. **Hypotension must be avoided**, as it may worsen ischemic deficits. Any reduction in blood pressure should be undertaken slowly and carefully. Cardiac monitoring is advised. **Nimodipine**, a calcium channel blocker, improves outcome in subarachnoid hemorrhage patients and seems to reduce the incidence of associated cerebral infarction with few side effects (*N. Engl. J. Med.* 308:619, 1983; *J. Neurosurg.* 68:505, 1988; *Br. Med. J.* 298:636, 1989). Recommended dosage is 60 mg PO q4h, for

21 days, initiated within 4 days of presentation. Volume expansion and induced hypertension can occasionally be used to reverse neurologic deterioration due to vasospasm. Aminocaproic acid (Amicar) increases the risk of complications without affecting outcome (*N. Engl. J. Med.* 311:432, 1984; *Neurology* 37:1586, 1987).

Seizures

Prolonged or recurrent generalized convulsions require prompt medical attention. Generalized seizure activity recurring before the patient's full recovery from the postictal state of the preceding seizure is referred to as generalized (tonic-clonic) status epilepticus. However, the patient with continual tonic-clonic activity clearly requires more aggressive treatment than the patient with two brief seizures separated by an hour. Other forms of status epilepticus do occur (simple partial, complex partial, absence) but are not life-threatening and are not discussed here. The goals of treatment of status epilepticus are to support vital functions, identify and treat the precipitating causes, treat or prevent complications of status epilepticus, and administer a full loading dose of a long-acting anticonvulsant. Rapid administration of a long-acting anticonvulsant drug requires intravenous administration, which has attendant risks. Patients not in status epilepticus should be given oral anticonvulsants. Thus, neither postictal lethargy following a single seizure nor recurrent seizures with intervening recovery of consciousness should be treated with intravenous anticonvulsants. (For a thorough discussion of the management of epilepsy, see T. R. Browne and R. G. Feldman. *Epilepsy: Diagnosis and Management.* Boston: Little, Brown, 1983.)

I. **Parenteral anticonvulsants**

   A. **Phenytoin** is the traditional drug of choice for treatment of status epilepticus due to its high efficacy, long duration of action, low incidence of serious complications, and frequent utility in chronic seizure management. **Intravenous phenytoin must be administered with a glucose-free solution to avoid precipitation.** The risk of soft-tissue injury can be minimized by using an IV site at the antecubital fossa or higher and infusing saline solution at a rapid rate during phenytoin administration. The infusion rate of phenytoin should not exceed 50 mg/minute for a total loading dose of 18–20 mg/kg. **Transient hypotension and heart block** may occur during intravenous phenytoin administration, particularly in elderly and debilitated patients; close monitoring of blood pressure and cardiac rhythm is necessary. These phenomena are a function of infusion rate and should not limit the total dose of phenytoin. Peak brain levels are achieved within 1 hour following administration. Daily maintenance dosage of phenytoin is 300–500 mg (4–8 mg/kg) PO or IV adjusted to maximize seizure control without toxicity. In most patients this can be accomplished with a plasma level of 10–20 µg/ml. Phenytoin should not be used in patients with known hypersensitivity.

   B. **Phenobarbital** may be used as an alternative for first-line treatment of status epilepticus (*Neurology* 38:202, 1988). It is also used when seizures recur despite a full loading dose of phenytoin; in this setting, patients should be intubated. Phenobarbital should be administered IV at a rate of 100 mg/minute to provide a loading dose of 10 mg/kg. For persistent seizures, additional phenobarbital may be given at a rate of 50 mg/minute IV to a maximum of 30 mg/kg. If phenobarbital is used as the first-line drug, adjunctive therapy with phenytoin is indicated if seizures persist. Arrhythmias and hypotension may occur, and the ECG and blood pressure should be continuously monitored during administration of phenobarbital. Peak plasma levels are achieved within 1 hour of intravenous administration. Maintenance dosages are 1–5 mg/kg/day PO or IV, to maintain a therapeutic plasma level of 15–40 mg/liter.

   C. **Diazepam** (5–10 mg IV) or lorazepam (2–4 mg IV), administered at a rate of 1–2 mg/minute, may be used to treat status epilepticus. They are used in patients with prolonged (over 5 minutes) generalized convulsive episodes and when loading doses of phenytoin and phenobarbital are unsuccessful. Brief, widely spaced convulsive episodes are not an indication for diazepam or lorazepam. Diazepam should not be mixed with IV fluids because of adherence to tubing.

D. When seizures persist despite the preceding measures, large doses of short-acting barbiturates should be given in consultation with an anesthesiologist. Pentobarbital, administered as a 15 mg/kg loading dose followed by 1 mg/kg/hour, is effective for the treatment of resistant status epilepticus (*Neurology* 38:395, 1988). Dopamine may be required to control drug-induced hypotension.

II. **Supportive measures.** Respiratory and cardiac functions must be monitored and supported. A soft, plastic oral or nasal airway should be placed atraumatically. Endotracheal intubation is often necessary, particularly when sedating anticonvulsants (e.g., diazepam and phenobarbital) are used. Care should be taken to prevent aspiration, suffocation, and self-inflicted trauma during convulsive episodes.

III. **Determination and treatment of the underlying cause.** A metabolic or structural abnormality can be identified in more than two thirds of cases of generalized status epilepticus. Common structural abnormalities include CNS tumor, posttraumatic injury, CNS infection, cerebral infarction, and perinatal brain injury. The most common precipitants of generalized status epilepticus are noncompliance with chronically administered oral anticonvulsants or intercurrent febrile illness. Other precipitants include alcohol and sedative drug withdrawal, drug intoxication (e.g., amphetamines, cocaine, isoniazid), electrolyte abnormalities (including hyponatremia and hypocalcemia), uremia, hypoglycemia, and anoxia. Prompt diagnosis and treatment of precipitating causes are mandatory to achieve seizure control and prevent brain damage.

IV. **Complications,** such as cerebral edema, aspiration, rhabdomyolysis, myoglobinuria, and hyperthermia, must be anticipated and treated as they arise.

Alcohol Withdrawal

Alcohol withdrawal has a significant risk of death and requires a high index of suspicion for diagnosis. **Manifestations** include tremulousness, hallucinosis, seizures, and delerium tremens. A reason for interruption of alcohol intake must be determined. Often, an illness (e.g., trauma, infection, pancreatitis, gastritis) has interfered with alcohol intake.

I. **Minor withdrawal** is characterized by tremulousness, irritability, anorexia, and nausea. Symptoms usually appear within a few hours after reduction or cessation of alcohol consumption and resolve within 48 hours. A well-lighted room, the presence of friends or relatives, and reassurance are important aspects of treatment. Many of the symptoms can be treated with **benzodiazepines,** including chlordiazepoxide, 25–100 mg PO q6h, or diazepam, 5–20 mg PO q6h. The goal of therapy is to sedate the patient until calm. The dosage must be titrated to the patient's clinical state. **Thiamine,** 100 mg IM qd for 3 days, followed by 100 mg PO qd, and multivitamins containing folic acid should be given. The patient should be observed for signs of major alcohol withdrawal; social circumstances dictate whether this should be done at home or in the hospital.

II. **Delirium tremens** is manifested by tremulousness, hallucinations, agitation, confusion, disorientation, and autonomic overactivity, including fever, tachycardia, and profuse perspiration. It usually occurs 72–96 hours after cessation of drinking and generally starts to resolve within 3–5 days. It is seen in 5–10% of cases of alcohol withdrawal and carries a mortality of 5%. Other causes of delirium must be considered in the differential diagnosis (see Acute Confusional States). Supportive management is identical to that for minor withdrawal. Physical restraints should be avoided if possible, but self-inflicted injury must be prevented.

A. **Chlordiazepoxide,** 100 mg IV or PO, repeated q2–6h as needed, with a maximum dose of 500 mg in the first 24 hours is an effective sedative in this situation. One-half the initial 24-hour dose may be administered over the next

24 hours; the dosage may be reduced by 25–50 mg/day each day thereafter. Liver dysfunction prolongs the half-life of chlordiazepoxide.

B. **Adjunctive antihypertensives** such as **clonidine and atenolol** may be used to attenuate withdrawal symptoms due to central noradrenergic overactivity (*Alcoholism* 9:238, 1985; *Acta Psychiatr. Scand.* [Suppl. 327] 73:131, 1986; *N. Engl. J. Med.* 313:905, 1985). Care must be taken to avoid hypotension. An initial dosage of clonidine, 0.1 mg PO qid, can be increased gradually to 0.2–0.4 mg qid if symptoms persist and blood pressure is stable. Atenolol is used in doses of 50–100 mg PO qd.

C. **Maintenance of fluid and electrolyte balance** is important, since these patients are susceptible to hypomagnesemia, hypokalemia, and hypoglycemia. Fluid losses may be considerable because of fever, diaphoresis, and vomiting. Other medical complications should be anticipated and treated.

III. **Withdrawal seizures.** Alcohol withdrawal seizures occur 12–48 hours after cessation of intake and are usually generalized motor seizures. Seizures are usually few in number and responsive to oral or intravenous benzodiazepines; if they are frequent, phenytoin or barbiturates can be effective in the acute setting (see Seizures, sec. I). Treatment of alcohol withdrawal seizures with chronic anticonvulsant drugs is not indicated. Neurologic and systemic illnesses that present with seizures, including head trauma, meningitis, and metabolic abnormalities, are common in alcohol abusers and must always be considered.

Acute Confusional States

Acute confusional states, also known as delirium or metabolic encephalopathy, are characterized by abnormal attention with perceptual, cognitive, and behavioral disturbances. They develop over hours to days and are characterized by fluctuations of consciousness, disorientation, incoherent speech, memory impairment, agitation, and altered circadian rhythms. Systemic causes include septicemia, drug intoxication, drug or alcohol withdrawal, thiamine deficiency, hepatic or renal failure, thyrotoxicosis or hypothyroidism, hypoxia, hypoglycemia, and electrolyte abnormalities. CNS infections (e.g., meningitis, encephalitis), subarachnoid hemorrhage, and head trauma can also present with delirium. A relatively mild systemic illness may produce delirium in a demented patient. Psychiatric illness generally does not cause severe confusion, disorientation, or an altered level of consciousness.

I. **Evaluation.** A detailed history and physical and neurologic examination must be performed. **Serum chemistries** should include electrolytes, ABGs, calcium, magnesium, ammonia, thyroid-stimulating hormone (TSH), BUN, and creatinine. **Toxicologic screening** of urine and blood should be performed. CT of the brain is needed when a structural lesion is indicated by the history (e.g., sudden onset indicating subarachnoid hemorrhage) or neurologic examination (e.g., focal signs). Lumbar puncture is indicated if fever is present or the cause of delirium is unclear. CT scan of the head should be performed prior to lumbar puncture if neurologic signs of increased intracranial pressure are present (see Increased Intracranial Pressure). The EEG shows slow activity with drug intoxication, encephalitis, and metabolic disturbances; low-voltage fast activity is seen in drug withdrawal. A radionuclide brain scan or MRI should be obtained when focal, cerebral encephalitis (e.g., from herpes simplex) is suspected.

II. **Treatment.** A quiet, well-lighted environment is best. Close observation is necessary. Sedatives can aggravate symptoms. If sedation is necessary, low doses of short-acting benzodiazepines or haloperidol may be used with caution. Haloperidol and phenothiazines may cause hypotension (especially in the elderly) and may lower the seizure threshold. Restraints are occasionally needed for patient safety. Care should be taken to avoid circulatory compromise from tight restraints.

Headache

Headache is a commonly treated outpatient problem. It can require emergency evaluation when (1) there is a debilitating sudden or recent change in the character or frequency of chronic headaches, (2) it coincides with the sudden onset of neurologic deficits or coma, (3) it occurs days to months after head trauma, or (4) it constitutes the "worst headache" ever experienced. Exacerbation of a primary headache syndrome must be differentiated from a secondary process.

I. **Etiology**

A. **Primary headache syndromes** include **migraines** with (classic) or without (common) aura, **tension headaches,** and **cluster headaches. Exertional headaches,** cough- and cold-induced headaches, and fleeting ice pick (stabbing) headaches are also considered within the same category after underlying structural lesions have been excluded. The etiology of primary headache syndromes is poorly understood. Some studies propose a disturbance in serotonergic neurotransmission as the etiology. (For a review of etiology, diagnosis, and treatment of headache, see Neil Raskin. *Headache.* New York: Churchill Livingstone, 1988; or *Neurol. Clin.* 8:4, 1990.)

B. **Secondary headache syndromes** can be caused by many disease processes. These are discussed in sec. **II.D.**

II. **Evaluation**

A. **Migraines** are commonly unilateral, pulsating or throbbing, with associated nausea, vomiting, and phonophotophobia. Duration varies from 4–72 hours. They tend to build over minutes to hours. Longer spells constitute intractable migraines or "status migrainosus." The aura of **classic migraine** is a transient visual, motor, sensory, cognitive, or psychic disturbance that usually lasts minutes and precedes or coincides with the headache. **Provoking factors** may be identified and include stress, hunger, fatigue, sleep deprivation or excess, physical exertion, bright light, alcohol, menstruation, pregnancy, oral contraceptives, foods (cheese, chocolate), and food additives (MSG, nitrites). Most migraine sufferers are female (> 60%) and have their first episode before 30 years of age.

B. **Muscle contraction or tension headache** is often diagnosed when headaches are chronic, bilateral, constricting, nonpulsatile, and associated with neck muscle rigidity. Stress and anxiety are common aggravating factors. Migrainous symptoms frequently overlap. Tension headaches typically occur daily, begin later in the day, and wax and wane in intensity.

C. **Cluster headaches** are more common in males, excruciatingly painful, unilateral, orbital and periorbital or temporal in location, and associated with unilateral autonomic dysfunction (lacrimation, ptosis, miosis, nasal congestion, or conjunctival injection). Alcohol and nitroglycerin are known precipitants during a cluster of headaches. Assuming an upright position may actually alleviate the discomfort (as opposed to napping in a darkened room with migraines). Periodicity is a hallmark of cluster headache, with pain often recurring daily at about the same hour. "Clusters" last days to weeks and recur at intervals of months to years.

D. **Secondary headache syndromes** have temporal profiles that depend on the underlying pathologic process. For example, subarachnoid hemorrhage causes the abrupt onset of severe pain, whereas cerebral tumors tend to cause a fluctuating, less severe pain of gradual onset, sometimes affected by posture. Age can also be helpful in defining the underlying disease process. The headache of temporal arteritis rarely begins before age 50, whereas the onset of migraines is uncommon after age 50. Focal neurologic signs beginning with or after the onset of headache or persistent neurologic signs suggest an underlying neurologic disorder. Those signs preceding a headache and resolving before or during the headache suggest classic migraine.

1. **Intracranial causes** include subdural hematoma, intracerebral hematoma, subarachnoid hemorrhage, arteriovenous malformation, brain abscess, men-

ingitis, encephalitis, vasculitis, obstructive hydrocephalus, post–lumbar puncture, and cerebral ischemia or infarction. Pain is due to traction on or inflammatory irritation of the pain-sensitive, large, intracranial vessels, basilar dura mater, and sensory cranial nerves. Headaches from intracranial disease do not follow any one stereotype.

2. **Extracranial causes** include sinusitis, disorders of the cervical spine, temporomandibular joint syndrome, giant cell arteritis, glaucoma, optic neuritis, and dental disease.

3. **Systemic causes** include fever, viremia, hypoxia, hypercapnia, systemic hypertension, allergy, anemia, caffeine withdrawal, and vasoactive chemicals, including nitrites and carbon monoxide.

4. **Depression** is a common cause of long-standing, treatment-resistant, daily headaches. Specific inquiry should be made about vegetative signs of depression.

5. **Examination** should reveal normal findings during asymptomatic intervals in patients with primary headache syndromes. Neurologic abnormalities should be presumed to indicate an underlying disorder that requires further investigation.

E. **Ancillary studies** are required when the history and examination indicate an underlying disorder.

III. **Treatment**

A. **Acute treatment** is aimed at aborting headache.

1. **Nonnarcotic analgesics.** Aspirin, nonsteroidal anti-inflammatory agents, or acetaminophen may abort a vascular or tension headache if taken early. Ketorolac tromethamine, 60 mg IM, is also effective. Naproxen sodium, 550 mg PR or PO bid–tid for migraines, and indomethacin, 50 mg PR or PO bid–tid for cluster headaches, are often helpful. The suppository forms are rapidly absorbed when nausea limits PO intake. Isometheptene mucate (Midrin) and butalbital with aspirin or acetaminophen (Fiorinal, Fibricet) have both sedative and analgesic properties.

2. **Ergotamine** is a vasoconstrictive agent that is effective in aborting primary vascular headaches, particularly if administered during the prodromal phase. Ergotamine should be taken at symptom onset in the maximum dose tolerated by the patient; nausea often limits the dose. The maximum dose is best determined during a headache-free interval. Efficacy depends on absorption rate; oral, sublingual, aerosol, and rectal preparations (in ascending order of efficacy) are available. Sublingual and oral forms are most convenient; an initial dose of 2–3 mg PO is appropriate. Additional doses of 1–2 mg can be taken q30min, up to a total dose of 8–10 mg, but these rarely succeed when an initial dose has failed. Rectal (2 mg) or aerosol (1–2 puffs) administration should be tried in patients unresponsive to sublingual or oral delivery or when emesis prevents oral administration. Dosages exceeding 16 mg/week should be used cautiously to avoid toxicity, which includes angina pectoris, limb claudication, and ergotamine headache and dependency.

3. **Dihydroergotamine (DHE)** is a potent venoconstrictor with minimal peripheral arterial constriction. It is an alternative to the ergots described above. Again, **cardiac precautions** are indicated in those with a history of angina, peripheral vascular disease, or greater than 60 years of age. A dose of 1–2 mg IM or SQ may abort a vascular headache before it reaches peak intensity. If an attack has climaxed, 5 mg of prochlorperazine may be given IV, followed immediately by 0.75 mg of DHE IV given over 3 minutes. If there is no relief in 30 minutes, another 0.5 mg of DHE IV is given. This relieves the primary headache in the majority of cases. For intractable migraines (status migrainosus), DHE can be given q8h with IV metoclopramide (see *Neurology* 36:995, 1986; *Neurol. Clin.* 8:587, 1990).

4. **Chlorpromazine,** 0.1 mg/kg IV q15min (up to 3 doses), or **prochlorperazine,** 10 mg IV, may terminate migraine. Acute dystonic reactions and hypotension are potential side effects. These drugs are especially useful in patients with severe nausea and emesis. Suppository forms are also available.

5. **Opioid analgesics,** such as codeine and meperidine, are sometimes required to abort severe headaches. Chronic, daily headaches should not be treated with narcotic analgesics in order to prevent habituation and loss of efficacy (see Chap. 1).

6. **Caffeine,** given as coffee, tea, or a tablet in combination with ergotamine (Cafergot), is a useful adjunct to migraine therapy.

7. **Environment** plays an important role in alleviating headache. A quiet, dark, noise-free environment can speed recovery. Sleep is often effective in aborting migraine.

8. **Sumatriptan** is also effective for acute management of vascular headaches (*N. Engl. J. Med.* 325:316, 1991).

B. **Prophylaxis** is used for recurrent headaches, particularly those not responsive to acute therapy.

1. **Tricyclic antidepressants** are effective in preventing migraine and tension headaches. The dose is titrated to patient tolerance and response, with an initial dosage of 10–25 mg of amitriptyline PO hs, for example. The effective dosage varies from 10–175 mg/day. Efficacy does not depend on the presence of depressive symptomatology.

2. **Propranolol** and beta antagonists can decrease the frequency of recurrent vascular headaches. Initial dosage of propranolol is 20 mg PO bid; effective dosage ranges widely among patients. Heart failure and bronchospasm are contraindications.

3. **Low-dose ergot preparations** may be used for migraine prophylaxis if amitriptyline and propranolol are ineffective or contraindicated. Ergonovine, 0.2 mg PO bid, or a combination of ergotamine, belladonna, and phenobarbital (Bellergal, 1–2 tablets PO bid) may be used.

4. **Prednisone** is a first-line drug in the treatment of cluster headache and is effective in most cases. An initial oral dosage of 60–80 mg/day for the first week should be followed by a rapid taper.

5. **Methysergide,** 2 mg PO qd–qid, is effective in the prevention of migraine and cluster headache. Retroperitoneal, pleural, and endocardial fibrosis are severe but reversible complications of chronic methysergide treatment that occur uncommonly (1 in 5,000 cases).

6. **Other pharmacotherapy** for refractory migraine includes phenelzine, a monoamine oxidase (MAO) inhibitor (45 mg/day), and calcium channel antagonists (sustained-release verapamil, 90–360 mg/day as tolerated and needed). Lithium, indocin, and verapamil are useful medications for cluster headache prophylaxis.

7. **Environmental prophylaxis** includes avoidance of precipitating foods, chemicals, activities, and situations. Relaxation training should be attempted for sufferers of recurrent stress-induced headaches.

Weakness

Weakness is a common complaint that may be due to dysfunction at any of five levels: (1) muscle, (2) neuromuscular junction, (3) peripheral nerve, (4) lower motor neuron, or (5) upper motor neuron. Identification of the level involved is crucial in forming the proper differential diagnosis. Several specific disorders may present as rapidly progressing, generalized weakness. Maintenance of respiration is essential (see Chap. 9), and aggressive supportive measures similar to those described for coma should be used if necessary (see Coma, sec. **IV**).

I. **Myasthenia gravis (MG)** is a disorder of the neuromuscular junction resulting from autoimmune damage to the nicotinic cholinergic receptor. It is often associated with abnormalities of the thymus and is characterized by weakness and fatigability. The weakness is typically worse after exercise and better after rest, but a constant weakness may occur. **Presenting signs** include ptosis, diplopia, dysarthria, dysphagia, extremity weakness, and respiratory difficulty. Women outnumber men with the disease; it tends to occur in young women (third decade) and older men (fifth to sixth decade). The clinical course is variable; spontaneous remissions and exacerbations occur. Progressive deterioration is more likely to occur in the first 3 years. The differential diagnosis includes botulism and the Eaton-Lambert syndrome, a neuromuscular defect associated with carcinoma.

A. **Diagnosis** is usually evident from the history and physical examination. Ancillary tests may be useful in confirming the diagnosis.

    1. **Edrophonium (Tensilon) test.** Edrophonium often produces a marked improvement of strength in myasthenic patients. **A test dose** of 2 mg IV is given; if no reaction occurs after 45 seconds, an additional 3 mg is injected. If no reaction occurs after 45 seconds, the remaining 5 mg is given, for a total dose of 10 mg. An extraocular palsy or the muscle action potential (which cannot be voluntarily influenced) should be observed before and after each injection. The response to edrophonium lasts approximately 5 minutes. Because edrophonium may produce **severe bradycardia**, atropine should be available for treatment and vital signs monitored during the test.

    2. **Electromyogram.** The myasthenic muscle action potential shows a decremental response to repetitive nerve stimulation. In botulism and the Eaton-Lambert syndrome, the response is incremental.

    3. **Antibody levels** (anti–acetylcholine receptor and antistriatal) lend further support to the diagnosis. Chest x-ray or CT of the thorax is necessary to exclude thymoma.

B. **Treatment of MG** follows no specific protocol. The clinician must choose among modalities based on symptoms, life-style, and response to treatment. A rapid deterioration in respiratory and swallowing functions necessitates aggressive support, therapy, and correction of precipitating causes (e.g., infection, thyroid dysfunction).

    1. **Anticholinesterase drugs** can produce symptomatic improvement in all forms of MG. Pyridostigmine should be started at 30–60 mg PO tid–qid and subsequently titrated to the minimum amount providing symptom relief. Occasional patients require dosing as frequently as q2–3h. Neostigmine methylsulfate, 0.5 mg IM q3–4h, can also be used.

    2. **Immunosuppressive drugs** are often effective when cholinesterase inhibitors alone fail. **Prednisone** is frequently used to alter the natural course of the disease. Improvement is more rapid with high-dose daily regimens, but an initial exacerbation of weakness occurs in many patients and hospitalization is advised. A dosage of 60–80 mg qd for 1–2 weeks, followed by an alternate-day regimen and slow (months) taper to the lowest effective dose, may be used. Initiation of therapy with alternate-day low-dose regimens may also be used; dosages of prednisone are then gradually increased as needed; onset of beneficial effect may be delayed, but there is reduced risk of early exacerbation. Hospitalization and close observation are advised when initiating steroids. Potential risks of steroid treatment (see Chap. 24) need to be weighed against observed clinical benefit on an individual basis. **Azathioprine,** 1–2 mg/kg PO qd, is an alternative drug for those who do not respond to steroids or cannot tolerate steroids. Onset of benefit is usually delayed for at least 2 months. **Side effects** include leukopenia, pancytopenia, infection, gastrointestinal irritation, and abnormal liver function tests (see Chap. 24). Cyclophosphamide, cyclosporine, and intravenous gamma globulin have been beneficial in select refractory patients.

    3. **Thymectomy** is effective treatment for generalized or disabling ocular MG and produces complete remission in many patients. Transsternal thymectomy should be carried out in patients with moderate to marked generalized myasthenia, early in the course of their disease, and especially if response to medical treatment is unsatisfactory. Thymoma is an absolute indication for surgery. Thymectomy is controversial in children, adults older than 60 years, and purely ocular myasthenia gravis.

    4. **Plasmapheresis** is used in the treatment of acute exacerbations, impending crisis, disabling myasthenia refractory to other therapies, and prior to surgery where postoperative deterioration is possible. Benefits are temporary,

and there is a lack of general agreement about exact indications and protocol. Hypotension and thromboembolism are potential complications.

  5. Precipitating factors should be treated. These include infection, pregnancy, thyroid dysfunction, and drug reaction. Quinidine, quinine, aminoglycosides, polymyxin, bacitracin, colistin, procainamide, phenytoin, propranolol, curare, and ether can worsen weakness in patients with MG.

- **C. Myasthenic crisis,** the need for assisted ventilation and/or airway protection, occurs in about 10% of patients with MG. Patients with bulbar and respiratory muscle weakness are particularly prone to respiratory failure. Respiratory infection and surgery (e.g., thymectomy) can precipitate crisis. Patients at risk should have pulmonary function closely monitored. Respiratory support follows the guidelines given in Chap. 9. Anticholinesterases should be temporarily withdrawn from patients receiving ventilation support; this avoids uncertainties about overdosage ("cholinergic crisis") and avoids cholinergic stimulation of pulmonary secretions. A 2-mg test dose of edrophonium IV should worsen symptoms due to cholinergic oversupply. Steroids or plasmapheresis may be helpful. Thymectomy is not part of emergency treatment of MG.

II. Guillain-Barré syndrome (GBS)

- **A. Presentation** is typically a rapidly progressive, ascending paralysis. Proximal weakness may be pronounced. Cranial nerves, especially the facial nerves, may be involved. Sensory symptoms may be present, but objective sensory loss is uncommon. Reflexes are usually hypoactive or absent. CSF protein is usually elevated (especially immunoglobulin G [IgG]), without pleocytosis. Lymphocytes, usually less than 20/μl, may be seen. Differential diagnosis includes arsenic exposure, acute porphyria, collagen vascular disease, tick paralysis, botulism, AIDS, and postdiphtheritic paralysis. A viral or diarrheal illness or exposure to Epstein-Barr virus, cytomegalovirus, *Campylobacter,* hepatitis, or HIV may precede this acute polyneuritis.

- **B. Treatment** is supportive (see Coma, sec. **IV**). Plasmapheresis is beneficial when carried out early in those who are severely compromised or worsening (loss of ambulation, respiratory failure). Indications for plasmapheresis in mild forms of stable and improving GBS are less clear (*Neurology* 35:1096, 1985; *Ann. Neurol.* 22:753, 1987; *Ann. Neurol.* 23:347, 1988). Corticosteroids, immunosuppressive drugs, and other agents are not of proven value in acute idiopathic demyelinating polyneuropathy (GBS).

  1. Respiratory function must be closely monitored. Respiratory assistance may be necessary and should be anticipated.

  2. Autonomic neuropathy can cause fatal overactivity or underactivity of autonomic functions. There is no uniform approach to the treatment of autonomic dysfunction; only general therapeutic guidelines can be given.

  a. Paroxysmal hypertension should be managed with short-acting agents that can be titrated against the patient's blood pressure (see Chap. 4). Hypotension is usually caused by decreased venous return and peripheral vasodilatation. Patients on respirators, who already have compromised venous return, are particularly prone to hypotension. Treatment consists of intravascular volume expansion with IV fluids. Occasionally, vasopressors may be required (see Chap. 8).

  b. Cardiac arrhythmias have been implicated as a significant cause of mortality in GBS; thus, cardiac monitoring is necessary. Bradyarrhythmias (sinus arrest or complete heart block) as well as tachyarrhythmias are frequent. Hypoxia and electrolyte abnormalities should be excluded as causes of cardiac arrhythmias.

III. Polymyositis and dermatomyositis may present with rapidly progressive, proximal muscle weakness. Less than one-half of patients with polymyositis have associated muscle pain, and approximately one-third have an elevated ESR. Other causes of acquired myopathies should be considered. In the initial evaluation, it is important to measure electrolytes, particularly potassium, calcium, and phosphate. Thyroid function, BUN, creatine kinase, and antinuclear antibodies should also be evaluated (see Chap. 24).

IV. Botulism is a disorder of the neuromuscular junction caused by ingestion of an exotoxin produced by *Clostridium botulinum*. The exotoxin interferes with release of acetylcholine from presynaptic terminals at the neuromuscular junction as seen with Eaton-Lambert syndrome.

    A. Symptoms begin within 12–36 hours of ingestion and include **autonomic dysfunction** (xerostomia, blurred vision, bowel and bladder dysfunction) followed by **cranial nerve palsies** and weakness.

    B. Management includes removing nonabsorbed toxin with **cathartics,** neutralizing absorbed toxin with **equine trivalent antitoxin,** 1 vial IV and 1 vial IM (after normal intradermal horse serum sensitivity test), and **supportive care.**

Tetanus

I. Definition. Tetanus is characterized by generalized (occasionally localized) muscle spasm (especially trismus) due to the exotoxin (tetanospasmin) of *Clostridium tetani.* The incubation period ranges from 2–54 days. In the majority of patients, the date of onset is within 14 days from the time of injury. Tetanus often follows puncture wounds, lacerations, and crush injuries but may also occur without a demonstrable wound. Tetanus may be seen in parenteral drug abusers, particularly heroin addicts who inject subcutaneously. Mortality may be as high as 50–60%; most deaths occur in the first 10 days.

II. Management. The goals of therapy are to remove the source of toxin, to neutralize toxin not yet fixed to the nervous system, to prevent respiratory compromise, and to treat muscle spasm. The intensity of muscle spasms begins to diminish during the second week. Complete recovery may take several months.

    A. Toxin production is eliminated by cleaning and debriding the infected site. Penicillin G, 2 million units IV q6h for 10 days, should be given. Tetracycline (2 g/day) or erythromycin may be used in patients allergic to penicillin.

    B. Toxin neutralization is achieved by administration of 3,000–10,000 units of human tetanus immune globulin distributed intramuscularly among several sites proximal to the suspected source of exotoxin. Active immunization is needed after the acute illness (see Appendix E, Tables E-1 and E-2).

    C. Muscle spasms are managed with diazepam and/or barbiturates or with chlorpromazine. The patient should be kept in quiet isolation. The optimum level of continuous sedation is achieved when the patient remains sleepy but can be aroused to follow commands. Refractory spasms may necessitate curariform drugs and ventilatory support. Painful tonic contractures require analgesia.

    D. Supportive measures include ECG monitoring, since cardiac arrhythmias and fluctuations in blood pressure occur. Endotracheal intubation or tracheostomy is needed to prevent asphyxiation during laryngospasm. Care of the immobile patient is outlined under Coma, sec. **IV.**

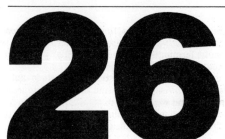

Medical Emergencies

Daniel Goodenberger

This chapter outlines an approach to medical urgencies and emergencies not covered elsewhere. Medical emergencies may not allow time for orderly information-gathering and formulation of a narrow differential diagnosis prior to initiation of therapy. **The first responsibility** is to provide basic life support (i.e., maintain an intact airway, adequate ventilation, and circulation).

Acute Upper Airway Obstruction

In the **conscious patient,** manifestations may include stridor, impaired or absent phonation, sternal or suprasternal retractions, display of the universal choking sign, and respiratory distress. Urticaria, angioedema, fever, or evidence of trauma may be present. The **unconscious patient** may have labored breathing or apnea. Airway obstruction should always be suspected in a nonbreathing patient whom rescuers find difficult to ventilate. **Differential diagnosis** includes trauma to the face and neck, foreign body, infection (croup, epiglottitis, Ludwig's angina, retropharyngeal abscess, and diphtheria), tumor, angioedema, laryngospasm, anaphylaxis, retained secretions, or blockage of the upper airway by the tongue in the unconscious patient. **Therapy** is directed at rapid relief of obstruction to prevent cardiopulmonary arrest and anoxic brain damage.

I. **Partial obstruction in the awake patient with adequate ventilation** requires rapid history-taking. A directed physical examination includes examination for airway swelling, trismus, pharyngeal obstruction, respiratory retractions, angioedema, stridor, wheezing, and grossly swollen lymph nodes and masses in the neck. Indirect laryngoscopy or fiberoptic nasopharyngolaryngoscopy may be performed if the patient is stable. Adults are unlikely to experience acute airway obstruction as the result of a careful examination. Soft tissue x-ray of the neck (posteroanterior and lateral view) is less sensitive and specific than direct examination but may be a valuable adjunct. It should be performed in the emergency department as a portable study, as the patient should not be left unattended. **Treatment** is aimed at the underlying disease process; the patient is carefully observed, and the physician must be prepared to intervene to maintain an airway.

II. **Airway obstruction in the awake patient without ventilation.** The most likely causes are a foreign body (usually food) and angioedema. Other causes include infection or posttraumatic hematoma. History is usually unavailable. The **Heimlich maneuver** (subdiaphragmatic abdominal thrust) should be performed repeatedly (6–10 times) (*J.A.M.A.* 255:2915, 1986). If this is unsuccessful, the patient will become unconscious (see sec. **III**).

III. **Airway obstruction in an unconscious patient without intact ventilation** may be seen in coma with obstruction of the upper airway by the tongue, foreign body, trauma, infection, or angioedema. A history is often unavailable except from paramedics or relatives. Examination reveals an unresponsive patient with no air movement or paradoxical respiratory efforts. **The first maneuver** should be head tilt with chin lift if cervical spine trauma is not suspected. This will clear the upper airway of the tongue and jaw. If cervical spine trauma is suspected, the best maneuver is application of a jaw thrust (see Chap. 8). If these maneuvers are effective and well tolerated, an oral or nasal airway may be placed. If they are ineffective, an attempt should be made to ventilate the patient with a bag-valve-mask apparatus. If this is unsuccessful, the oro- and hypopharynx should be rapidly examined. A blind finger sweep should be avoided in a well-equipped emergency department or hospital. **Direct examination** using a laryngoscope and McGill forceps should be undertaken. The supine Heimlich maneuver (straddling the supine patient and applying 6–10 subdiaphragmatic thrusts) may be attempted (*J.A.M.A.* 255:2915, 1986) if laryngoscopy cannot be performed immediately or a foreign body is suspected. If this fails, direct laryngoscopy and endotracheal intubation should be attempted. If the patient cannot be intubated, establishing a surgical airway becomes crucial. If a surgeon is not immediately available, needle cricothyrotomy using a 12- to 16-gauge over-the-needle catheter may be performed. A standard pediatric endotracheal tube adaptor will fit in the hub of the catheter, but it is difficult to provide adequate tidal volumes with a resuscitation bag. A high-flow oxygen source (50 psi) may be successful in ventilating the patient (*Ann. Emerg. Med.* 17:690, 1988). However, inappropriate catheter placement or high airway pressures may result in pneumomediastinum and tension pneumothorax. Surgical cricothyrotomy is rapid and simple, can be performed by nonsurgical physicians with appropriate training, and is the procedure of choice (*Textbook of Advanced Cardiac Life Support,* American Heart Association, 1987). An endotracheal tube may be placed through the incision. Emergency tracheostomy is inappropriate for management of complete airway obstruction.

Shock

Shock is a state of inadequate tissue perfusion and rapidly results in death if untreated. While systolic blood pressure may vary, it is most often below 80 mm Hg. Shock may be diagnosed at higher pressures when there are clinical signs of poor organ perfusion, including cool, clammy skin, altered mental status (ranging from confusion to coma), diminished urine flow, and poor capillary refill.

I. **Causes** can be conveniently categorized into several groups.
   A. **Cardiogenic shock** is the result of poor pump function and may be due to myocardial infarction, acute valvular dysfunction, acute ventricular septal defect, and dysrhythmias.
   B. **Extracardiac obstructive shock** occurs with pulmonary embolus and cardiac tamponade.
   C. **Oligemic shock** is the result of hemorrhage, gastrointestinal fluid loss (e.g., from dysentery), and other causes of dehydration (acute burns, diabetes insipidus).
   D. **Distributive shock** is due to diminished systemic vascular resistance with a normal or increased cardiac output. This may occur with sepsis, anaphylaxis, spinal shock, neurogenic shock, or drug overdose. Diabetic ketoacidosis, adrenal insufficiency, and hypopituitarism can also cause shock.

II. **Diagnostic studies** may include CBC, electrolytes, creatinine, coagulation studies, type and cross match, arterial blood gases, electrocardiogram, examination of the stool and nasogastric contents for blood, cultures of appropriate body fluids, appropriate endocrine studies, ventilation-perfusion lung scan, and echocardiogram. Hemodynamic monitoring may be useful in management.

III. **Therapy.** Maintenance of airway and ventilation is essential. Patients in shock should be managed in an intensive care unit, with appropriate cardiac and hemodynamic monitoring.
   A. **Volume resuscitation** must be undertaken promptly in all cases except for cardiogenic shock.
      1. **The pneumatic antishock garment (PASG),** with sequential inflation of legs and abdominal compartments to 15–40 mm Hg, may be temporizing in extracardiac, oligemic, distributive, and mixed states of shock. **PASG is contraindicated in cardiogenic shock.** Its beneficial effects are due to an increase in peripheral systemic vascular resistance (*Ann. Emerg. Med.* 11:409, 1982; *Ann. Emerg. Med.* 15:886, 1986; *Am J. Emerg. Med.* 1:7, 1983; *J. Trauma* 21:931, 1981).

    2. Trendelenburg's position increases venous return and cardiac index (*J. Trauma* 26:718, 1986).

    3. Fluid resuscitation must be prompt and should be given through large-bore catheters placed in large peripheral veins. Placement of central venous catheters may cause a delay in venous access. In the absence of overt signs of congestive heart failure, the patient should receive a 500-ml initial bolus of normal saline, with further infusions adjusted to achieve adequate blood pressure and tissue perfusion. There is no clear advantage of colloid over crystalloid for intravascular volume expansion; however, this may require more than 4 times as much Ringer's lactate as albumin (*Crit. Care Med.* 17:1078, 1989). When shock is due to hemorrhage, packed red blood cells should be given as soon as feasible. When hemorrhage is massive, type-specific unmatched blood can be given safely. Rarely, type O blood may be needed. Clotting factors should be replaced as needed with fresh frozen plasma. When hemorrhage causes shock, initial volume requirements may be large.

B. Vasopressors (see Appendix C) are indicated for obvious cardiogenic or anaphylactic shock and for patients in shock who fail to respond to volume administration (see Chap. 6).

    1. Dopamine (see Chap. 6) is the pressor of first choice except in cyclic antidepressant and phenothiazine overdoses.

    2. Norepinephrine (2–8 μg/minute) has predominantly alpha-adrenergic effects that result in peripheral vasoconstriction and lesser chronotropic and inotropic response. Side effects include dysrhythmias and peripheral ischemia.

    3. Dobutamine (1–10 μg/kg/minute) is the agent of choice to increase cardiac output in a low cardiac output state.

    4. Amrinone (an alternative to dobutamine) is prepared by adding 500 mg to 150 ml of normal saline for a final volume of 250 ml. A loading dose of 0.75 mg/kg is given over 2–3 minutes, with infusion following at 5–10 μg/kg/minute.

    5. Isoproterenol (1–4 μg/minute) should be **used only for profound atropine-unresponsive bradycardia pending pacemaker placement** (see Chap. 7 for other indications for isoproterenol). It is associated with substantial side effects, including dysrhythmias and reduction in coronary perfusion due to peripheral vasodilation.

C. Sodium bicarbonate should be used only when a pH of less than 7.2 interferes with the effectiveness of vasopressors. Inappropriate bicarbonate use may diminish peripheral tissue oxygen delivery and contribute to central nervous system acidosis.

D. Antibiotics should be administered empirically when sepsis is suspected, and **glucocorticoids** should be given when adrenal insufficiency is suspected, after baseline cortisol levels are drawn.

Anaphylaxis and Anaphylactoid Reactions

Anaphylaxis is the result of an IgE-mediated acute allergic reaction in a sensitized individual. Death from anaphylaxis occurs; penicillin (parenteral) and Hymenoptera stings are the most common causes. Other causes include local anesthetics, other antibiotics, serum, and food products. **Anaphylactoid reactions** result from the direct release of mediators. Responsible agents include intravenous radiographic contrast reagents, salicylates, and other nonsteroidal anti-inflammatory drugs.

I. Clinical manifestations are the same for both mechanisms. Onset may be immediate or delayed. Manifestations include pruritus, urticaria, angioedema, respiratory distress (due to laryngeal edema, laryngospasm, or bronchospasm), hypotension, and abdominal pain. Hypotension and shock may be due to hypoxemia, vasodilation, and capillary leak. The most common mode of death is airway obstruction, followed by hypotension.

II. Treatment
   A. Management of the airway is the first priority. If the patient cannot be ventilated, an endotracheal tube should be placed and ventilation begun with 100% oxygen. If laryngeal edema is not rapidly responsive to epinephrine and endotracheal intubation is unsuccessful, surgical airway management may be necessary (see Acute Upper Airway Obstruction).

   B. Epinephrine is the cornerstone of therapy and is given in a dosage of 0.3–0.5 mg (0.3–0.5 ml of 1:1,000 solution) SQ and repeated twice at 20-minute intervals if necessary. Patients with major airway compromise or hypotension may be given epinephrine sublingually (0.5 ml of 1:1,000), in a femoral or internal jugular vein (3–5 ml of 1:10,000), or via endotracheal tube (3–5 ml of 1:10,000). For severe reactions not immediately responsive to these measures, an epinephrine drip may be useful. One milligram is diluted in 250 ml D5W, and the infusion is begun at 0.1 μg/kg/minute, titrating to blood pressure. Patients taking beta-adrenergic antagonists may require glucagon (see sec. **II.I**).

   C. Volume expansion with 500–1000 ml of crystalloid or colloid, followed by titration to blood pressure and urine output, may be used in addition to epinephrine and glucagon to treat hypotension. The **PASG** may also be useful when the blood pressure is persistently less than 80 mm Hg (*Ann. Emerg. Med.* 13:189, 1989).

   D. Inhaled beta-agonists. Metaproterenol, 0.3 ml, or albuterol, 0.5 ml in 2.5 ml normal saline should be used to treat resistant bronchospasm.

   E. Aminophylline is a second-line drug (see Appendix C).

   F. General measures include delay of absorption of the offending antigen. When the allergen has been injected, slight constriction (constricting pressure less than arterial pressure) and local epinephrine injection at the affected site may be useful. The patient should be carefully examined; honeybee stingers are removed by gentle scraping, not squeezing. For orally ingested antigens, activated **charcoal** (50–100 g) with 1–2 g/kg (maximum 150 g) of sorbitol or 300 ml of magnesium citrate may decrease absorption of the antigen from the gastrointestinal tract. **Emesis is not indicated.**

   G. Antihistamines (e.g., diphenhydramine, 25–50 mg PO or IM q6h) do not have an immediate effect, but they may shorten the duration of the reaction. For persistent or recurrent symptoms, addition of an H_2-antagonist (e.g., cimetidine, 300 mg q6h IV) may be useful.

   H. Glucocorticoids have no significant effect for 6–12 hours. However, they may prevent recurrence or relapse of severe reactions. Hydrocortisone, 125 mg IV q6h, is an adequate dosage.

   I. Glucagon, given as a 10-mg bolus followed by a drip of 2–8 mg/hour, provides direct inotropic support for patients taking beta-antagonists (*Ann. Intern. Med.* 105:65, 1986; *Am. J. Emerg. Med.* 2:518, 1984). **Beta-adrenergic antagonist** therapy increases the risk of anaphylaxis and anaphylactoid reactions and makes the anaphylactic state more resistant to beta-adrenergic therapy (*Ann. Intern. Med.* 115:270, 1991; *J. Allergy Clin. Immunol.* 68:125, 1981; *Ann. Allergy* 47:35, 1981). Alpha-agonist vasopressors should be avoided, as they may prolong the anaphylactic state.

III. Observation.
Patients with mild to moderate reactions (urticaria or very mild bronchospasm) should be observed for a minimum of 6 hours. Patients with moderate to severe reactions (especially with orally ingested antigens) may relapse and should be **admitted to the hospital** (with close monitoring if there has been severe bronchospasm, laryngeal edema, hypotension, or rhythm disturbances).

IV. Prevention of recurrence.
If the allergen is identified, it should be avoided in the future. Patients who require **radiocontrast administration** despite a previously documented reaction should be given low ionic strength contrast. In addition, the patient should receive prednisone, 50 mg PO q6h for 3–4 doses (the last taken 1 hour before the procedure), and diphenhydramine, 50 mg PO 1 hour before the procedure. Advanced cardiac life support capability must be present in the radiology suite. Those who have had severe Hymenoptera reactions should receive epinephrine self-injection kits with adequate instructions. The patient should be referred to an allergist for evaluation and potential desensitization.

Near-Drowning

Drowning accounts for approximately 8,000 deaths/year, 40% of which occur in children less than 4 years of age. **Predisposing factors** include youth, inability to swim, alcohol and drug use, barotrauma (in scuba diving), head and neck trauma, and loss of consciousness associated with epilepsy, diabetes, syncope, or dysrhythmias. Near-drowning, defined as survival for at least 24 hours after submersion in a liquid medium, is more common.

I. **Pathophysiology.** Electrolyte abnormalities, hemoglobin concentration, volume status, and frequency of lung injury are similar for fresh- and salt-water drownings (*Chest* 70:231, 1976). **Major insults** (i.e., hypoxemia and tissue hypoxia, acidosis, and hypoxic brain injury with cerebral edema) are common to both. Hypothermia, pneumonia, and, rarely, disseminated intravascular coagulation (DIC), acute renal failure, and hemolysis also occur.

II. **Treatment** begins with resuscitation, focusing on airway management and ventilation with 100% oxygen. An IV should be established with normal saline or Ringer's lactate. The Heimlich maneuver is not indicated unless upper airway obstruction is present.

A. **The cervical spine should be immobilized,** since trauma may be present.

B. **Hypothermia** should be vigorously treated (see Environmental Illness).

C. **Management of pulmonary complications** includes administration of 100% oxygen, with titration by arterial blood gases. Endotracheal intubation and mechanical ventilation, positive end-expiratory pressure, and bronchodilators should be used if needed. Bronchoscopy is not routinely needed.

D. **Antibiotics should be reserved for documented infection.** Prophylactic glucocorticoids have no role (*Heart Lung* 16:474, 1987).

E. **Metabolic acidosis** is managed with mechanical ventilation, sodium bicarbonate (for a persistent pH less than 7.2), and blood pressure support.

F. **Cerebral edema** may occur suddenly within the first 24 hours and is a major cause of death. Although treatment of cerebral edema does not appear to increase survival (*Crit. Care Med.* 14:529, 1986), intracranial pressure monitoring is recommended if there is CT evidence of cerebral edema or if the Glasgow coma scale is 7 or below (see Chap. 25). There is no evidence supporting use of glucocorticoids, and extrapolation of data from head trauma patients argues against their routine administration. Induction of a barbiturate "coma" in near-drowning is not supported by data.

III. **Observation.** Patients who have survived severe episodes of near-drowning should be admitted to an intensive care unit. Those with less severe initial immersions may still develop noncardiogenic pulmonary edema. Any pulmonary signs or symptoms mandate admission, including cough, bronchospasm, abnormal arterial blood gas, or abnormal chest x-ray. The asymptomatic patient with a questionable or brief episode may be observed for 4–6 hours and discharged if chest x-ray and arterial blood gas are normal. However, if there is a documented long submersion, initial cyanosis or apnea, or even brief requirement for resuscitation, the patient must be **admitted for at least 24 hours.**

Environmental Illness

I. **Heat illness** is due to exposure to increased ambient temperature under conditions in which the body is unable to maintain appropriate homeostasis. The milder syndromes are exertional; the most severe may occur without exercise.

A. **Heat cramps** occur in unacclimatized individuals engaging in vigorous exercise in the heat. They are caused by salt depletion with hypotonic fluid replacement. Cramps occur in large muscle groups that have been in use, most often in the legs. Examination of the patient reveals moist, cool skin, a normal body temperature, and minimal distress. **Treatment** includes rest in a cool environment and salt replacement with a 650-mg sodium chloride tablet in 500 ml of water PO or a commercially available, oral, balanced electrolyte replacement solution. Intravenous therapy is rarely required, but 2 liters of normal saline administered over several hours will cure the syndrome.

B. Heat exhaustion occurs in an unacclimatized individual exercising in the heat and results from loss of both salt and water. The patient complains of headache, nausea, vomiting, dizziness, weakness, irritability, or cramps, is sweating, and has normal or minimally increased core temperature. **Therapy** consists of rest in a cool environment, acceleration of heat loss by fan evaporation, and fluid repletion with salt-containing solutions. If the patient is not vomiting and the blood pressure is stable, an oral, commercial balanced salt solution is adequate. If vomiting occurs or hemodynamic status is unstable, electrolytes should be checked and 1–2 liters of intravenous normal saline given. The patient should avoid exercise in a hot environment for 2–3 additional days.

C. Heat stroke causes 4,000 deaths/year in the United States; 80% occur in those greater than age 50. High core temperature causes direct thermal tissue injury; secondary effects include acute renal failure from rhabdomyolysis. Even with rapid therapy, mortality may be as high as 76% for body temperatures greater than or equal to 106°F (41.1°C) (*D. M.* 35:301, 1989).

  1. **Classic heat stroke** occurs after several days of heat exposure in individuals at risk. Risk factors include chronic illness, old age, high humidity, obesity, chronic cardiovascular disease, poverty, urban upper-story residence, lack of air-conditioning, dehydration, alcohol abuse, and use of sedatives, hypnotics, anticholinergics, or antipsychotics. Typically, such patients have core temperatures greater than 105°F (40.5°C) and are comatose and anhydrotic.

  2. **Exertional heat stroke** occurs rapidly in unacclimatized individuals exercising in conditions of high ambient temperature and humidity. Those at risk include athletes (especially long-distance runners and football players), soldiers, and laborers without access to adequate water. Some of the risks associated with classic heat stroke may also be present, and certain congenital diseases that impair sweating may contribute. The core temperature may be less than 40.5°C; 50% of patients are still sweating at presentation. Individuals with exertional heat stroke are more likely to have **disseminated intravascular coagulation, lactic acidosis, and rhabdomyolysis** than those with classic heat stroke.

  3. **Diagnosis** is based on the history of exposure, a core temperature usually 105°F (40.5°C) or above, and changes in mental status ranging from confusion to delirium and coma. Differential diagnosis includes malignant hyperthermia, neuroleptic malignant syndrome, severe hyperthyroidism, sepsis, meningitis, Rocky Mountain spotted fever, and cerebral malaria.

  4. **Therapy**
     a. **Immediate cooling.** Constant misting of the patient with 20–25°C tepid water is very effective if the patient is continuously cooled by a large electric fan, especially with maximum body surface exposure. Ice packs at points of major heat transfer, such as the groin, the axilla, and the chest, may speed cooling. Ice-water immersion is difficult to arrange, results in inappropriate vasoconstriction, and interferes with other resuscitative maneuvers and therefore should not be employed. For severely elevated core temperature not responsive to the above maneuvers, gastric lavage with ice water may be helpful. **Dantrolene sodium does not appear to be effective** (*Crit. Care Med.* 19:176, 1991). Shivering and vasoconstriction impair cooling and may be prevented by administration of **chlorpromazine,** 10–25 mg IM. Core temperatures should be constantly monitored by rectal probe or tympanic membrane thermistor. Cooling measures should be discontinued at a core temperature of 39°C (102.2°F).

     b. **Baseline laboratory studies** include CBC, platelets, partial thromboplastin time (PTT), prothrombin time (PT), fibrin degradation products (FDP), electrolytes, BUN, creatinine, glucose, calcium, creatine kinase (CK), liver function tests (LFTs), arterial blood gases (ABGs), urinalysis, and ECG.

    c. Hypotension unresponsive to crystalloids may require vasopressors and hemodynamic monitoring (avoiding alpha-adrenergic agents as they cause vasoconstriction and impair cooling). Crystalloids should be administered cautiously to the normotensive patient.

    d. Rhabdomyolysis (or urine output less than 30 ml/hr) should be treated with adequate volume replacement, mannitol, 12.5–25.0 g, and bicarbonate, 44 mEq/liter in one half normal saline, to promote osmotic diuresis and urine alkalinization. **Renal failure** may still occur in 5% of patients with classic heat stroke and in 25% with exertional heat stroke.

    e. Hypoxemia and adult respiratory distress syndrome may require administration of oxygen, mechanical ventilation, and positive end-expiratory pressure.

    f. Other complications. Seizures are treated with diazepam and phenytoin. Hepatic injury, congestive heart failure, and coagulopathy may occur.

II. Cold injury. Exposure to the cold may result in several different forms of injury. An important risk factor is accelerated heat loss, which may be promoted by exposure to high wind or by immersion. Extended cold exposure may result from alcohol or drug abuse, injury or immobilization, and mental impairment.

    A. Chilblains are among the mildest form of cold injury and result from exposure of bare skin to a cold, windy environment (33–60°F). The ears, fingers, and tip of the nose are typically injured, with itchy, painful erythema on rewarming. Treatment consists of rapid rewarming, analgesics, and avoidance of recurrence.

    B. Immersion injury (trench foot) is caused by prolonged immersion (greater than 10–12 hours at ≤ 50° F). Treatment includes removal from exposure, rewarming, dry dressings, and treatment of secondary infections.

    C. Frostnip is the mildest form of frostbite and occurs most frequently on the distal extremities, the nose, or the ear. It is marked by tissue blanching and decreased sensitivity. **Rapid rewarming, in a water bath at 104–106°F,** is the treatment of choice of all forms of frostbite. The water temperature should never be hotter than 112°F.

    D. Superficial frostbite involves the skin and subcutaneous tissues, which are white, waxy, and anesthetic, have poor capillary refill, and are painful on thawing. No deep injury occurs and healing occurs in 3–4 weeks.

    E. Deep frostbite involves death of skin, subcutaneous tissue, and muscle (third degree) or deep tendons and bones (fourth degree). The tissue appears frozen and hard. Upon rewarming there is no capillary filling. Healing is very slow, and demarcation of tissue with autoamputation may occur. Diabetes mellitus, peripheral vascular disease, outdoor life-style, high altitude, and being non-white are all additional risk factors. Greater than 90% of deep frostbite occurs at temperatures less than 6.7°C (44°F) with exposures greater than 7–10 hours. **Initial treatment** consists of rapid rewarming. Refreezing must not be allowed. Analgesics (intravenous opioids) are given as needed. The patient should be admitted to a surgical service, with elevation of the affected extremity, non–weight-bearing, separation of affected digits by cotton wool, prevention of tissue maceration with a blanket cradle, and no smoking. Tetanus immunization should be updated if necessary. Intraarterial reserpine, heparin, dextran, prostaglandin inhibitors, thrombolytics, and sympathectomy are not routinely justified. Amputation is undertaken only after full demarcation has occurred.

    F. Hypothermia is defined as a core temperature less than 35°C (95°F). Hypothermia is defined as mild at 34–35°C, moderate at 30–34°C, and severe at less than 30°C. The most common cause of hypothermia in the United States is cold exposure due to alcohol intoxication. Another common cause is cold-water immersion. Differential diagnosis and other risk factors include extremes of age, cerebrovascular accident, subdural hematoma, drug use, diabetic ketoacidosis, uremia, adrenal insufficiency, and myxedema.

    1. Diagnosis. A standard oral thermometer registers only to a lower limit of 35°C. Therefore, the patient should be continuously monitored with either a rectal probe with a full range of 20–40°C, or with an ear thermistor.

    2. Signs and symptoms vary with the temperature of the patient at presentation.

a. **All organ systems** are involved. At temperatures 35°C or below, mental processes are slowed and the affect is flattened. At temperatures less than 32.2°C (90°F), the ability to shiver is lost, and deep tendon reflexes are diminished. At 28°C, coma often supervenes. At 18°C or below, the electroencephalogram is flat. Upon rewarming from severe hypothermia, central pontine myelinolysis may develop.

b. **Cardiovascular effects.** After an initial increased release of catecholamines, there is a decrease in cardiac output and heart rate with relatively preserved mean arterial pressure. ECG changes, manifest initially as sinus bradycardia with T-wave inversion and QT-interval prolongation, may progress to atrial fibrillation at temperatures below 32°C. Osborne waves (J-point elevation) may be visible, particularly in leads II and V6. There is an increased susceptibility to ventricular arrhythmias at temperatures below 32°C. At about 28–30°C, the susceptibility to ventricular fibrillation is significantly increased, and unnecessary manipulation, jostling, and esophageal and tracheal manipulation should be avoided. At 29°C or less, a decrease in mean arterial pressure may occur. At temperatures below 28°C, progressive bradycardia supervenes. At about 22°C, maximum ventricular fibrillation susceptibility occurs, and at temperatures below 18°C, asystole may supervene.

c. **Respiratory complications.** After an initial increase in minute ventilation, respiratory rate and tidal volume decrease progressively with decreasing temperature. **Arterial blood gases measured with the machine set at 37°C should serve as the basis for therapy without correction of pH and PCO$_2$** (as is done by many cardiac anesthesiologists in hypothermic cardiac surgery). Supplemental oxygen should be supplied (*Ann. Emerg. Med.* 18:72, 1989; *Arch. Intern. Med.* 148:1643, 1988; *Anesthesiology* 56:41, 1982).

d. **Renal manifestations** include cold diuresis as well as tubular concentrating defects.

3. **Laboratory evaluation** includes CBC, electrolytes, BUN, creatinine, glucose, coagulation studies, CK, liver function tests, calcium, magnesium, amylase, urinalysis, arterial blood gases, and ECG. All patients with a history of trauma or immersion injury should be evaluated with a chest x-ray, abdominal film, and cervical spine films. Electrolyte abnormalities are common. Potassium is often increased. Elevated serum amylase may reflect underlying pancreatitis. Hyperglycemia may be noted but should not be treated, as there may be rebound hypoglycemia with rewarming. DIC may be present.

4. **Therapy.** Attention should be directed toward maintaining an airway and oxygenation. **Intubation,** when indicated, should be done by the most experienced operator in the most gentle fashion possible (see Sec. **II.F.2.b**).

a. **Cardiopulmonary resuscitation (CPR)** is carried out in standard fashion with simultaneous vigorous core rewarming, as the patient should not be considered unresuscitatable as long as the core temperature is severely decreased. Reliable defibrillation requires a core temperature greater than or equal to 32°C. CPR should not be undertaken if an organized electrocardiographic rhythm is present because inability to detect peripheral pulses may be due to vasoconstriction and CPR may precipitate ventricular fibrillation. When ventricular fibrillation is present, bretylium (5 mg/kg IV) is the agent of choice; lidocaine is an alternative. Procainamide should be avoided because it may precipitate ventricular fibrillation and increase the temperature necessary to defibrillate the patient successfully. Patients with an intact circulation should have electrocardiographic rhythm, urine output, and possibly central venous pressure monitoring. Swan-Ganz catheterization should not be performed because it may precipitate ventricular fibrillation.

b. **Rewarming** should be done with the goal of increasing the temperature by 0.5–2.0°C/hour. Recommendations on rewarming are based on general consensus and clinical experience.

    (1) Passive external rewarming depends on the patient's ability to shiver and thus generate heat. It is effective only at core temperatures greater than or equal to 32°C. The patient is covered with blankets, placed in a warm environment, and monitored.

    (2) Active external rewarming includes application of heating blankets (40–45°C) or warm bath immersion. This may cause paradoxical core acidosis, hyperkalemia, and decreased core temperature, as cold stagnant blood returns to the central vasculature. For this reason, active rewarming should be used only on the trunk of a young, previously healthy patient with acute hypothermia and minimal pathophysiologic derangement.

    (3) Active core rewarming is preferred for treatment of severe hypothermia. Heated oxygen is the initial therapy of choice for the patient whose cardiovascular status is stable. It can be expected to raise core temperatures by 1–2°C/hour (*Am. J. Emerg. Med.* 2:533, 1984). Heated oxygen is administered through a cascade humidifier at a temperature less than or equal to 43°C. Intravenous fluids may be heated in a microwave oven (*Am. J. Emerg. Med.* 3:316, 1985) or delivered through a blood warmer and should be given only through peripheral IVs. Heated nasogastric or bladder lavage should be reserved for the patient with cardiovascular collapse. Heated peritoneal lavage is more effective than heated aerosol inhalation (*Am. J. Emerg. Med.* 2:210, 1984) but should be performed only for patients with cardiovascular collapse, by those experienced in its use, and in combination with other modes of rewarming. Extracorporeal circulation (cardiac bypass) is reserved for hypothermic individuals with cardiac arrest. It may raise the temperature as rapidly as 10–12°C/hour and must be performed in an intensive care unit or operating room.

  c. Medications. Most patients with exposure should receive thiamine. Administration of antibiotics is an unsettled issue; many authorities recommend antibiotic administration for 72 hours, pending cultures. In general, those with hypothermia due to exposure and alcohol intoxication are less likely to have a seriously underlying infection than those who are elderly or have an underlying medical illness.

  d. Observation. Patients with an underlying disease, physiologic derangement, or core temperature less than 32°C should be admitted, preferably to an intensive care unit. Those with mild hypothermia (32–35°C) and no predisposing medical conditions or complications may be discharged when they are normothermic if an adequate home environment can be ensured.

High-Altitude Illness

Acute high-altitude illness typically occurs in individuals unacclimatized to altitude who ascend to more than 2,000 meters (7,200 feet) in less than 1–2 days. Symptoms usually occur within 24 hours of ascent. **Risk factors** include a prior history of altitude illness, lack of acclimatization, rapid ascent, drugs that diminish ventilatory response to hypoxia, young age, vigorous exercise, preexisting history of pulmonary disease, and alcohol use.

I. Acute mountain sickness is the most common manifestation. Symptoms include headache, nausea, vomiting, anorexia, dyspnea, lethargy, sleep disturbance, vertigo, palpitations, and difficulty concentrating. It typically is worst on the second to third day. **Treatment** consists of liberal fluids, mild analgesics for headache (acetaminophen, 650 mg), compazine, 10 mg IM q6h for nausea, and, for severe symptoms, oxygen at 2–3 liters/minute and descent of 3,000–4,500 feet (1,000–1,500 meters). **Acetazolamide,** 250 mg PO bid, may abort the illness and speed acclimatization. **Dexamethasone,** 4 mg PO or IM q6h, may be effective for severe headaches, vomiting, and neurologic symptoms (*Aviat. Space Environ. Med.* 59:950, 1988).

II. **High-altitude pulmonary edema** is most common in the young, vigorously active individual and may be fatal. Symptoms include dyspnea, cough, weakness, lethargy, tachycardia, and frothy, bloody sputum. Rales are heard on chest examination, and chest x-ray shows pulmonary edema. **Treatment is urgent descent** of at least 3,000 to 4,000 feet. **Oxygen** is administered at high flow rates. For the severely ill, continuous positive airway pressure by mask or mechanical ventilation with positive end-expiratory pressure may be lifesaving. Furosemide and morphine sulfate (in the absence of central nervous system manifestations) may be used but are unlikely to be effective.

III. **High-altitude cerebral edema** is rare and ordinarily occurs only at very high altitudes, usually greater than 3,500 meters (14,400 feet). Its symptoms include severe headache, ataxia, confusion, emotional lability, and hallucinations. Papilledema may be present. Untreated, it progresses to coma and death. The primary **treatment is emergency descent, with oxygen** administration at 2–4 liters/minute in the meantime. If possible, endotracheal intubation with hyperventilation is indicated. Furosemide, 20–40 mg IV, and dexamethasone, 10 mg IV followed by 4 mg IV q6h, are recommended.

IV. **Prevention of high-altitude illness** depends on slow ascent and graded exercise. Those planning on undertaking travel should not go from 0–7,500 feet in 1 day. At least one night should be spent at an intermediate altitude. **Acetazolamide,** 125–150 mg PO bid or tid or 500 mg sustained release PO q12–24h, may be useful in prophylaxis. **Dexamethasone,** 4 mg PO q6h for 48 hours prior to ascent and during altitude exposure, is also effective (*N. Engl. J. Med.* 310:683, 1984); smaller doses are less useful (*Chest* 95:568, 1989).

Overdosage

Recognition of poisoning and medication overdose requires a high index of suspicion and careful clinical evaluation. Up to 50% of all initial poisoning histories may be incorrect. Identification of the drug or drugs ingested and their dosages should be sought from the patient's family or friends, private physician, pharmacist, and paramedical personnel. Supporting materials (e.g., pill bottles) should be sought, as should clues regarding timing of ingestion. Recognition of specific toxic syndromes is often helpful in directing initial management (Table 26-1). Vital signs, neurologic status, pupillary reactions, cardiovascular response, abdominal findings, and unusual odors and excreta, as well as evaluation of ABGs, serum electrolytes, and acid-base abnormalities, may suggest a particular toxicity. Screening of blood, urine, or gastric aspirate for specific agents is important, but in most cases, therapy must proceed before such results are available. Abdominal radiography may be useful in detecting retained pills (such as iron). While a computerized Poisindex system is helpful, specific advice should be sought from the regional poison control center.

I. **Supportive care** is crucial. A patent airway and adequate ventilation must be maintained. Endotracheal intubation may be required to protect the airway. Hypotension usually responds to intravenous fluid therapy, although vasopressors may be required in refractory cases or in the presence of pulmonary edema (see Chap. 6). Dopamine is used in most situations; norepinephrine is preferred in overdoses with alpha-antagonists (phenothiazines) and tricyclic antidepressants (due to the proarrhythmic effect of dopamine). **Arrhythmias** may be related to cardiac or autonomic effects; treatment may vary depending on the toxin. Central nervous system depression or coma occurs frequently and should prompt the administration of naloxone (2 mg IV) for possible narcotic overdose, 50% dextrose (50 ml IV) for hypoglycemia, thiamine (100 mg IV) for Wernicke-Korsakoff syndrome, flumazenil (0.2 mg IV; see Sec. **VI.L.2.b**) for benzodiazepine overdose, and oxygen for carbon monoxide intoxication.

II. **Prevention of further drug absorption** may be facilitated by gastric lavage, induced

Table 26-1. Toxic syndrome and possible causes

Syndrome	Manifestations	Possible causes
Acquired hemoglobinopathies	Dyspnea, cyanosis, confusion or lethargy, headache	Carbon monoxide Methemoglobinemia (nitrites, phenazopyridine) Sulfhemoglobinemia
Anion gap metabolic acidosis	Variable	Methanol Ethanol Ethylene glycol Paraldehyde Iron Isoniazid Salicylate Vacor Cyanide
Anticholinergic	Dry mouth and skin, blurred vision; mydriasis; tachycardia; generalized sunburn-like rash or flushing of skin; hyperthermia; abdominal distention; urinary urgency/retention; confusion, hallucinations, delusions, excitation, or coma	Atropine and other belladonna alkaloids Antihistamines Tricyclics Phenothiazines Jimson seeds
Cholinergic	Hypersalivation, bronchorrhea, bronchospasm, urination/defecation, neuromuscular failure, lacrimation	Acetylcholine Organophosphate insecticides Bethanechol Methacholine Wild mushrooms (usually *Amanita* sp.)
Cyanide	Nausea, vomiting, collapse, coma, bradycardia, no cyanosis, decreased AV O_2 difference with severe metabolic acidosis	Cyanide Amygdalin
Extrapyramidal	Dysphoria and dysphagia, trismus, oculogyric crisis, rigidity, torticollis, laryngospasm	Phenothiazines and other antipsychotics

Narcotic	Central nervous system depression, respiratory depression, miosis, hypotension	Morphine and heroin Codeine Propoxyphene Other synthetic and semisynthetic opiates
Salicylism	Fever, hyperpnea, respiratory alkalosis or mixed acid-base disturbance, hypokalemia, tinnitus	Aspirin Other salicylate products
Sympathomimetic	Excitation, hypertension, cardiac arrhythmias, seizures	Amphetamines Cocaine Caffeine Aminophylline β-Agonists, inhaled or injected

Source: Modified from G. Quick and P. J. Crocker. Toxic emergency: Agent unknown. *Emerg. Decisions* 7:44, 1986.

emesis, or administration of activated charcoal. Gastric emptying procedures should be initiated within 1 hour of the ingestion (*Ann. Emerg. Med.* 14:562, 1985). Because most adult overdose patients present several hours after toxic ingestion and because the use of syrup of ipecac may delay subsequent therapy, the use of activated charcoal is recommended as the primary gastrointestinal decontamination procedure for most patients (*Ann. Emerg. Med.* 16:838, 1987). Gastric emptying should be performed for phenothiazine overdose and ingestion of rapidly absorbed agents, such as strychnine and cyanide.

A. Activated charcoal absorbs most drugs, preventing further absorption from the gastrointestinal tract. Exceptions include alkalis, cyanide, ferrous sulfate, and mineral acids. It may also promote efflux of selected drugs (theophylline, phenobarbital, and carbamazepine) from the blood into the bowel lumen. **Activated charcoal should not be given in conjunction with an oral antidote, as it may bind and inactivate these agents;** it may be given 2 hours later, however. It is preferable not to give it simultaneously with ipecac, as it obscures gastric contents, and it should not be used when endoscopy is contemplated. Activated charcoal, 50–100 g diluted in water or sorbitol, should be given as soon as possible after the toxic ingestion; prehospital administration further enhances drug recovery. Repeated dosing (without sorbitol) also improves efficacy.

B. Gastric emptying may be utilized in obtunded patients presenting soon after ingestion and in other situations (see Sec. II). **The airway must be protected;** an endotracheal tube may be necessary. If the patient is awake and alert, **ipecac,** 30 ml, repeated once in 20 minutes if necessary, is a useful emetic. Additional ingestion of water is not needed and may prompt inappropriate antegrade gastric emptying. Contraindications to ipecac include decreased level of consciousness, absent gag reflex, caustic ingestion, convulsions, or exposure to a substance likely to cause convulsions, and medical conditions making emesis unsafe. If no response is achieved after the second ipecac dose, the patient should undergo gastric lavage. A large orogastric tube (greater than 28 French, preferably greater than 36 French) is the preferred method for patients with a decreased gag reflex **after endotracheal intubation.** Lavage with 200-ml boluses of warm saline, repeated until the effluent is clear, is followed by instillation of activated charcoal and a single dose of cathartic. The added efficacy of a **cathartic** is not clear, but it does decrease transit time through the intestine. Acceptable forms include magnesium citrate, 4 ml/kg (300 ml maximum), sorbitol, 1–2 g/kg (150 g maximum), and magnesium or sodium sulfate, 25–30 g. Magnesium salts should not be given in renal failure. Sorbitol premixed with charcoal is available commercially. Intestinal lavage with commercially available bowel preparation materials is not routinely recommended (*Ann. Emerg. Med.* 17:681, 1988); iron ingestion with radiographically persistent tablets in the gastrointestinal tract may be an exception (*Clin. Toxicol.* 23:177, 1985).

III. Removal of absorbed drugs. Enhancement of renal excretion and extracorporeal methods may be used. Increased urinary pH may increase elimination of weak acids.

A. Forced diuresis should be used only when specifically indicated because of the risk of causing acid-base disturbances, electrolyte abnormalities, and cerebral or pulmonary edema. It should not be attempted in patients with renal insufficiency, cardiac disease, or existing electrolyte abnormalities. Little data exist about its efficacy in improving survival.

1. Forced alkaline diuresis, achieving a urinary pH of 7.5–9.0, promotes excretion of drugs that are weak acids, such as salicylates, barbital, and phenobarbital. A solution of sodium bicarbonate, 50–100 mEq, added to 1 liter of 0.45% saline, may be administered at 250–500 ml/hour for the first 1–2 hours. Great care must be exercised to avoid overhydration, especially in the elderly. Maintenance alkaline solution and diuretics should be administered to maintain a urinary output of 2–3 ml/kg/hour. In salicylate poisoning, potassium supplementation will almost always be required.

2. Forced acid diuresis is no longer recommended for any agent.

B. Extracorporeal removal of specific toxins by dialysis or hemoperfusion is used when (1) there is clinical deterioration despite intensive supportive therapy, (2) blood levels reach potentially lethal concentrations, (3) there is a risk of lethal delayed effects, and (4) renal or hepatic failure impairs clearance of toxin.

  1. **Peritoneal or hemodialysis** is most useful for low-molecular-weight, water-soluble toxins that are minimally bound to plasma proteins (e.g., ethanol, ethylene glycol, lithium, methanol, and salicylates). It is also used for heavy-metal intoxication in patients with renal failure. Dialysis also corrects electrolyte, acid-base, and osmolar derangements that may accompany toxic ingestions.
  2. **Hemoperfusion** removes toxins by direct adsorption and is generally more effective than either peritoneal or hemodialysis. It is useful in overdoses with barbiturates, sedative-hypnotics, and lipid-soluble drugs. It may be helpful in theophylline intoxications but is of marginal help in cyclic antidepressants.

IV. **Specific antidotes** are available that neutralize or prevent the toxic effect of certain drugs (Table 26-2). The regional poison control center should be contacted immediately if it is known what drug was ingested; information on specific treatment and the pharmacokinetics of the drug can often be provided.

V. **Disposition.** Patients with apparently trivial overdoses of potentially toxic agents should be observed for at least 4 hours before contemplation of discharge. No patient who has taken an intentional overdose should be discharged from the emergency department without formal psychiatric consultation and disposition. Individuals suffering inadvertent recreational drug overdose require referral for counseling and possibly detoxification. All symptomatic (and some asymptomatic) patients require admission. Patients considered to be potentially suicidal require one-to-one constant supervision while on the medical service.

VI. **Specific agents**
  A. **Acetaminophen** is a common ingredient in many analgesic and antipyretic preparations. Hepatic toxicity is due to depletion of hepatic glutathione and subsequent accumulation of a toxic intermediate metabolite, N-acetyl-p-benzoquinonimine. Toxicity usually occurs after ingestion of greater than 140 mg/kg. Precise determination of probable toxicity can be obtained by plotting a plasma acetaminophen level (drawn at least 4 hours after ingestion) versus time since ingestion on a nomogram (Fig. 26-1).

  1. **Symptoms** over the first 24 hours include anorexia, vomiting, and diaphoresis. Hepatic enzymes begin to rise 48 hours after ingestion and peak 72–96 hours after ingestion. Recovery starts after approximately 4 days unless hepatic failure develops.

  2. **Treatment** includes supportive measures and induced emesis or gastric lavage. **Acetylcysteine (Mucomyst)**, a specific antidote that acts as a glutathione substrate, should be given within 8 hours of ingestion to prevent hepatic toxicity but may be effective when administered up to 36 hours after ingestion (*Lancet* 335:1572, 1990). **The initial dosage** is 140 mg/kg PO or by gastric tube; subsequent administration (70 mg/kg q4h for a total of 17 doses) is directed by plasma acetaminophen levels. If toxic levels are detected, the full 17 doses are given; if not, no further antidote is indicated. If vomiting occurs less than 1 hour after administration of antidote, the dose should be repeated. If vomiting is repetitive and interferes with acetylcysteine administration, metoclopramide or droperidol may be used, or acetylcysteine may be administered via fluoroscopically placed nasoduodenal drip over a period of 30–60 minutes. Baseline AST, ALT, bilirubin, BUN, and prothrombin time should be drawn and repeated at least daily for 3 days (see Chap. 16). If activated charcoal is administered less than 1 hour before acetylcysteine, any residual charcoal should be removed by gastric lavage. If a mixed overdose requires multidose charcoal for another agent, it should be given 2 hours after each dose of acetylcysteine with lavage before each subsequent acetylcysteine dose. **Intravenous acetylcysteine** is available at a limited number of participating centers for those who cannot or will not take oral acetylcysteine (Rocky Mountain Poison Center, 1-800-525-6115). Side effects include bronchospasm, rash, flushing, and anaphylactoid reaction.

Table 26-2. Antidotes

Poison/toxic sign	Antidote	Adult dosage
Acetaminophen	*N*-Acetylcysteine	140 mg/kg PO, followed by 70 mg/kg q4h × 17 doses
Anticholinergics	Physostigmine sulfate	0.5–2.0 mg IV (IM) over 2 min q30–60min prn
Anticholinesterases	Atropine sulfate	1–5 mg IV (IM, SQ) q15min prn to drying of secretions
	Pralidoxime (2-PAM) chloride[a]	1 g IV (PO) over 15–30 min q8–12h × 3 doses prn
Carbon monoxide	Oxygen	100%, hyperbaric
Cyanide	Amyl nitrite[b] *followed by*	Inhalation perles for 15–30 sec qmin
	Sodium nitrite[b]	300 mg (10 ml of 3% solution) IV over 3 min, repeated in half dosage in 2 hr if persistent or recurrent signs of toxicity
	Followed by	
	Sodium thiosulfate	12.5 g (50 ml of a 25% solution) IV over 10 min, repeated in half dosage in 2 hr if persistent or recurrent signs of toxicity
Digoxin	Antidigoxin (Fab' fragments)	Number of vials (40 mg/vial) = $\dfrac{\text{serum digoxin level (ng/ml)} \times \text{weight (kg)}}{100}$
Ethylene glycol	Ethanol[d]	0.6 g/kg of ethanol in D5W IV (PO) over 30–45 min, followed initially by 110 mg/kg/hr to maintain a blood alcohol level of 100–150 mg/dl
Extrapyramidal signs	Diphenhydramine hydrochloride	25–50 mg IV (IM, PO) prn
	Benztropine mesylate	1–2 mg IV (IM, PO) prn
Heavy metals (e.g., arsenic, copper, gold, lead, mercury)	Chelators[c] Calcium disodium edetate (EDTA)	1 g IM or IV in normal saline over 1 hr q12h
	Dimercaprol (BAL)	2.5–5.0 mg/kg IM q4–6h
	Penicillamine	250–500 mg PO q6h
	2,3-dimercaptosuccinic acid (DMSA, Succimer)	10 mg/kg PO tid × 5 days, then bid × 14 days
Iron	Deferoxamine mesylate	1 g IM (IV at a rate ≤ 15 mg/kg/hr if hypotension) q8h prn

Isoniazid	Pyridoxine	Amount equal to estimated INH ingestion up to 5 g over 30–60 min; any remainder by IV drip over 1–2 hr
Methanol	Ethanol[d]	See Ethylene glycol
Methemoglobinemia	Methylene blue	1–2 mg/kg (0.1–0.2 ml/kg of 1% solution) IV over 5 min, repeated in 1 hr prn
Opioids	Naloxone hydrochloride	0.4–2.0 mg IV (IM, SQ, endotracheally) prn
Warfarin and related drugs	Vitamin K_1	10 mg IM, SQ, or IV[e]
	Fresh frozen plasma	Variable

[a] Pralidoxime is indicated in severe organophosphate poisoning with muscle weakness, fasciculations, or respiratory depression.

[b] Nitrites probably have an antidotal effect in hydrogen sulfide poisoning.

[c] The use of a specific chelating agent or combination of agents will depend on the heavy metal involved and on the clinical situation.

[d] The requisite ethanol dose will depend on prior alcohol use, liver function, and dialysis. Consult the regional poison control center for assistance.

[e] Caution should be used when giving vitamin K_1 IV. It should be given over 20 min.

Note: This table is only a guide. Antidote usage and dosage will depend on the specific clinical situation. The regional poison control center should be contacted for specific therapeutic recommendations.

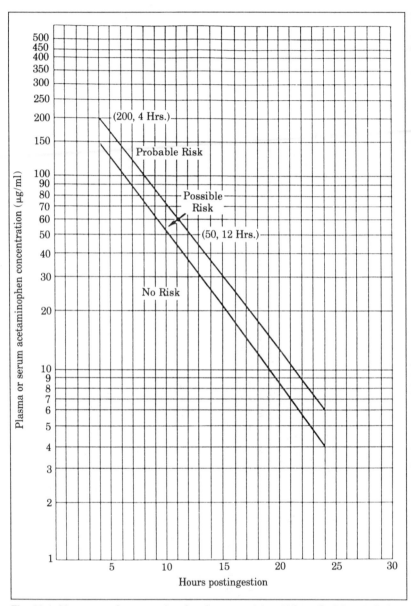

Fig. 26-1. Nomogram for acetaminophen hepatotoxicity. (Adapted with permission from B.H. Rumack et al., Acetaminophen overdose: 662 cases with evaluation of oral acetylcysteine treatment. *Arch. Intern. Med.* 141:380, 1981.)

B. Caustic ingestions

1. **Alkaline ingestions** may be either accidental or suicidal. Liquid and crystalline lye, automatic dishwater detergents, Clinitest tablets, and some toilet bowl cleaners are alkaline. Strong alkali solutions, such as liquid drain cleaner, are the agents most commonly associated with injury.

   a. **Deep tissue injury in the aerodigestive tract is common.** Oral burns are common; drooling may be a manifestation of this. Studies of whether the absence of oral burns correlates with infrequent esophageal injuries are conflicting (*Am. J. Surg.* 157:116, 1980; *Arch. Intern. Med.* 140:501, 1980). The overall rate of esophageal injury for all alkali ingestions is 30–40% and is suggested by vomiting, drooling, or stridor. Subsequent esophageal stricture may occur, especially with liquid lye (*Am. J. Surg.* 157:116, 1989). Gastric injury with perforation may occur and is much more likely with liquid lye ingestions, since they pass rapidly into the stomach. Alkaline ingestions may cause severe upper airway injury, with stridor and airway obstruction requiring rapid intervention. Symptoms include oral pain, odynophagia, stridor, chest pain, abdominal pain, nausea, and vomiting.

   b. **Therapy** includes immediate rinsing of the oral cavity with copious cold water. **Emesis should not be induced** because it may increase injury; charcoal administration, cathartic administration, and lavage are not indicated. Administration of milk obscures anatomic detail for subsequent endoscopy. Diluents are controversial and may induce emesis (*Vet. Hum. Toxicol.* 31:338, 1989). *Poisindex* currently recommends administration of diluents (*Poisindex* Editorial Board Consensus Opinion, December 1988). Attempting to neutralize the alkaline agent with a weak acid will result in an exothermic reaction and increase tissue damage. The **airway** should be rapidly ensured, oxygen administered, and fluids given as appropriate. Endotracheal intubation or early tracheostomy may be required. Examination and appropriate radiographs for evidence of perforation should be obtained. **Endoscopy** should be performed immediately when the patient has drooling, stridor, or odynophagia; it may be deferred 12–24 hours otherwise. Glucocorticoid treatment of esophageal burns for the prevention of stricture is controversial. Prednisone, 1–2 mg/kg/day, or the equivalent is currently recommended for deep or circumferential burns, with tapering over 3 weeks. Surgical consultation should be obtained. Prophylactic antibiotics are not appropriate. Barium swallow should be performed at 2–4 weeks (*South. Med. J.* 81:724, 1988) to assess for esophageal stricture.

2. **Acids.** Tissue injury is less deep than that produced by alkaline agents. Gastric injury may be more common than esophageal injury due to rapid transit of liquid and resistance of squamous esophageal epithelium to acid injury.

   a. **Symptoms** and signs include oral pain, drooling, odynophagia, and abdominal pain. Occasionally respiratory distress, DIC, hemolysis, and systemic acidosis may occur.

   b. **Therapy** consists of airway maintenance and circulatory support. Diluent administration has no demonstrated clinical efficacy. The mouth should be copiously washed with cold water. Neutralization with a weak base is contraindicated, as it may cause an exothermic tissue reaction. **Induction of emesis, lavage, or charcoal administration is contraindicated,** and a nasogastric tube should probably not be placed. Sucralfate may decrease symptoms but does not appear to decrease complications or perforation. Unsuspected esophageal and gastric burns and duodenal injury are commonly seen with endoscopy. The likelihood of stricture formation (gastric or esophageal) and perforation depends on the severity of ingestion (*Gastroenterology* 97:702, 1989). Surgical consultation should be obtained. The administration of glucocorticoids is controversial; prednisone, 1–2 mg/kg/day or the equivalent, is generally given, with tapering over 3 weeks. Prophylactic antibiotics are not recommended. Upper GI x-ray should be obtained in 2–4 weeks.

C. Ethanol and other alcohols

1. **Ethanol.** The toxicity of ethanol (EtOH) is dose-related, but tolerance varies widely among individuals. Blood levels greater than 100 mg/dl define legal intoxication and are typically associated with ataxia, while at 200 mg/dl patients are drowsy and confused. At levels greater than 400 mg/dl there is often respiratory depression, and death is possible.

   a. **Laboratory studies** should include electrolytes, glucose, serum osmolality, and blood EtOH level. The blood EtOH level may be rapidly estimated by calculating the **osmolal gap** (measured osmolality minus calculated osmolality).

   $$2[Na^+] + \frac{BUN}{2.8} + \frac{[glucose]}{18} \approx \text{calculated osmolality}$$

   The blood alcohol level (BAL) in milligrams per deciliter divided by 4.3 equals the osmolal gap, in the absence of other low-molecular-weight toxins (*Am. J. Clin. Pathol.* 60:690, 1973):

   $$\frac{BAL\ mg/dl}{4.3} = \text{measured osmolality} - \left(2[Na^+] + \frac{BUN}{2.8} + \frac{[glucose]}{18}\right)$$

   b. **Therapy.** If the patient's mental status is severely depressed, an endotracheal tube should be placed followed by gastric lavage. Charcoal is not helpful due to the rapid absorption of EtOH from the stomach (*Clin. Toxicol.* 24:225, 1986). For life-threatening overdoses, hemodialysis may be useful. **In the comatose alcoholic,** 50 ml of 50% dextrose should be administered IV after 100 mg of thiamine IV. Patients with alcohol intoxication should be admitted when there is severe underlying illness or requirement for ventilatory support. Other patients should be observed until they are sober (BAL < 100 mg/dl).

2. **Isopropyl alcohol** (IPA). Rubbing alcohol is 70% IPA. It has more toxicity than EtOH at any blood level (50 mg/dl = intoxication, 100–200 mg/dl = stupor and coma). Respiratory depression and hypotension occur at high blood levels. Nausea, vomiting, and abdominal pain occur frequently.

   a. **Laboratory evaluation** commonly reveals ketosis without acidosis (IPA is metabolized to acetone). Metabolic acidosis is usually related to associated hypotension. IPA concentration in the blood may be measured directly or may be estimated in the same fashion as for EtOH, substituting a denominator of 5.9 for 4.3 (*Top. Emerg. Med.*, July 1984, pp. 14–29).

   b. **Therapy.** Emesis is not recommended, as mental status may decline rapidly, with subsequent aspiration. For cutaneous exposures, the skin should be washed and contaminated clothes should be removed (*Vet. Hum. Toxicol.* 28:233, 1986). An adequate airway and blood pressure must be maintained. Hemodialysis is reserved for patients with hypotension.

3. **Methanol** (MeOH) is in gas-line antifreeze and windshield washer fluid. Sterno contains MeOH, and the EtOH present results in delayed manifestation of MeOH toxicity. The toxicity of MeOH is due to its conversion by alcohol dehydrogenase to formaldehyde and formic acid. EtOH delays this metabolism by competing for this enzyme. The patient may have initial symptoms of lethargy and confusion, followed by an apparent "hangover." Delayed toxic symptoms consisting of headache, visual symptoms, nausea, vomiting, abdominal pain, tachypnea, and respiratory failure may ensue. Coma and convulsions may occur in severe cases.

   a. **Examination** typically reveals an uncomfortable patient who may be remarkably tachypneic with decreased visual acuity; optic disc hyperemia may be hard to appreciate. Laboratory studies should include CBC, electrolytes, BUN, creatinine, amylase, EtOH level, MeOH level, and

Table 26-3. Maintenance ethanol dosage regimens for ethylene glycol and methanol intoxication

	10% ethanol IV	40% ethanol PO	95% ethanol PO	Hemodialysis with 10% ethanol IV*
Moderate drinker	1.39 ml/kg/hr	0.29 ml/kg/hr	0.15 ml/kg/hr	3.29 ml/kg/hr
Chronic drinker	1.95 ml/kg/hr	0.41 ml/kg/hr	0.21 ml/kg/hr	3.85 ml/kg/hr
Nondrinker	0.83 ml/kg/hr	0.17 ml/kg/hr	0.09 ml/kg/hr	2.73 ml/kg/hr

* Dialysate bath concentration of 100 mg/dl is preferable.
Source: Modified from J. P. Duffy. Methanol (Management/Treatment Protocol). In B. H. Rumack and D. G. Spoerke (eds.), *Poisindex Information System.* Denver: Micromedex, 1991.

ABGs, which will reveal a severe anion gap metabolic acidosis. The range of toxic ingestion is 15–400 ml. In general, pH and acid-base status are better predictors of toxicity than absolute level. The MeOH level in mg/dl may be estimated in the same way as for EtOH, substituting a denominator of 2.6 for 4.3.

  b. Therapy of MeOH intoxication includes gastric lavage and charcoal administration. A cathartic may be given once.

    (1) Folinic acid (leucovorin), 1 mg/kg (maximum 50 mg) IV, with folic acid, 1 mg/kg IV q4h for 6 doses, increases the metabolism of formate.

    (2) 4-Methylpyrazole (an alcohol dehydrogenase antagonist) is not yet available in the United States (*J. Emerg. Med.* 8:455, 1990).

    (3) EtOH should be administered for any peak MeOH level greater than 20 mg/dl, for a suspicious ingestion while awaiting levels, for a suspicious anion gap metabolic acidosis, or to any symptomatic patient with an appropriate history. The **loading dose of EtOH** is 7.6–10.0 ml/kg of a 10% solution given IV or 0.8–1.0 ml/kg of 95% alcohol, administered PO in orange juice. Maintenance dosage varies depending on previous alcohol exposure (Table 26-3). The goal is achievement of a blood alcohol level of 100–150 mg/dl to saturate the available alcohol dehydrogenase and prevent formation of MeOH's toxic metabolites. EtOH is administered continuously until the MeOH level is less than 10 mg/dl, the formate level is less than 1.2 mg/dl, there is resolution of acidosis, CNS symptoms abate, and normal anion gap is restored. If MeOH levels cannot be readily measured, EtOH should be administered for at least 5 days without dialysis or 1 day with dialysis and until clinical findings resolve (*Poisindex,* 1992).

    (4) Hemodialysis is generally indicated for a MeOH level greater than 50 mg/dl, severe and resistant acidosis, renal failure, or visual symptoms.

D. Glycols. Ethylene glycol (EG) and **diethylene glycol** are commonly used in antifreeze and windshield de-icer. Various metabolites are responsible for toxicity. **Initial symptoms** resemble alcohol intoxication. Vomiting is common. CNS depression or coma may be seen. Congestive heart failure and pulmonary edema may occur 12–36 hours after ingestion. Death is most likely in this stage. Oliguric renal failure (from oxalate crystal deposition) may be seen 36–72 hours after ingestion. Associated flank pain may be prominent.

  1. Laboratory findings include a severe metabolic acidosis with an anion gap, an osmolal gap, and oxalate and hippurate crystalluria. Fluorescein is often added to antifreeze, and urine fluorescence detected with a Wood's lamp is diagnostic (*Ann. Emerg. Med.* 19:663, 1990).

  2. Treatment is supportive (e.g., correction of acidosis with intravenous sodium bicarbonate).

a. **Emesis** should be induced within 30 minutes of ingestion followed by charcoal and a single dose of nonmagnesium-containing cathartic.

b. **Indications for intravenous EtOH** (see sec. **VI.C.3.b**) include an EG level greater than 20 mg/dl, suspicion of ingestion pending level, or an EG level below 20 mg/dl in the setting of an anion gap metabolic acidosis. An EtOH level of at least 100 mg/dl should be maintained.

c. **Pyridoxine** (100 mg IV qd) and **thiamine** (100 mg IV qd) promote the conversion of glyoxylate to glycine.

d. **Dialysis** is highly effective in severe cases; EtOH infusion should be continued during dialysis. Indications for dialysis include a glycol level greater than 50 mg/dl, congestive heart failure, renal failure, or severe persistent acid-base abnormalities. Dialysis may be discontinued when the glycol level is less than 10 mg/dl, the glycolic acid level is non-detectable, and the acidosis, clinical status, and anion gap have returned to normal. When levels cannot be measured easily, EtOH administration should continue for at least 3 days without hemodialysis or 1 day with hemodialysis and until clinical findings resolve, whichever is longer (*Poisindex,* 1992).

e. **4-Methylpyrazole** is not yet available in the United States (*N. Engl. J. Med.* 319:97, 1988).

E. **Hydrocarbon ingestions** (e.g., petroleum products, kerosene, turpentine, mineral spirits, and mineral seal oil) are characterized by gastrointestinal upset, pulmonary aspiration, and CNS alterations. Morbidity and mortality are usually attributed to pulmonary aspiration. Motor oil, transmission oil, mineral oil, baby oil, and suntan oil are usually nontoxic.

1. **Clinical manifestations** are usually apparent within the first 6 hours and include vomiting, chest or abdominal pain, cough, dyspnea, low-grade fever, arrhythmias, seizures, an altered sensorium, and radiographic evidence of aspiration pneumonitis or pulmonary edema.

2. **Treatment of nontoxic hydrocarbon** ingestion is not required in the absence of symptoms. Gastric emptying is never required, and chest x-rays are obtained only in patients with pulmonary symptoms. Those with an abnormal chest x-ray and/or arterial blood gas should be hospitalized and treated supportively. **Treatment of toxic hydrocarbon** ingestion is initiated by removing contaminated clothing and washing the affected skin to prevent dermatitis and percutaneous absorption. Supplemental oxygen is indicated in all significant aspiration injuries. Gastric emptying, followed by administration of activated charcoal, although controversial, is recommended for ingestion of toxic hydrocarbons, particularly halogenated hydrocarbons, or those containing toxic additives (e.g., heavy metals, insecticides, nitrobenzene, or camphor). In alert patients, gastric emptying should be performed by emesis induced with ipecac. In patients with CNS depression, a depressed gag reflex, or seizures, gastric lavage is indicated but should be performed only after a cuffed endotracheal tube is in place. Following gastric decontamination, observation for at least six hours is required. Hospitalization is recommended for patients who are symptomatic (including cough), have an abnormal pulmonary examination, are lethargic, or have an abnormal arterial blood gas or chest radiograph. Prophylactic antibiotics or glucocorticoids are not indicated; seizures may be managed with diazepam and phenytoin.

F. **Methemoglobinemia** may be caused by nitrites, nitroprusside, nitroglycerin, chlorates, sulfonamides, aniline dyes, nitrobenzene, antimalarials, sexual stimulant inhalants (containing butyl or amyl nitrite), and phenazopyridine. Symptoms include headache, fatigue, dyspnea, tachycardia, and dizziness.

1. **The diagnosis** is suggested in patients with a normal PO_2 and generalized cyanosis (suggesting a methemoglobin level of 15%) that does not respond to oxygen. Final confirmation rests with measurement of a methemoglobin level. Blood levels greater than 50% indicate severe toxicity, often associated with CNS depression, seizures, coma, and arrhythmias; levels greater than 70% are often fatal.

2. **Treatment** includes supplemental oxygen and administration of **methylene blue,** 1–2 mg/kg in a 1% solution given IV over 5 minutes, if there are signs of hypoxia or if the methemoglobin level exceeds 30%; the dose may be repeated in 1 hour if there are persistent signs of hypoxia and q4h thereafter to a total dose of 7 mg/kg. The patient should be hospitalized if there are symptoms or if the methemoglobin level is greater than 20%.

G. **Organophosphates.** Parathion and malathion are the most common insecticides involved in human poisonings; they are often contained in hydrocarbon solvent. Suicidal ingestion and agricultural exposure occur.

   1. **Diagnosis and routine laboratory measurements.** Nonketotic hyperglycemia and glucosuria are common. Hyperamylasemia may reflect pancreatitis. Red cell cholinesterase and plasma pseudocholinesterase levels are decreased; depression of greater than 50% from baseline is associated with poor outcome. **Toxic manifestations** are due to inhibition of acetylcholinesterase in the nervous system. **Muscarinic** manifestations include miosis, increased lacrimation, bronchospasm, bronchorrhea, diaphoresis, salivation, bradycardia, hypotension, blurred vision, urinary incontinence, and increased gastrointestinal motility. **Nicotinic** manifestations include fasciculations, muscle weakness, hypotension, cramps, and respiratory paralysis. CNS toxicity includes anxiety, slurred speech, mental status changes (e.g., delirium, coma, and seizures), and respiratory depression. Complications of ingestion include pulmonary edema, aspiration pneumonia, chemical pneumonitis, and the adult respiratory distress syndrome.

   2. **Treatment** includes measures to support ventilation and circulation, decontamination of the skin, and gastric emptying by lavage (only with a cuffed endotracheal tube when there is respiratory depression). This should be followed with activated charcoal.

      a. **Atropine** (preservative-free) is the drug of choice in organophosphate toxicity. An initial dose of 2 mg IV is given and repeated in 15 minutes if there are no adverse effects. The dose is repeated every 15 minutes until atropinization (as manifested by flushing, dry mouth, and dilated pupils) occurs. The average patient requires approximately 40 mg/day (*Ann. Emerg. Med.* 16:193, 1987), but larger doses (500–1500 mg/day) may be required. Intermittent administration may need to be continued for at least 24 hours until the organophosphate is metabolized. Atropine will not reverse the muscle weakness.

      b. **Pralidoxime,** 1 g IV given over 30 minutes, reactivates the cholinesterase and counteracts weakness, muscle fasciculations, and respiratory depression. It may be repeated q6–12h to a maximum of 12 g in 24 hours.

      c. **Hemoperfusion** should be considered for severe parathion overdoses.

H. **Opioids**

   1. **Symptoms.** Overdosage causes respiratory depression, depressed level of consciousness, and miosis. However, the pupils may be dilated with acidosis or hypoxia or following overdoses with meperidine and diphenoxylate plus atropine. Less common complications include hypotension, bradycardia, and pulmonary edema.

   2. **Treatment** includes airway maintenance, ventilatory and circulatory support, and prevention of further drug absorption by gastric emptying and charcoal administration. **Naloxone hydrochloride** specifically reverses opioid-induced respiratory and CNS depression and hypotension. The initial dose is 2 mg IV; large doses may be required to reverse the effects of propoxyphene, diphenoxylate, or pentazocine. In the absence of an intravenous line, it can be administered sublingually (*Ann. Emerg. Med.* 16:572, 1987) or via endotracheal tube. Isolated opioid overdose is unlikely if there is no response after a total of 10 mg of naloxone. Repetitive doses may be required, and this should prompt hospitalization despite return to an alert status. A continuous IV drip providing two-thirds of the initial dose hourly, diluted in 5% dextrose, may be necessary to maintain an alert state (*Ann. Emerg. Med.* 15:566, 1986).

I. Phencyclidine (PCP) is a dissociative anesthetic and is available on the street mislabeled as LSD, mescaline, psilocybin, and THC.
  1. **Symptoms** include agitation, bizarre or violent behavior, hypertension, tachycardia, and horizontal or vertical nystagmus when ingested in small amounts. Patients are relatively impervious to pain and may be catatonic or self-destructive and difficult to subdue (*Ann. Emerg. Med.* 10:290, 1981). Stupor progressing to coma, hypertension, hyperpyrexia, hypertonicity, and bronchospasm characterize moderate ingestions. Massive ingestions may lead to hypotension, respiratory failure, rhabdomyolysis, and acute tubular necrosis. Hypoglycemia is frequent. Death may occur (*Ann. Emerg. Med.* 10:237, 1981).
  2. **Treatment** is primarily supportive. Sensory input should be minimized and potentially injurious objects removed from the area. Haloperidol or diazepam may be used to control agitation; dystonic reactions may be treated with diphenhydramine. Adrenergic manifestations (e.g., hypertension) may be controlled with beta-adrenergic blockade if bronchospasm is not present; sodium nitroprusside may be required in severe cases. Gastric emptying may provoke violent behavior and is recommended only in severe poisonings and only after the airway is protected. In that case, repeated charcoal administration is also recommended. Restraints are avoided as they may increase rhabdomyolysis (*J. Clin. Psychiatry* 44:184, 1983). Patients with low-dose intoxication can be discharged from the emergency department after symptoms resolve and psychiatric consultation is obtained. More severe intoxication requires hospitalization.

J. Phenothiazines. Chlorpromazine, thioridazine, prochlorperazine, haloperidol, and thiothixene are the most common agents.
  1. **Overdoses** are characterized by agitation or delirium, which may rapidly progress to coma. Pupils are miotic, and deep tendon reflexes are depressed. Seizures and disorders of thermoregulation may occur. Hypotension (due to strong alpha-adrenergic antagonism), tachycardia, arrhythmias, and depressed cardiac conduction occur. Measuring blood levels is not helpful. X-rays may reveal pill concretions present in the stomach despite apparently effective gastric emptying.
  2. **Treatment** includes airway protection, respiratory and hemodynamic support, and gastric emptying followed by administration of activated charcoal. Ipecac may be given within 30 minutes of the ingestion; after that point, the onset of dystonic effects may result in aspiration of vomitus (Poisindex, 1991). When treatment is more delayed, the stomach should be emptied by gastric lavage, which may be effective hours later due to delay in gastric emptying caused by the phenothiazines. Arrhythmias are treated with lidocaine and phenytoin; type I agents (e.g., procainamide, quinidine, disopyramide) are contraindicated. Hypotension is treated by fluid administration and alpha-adrenergic vasopressors (norepinephrine). Paradoxic vasodilation may occur in response to epinephrine administration because of unopposed beta-adrenergic response in the setting of strong alpha-adrenergic antagonism. Recurrent ventricular tachycardia, especially with prolonged QT interval, may require isoproterenol or pacemaker placement. Seizures are treated with diazepam and phenytoin. Hemodialysis is not useful. Patients with significant overdosage require cardiac monitoring for at least 48 hours.

K. Salicylate toxicity may result from acute ingestion or chronic intoxication. Toxicity is mild for acute ingestions less than 150 mg/kg, moderate for ingestions of 150–300 mg/kg, and generally severe at levels of 300–500 mg/kg. Toxicity from chronic ingestion is typically due to ingestions of more than 100 mg/kg/day over a period of several days and usually occurs in elderly patients with chronic underlying illness. Diagnosis is often delayed in this group of patients, and mortality is about 25% (*Ann. Intern. Med.* 85:745, 1976). Significant toxicity due to chronic ingestion may be present at blood levels lower than those associated with acute ingestions.
  1. **Symptoms** include nausea, vomiting, tinnitus (implying levels greater than

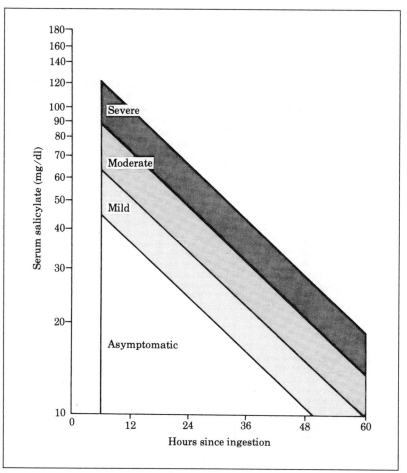

Fig. 26-2. Severity of salicylate intoxication. (Adapted with permission from A. K. Done. Salicylate intoxication. *Pediatrics* 26:800, 1960.)

30 mg/dl), and malaise. Fever may occur and is a bad prognostic sign in adults. More severe intoxications are associated with lethargy, convulsions, and coma. Noncardiogenic pulmonary edema may occur in up to 30% of adults and is more common with chronic ingestion, cigarette smoking, neurologic symptoms, and older age (*Ann. Intern. Med.* 95:405, 1981).

2. **Laboratory data** should include CBC, electrolytes, BUN, creatinine, blood glucose, and coagulation parameters. Arterial blood gases may reveal an early respiratory alkalosis, followed by metabolic acidosis. Approximately 20% of patients will have either respiratory alkalosis or metabolic acidosis alone (*J. Crit. Illness* 1:77, 1986). Most adults with pure salicylate overdose have both a primary metabolic acidosis and a primary respiratory alkalosis. Following mixed overdoses, respiratory acidosis may become prominent (*Arch. Intern. Med.* 138:1481, 1978). Blood levels must be drawn 6 hours or more after ingestion to allow prediction of severity and disposition (Fig. 26-2). Earlier levels are appropriate in severely intoxicated patients to guide intervention. Levels greater than 70 mg/dl at any time represent moderate to

severe intoxication; levels greater than 100 mg/dl are very serious and often fatal. This information is of use only for acute overdoses; estimation of severity is invalidated by the use of enteric-coated aspirin or chronic ingestion.

3. **Therapy** includes induced emesis followed by administration of charcoal and cathartic. Multidose charcoal may be of some use in severe overdose (*Pediatrics* 85:594, 1990). **Alkaline diuresis** is indicated for levels above 40 mg/dl and is achieved by administering 88 mEq of sodium bicarbonate in 1,000 ml D5W at a rate of 10–15 ml/kg/hour if the patient is clinically dehydrated, until urine flow is achieved. Alkalinization is maintained using the same solution at two to three times maintenance fluid requirement, following urine output, urine pH (target 7–8), and serum potassium. Achievement of alkaline diuresis often requires the simultaneous administration of at least 20 mEq/liter of potassium chloride. Vigorous fluid therapy is problematic in the elderly, as it may promote pulmonary edema. Although acetazolamide will cause urine alkalinization, the associated acidemia increases salicylate toxicity, and it should not be used. **Hemodialysis** is indicated for levels greater than 100–130 mg/dl but may be useful in chronic overdoses at levels as low as 40 mg/dl, if other indications for dialysis exist, including refractory acidosis, severe CNS symptoms, progressive clinical deterioration, pulmonary edema, and renal failure. In addition to dialysis, treatment of pulmonary edema may require mechanical ventilation with high fractions of inspired oxygen and positive end-expiratory pressure (PEEP). Cerebral edema is treated with hyperventilation and osmotic diuresis. Patients with minor symptoms (nausea, vomiting, tinnitus), an acute ingestion less than 150 mg/kg, a first blood level less than 65 mg/dl, and documented subsequent decline in blood level may be treated in the emergency department; these patients are often medically stable for discharge, and disposition should be determined based on psychiatric evaluation. Moderate symptomatology mandates admission for at least 24 hours; severe overdoses, manifested by tachypnea, dehydration, altered mental status, or a total dose greater than 300 mg/kg, require admission, usually to the intensive care unit. The elderly are at high risk and should be treated as such.

L. **Sedative-hypnotics** include a diverse spectrum of frequently abused compounds.

1. **Barbiturates.** Toxic manifestations of barbiturates vary with the amount of ingestion, type of drug, and length of time since ingestion. Short-acting barbiturates (e.g., amobarbital, secobarbital, and pentobarbital) generally cause toxicity with lower doses than the long-acting barbiturates (e.g., phenobarbital and barbital), but fatalities are more common with the latter.

   a. **Clinical manifestations.** Mild intoxication resembles alcohol intoxication. Moderate intoxication is characterized by greater depression of mental status, response only to painful stimuli, decreased deep tendon reflexes, and slow respirations. Severe intoxication causes coma and a loss of all reflexes (except pupillary light reflex). Plantar reflexes are extensor. Characteristic bullae ("barb burns") may be seen over pressure points, as well as on the dorsum of the fingers (*Br. Med. J.* 1:835, 1965). Hypothermia and hypotension may occur. In severe cases, there is no electrical activity seen on an EEG.

   b. **Treatment.** Maintenance of a patent airway and adequate ventilation and tissue perfusion are essential. Longer-acting barbiturate overdoses should be treated by **gastric emptying** and **activated charcoal** administration. Multidose activated charcoal (50 g PO or per gastric tube q4h) markedly decreases the half-life of phenobarbital (*J.A.M.A.* 251:3104, 1984; *Q. J. Med.* 235:997, 1986). A single dose of cathartic may be useful. Pill concretions may require repeated lavage. **Forced alkaline diuresis,** similar to that used for salicylate intoxication, and hemoperfusion are effective. Charcoal or resin **hemoperfusion** should be used for stage IV coma with high blood levels and is more effective than hemodialysis. Norepinephrine or dopamine may be necessary to correct hypotension, although fluid administration is usually effective. For short-acting barbiturates, charcoal or resin hemoperfusion appears to be more effective than hemo-dialysis. Multidose activated charcoal and alkalinization have not shown any benefit.

2. **Benzodiazepines** depress mental and respiratory function when taken in overdose. Fatalities are rare (*J. Intern. Med.* 226:117, 1989). Mixed overdoses are commmon.

   a. **Symptoms** include drowsiness, dysarthria, ataxia, and confusion.

   b. **Treatment** should include gastric emptying, activated charcoal administration, cathartic, and general supportive measures. Rarely, respiratory depression may require intubation. **Flumazenil,** a benzodiazepine antagonist, reverses toxicity without causing respiratory depression (*Eur. J. Anaesth.* 2[Suppl.]:295, 1988); 0.2 mg (2 ml) is administered IV over 30 seconds followed by 0.3 mg at 1 minute, 0.5 mg at 2 minutes, and repeated doses of 0.5 mg each minute to a total dose of 3 mg. If, at this point, no response has been observed, benzodiazepines are unlikely to be the cause of the sedation. If a partial response has occurred, further 0.5-mg increments may be given to a total of 5 mg. Recurrence of sedation and/or respiratory depression may be treated by repeating the above regimen or by continuous infusion of 0.1–0.5 mg/hour.

3. **Nonbarbiturate sedative-hypnotics.** Toxicities are similar to barbiturates.

   a. **Nonspecific manifestations** of mild intoxication include drowsiness, nystagmus, slurred speech, and ataxia. Severe overdoses cause respiratory and CNS depression. Hypothermia, seizures, and pulmonary edema may occur.

   b. **Specific toxicities**

      (1) **Methaqualone** causes pyramidal tract signs, including hypertonicity, myoclonus, and hyperreflexia. Cardiovascular and respiratory depression are generally less severe than with the other agents.

      (2) **Glutethimide** produces more pronounced anticholinergic effects than the other agents. Additionally, coma may be prolonged and may recur despite initial improvement. Cerebral edema and papilledema may occur, presumably secondary to cerebral hypoxia.

      (3) **Ethchlorvynol** imparts a pungent aromatic odor to the breath. Bradycardia may be a prominent component in severe toxicity. Noncardiogenic pulmonary edema may occur.

      (4) **Chloral hydrate** has a negative inotropic effect that exacerbates the hypotension characteristic of the sedative-hypnotics. Ventricular and supraventricular arrhythmias may occur with severe overdoses.

   c. **Treatment** includes support of respiration and circulation along with activated charcoal administration. Hemoperfusion may be used for severe overdoses. Hospitalization is recommended in all cases because of the prolonged duration of action of drugs in this class.

M. **Stimulants** include amphetamines and cocaine.

   1. **Amphetamine** toxicity is manifested by hyperactivity, irritability, delirium, hallucinations, psychosis, mydriasis, hyperpyrexia, hypertension, arrhythmias, vomiting, and diarrhea. Less common manifestations include acute renal failure secondary to rhabdomyolysis, seizures, CNS hemorrhage, coma, and circulatory collapse. **Treatment** includes early administration of activated charcoal and cathartic. **Emesis is contraindicated,** as it may induce seizures. Hemodialysis is not clearly effective. Agitation and psychosis are treated with haloperidol or chlorpromazine, which may also be useful in treating hypertension. Severe hypertension may require administration of nitroprusside or a beta-adrenergic antagonist. Diazepam is the drug of choice for seizures. Arrhythmias usually respond to propranolol or lidocaine. Hyperthermia may require cooling blankets or paralysis.

   2. **Cocaine**

      a. **Symptoms.** Cocaine causes short-lived CNS and sympathetic stimulation, hypertension, tachypnea, tachycardia, and mydriasis. Depression of the higher nervous centers follows rapidly and may result in death. Mortality may also result from drug-induced seizures, subarachnoid hemorrhage, stroke, or direct cardiac effects (e.g., coronary artery spasm, myocardial injury, and precipitation of lethal arrhythmias) (*N. Engl. J. Med.* 315:1495, 1986). **Myocardial infarction** may be precipitated in individuals without underlying heart disease. Rhabdomyolysis may occur. **Pulmonary edema** may develop abruptly after smoking the alkaloidal form ("crack"). Pneumomediastinum may occur after smoking crack and may progress to pneumothorax. Other pulmonary complications include alveolar hemorrhage, obliterative bronchiolitis, hypersensitivity pneumonitis, and asthma (*Am. J. Med.* 87:664, 1989).

   b. Treatment includes maintenance of a patent airway and support of respiration and circulation. Myocardial infarction should be managed as outlined in Chap. 5; calcium channel antagonists and nitrates may be useful for coronary artery spasm. Beta-adrenergic antagonists should be avoided, as they allow unopposed alpha-adrenergic vasospasm. Urgent catheterization and thrombolysis may be necessary. Benzodiazepines are helpful in decreasing the stimulatory effect of cocaine and should be used to treat seizures. Noncoronary manifestations of adrenergic stimulation may be treated with labetalol; severe or sustained hypertension may require treatment with nitroprusside. Rhabdomyolysis and hypotension are treated supportively. Hyperthermia may require a cooling blanket, sedation, or paralysis. Patients with marked toxicity require hospitalization for observation. Suspected patients should be x-rayed for continued presence of cocaine-containing condoms in their intestinal tract (*Gastrointest. Radiol.* 11:351, 1986). If present, gentle catharsis with charcoal and mineral oil should be performed (*Ann. Intern. Med.* 100:73, 1984). Whole bowel irrigation and surgery are probably not necessary, but intensive care unit admission and monitoring are. With appropriate care, mortality is less than 1% (*Am. J. Med.* 88:325, 1990).

N. Cyclic antidepressants. Traditional tricyclics include amitriptyline, imipramine, desipramine, nortriptyline, doxepin, and protriptyline. Pharmacologic actions include central and peripheral anticholinergic activity, depression of myocardial contractility, slowing of intraventricular and atrioventricular conduction, and CNS effects similar to phenothiazines. Newer cyclic antidepressants include amoxapine and loxapine (tricyclics with diminished cardiovascular toxicity but increased propensity to severe seizures), maprotiline (a tetracyclic with seizure proclivity and cardiovascular toxicity similar to older tricyclics), and trazodone (a noncyclic with minimal cardiovascular and CNS toxicity). Overdose with cyclic antidepressants is the leading cause of drug-related death in the United States. Overdoses less than 20 mg/kg cause few fatalities; 35 mg/kg is the approximate median lethal dose; and overdoses greater than 50 mg/kg are likely to cause death.

   1. Clinical manifestations include evidence of cholinergic blockade (mydriasis, ileus, urinary retention, and hyperpyrexia). **Cardiovascular toxicity** occurs as a result of anticholinergic, catecholamine-related, quinidine-like, and alpha-antagonist effects; these include supraventricular and ventricular arrhythmias, conduction blocks, hypotension, hypoperfusion, and pulmonary edema. **CNS manifestations** range from initial agitation to confusion, stupor, and coma. Seizures may occur, and the resultant metabolic acidosis may worsen cardiac toxicity.

   2. Laboratory evaluation. Plasma levels correlate poorly with severity of symptoms, although blood levels greater than 1,000 ng/ml have a higher risk of cardiac toxicity. ABGs are useful for ensuring adequate gas exchange and monitoring alkalinization. ECGs showing limb lead QRS duration greater than 100 msec are predictive of seizures and cardiac toxicity; a terminal 40-msec QRS axis greater than 120 degrees is even more sensitive (*N. Engl. J. Med.* 313:474, 1985; *Ann. Emerg. Med.* 18:348, 1989).

   3. Treatment includes supportive measures and gastrointestinal decontamination. Ipecac syrup is not recommended, as obtundation may occur rapidly and promote aspiration. **Gastric lavage** should be performed regardless of time of presentation, as gastric emptying is delayed by the drug. Repetitive administration of activated charcoal, 50 g PO or per tube q2–4h, is useful. One dose of cathartic should be given. Charcoal given q1h may reduce the half-life from 36 to 4 hours. Gastric suction between charcoal instillations may promote further removal. Forced diuresis and hemodialysis are not indicated. **Resin or charcoal hemoperfusion** removes less than 1–3% of body burden, but this reduction may be associated with improvement of life-threatening cardiac or CNS complications.

- a. **Cardiac toxicity. Continuous cardiac monitoring is mandatory.** Cyclic antidepressants are protein-bound in an alkaline environment and are toxic in an acid environment. Cardiac (and CNS) toxicity is therefore enhanced by metabolic or respiratory acidosis. Treatment should be initiated prophylactically, as toxic complications are often refractory to therapy once they have developed. **Alkalinization** with IV sodium bicarbonate, 1–2 mEq/kg, to maintain an arterial pH of 7.45–7.55, is effective in preventing and treating hypotension, arrhythmias (including ventricular and supraventricular arrhythmias), and conduction disturbances. For the intubated patient, hyperventilation to a PCO_2 equal to or greater than 25 and arterial pH of 7.45–7.55 is an effective means of alkalinization and avoids the administration of large amounts of sodium. Physostigmine, because of its narrow margin of safety, should virtually never be used to treat dysrhythmias. Refractory ventricular arrhythmias may be managed with lidocaine or phenytoin. **Type I antiarrhythmics** (procainamide, quinidine, or disopyramide) **are contraindicated** because of additive toxicity. Phenytoin's ability to reverse heart conduction abnormalities is largely anecdotal, and objective studies do not support its use (*Ann. Emerg. Med.* 15:876, 1986). Temporary ventricular pacing is used for complete heart block. Hypotension unresponsive to alkalinization and fluid administration should be treated with norepinephrine.
- b. **CNS complications.** Alkalinization does not reverse CNS complications. Physostigmine (2 mg IV over 1 minute) reverses CNS depression rapidly in patients with pure cyclic antidepressant overdose. However, because repeated doses are necessary and physostigmine may cause seizures, its use is generally not recommended. Supportive care of coma is usually adequate. Seizures may be treated with diazepam and phenytoin; status epilepticus (particularly common with amoxapine) should be treated aggressively, including high-dose barbiturates, paralysis, and general anesthesia, to prevent permanent neurologic damage (*J.A.M.A.* 250:1069, 1983).
- c. **Respiratory depression is common** and is treated with mechanical ventilation. Pulmonary edema and aspiration are common (*Clin. Toxicol.* 25:443, 1987) as is charcoal aspiration (*Chest* 96:852, 1989).
4. **Disposition.** Patients who have a depressed level of consciousness, respiratory depression, hypotension, arrhythmia, conduction blocks (including QRS > 100 msec), or seizures must be admitted to an intensive care unit. Asymptomatic individuals with a normal ECG may be observed in the emergency department with cardiac monitoring for 6 hours following intestinal decontamination and repeated charcoal. If they remain asymptomatic, the ECG remains normal, and they have normal bowel sounds, they may undergo psychiatric disposition (*J.A.M.A.* 257:521, 1987; *J. Emerg. Med.* 6:121, 1988). If any signs or symptoms are present, they must be admitted. Caution is imperative; 25% of fatal cases are awake and alert at the time of presentation, and three-fourths of those are in normal sinus rhythm. After admission, criteria for discharge from an intensive care unit include lack of all cyclic antidepressant symptoms, normal mental status, and no ECG abnormalities (including sinus tachycardia) for 24 hours. Patients fully meeting these criteria rarely develop subsequent significant arrhythmias.

Toxic Inhalants

Toxic inhalants comprise a variety of noxious gases and particulate matter capable of producing local irritation, asphyxiation, and systemic toxicity. In managing exposure victims, it is important to identify the offending agent and contact the regional poison control center for specific therapeutic guidelines.

I. **Irritant gases** produce cutaneous burns, mucosal irritation, laryngotracheitis, bronchitis, pneumonitis, bronchospasm, and pulmonary edema (which may be delayed up to 24 hours after exposure). The more water-soluble gases (e.g., chlorine, ammonia, formaldehyde, sulfur dioxide, ozone) primarily produce inflammation of the eyes, throat, and upper respiratory tract, whereas the less soluble gases (e.g., phosgene, nitrogen dioxide) tend to cause more damage to the terminal airways and alveoli. Household exposure may result from inadvertent mixture of bleach (sodium hypochlorite) with toilet bowl cleaner (sulfuric acid), producing chlorine gas, or bleach with ammonia, producing chloramine gas.

   A. **Treatment.** A patent airway and adequate oxygenation are essential. Bronchospasm should be treated with bronchodilators. Noncardiogenic pulmonary edema should be treated with oxygen, mechanical ventilation, and positive end-expiratory pressure as needed (see Chap. 9). Skin burns are treated by copious irrigation, removal of contaminated clothing, and tetanus prophylaxis (see Appendix E), if needed. Chemical contact with the eyes requires immediate, copious irrigation with water or saline. Ophthalmologic consultation is recommended for caustic eye burns.

   B. **Disposition.** Because pulmonary edema may develop, asymptomatic patients with normal ABGs and chest radiographs should be observed for at least 6 hours. Patients with symptoms or signs of upper airway edema or pulmonary involvement warrant hospitalization.

II. **Simple asphyxiants** (e.g., acetylene, argon, ethane, helium, hydrogen, nitrogen, methane, butane, neon, carbon dioxide, natural gas, and propane) cause hypoxia by displacing oxygen from the inspired air. Morbidity and mortality are related to the extent and duration of the hypoxia. **Treatment** consists of supplemental oxygen for symptomatic patients and supportive care.

III. **Systemic toxic inhalants** are those gases capable of producing prominent systemic toxicity, including hydrogen sulfide, methyl bromide, organophosphates (see Overdosage, sec. **VI.G**), carbon monoxide, and hydrogen cyanide. Treatment consists of supportive care and specific therapy directed toward the offending agent.

   A. **Carbon monoxide** displaces oxygen from hemoglobin, shifts the oxyhemoglobin dissociation curve to the left, and depresses cellular respiration by inhibiting the cytochrome oxidase system. Direct binding to cardiac myoglobin depresses cardiac function. Toxic manifestations are a consequence of tissue hypoxia. Poisoning usually occurs in poorly ventilated areas in which carbon monoxide is released by fires, combustion engines, or faulty stoves or heating systems. **Arterial PO_2 is usually normal; thus the diagnosis of carbon monoxide poisoning requires a high level of suspicion and direct measurement of arterial oxygen saturation or carbon monoxide (carboxyhemoglobin) levels.**

      1. **Symptoms,** in general, correlate with the carbon monoxide level. Levels of 20–40% are associated with dizziness, headache, weakness, disturbed judgment, nausea and vomiting, and diminished visual acuity. Examination may reveal retinal hemorrhages. Levels of 40–60% are associated with tachypnea, tachycardia, ataxia, syncope, and seizures. The ECG may reveal ST segment changes, conduction blocks, and atrial or ventricular arrhythmias. Levels greater than 60% are associated with coma and death. Cherry-red coloration of the lips or skin is a relatively rare, late manifestation. Late complications include basal ganglia infarction and parkinsonism. Less severe, delayed neuropsychiatric symptoms may also occur.

      2. **Treatment** consists of supportive care and administration of **100% oxygen** delivered by tight-fitting mask or endotracheal tube. The latter ensures tissue oxygen delivery and decreases the half-life of carboxyhemoglobin to 90

minutes from 4–5 hours. Carboxyhemoglobin levels should be measured q2–4h, and oxygen should be continued until blood levels are less than 10%. **Hyperbaric oxygen** (3 atm) is strongly recommended for patients who present with neurologic signs or symptoms, ECG changes consistent with ischemia, severe metabolic acidosis, pulmonary edema, or shock. It is also recommended for carboxyhemoglobin levels greater than 25–30%, but this is controversial. Transfer to a hyperbaric oxygen facility should occur only after the patient is stabilized. Seizures are treated with diazepam and phenytoin.

B. Hydrogen cyanide may be present in industrial fumigants, insecticides, and products of combustion of synthetics and plastics from house fires. The gas has a characteristic "bitter almond" odor, which many people are unable to smell. Toxic amounts are rapidly absorbed through the bronchial mucosa and alveoli, and symptoms usually appear seconds after inhalation. Concentrations of 0.2–0.3 mg/liter of air are almost immediately fatal. Oral exposures to **potassium cyanide** may occur with rodenticides, insecticides, silver polish, artificial fingernail remover (acetonitrile), film developer, laboratory reagents, and amygdalin (*N. Engl. J. Med.* 300:238, 1979).

    1. Toxic manifestations are due to inhibition of cytochrome oxidase and include palpitations, dyspnea, and mental status depression, which may quickly progress to coma and death. ECG changes include atrial fibrillation, ventricular ectopy, and abnormal ventricular repolarization. Severe lactic acidosis is present, and venous oxygen content is approximately equal to arterial oxygen content. Measurement of whole blood cyanide levels will delay therapy for at least 2 hours.

    2. Therapy. Specific antidote kits are available to treat cyanide poisoning. **Amyl nitrite** (one perle held under the nostril for 15–30 seconds/min, repeated every minute with a new perle) produces a methemoglobin level of approximately 5% and should be followed by 10 ml of 3% **sodium nitrite** (0.3 g IV over 3–5 minutes). This also converts hemoglobin to methemoglobin, which binds to the cyanide ion, sparing vital oxidative enzymes. One-half of this dose of sodium nitrite may be repeated in 30 minutes if there is an inadequate response. The goal is a measured methemoglobin level of 30%. Methylene blue should not be given. **Sodium thiosulfate** (50 ml of a 25% solution IV) converts the cyanide into thiocyanate. One-half the dose may be repeated in 30 minutes if there is an inadequate response. **Oxygen (100%)** must be administered at all times during treatment to ensure adequate tissue oxygen delivery despite methemoglobinemia. Continuous ECG monitoring is mandatory. Endotracheal intubation will protect the airway; mechanical ventilation may be needed. **Sodium bicarbonate,** 1 mEq/kg, is administered after the above measures are undertaken for severe, persistent acidosis (pH less than 7.2). Seizures are treated with diazepam and phenytoin. In the event of an oral ingestion, the stomach should be emptied after the above measures have been undertaken, and activated charcoal should be administered. The efficacy of **hyperbaric oxygen** is controversial but may be considered for those who respond poorly to the above. **Hydroxycobalamin** binds cyanide but is not currently available in the United States.

C. Hydrogen sulfide is a colorless gas with a characteristic "rotten egg" odor. It is found in mines and sewers as well as petrochemical, agricultural, and tanning industries. As with hydrogen cyanide, toxicity is secondary to inhibition of cytochrome oxidase.

    1. Symptoms. Exposure to low concentration causes eye irritation and visual changes, including blurred vision and scotomata. Higher concentrations cause cyanosis, confusion, pulmonary edema, coma, and convulsions. Rapid death occurs in approximately 6%.

    2. Treatment is similar to that used for hydrogen cyanide. Oxygen (100%) and nitrites are used; thiosulfate is not. The efficacy of nitrites is controversial.

IV. Smoke inhalation. Smoke is a suspension of small particles in a heated gas. Greater than 50% of fire-related deaths are due to smoke inhalation. Thermal injury is usually confined to the upper airway because of the rapid cooling of inhaled gases that occurs proximal to the larynx. Toxic gases released by pyrolysis include carbon dioxide, carbon monoxide, hydrogen chloride, phosgene, chlorine, benzene, isocyanate, hydrogen cyanide, aldehydes, oxides of sulfur and nitrogen, ammonia, and numerous organic acids. Carbon monoxide accounts for 80% of mortality in the first 12 hours. The other toxins produce epithelial injury resulting in airway edema, increased capillary permeability, and mechanical obstruction from desquamated tissue and secretions. Patients who have been exposed to a large quantity of smoke in a closed space, had prolonged inhalation, had steam exposure, were involved in an explosion, were with other persons who died or were severely injured, or have sustained facial burns or singed nasal vibrissae are at risk for developing respiratory complications, which may be delayed in onset for up to 3 days. High-risk patients should undergo upper airway endoscopy to rule out immediately life-threatening airway injury; bronchoscopy or Xenon lung scanning is useful in confirming the diagnosis. A positive Xenon scan predicts increased mortality. Carboxyhemoglobin levels greater than 15% are indicative of severe exposure.

A. **Clinical manifestations.** Asphyxiation, expectoration of carbonaceous sputum, hoarseness, dyspnea from upper airway edema, stridor, bronchospasm, and noncardiogenic pulmonary edema are characteristic features of smoke inhalation. Upper airway burns may also be noted. Late complications include bacterial pneumonia and pulmonary embolism.

B. **Treatment. Scrupulous airway care is essential,** with frequent suctioning as needed. Endotracheal intubation is required in patients with evidence of significant upper airway edema or respiratory insufficiency. Bronchoscopy may be necessary to remove endotracheal debris. **Humidified oxygen** should be administered to all patients. Bronchodilators are indicated for bronchospasm. For those who develop adult respiratory distress syndrome, mechanical ventilation with PEEP is indicated. Prophylactic antibiotics and glucocorticoids are not indicated. Specific toxins, such as cyanide, carbon monoxide, and so on, should be treated (see sec. **III**).

C. **Disposition.** Patients who have minor smoke inhalation and are asymptomatic at 4–6 hours with none of the above noted risk factors may be safely discharged home. Patients who are asymptomatic but have any of the above noted risk factors should be admitted for a minimum of 24 hours. Patients who have symptoms, significant laboratory abnormalities, or abnormal A-a gradient should be admitted to an intensive care unit.

Barnes Hospital Laboratory Reference Values

Richard D. Hockett, Jr., and
Eric D. Green

Reference values for the more commonly used laboratory tests are listed in the following table. The reference values are given in the units currently used at Barnes Hospital and in Systeme International (SI) units, which are used in many areas of the world. Individual reference values can be population- and method-dependent. Footnotes and a key to abbreviations appear on pages 522–523.

Test	Current units	Factor[a]	SI units
Common Serum Chemistries			
Albumin	3.6–5.0 g/dl	10	36–50 g/L
Ammonia (plasma)	19–43 μmol/L	1	19–43 μmol/L
Bilirubin			
Total[b]	0.2–1.3 mg/dl	17.1	3.4–22.2 μmol/L
Direct	0–0.2 mg/dl	17.1	0–3.4 μmol/L
Blood gases (arterial)			
pH	7.35–7.45	1	7.35–7.45
PO_2	80–105 mm Hg	0.133	10.6–14.0 kPa
PCO_2	35–45 mm Hg	0.133	4.7–6.0 kPa
Calcium			
Total	8.9–10.3 mg/dl	0.25	2.23–2.57 mmol/L
Free	4.6–5.1 mg/dl	0.25	1.15–1.27 mmol/L
CO_2 content (plasma)	22–31 mmol/L	1	22–31 mmol/L
Ceruloplasmin	21–53 mg/dl	0.063	1.3–3.3 μmol/L
Chloride	97–110 mmol/L	1	97–110 mmol/L
Cholesterol[c]			
Desirable level	<200 mg/dl	0.0259	<5.18 mmol/L
Borderline high	200–239 mg/dl	0.0259	5.18–6.19 mmol/L
High	≥240 mg/dl	0.0259	≥6.22 mmol/L
HDL cholesterol[b]	27–98 mg/dl	0.0259	0.70–2.54 mmol/L
Copper (total)	70–155 μg/dl	0.157	11.0–24.3 μmol/L
Creatinine[b]	0.5–1.7 mg/dl	88.4	44–150 μmol/L
Ferritin			
Male, adult	36–262 ng/ml	2.25	81–590 pmol/L
Female, adult	10–155 ng/ml	2.25	23–349 pmol/L
Folate			
Plasma	1.7–12.6 ng/ml	2.27	3.9–28.6 nmol/L
Red cell	153–602 ng/ml	2.27	347–1367 nmol/L
Glucose, fasting (plasma)	65–110 mg/dl	0.055	3.58–6.05 mmol/L
Glycated hemoglobin	4.4–6.3%	0.01	0.044–0.063
Haptoglobin	44–303 mg/dl	0.01	0.44–3.03 g/L
Iron (total)	50–175 μg/dl	0.179	9.0–31.3 μmol/L
Binding capacity	250–450 μg/dl	0.179	44.8–80.6 μmol/L
Transferrin saturation	20–50%	0.01	0.20–0.50

Test	Current units	Factor[a]	SI units
Common Serum Chemistries (continued)			
Lactate (plasma)	0.3–1.3 mmol/L	1	0.3–1.3 mmol/L
Magnesium	1.3–2.2 mEq/L	0.5	0.65–1.1 mmol/L
Osmolality	270–290 mOsm/kg	1	270–290 mmol/kg
Phosphate	2.5–4.5 mg/dl	0.323	0.81–1.45 mmol/L
Potassium (plasma)	3.3–4.9 mmol/L	1	3.3–4.9 mmol/L
Protein, total	6.5–8.5 g/dl	10	65–85 g/L
Sodium	135–145 mmol/L	1	135–145 mmol/L
Triglycerides, fasting[c]	<250 mg/dl	0.113	<2.83 mmol/L
Urea nitrogen	8–25 mg/dl	0.357	2.9–8.9 mmol/L
Uric acid[b]	3.0–8.0 mg/dl	59.5	179–476 μmol/L
Vitamin B_{12}	200–800 pg/ml	0.738	148–590 pmol/L
Common Serum Enzymatic Activities			
Aminotransferases			
Alanine (ALT, SGPT)	7–53 IU/L	0.01667	0.12–0.88 μkat/L
Aspartate (AST, SGOT)	11–47 IU/L	0.01667	0.18–0.78 μkat/L
Amylase	35–118 IU/L	0.01667	0.58–1.97 μkat/L
Creatine kinase			
Male	30–220 IU/L	0.01667	0.5–3.67 μkat/L
Female	20–170 IU/L	0.01667	0.33–2.83 μkat/L
MB fraction	0–12 IU/L	0.01667	0–0.20 μkat/L
γ-Glutamyl transpeptidase			
Male	20–76 IU/L	0.01667	0.33–1.27 μkat/L
Female	12–54 IU/L	0.01667	0.2–0.9 μkat/L
Lactate dehydrogenase[b]	90–280 IU/L	0.01667	1.50–4.67 μkat/L
Lipase	2.3–20 IU/dl	0.1667	0.38–3.33 μkat/L
5'-Nucleotidase	2–16 IU/L	0.01667	0.03–0.27 μkat/L
Phosphatase, acid	0–0.7 IU/L	16.67	0–11.6 nkat/L
Phosphatase, alkaline[d]	38–126 IU/L	0.01667	0.63–2.10 μkat/L
Common Serum Hormone Values[e]			
ACTH, fasting (8 A.M., supine)[f]	<60 pg/ml	0.22	<13.2 pmol/L
Aldosterone[f]	10–160 ng/L	2.77	28–443 mmol/L
Cortisol (plasma, morning)	8–25 μg/dl	0.027	0.22–0.68 μmol/L
FSH			
Male	2.4–19.9 IU/L	1	2.4–19.9 IU/L
Female			
Follicular	3.1–19.7 IU/L	1	3.1–19.7 IU/L
Luteal	10.4–23.1 IU/L	1	10.4–23.1 IU/L

Test	Current units	Factor[a]	SI units
Common Serum Hormone Values[e] (continued)			
Midcycle	1.7–11.2 IU/L	1	1.7–11.2 IU/L
Postmeno-pausal	18–126 IU/L	1	18–126 IU/L
Gastrin, fasting	0–130 pg/ml	1	0–130 ng/L
Growth hormone, fasting	<8 ng/ml	1	<8 µg/L
17-Hydroxy-progesterone			
Prepubertal	3–90 ng/dl	0.03	0.1–2.7 nmol/L
Male, adult	27–199 ng/dl	0.03	0.8–6.0 nmol/L
Female			
Follicular	15–70 ng/dl	0.03	0.5–2.1 nmol/L
Luteal	35–290 ng/dl	0.03	1.1–8.8 nmol/L
Insulin, fasting	5–25 mU/L	7.18	36–180 pmol/L
LH			
Male	0–8.9 IU/L	1	0–8.9 IU/L
Female			
Follicular	1.4–11.5 IU/L	1	1.4–11.5 IU/L
Luteal	0.1–16.1 IU/L	1	0.1–16.1 IU/L
Midcycle	20.1–73.9 IU/L	1	20.1–73.9 IU/L
Postmeno-pausal	8.4–46.5 IU/L	1	8.4–46.5 IU/L
Parathyroid hor-mone	4–9 µEq/ml		
Progesterone			
Male	<0.5 ng/ml	3.18	<1.6 nmol/L
Female			
Follicular	0.1–1.5 ng/ml	3.18	0.32–4.8 nmol/L
Luteal	2.5–28 ng/ml	3.18	8–89 nmol/L
1st trimester	9–47 ng/ml	3.18	29–149 nmol/L
3rd trimester	55–255 ng/ml	3.18	175–811 nmol/L
Postmeno-pausal	<0.5 ng/ml	3.18	<1.6 nmol/L
Prolactin			
Male	2–12 ng/ml	1	2–12 µg/L
Female	2–20 ng/ml	1	2–20 µg/L
Renin activity (plasma)[g]	0.9–3.3 ng/ml/hr	0.278	0.25–0.91 ng/(L × s)
Testosterone, to-tal			
Male	300–1200 ng/dl	0.0346	10.4–41.5 nmol/L
Female	30–120 ng/dl	0.0346	1–4 nmol/L
Testosterone, free			
Male	52–280 pg/ml	3.46	180–970 pmol/L
Female	1.1–6.3 pg/ml	3.46	4.0–22 pmol/L
Thyroxine, total (T_4)	3–12.0 µg/dl	12.9	39–155 nmol/L
Thyroxine, free	1.0–2.3 ng/dl	12.9	13–30 pmol/L
T-uptake[h]	20–40%	0.01	0.2–0.4
Triiodothyronine (T_3)	80–200 ng/dl	0.0154	1.2–3.1 nmol/L
T_4 index[i]	0.85–3.5	1	0.85–3.5
TSH	0.45–6.20 µU/ml	1	0.45–6.20 mU/L

Test	Current units	Factor[a]	SI units
Common Serum Hormone Values[e] (continued)			
Vitamin D, 1,25 dihydroxy	20–76 pg/ml	2.40	48–182 pmol/L
Vitamin D, 25 hydroxy	15–30 ng/ml	2.49	37–75 nmol/L
Common Urinary Chemistries			
δ-Aminolevulinic acid	1.3–7.0 mg/day	7.6	9.9–53 μmol/day
Amylase	0.04–0.30 IU/min	16.67	0.67–5.00 nkat/min
Calcium	0–250 mg/day	0.025	0–6.25 mmol/day
Catecholamines	<540 μg/day		
Dopamine	<85 μg/day		
Epinephrine	0–13 μg/day	5.5	0–71 nmol/day
Norepinephrine	11–86 μg/day	5.9	65–507 nmol/day
Copper	15–50 μg/day	0.0157	0.24–0.78 μmol/day
Cortisol, free	20–90 μg/day	2.76	55–248 nmol/day
Creatinine			
Male	1.0–2.0 g/day	8.84	8.8–17.7 mmol/day
Female	0.6–1.5 g/day	8.84	5.3–13.3 mmol/day
5-Hydroxyindole-acetic acid	0.2–5.7 mg/day	5.23	1.0–30 μmol/day
Hydroxyproline, total	25–77 mg/day	7.63	191–588 μmol/day
Metanephrine	0–1.0 mg/day	5.46	0–5.46 μmol/day
Oxalate	10–40 mg/day	11.4	114–456 μmol/day
Porphyrins			
Coproporphyrin	0–72 μg/day	1.53	0–110 nmol/day
Uroporphyrin	0–27 μg/day	1.2	0–32 nmol/day
Protein	0–150 mg/day	0.001	0–0.150 g/day
Vanillylmandelic acid (VMA)	2–10 mg/day	5.05	10–51 μmol/day
Common Hematologic Values			
Coagulation studies			
Bleeding time[j]	2.5–9.5 min	60	150–570 sec
Fibrin degradation products	<8 mg/ml		
Fibrinogen[k]	150–360 mg/dl	0.01	1.5–3.6 g/L
Partial thromboplastin time (activated)	25–36 sec	1	25–36 sec
Prothrombin time	11.0–14.0 sec	1	11.0–14.0 sec
Thrombin time	11.3–18.5 sec	1	11.3–18.5 sec

Test	Current units	Factor[a]	SI units
Common Hematologic Values (continued)			
Complete blood count			
Hematocrit			
Male	40.7–50.3%	0.01	0.407–0.503
Female	36.1–44.3%	0.01	0.361–0.443
Hemoglobin			
Male	13.8–17.2 g/dl	0.620[l]	8.56–10.7 mmol/L
Female	12.1–15.1 g/dl	0.620	7.50–9.36 mmol/L
Erythrocyte count			
Male	$4.5–5.7 \times 10^6/\mu l$	1	$4.5–5.7 \times 10^{12}/L$
Female	$3.9–5.0 \times 10^6/\mu l$	1	$3.9–5.0 \times 10^{12}/L$
Mean corpuscular hemoglobin	26.7–33.7 pg/cell	0.062	1.66–2.09 fmol/cell
Mean corpuscular hemoglobin concentration	32.7–35.5 g/dl	0.620	20.3–22.0 mmol/L
Mean corpuscular volume	$80.0–97.6 \ \mu m^3$	1	80.0–97.6 fl
Red cell distribution width	11.8–14.6%	0.01	0.118–0.146
Leukocyte profile			
Total	$3.8–9.8 \times 10^3/\mu l$	1	$3.8–9.8 \times 10^9/L$
Lymphocytes	$1.2–3.3 \times 10^3/\mu l$	1	$1.2–3.3 \times 10^9/L$
Mononuclear cells	$0.2–0.7 \times 10^3/\mu l$	1	$0.2–0.7 \times 10^9/L$
Granulocytes	$1.8–6.6 \times 10^3/\mu l$	1	$1.8–6.6 \times 10^9/L$
Platelet count	$190–405 \times 10^3/\mu l$	1	$190–405 \times 10^9/L$
Sedimentation rate	0–30 mm/hr		
Reticulocyte count	0.5–1.5%	0.01	0.005–0.015
Immunology Testing			
Complement (total hemolytic)[m]	118–226 CH_{50} U/ml		
C3	77–156 mg/dl	0.01	0.71–1.56 g/L
C4	15–39 mg/dl	0.01	0.15–0.39 g/L
Immunoglobulin			
IgA	91–518 mg/dl	0.01	0.91–5.18 g/L
IgM	61–355 mg/dl	0.01	0.61–3.55 g/L
IgG	805–1830 mg/dl	0.01	8.05–18.3 g/L
Therapeutic Agents			
Amitriptyline (+ Nortriptyline)	100–250 μg/L		
Carbamazepine	4–10 mg/L	4.23	17–42 μmol/L
Clonazepam	10–80 ng/ml	3.17	32–254 nmol/L
Cyclosporine (whole blood)	125–300 ng/ml		

Test	Current units	Factor[a]	SI units
Therapeutic Agents (continued)			
Digoxin	0.5–2.0 µg/L	1.28	0.6–2.6 nmol/L
Disopyramide	2–5 mg/ml	2.95	6–15 µmol/L
Ethosuximide	40–100 mg/ml	7.08	283–708 µmol/L
Imipramine			
Imipramine	150–300 µg/L	3.57	536–1071 nmol/L
Desipramine	100–300 µg/L	3.75	375–1125 nmol/L
Lithium	0.6–1.2 mmol/L	1	0.6–1.2 mmol/L
Nortriptyline	50–175 µg/L	3.80	190–665 nmol/L
Phenobarbital	10–40 mg/L	4.30	43–172 µmol/L
Phenytoin (diphe-nylhydantoin)	10–20 mg/L	3.96	40–79 µmol/L
Primidone			
Primidone	5–15 mg/L	4.58	23–69 µmol/L
Phenobarbital	10–40 mg/L	4.30	43–172 µmol/L
Procainamide			
Procainamide	4–8 mg/L	4.23	17–34 µmol/L
Procainamide + N-Acetyl-procainamide	5–30 mg/L		
Quinidine	1.7–6.1 mg/L	3.08	5.2–18.8 µmol/L
Salicylate[n]	20–290 mg/L	0.0072	0.14–2.1 mmol/L
Theophylline	10–20 mg/L	5.5	55–110 µmol/L
Valproic acid	50–100 mg/L	6.93	346–693 µmol/L
Antimicrobials			
Amikacin			
Trough	5–10 mg/L	1.71	8.6–17 µmol/L
Peak	20–30 mg/L	1.71	34–51 µmol/L
5-Fluorocytosine			
Trough	20–60 mg/L		
Peak	50–100 mg/L		
Gentamicin			
Trough	<2 mg/L	2.09	<4.2 µmol/L
Peak	4–8 mg/L	2.09	8.4–16.7 µmol/L
Ketoconazole			
Trough	≤1 mg/L		
Peak	1–4 mg/L		
Sulfamethoxazole			
Trough	75–120 mg/L		
Peak	100–150 mg/L		
Tobramycin			
Trough	<2 mg/L	2.14	<4.3 µmol/L
Peak	4–8 mg/L	2.14	8.6–17 µmol/L
Trimethoprim			
Trough	2–8 mg/L		
Peak	5–15 mg/L		
Vancomycin			
Trough	5–10 mg/L		
Peak	20–35 mg/L		

[a] A more complete list of multiplication factors for converting conventional units to SI units can be found in *Ann. Intern. Med.* 106:114, 1987; and in *The SI for the Health Professions,* World Health Organization, 1977.

[b] Variation occurs with age and sex. This range includes both sexes and persons older than 5 years.
[c] Guidelines of the Adult Treatment Panel of the National Cholesterol Education Program (*Arch. Intern. Med.* 148:36, 1988).
[d] Higher values (up to 250 mU/ml) can be normal in persons younger than 20 years.
[e] Since most hormones are measured by immunologic techniques and because hormones may vary in molecular weight (e.g., gastrin), most are expressed as mass/liter. The reference ranges are highly method-dependent.
[f] Supine, normal salt diet; in the upright position, the reference range is 40–310 ng/liter.
[g] High-sodium diet, supplemented with sodium 3 g/day.
[h] Replaces T_3 resin uptake.
[i] $T_4 \times$ (T-uptake).
[j] Template modified after Ivy.
[k] Determined by the Clauss method (see Chap. 17).
[l] This factor assumes a unit molecular weight of 16,000; assuming a unit molecular weight of 64,500, the multiplication factor is 0.155.
[m] CH_{50} = reciprocal of dilution of sera required to lyse 50% of sheep erythrocytes.
[n] Therapeutic range for treatment of rheumatoid arthritis (see Chap. 24).

Key to abbreviations
dl = deciliter
fl = femtoliter
fmol = femtomole
hr = hour
g = gram
Hg = mercury
IU = international unit
katal = mole/sec
kPa = kilopascal
kg = kilogram
L = liter
μg = microgram
μkat = microkatal
μl = microliter
μm^3 = cubic micron
μmol = micromole
μU = microunit
mEq = milliequivalent
mg = milligram
min = minute
ml = milliliter
mm = millimeter
mmol = millimole
mOsm = milliosmole
mU = milliunit
ng = nanogram
nkat = nanokatal
nmol = nanomole
pg = picogram
pmol = picomole
sec = second
SGOT = serum glutamic oxaloacetic transaminase
SGPT = serum glutamic pyruvic transaminase
U = unit

B

Drug Interactions of Commonly Prescribed Medications

Anne M. Pittman

Medication	Increases level or effect of:	Decreases level or effect of:	Potentiates side effect or toxicity of:
Acetazolamide	Quinidine		Phenytoin
Allopurinol	Azathioprine, cyclophosphamide, 6-mercaptopurine, warfarin		
Aminoglycosides	Neuromuscular blocking agents		Ethacrynic acid
Amiodarone	Digoxin, quinidine, warfarin		
Antacids	Quinidine	Cimetidine, iron supplements, isoniazid, salicylates, tetracycline	
Barbiturates	CNS depressants	Chloramphenicol, griseofulvin, oral contraceptives, quinidine, tetracycline, warfarin, beta antagonists	
Benzodiazepines	CNS depressants		
Beta antagonists	Chlorpromazine		
Captopril	K$^+$ supplements		
Carbamazepine	Isoniazid metabolites, lithium	Theophylline, warfarin	
Chloral hydrate	Ethanol, warfarin		
Chloramphenicol	Barbiturates, phenytoin, oral hypoglycemic agents, warfarin		
Chlorpromazine	Beta antagonists		
Cimetidine	Benzodiazepines, beta antagonists, CNS depressants, procainamide, quinidine, theophylline, tricyclic antidepressants, warfarin	Antacids	
Ciprofloxacin	Theophylline		
Clofibrate	Oral hypoglycemic agents, warfarin		
Clonidine			Beta antagonists

Medication	Increases level or effect of:	Decreases level or effect of:	Potentiates side effect or toxicity of:
CNS depressants	Anticonvulsants, barbiturates, benzodiazepines, beta antagonists, cimetidine, ethanol, MAO inhibitors, narcotic analgesics, phenothiazine		Lithium, muscle relaxants
Cyclophosphamide	Allopurinol		
Digoxin	Amiodarone		
Disulfiram	Benzodiazepines, phenytoin, warfarin		
Erythromycin	Carbamazepine, theophylline, warfarin		Terfenadine
Ethacrynic acid	Warfarin, glucocorticoids, aminoglycosides, digoxin		
Furosemide	Digoxin		
Griseofulvin		Warfarin, barbiturates	
Indomethacin/ibuprofen	Lithium, methotrexate	Captopril, furosemide	Triamterene
Isoniazid	Carbamazepine, phenytoin		
Ketoconazole	Warfarin, cyclosporine		Terfenadine
Lidocaine	Cimetidine	Phenytoin	
MAO inhibitors	CNS depressants, oral hypoglycemic agents, sympathomimetic agents		
Methotrexate	Sulfonamides		
Methyldopa	Lithium, MAO inhibitors		
Metronidazole	Disulfiram, warfarin		
Muscle relaxants	CNS depressants, neuromuscular blocking agents		
Oral contraceptives	Benzodiazepines		
Oral hypoglycemic agents	Clofibrate, MAO inhibitors, warfarin		
Phenytoin	Chloramphenicol	Quinidine, theophylline, warfarin	

Medication	Increases level or effect of:	Decreases level or effect of:	Potentiates side effect or toxicity of:
Probenecid Propoxyphene Quinidine	Methotrexate Carbamazepine Digoxin, muscle relaxants, warfarin	Salicylates	
Rifampin		Beta antagonists, benzodiazepines, digoxin, disopyramide, oral hypoglycemic agents, quinidine, warfarin	
Salicylates	Methotrexate, oral hypoglycemic agents, warfarin		
Sulfonamides	Barbiturates, oral hypoglycemic agents, phenytoin, warfarin		
Theophylline		Lithium	
Thiazides	Digoxin, lithium		
Trazadone	Digoxin, phenytoin	Clonidine	
Triamterene	Potassium, indomethacin		
Tricyclic antidepressants		Clonidine	
Verapamil	Digoxin		

C

Intravenous Admixture Preparation and Administration Guide*

John R. Onufer and Robyn Burns Schaiff

Aminophylline
  Diluent: D5W, NS
  Concentration: 1 g/500 ml = 2 mg/ml
  Initial dosage: Loading dose 6 mg/kg over 20 minutes
  Infusion rate:
    Adult nonsmokers: 0.4 mg/kg/hr (28 mg or 14 ml/hr for 70-kg patient)
    Adult smokers: 0.7 mg/kg/hr (49 mg or 25 ml/hr for 70-kg patient)
    In CHF: 0.2 mg/kg/hr (14 mg or 7 ml/hr for 70-kg patient)
Bretylium (Bretylol)
  Diluent: NS, D5W
  Concentration: 2 g/500 ml = 4 mg/ml
  Drip rate:
    1 mg/min = 15 ml/hr
    2 mg/min = 30 ml/hr
    3 mg/min = 45 ml/hr
    4 mg/min = 60 ml/hr
Dobutamine (Dobutrex)
  Diluent: NS, D5W
  Concentration: 500 mg/500 ml = 1,000 μg/ml
  Drip rate: Usually starting at 3 μg/kg/min
    (Example: For a 70-kg patient to receive 3 μg/kg/min, the drip rate should be 13 ml/hr.)
Dopamine (Intropin)
  Diluent: NS, D5W
  Concentration: 800 mg/500 ml = 1,600 μg/ml (premix)
  Drip rate: Usually starting at 3 μg/kg/min
    (Example: For a 70-kg patient to receive 3 μg/kg/min, the drip rate should be 8 ml/hr.)
Isoproterenol (Isuprel)
  Diluent: NS, D5W
  1 amp = 1 mg
  Concentration: 2 mg/500 ml = 4 μg/ml
  Drip rate:
    1 μg/min = 15 ml/hr
    2 μg/min = 30 ml/hr
Levophed (see *Norepinephrine*)
Lidocaine
  Diluent: NS, D5W
  Concentration: 2 g/500 ml (premix) = 4 mg/ml
  Drip rate:
    1 mg/min = 15 ml/hr
    2 mg/min = 30 ml/hr
    3 mg/min = 45 ml/hr
Neo-Synephrine (see *Phenylephrine*)
Nitroglycerin
  Diluent: NS, D5W (glass bottles only, use special nitroglycerin tubing)
  1 vial = 50 mg
  Concentration: 50 mg/250 ml = 200 μg/ml
  Drip rate:
    10 μg/min = 3 ml/hr
    20 μg/min = 6 ml/hr

527

30 μg/min = 9 ml/hr
40 μg/min = 12 ml/hr

Nitroprusside (*Nipride*)
  Diluent: D5W **only**
  1 amp = 50 mg
  Concentration: 50 mg/250 ml = 200 μg/ml
  Drip rate:
    10 μg/min = 3 ml/hr
    20 μg/min = 6 ml/hr
    30 μg/min = 9 ml/hr

Norepinephrine (*Levophed*)
  Diluent: D5W **only**
  1 amp = 4 mg
  Concentration: 8 mg/500 ml = 16 μg/ml
  Drip rate:
    2 μg/min = 8 ml/hr (usual starting dose)
    3 μg/min = 11 ml/hr
    4 μg/min = 15 ml/hr

Phenylephrine (*Neo-Synephrine*)
  Diluent: NS, D5W
  Concentration: 10 mg/250 ml = 0.04 mg/ml
  Drip rate:
    0.04 mg/min = 60 ml/hr
    0.06 mg/min = 90 ml/hr
    0.08 mg/min = 120 ml/hr

Procainamide (*Pronestyl*)
  Diluent: NS, D5W
  Concentration: 2 g/500 ml = 4 mg/ml
  Drip rate:
    1 mg/min = 15 ml/hr
    2 mg/min = 30 ml/hr
    3 mg/min = 45 ml/hr

Theophylline (see *Aminophylline*)

---

* To determine drip rate:

$$\text{Concentration of solution} \left(\frac{\mu g}{ml}\right) \times \text{Drip rate} \left(\frac{ml}{min}\right) =$$

$$\text{Desired concentration of infusion} \left(\frac{\mu g}{min}\right)$$

$$\text{Drip rate} \left(\frac{ml}{min}\right) = \frac{\text{Desired concentration infused } (\mu g/kg/min) \times \text{weight in kg}}{\text{Concentration of solution } (\mu g/ml)}$$

Drip rate (gtt/min) = (60 gtt/ml) × (drip rate ml/min) **(if using microtubing)**

Dosage Adjustments of Drugs in Renal Failure

Steven B. Miller

Name	Route of elimination	Adjusted dosing interval (hr) or dose % for GFR (ml/min)			Supplement after dialysis
		>50	10–50	<10	
Aminoglycosides					
Amikacin*	R	12	12–18	>24	HD, PD
Gentamicin*	R	8–12	12	>24	HD, PD
Netilmicin*	R	8–12	12	>24	HD, PD
Tobramycin*	R	8–12	12	>24	HD, PD
Penicillins					
Ampicillin	R,H	6	6–12	12–16	HD
Carbenicillin	R,H	8–12	12–24	24–48	HD, PD
Dicloxacillin	R,H	N	N	N	N
Mezlocillin	R,H	4–6	6–8	8–12	HD
Oxacillin	R,H	N	N	N	N
Penicillin G	R,H	N	75%	25–50%	HD
Piperacillin	R,H	4–6	6–8	8	HD
Ticarcillin	R	8	8–12	24	HD
Cephalosporins					
Cefamandole	R	6	6–8	8–12	HD
Cefazolin	R	8	12	24–48	HD
Cefixime	R	12–24	75%	50%	N
Cefoperazone	H	N	N	N	N
Cefotaxime	R,H	6–8	8–12	24	HD
Cefotetan	R	12	24	24	HD, PD
Cefoxitin	R	8	8–12	24–48	HD
Ceftazidime	R	8–12	24–48	48–72	HD
Ceftizoxime	R	8–12	36–48	48–72	HD
Ceftriaxone	R,H	N	N	24	N
Cefuroxime	R	N	12	24	HD
Cephalexin	R	6	6	8–12	HD, PD
Cephalothin	R	6	6–8	12	HD, PD
Quinolones					
Ciprofloxacin	R	N	12–24	24	N
Norfloxacin	R	N	12–24	A	N
Ofloxacin	R	N	12–24	24	N
Other Antibacterial Agents					
Aztreonam	R	N	50–75%	25%	HD, PD
Chloramphenicol	R,H	N	N	N	N
Clindamycin	H	N	N	N	N
Doxycycline	R,H	12	12–18	18–24	N
Erythromycin	H	N	N	N	N

| Name | Route of elimination | Adjusted dosing interval (hr) or dose % for GFR (ml/min) | | | Supplement after dialysis |
		>50	10–50	<10	
Other Antibacterial Agents (continued)					
Imipenem	R	N	50%	25%	HD
Metronidazole	R,H	N	N	50%	HD
Minocycline	H	N	N	N	N
Pentamidine	?	N	N	24–48	N
Sulfamethoxazole	R,H	12	18	24	HD
Sulfisoxazole	R	6	8–12	12–24	HD, PD
Tetracycline	R,H	12	12–18	18–24	N
Trimethoprim	R,H	12	18	24	HD
Vancomycin* (IV)	R	24–72	72–240	240	N
Antifungal Agents					
Amphotericin B	N	24	24	24–36	N
Fluconazole	R,H	N	50%	25%	HD
Flucytosine	R	6	24	24–48	HD, PD
Ketoconazole	H	N	N	N	N
Miconazole	H	N	N	N	N
Antimycobacterial Agents					
Ethambutol	R	24	24–36	48	HD, PD
Isoniazid	H,R	N	N	N	HD, PD
Pyrazinamide	H,R	N	N	50%	HD, PD
Rifampin	H	N	N	N	N
Antiviral Agents					
Acyclovir (IV)	R	8	24	48	HD
Acyclovir (PO)	R	N	12–24	24	HD
Amantadine	R	12–24	24–72	72–168	N
Ganciclovir	R	12	24	24	HD
Zidovudine	H	N	N	N	HD
Nonsteroidal Anti–Inflammatory Drugs					
Acetaminophen	H	4	6	8	HD
Aspirin	H,R	4	4–6	A	HD
Ibuprofen	H	N	N	N	N
Indomethacin	H,R	N	N	N	N
Ketorolac (IM)	H,R	N	N	50%	N
Naproxen	H	N	N	N	N
Piroxicam	H	N	N	N	N
Sulindac	H,R	N	N	50%	N
Opioid Analgesic Drugs					
Codeine	H	N	75%	50%	N
Meperidine	H	N	75%	50%	N
Morphine	H	N	75%	50%	N

Name	Route of elimination	Adjusted dosing interval (hr) or dose % for GFR (ml/min)			Supplement after dialysis
		>50	10–50	<10	

Antihypertensive Drugs (see Angiotensin-Converting Enzyme Inhibitors, Beta-Adrenergic Antagonists, and Calcium Antagonists)

Name	Route of elimination	>50	10–50	<10	Supplement after dialysis
Clonidine	R	N	N	N	N
Doxazosin	H	N	N	N	N
Guanfacine	H	N	N	N	N
Hydralazine (PO)	H	8	8	8–16	N
Methyldopa	R,H	8	8–12	12–24	HD, PD
Minoxidil	H	N	N	N	HD
Nitroprusside	N	N	N	N	N
Prazosin	H,R	N	N	N	N

Angiotensin-Converting Enzyme Inhibitors

Name	Route of elimination	>50	10–50	<10	Supplement after dialysis
Captopril	R,H	N	N	50%	HD
Enalapril	H	N	N	50%	HD
Fosinopril	R,H	N	N	N	N
Lisinopril	R	N	50%	25%	HD
Ramipril	R,H	N	50%	50%	HD

Beta-Adrenergic Antagonists

Name	Route of elimination	>50	10–50	<10	Supplement after dialysis
Acebutolol	R,H	N	50%	25%	N
Atenolol	R	N	50%	25%	HD
Betaxolol	H,R	N	N	50%	N
Labetalol	H	N	N	N	N
Metoprolol	H	N	N	N	HD
Nadolol	R	N	50%	25%	HD
Pindolol	H,R	N	N	N	?
Propranolol	H	N	N	N	N
Timolol	H	N	N	N	N

Calcium Antagonists

Name	Route of elimination	>50	10–50	<10	Supplement after dialysis
Diltiazem	H	N	N	N	N
Isradipine	H	N	N	N	N
Nicardipine	H	N	N	N	N
Nifedipine	H	N	N	N	N
Verapamil	H	N	N	50–75%	N

Diuretics

Name	Route of elimination	>50	10–50	<10	Supplement after dialysis
Acetazolamide	R	6	12	A	
Bumetanide	R,H	N	N	N	
Furosemide	R	N	N	N	
Indapamide	H	N	N	N	
Metolazone	R	N	N	N	
Spironolactone	R	6–12	12–24	A	
Thiazide	R	N	N	A	

Antiarrhythmic Drugs

Name	Route of elimination	>50	10–50	<10	Supplement after dialysis
Amiodarone	H	N	N	N	N
Bretylium	R,H	N	25–50%	A	?
Digoxin*	R	24	36	48	N

Name	Route of elimination	Adjusted dosing interval (hr) or dose % for GFR (ml/min)			Supplement after dialysis
		>50	10–50	<10	
Antiarrhythmic Drugs (continued)					
Disopyramide*	R,H	75%	25–50%	10–25%	HD
Flecainide*	R,H	N	50%	50%	N
Lidocaine*	H,R	N	N	N	N
Mexiletine	H,R	N	N	50–75%	HD
Moricizine	H	N	N	50–75%	N
Procainamide*	R,H	4	6–12	12–24	HD
Propafenone	H	N	N	50–75%	N
Quinidine*	H,R	N	N	N	HD, PD
Tocainide*	R,H	N	N	50%	HD
Sedative Drugs					
Alprazolam	H	N	N	N	N
Chlordiazepoxide	H	N	N	50%	N
Diazepam	H	N	N	N	N
Flurazepam	H	N	N	N	N
Lorazepam	H	N	N	N	N
Midazolam	H	N	N	50%	N
Temazepam	H	N	N	N	N
Antidepressant Drugs					
Amitriptyline	H	N	N	N	N
Doxepin	H	N	N	N	N
Fluoxetine	H	N	N	N	N
Imipramine	H	N	N	N	N
Nortriptyline	H	N	N	N	N
Trazodone	H	N	N	N	N
Other Psychoactive Drugs					
Buspirone	H,R	N	N	25–50%	HD
Chlorpromazine	H	N	N	N	N
Haloperidol	H	N	N	N	N
Lithium*	R	N	50–75%	25–50%	HD, PD
Anticonvulsant Drugs					
Carbamazepine*	H,R	N	N	75%	N
Ethosuximide*	H,R	N	N	75%	HD
Phenobarbital*	H,R	N	N	12–16	HD, PD
Phenytoin*	H	N	N	N	N
Primidone*	H,R	8	8–12	12–24	HD
Valproic acid*	H	N	N	75%	N
Gastrointestinal Drugs					
Cimetidine	R	6	8	12	N
Famotidine	R,H	N	N	50%	N
Metoclopramide	R,H	N	75%	50%	N
Misoprostol	R	N	N	N	N
Nizatidine	H	N	24	48	N

Name	Route of elimination	Adjusted dosing interval (hr) or dose % for GFR (ml/min)			Supplement after dialysis
		>50	10–50	<10	
Gastrointestinal Drugs (continued)					
Omeprazole	H	N	N	N	?
Ranitidine	R	N	18–24	24	HD
Sucralfate	N	N	N	N	N
Antilipemic Drugs					
Clofibrate	H	6–12	12–24	24–48	N
Gemfibrozil	R,H	N	50%	25%	N
Lovastatin	H	N	N	N	N
Probucol	?	N	N	N	N
Hypoglycemic Drugs					
Acetohexamide	H	12–24	A	A	N
Chlorpropamide	?	24–36	A	A	N
Glipizide	H	N	N	N	N
Glyburide	H	N	N	N	N
Insulin	H	N	75%	50%	N
Tolazamide	H	N	N	N	N
Tolbutamide	H	N	N	N	N
Anticoagulant Drugs					
Heparin	H	N	N	N	N
Warfarin	H	N	N	N	N
Other Drugs					
Allopurinol	R	N	50%	10–25%	HD
Colchicine (PO)	R,H	N	N	50%	N
Dipyridamole	H	N	N	N	N
Glucocorticoids	H	N	N	N	?
Nitrates	H	N	N	N	N
Terbutaline	H,R	N	50%	A	?
Theophylline	H	N	N	N	HD, PD

* Serum levels should be used to determine exact dosing.
Key: GFR = glomerular filtration rate; R = renal; HD = hemodialysis; PD = peritoneal dialysis; H = hepatic; N = none; % = percent of the normal dose; A = should be avoided.
Source: Data from G. K. McEvoy (ed.). *American Hospital Formulary Service Drug Information.* Bethesda: American Society of Hospital Pharmacists, 1991; W. M. Bennett. Guide to drug dosing in renal failure. *Clin. Pharmacokinet.* 15:3226, 1988; R. W. Schrier and J. G. Gambertoglio (eds.). *Handbook of Drug Therapy in Liver and Kidney Disease.* Boston: Little, Brown, 1991.

E

Immunizations

Victoria J. Fraser

Table E-1. Routine adult immunization information

Vaccine	Indicated for	Dosage	Adverse effects	Contraindications
Tetanus-diphtheria (adult Td)[a] Adsorbed tetanus and diphtheria toxoids	Everyone	Unimmunized; 2 doses 0.5 ml IM 1–2 months apart, then 1 dose 6–12 months later; booster every 10 years	Local pain and swelling, rare hypersensitivity	Neurologic or hypersensitivity reaction to previous dose
Influenza Inactivated subunit or whole virus grown in chick embryo cells	High-risk patients,[b] health care workers, and everyone over 65 years of age	1 dose 0.5 ml IM annually in the fall	Fever, chills, myalgia, malaise	Anaphylactic hypersensitivity to eggs
Pneumococcal Capsular polysaccharides from 23 types	High-risk patients[c] and everyone over 65 years of age	1 dose 0.5 ml IM	Local soreness	Previous pneumococcal vaccine
Hepatitis B Recombinant HBsAg Plasma-derived inactivated HBsAg	High-risk patients[d] and health care workers	3 doses each 1 ml IM *in the deltoid,* at 0, 1, and 6 months, higher doses for dialysis patients and immunocompromised patients[e]	Local soreness	None
Measles[f] Attenuated live virus	Unimmunized born after 1956 Previously immunized: entering college, health care workers, foreign travel	2 doses 0.5 ml SQ at least 1 month apart 1 dose 0.5 ml SQ	Low-grade fever	Pregnancy, history of anaphylaxis to eggs or neomycin, significant immunosuppression (except those with HIV)

| Rubella[f] | Attenuated live virus | Nonimmune health care workers and women of child-bearing age | 1 dose 0.5 ml SQ | Low-grade fever, rash, arthralgia and arthritis in up to 40% of nonimmune adults | Pregnancy, significant immunosuppression (not HIV), hypersensitivity to neomycin |

[a] Guidelines for tetanus prophylaxis in wound management are given in Table E-2.

[b] The population at risk for severe influenza includes those with acquired or congenital heart disease, chronic lung disease, chronic renal disease or nephrotic syndrome, sickle cell disease, diabetes mellitus, and immunocompromised patients.

[c] Populations at increased risk for pneumococcal pneumonia or complications thereof include people with diabetes mellitus, anatomic or functional asplenia, people with chronic lung, cardiac, renal, or hepatic disease or CSF leaks.

[d] High-risk patients for hepatitis B include IV drug users, sexually active adults with multiple partners, homosexual/bisexual men, dialysis patients, and sex partners or household contacts of hepatitis B carriers.

[e] Compromised hosts or dialysis patients should receive *twice* the recommended dose of plasma-derived HB vaccine.

[f] Available as a monovalent (measles only) or in combination (measles-rubella [MR] and measles-mumps-rubella [MMR]) vaccines.

Table E-2. Guidelines for tetanus prophylaxis in wound management

History of tetanus immunization (doses)	Clean minor wounds		Other wounds	
	Give Td	Give TIG*	Give Td	Give TIG*
Unknown or less than 3	Yes	No	Yes	Yes
3 doses or more	No (Yes if > 10 years since last dose)	No	No (Yes if > 5 years since last dose)	No

* TIG (tetanus immune globulin) given concurrently with toxoid at separate sites, 250 units IM.

Table E-3. Passive immunization

Disease	Dosage
Diphtheria	Diphtheria antitoxin (DAT), equine source; 20,000–120,000 units IV as specific therapy for diphtheria
Hepatitis B	Hepatitis B immune globulin (HBIG); 0.06 ml/kg IM as soon as possible after exposure; second dose 1 month later unless vaccine given
Measles	Immunoglobulin, 0.25 ml/kg IM (maximum dose of 15 ml) when live virus vaccine cannot be given to persons exposed to measles, or when close exposure has occurred within 6 days; especially immunocompromised persons
Rabies	Rabies immune globulin (RIG); 20 IU/kg (one-half dose IM and one-half infiltrated at wound site)
Tetanus	Tetanus immune globulin, human (TIG); 3,000–6,000 units IM with part of dose infiltrated around the wound Equine tetanus antitoxin (TAT); 50,000–100,000 units (20,000 IV and the rest IM) if TIG unavailable

Table E-4. Postexposure antirabies treatment guide[a]

Species	Condition of animal at time of attack	Treatment of exposed person
Domestic cat, dog	Healthy and available for 10 days of observation	None unless animal develops rabies[b]
	Rabid or suspected rabid Unknown	RIG and HDCV[c] Contact Public Health Department
Wild skunk, bat, fox, coyote, raccoon, or other carnivore	Regard as rabid unless proved negative by laboratory tests	RIG and HDCV

[a] This guide should be applied in conjunction with knowledge of the animal species involved, circumstances of the bite, vaccination status of the animal, and prevalence of rabies in the region.
[b] Begin RIG and HDCV at first sign of rabies in animal under observation.
[c] Discontinue vaccine if fluorescent antibody test results in the animal are negative.

Table E-5. Rabies immunization and treatment recommendations

Vaccine/passive immunization	Indications	Dosage	Adverse effects
HDCV (human diploid cell vaccine) inactivated virus	Preexposure: veterinarians, animal handlers, people staying > 1 month in endemic rabies areas	3 doses of HDCV (0.1 ml ID or 1 ml IM) day 0, 7, and 28; booster every 2 years	Rare anaphylactic and allergic reactions
	Postexposure: Combined passive (RIG) and active (HDCV) treatment recommended for those exposed to animals suspected of being rabid (see Table E-4)	RIG, 20 IU/kg (½ dose IM and ½ infiltrated at wound site) Five 1-ml doses of HDCV IM; first dose immediately with RIG at different site; then day 3, 7, 14, and 28 after first dose If previously immunized, give booster HDCV on days 0 and 3	

F

Infection Control and Isolation Recommendations

Marilyn Jones and
Victoria J. Fraser

I. **Body substance isolation (BSI)** should be practiced on **all patients at all times.** All moist body substances should be considered potentially infectious. **Barrier protection (gloves, masks, goggles) should be used to prevent direct contact with moist body substances.** The use of BSI for all patients eliminates the need for disease-specific categories of isolation except for airborne or respiratory precautions. BSI helps to prevent transmission of hospital infections and helps protect health care workers from communicable diseases (*Am. J. Infect. Control* 18:1, 1990).

Specific recommendations:

  A. **Wear gloves** when direct contact with moist body substances (e.g., pus, sputum, urine, feces, blood) from any patient is anticipated.

  B. **Wear a gown** when clothing is likely to be soiled by any patient's body fluids.

  C. **Wear masks and goggles/glasses** when splashes from any patient's body fluids are anticipated.

II. **Respiratory isolation** should be provided for patients with communicable diseases with airborne transmission. Infection Control should be notified and a private room and masks required.

Diseases	Duration of Airborne Precautions
Anthrax	Duration of illness
Chickenpox (varicella)*	Until all lesions are crusted
Diphtheria	Until cultures are negative (at least 24 hours after stopping antibiotics)
Hemorrhagic fevers	Duration of illness
Herpes zoster (varicella)* **localized in immunocompromised patients or disseminated disease**	Until all lesions are crusted
Measles (rubeola)*	For 4 days after rash starts Immunocompromised patients may remain contagious for the duration of illness
Meningitis (*Haemophilus influenzae* or *Neisseria meningitidis;* known or suspected)	For 24 hours after start of effective antibiotic therapy
Meningococcal pneumonia or sepsis	For 24 hours after start of effective antibiotic therapy
Mumps*	For 9 days after onset of swelling
Pertussis (whooping cough)	For 7 days after start of effective antibiotic therapy
Rubella (German measles)*	For 7 days after rash appears
Tuberculosis, pulmonary (confirmed or suspected)	Usually 2–3 weeks after therapy begins; duration may be guided by clinical response and a reduction in number of AFB on smears

* People who are not immune to these diseases should not enter the room.

G

Partial List of Drugs Used During Pregnancy at Barnes Hospital

Anne M. Pittman

Type of medication	Safe to use in pregnancy[a]	Limited information, relatively safe[b]	Risks associated with use[c]	Avoid in pregnancy[d]
Analgesics	Acetaminophen	Hydromorphone[e] Codeine[e] Meperidine[e] Oxycodone with aspirin[e] Morphine[e]	Salicylates Ibuprofen Indomethacin	
Antibiotics	Ampicillin Erythromycin Penicillin Carbenicillin	Amikacin Amphotericin B Nitrofurantoin Ampicillin with sublactam Amoxicillin with clavulanic acid Miconazole Aztreonam Ticarcillin Oxacillin Methicillin Cephalosporins Clindamycin Gentamicin Tobramycin	Chloramphenicol Metronidazole Isoniazid Streptomycin Sulfonamides Rifampin Trimethoprim Kanamycin	Chloroquine Ciprofloxacin Norfloxacin Tetracyclines
Anticoagulants		Dipyridamole Heparin		Warfarin
Antiemetics		Meclizine Trimethobenzamide Metoclopramide	Thiethylperazine Prochlorperazine	
Antiepileptics		Ethosuximide	Clonazepam Phenytoin Valproic acid Primidone Phenobarbital	
Antihistamines	Tripelennamine		Brompheniramine Terfenadine Astemizole Diphenhydramine	Hydroxyzine

Type of medication	Safe to use in pregnancy[a]	Limited information, relatively safe[b]	Risks associated with use[c]	Avoid in pregnancy[d]
Antihypertensives		Hydralazine Methyldopa Clonidine Metoprolol Prazosin	Atenolol Nitroprusside Diazoxide Labetalol Timolol Propranolol Nadolol	Captopril Reserpine Enalapril Lisinopril
Asthma preparations		Beclomethasone Aminophylline Cromolyn sodium Terbutaline Ipratropium bromide	Albuterol Isoproterenol Metaproterenol	
Cardiac drugs	Digoxin	Procainamide Atropine Quinidine Lidocaine Verapamil Disopyramide	Diltiazem Nifedipine	
Cough preparations		Terpin hydrate Guaifenesin		
Diuretics[f]		Furosemide	Bumetanide Ethacrynic acid Acetazolamide Hydrochlorothiazide	
Hypoglycemics[g]	Insulin			Chlorpropamide Tolbutamide Glyburide
Laxatives	Milk of magnesia Psyllium	Docusate		
Sedatives				Barbiturates Benzodiazepines
Thyroid preparations	Thyroxine		Methimazole Propylthiouracil Iodide	

Type of medication	Safe to use in pregnancy[a]	Limited information, relatively safe[b]	Risks associated with use[c]	Avoid in pregnancy[d]
Other drugs	Ferrous sulfate Kaopectate Probenecid Antacids	Allopurinol Clofibrate H$_2$ antagonists Vaccines (influenza, polio, rabies, tetanus)	Glucocorticoids Amphetamines EDTA General anesthesia drugs Haloperidol Penicillamine Phenothiazines	Antineoplastic agents Bromocriptine Lithium Disulfiram Estrogens, DES Isotretinoin Quinine Tricyclic antidepressants Vaccines (rubella, mumps, measles, smallpox) Misoprostol

[a] Although no drug can be used with certainty that there will be no adverse effects, drugs listed in this column are used at Barnes Hospital.

[b] Many drugs in this column are new and data are limited, but no consistent adverse effect has been attributed to their use.

[c] These drugs have some associated risk when used in pregnancy. The potential benefit must be weighed against possible adverse effects.

[d] These drugs have been well documented to produce adverse fetal effects. They should not be used in pregnancy.

[e] Possible neonatal addiction and withdrawal may occur after long-term use. Neonatal depression may occur with intrapartum use.

[f] Diuretics can deplete maternal intravascular volume and, in rare instances, can be associated with neonatal thrombocytopenia. Diuretics are not indicated in pregnancy-induced hypertension as first-line agents.

[g] There is no place for oral hypoglycemic agents in the treatment of diabetes in pregnancy. Oral hypoglycemic agents have been associated with prolonged hypoglycemia in newborn infants. Insulin and dietary control are indicated to bring blood sugar under rigid control.

Barnes Hospital Parenteral Nutrition Order Form

Date due _____ Bag # _____ Calories to the nearest 100 kcals per
24 hours _____ Hang time _____

Check one	Central formulas[a]	% Total cals provided as CHO/AA/Fats	Grams/1000 kcal of CHO/AA/Fat	~ ml/1000 kcal
▨	Intermediate nitrogen			
	A. Standard CHO	60/16/24	176/40/24	771 ml
	B. Intermediate CHO	49/16/35	144/40/35	780
	C. Low CHO, high fat	42/16/42	123/40/42.5	787
	D. Standard, no fat	84/16/—	247/40/—	752
▨	High nitrogen			
	Standard CHO, high nitrogen	60/20/20	176/50/20	850
	Intermediate CHO	50/20/30	147/50/30	860
	High nitrogen, no fat	80/20/—	235/50/—	836
	Very high nitrogen	56/24/20	165/60/20	935
▨	Low nitrogen			
	Standard CHO, low nitrogen	65/12/23	191/30/23	688
	Intermediate CHO	55/12/33	162/30/33	696
	Low nitrogen, high fat	50/10/40	147/25/40	660
	Peripheral formula	32/16/52	94/40/52	1429
	Special requests: Dextrose/AA	10% AA _____ ml 70% CHO _____ ml/24 hour		
	Lipids (as separate infusion)	circle one: 100 ml, 250 ml, 350 ml, 500 ml; 20% intralipid rate _____ ml/hour		

Electro-lytes	Daily suggested amount	Quantity ordered (mEq)	Other Additives	Suggested Amount	Quantity ordered
Na	60–80		MVI-12[b]	10 ml/day	ml
K[b]	30–60		Trace elements[b]	1 ml/day	ml
Cl[c]	80–100		Insulin	Reg. humulin only	units
Acetate[c]	(see below)	Balance	Vitamin K₁	10 mg/ Monday	mg
Ca⁺⁺	4.6–9.2 mEq				
Mg⁺ᵇ	8.1–20 mEq				
PO₄ᵇ	12–24 mmol				

[a] Other amino acids may be added in consultation with the nutrition department.
[b] Usually modified for renal failure.

[c] The total quantity of sodium and potassium must be balanced by equal amounts of anions (chloride and acetate). In patients with normal serum electrolytes, chloride should compose two-thirds of this total. Too little chloride may result in excessive acetate and a metabolic alkalosis.

Key: CHO = carbohydrate; AA = amino acids.

Source: Adapted from Barnes Hospital Parenteral Nutrition Order Form.

Basal Metabolic Rate

The basal metabolic rate (BMR) is the energy requirement at rest and correlates with body surface area. The daily energy expenditure related to the BMR can be estimated using the Harris-Benedict equations:

Energy requirement from BMR (kcal/day):

For women = $655 + (9.6 \times W) + (1.8 \times H) - (4.7 \times A)$

For men = $66 + (13.7 \times W) + (5 \times H) - (6.8 \times A)$

where W = actual weight (kg), H = height (cm), and A = age (years).

Index

Index

Abdominal thrusts, in basic life support, 167
Abscess
  brain, 258–259
  hepatic, 319
  lung, 208
  pancreatic, 307
  perirectal, 306
  in peritonitis, 265
  skin, in diabetes mellitus, 380
Accelerated idioventricular rhythm, 96
Accessory pathways, 133
  ablation of, 143
  concealed, 133, 142
  manifest, 133
Acebutolol
  in angina pectoris, 83
  in hypertension, 72
  in renal failure, 531
Acetaminophen, 2
  antidote to, 499, 500
  dosage in renal failure, 530
  in headaches, 481
  hepatotoxicity of, 499, 502
  overdose of, 499
  oxycodone with, 4
  propoxyphene with, 4
Acetazolamide
  dosage in renal failure, 531
  in glaucoma, 22
  interactions with other drugs, 524
  in metabolic acidosis, 59
  in mountain sickness, 494
  in uric acid nephropathy prevention, 219
Acetohexamide, 381
Acetylcholine, toxic effects of, 496
N-Acetylcysteine, in acetaminophen poisoning, 499, 500
Acetylsalicylic acid, 447. See also Aspirin; Salicylates
Acid–base disorders, 54–61. See also Acidosis; Alkalosis
  compensatory responses in, 55
  in mechanical ventilation, 190–191
  mixed, 61
Acid ingestions, 503–504
Acid phosphatase levels, in serum, 518
Acidemia from transfusions, 355
Acidosis. See also Acid–base disorders; pH
  bedside interpretation of, 55

  in chronic renal failure, 226
  ketoacidosis
    alcoholic, 57
    diabetic, 387–389
      bicarbonate therapy in, 388–389
      complications of, 390
      dextrose in, 389
      diagnosis of, 387–388
      fluid management in, 388
      insulin in, 389
      monitoring of therapy in, 388
      phosphate in, 389
      potassium replacement in, 389
      in pregnancy, 394
      prevention of recurrences, 390
  lactic acid, 57–58
    in diabetic ketoacidosis, 390
  metabolic, 56–59
    acute, 56–57
    in acute renal failure, 221
    anion gap, 56, 57–58
    chronic, 57
    compensatory responses in, 55
    hypokalemia with, 51
    in near-drowning, 490
    osmolal gap in, 58
  renal tubular, 58–59
    hyperkalemic distal, 58–59
    hypokalemic, 58
  respiratory, 56, 60
    compensatory responses in, 55
Acinetobacter infections, imipenem in, 239
ACLS. See Advanced cardiac life support
Acne vulgaris, 14
Acquired immunodeficiency syndrome. See AIDS; Human immunodeficiency virus infection
Acromegaly, 409
ACTH, 408
  ectopic secretion of, 417
  serum levels, 518
  stimulation test, 415
Actinomycosis, 274
Activated charcoal, for poisoning, 498
Acute renal failure. See Renal failure
Acyclovir, 246
  dosage in renal failure, 530
  in herpes simplex infection, 271
  in herpes zoster ophthalmicus, 23
Adams-Stokes attacks, 141

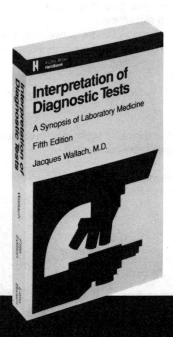

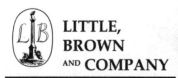

The Little, Brown Spiral® Manual Series
The Little, Brown Handbook Series
AVAILABLE AT YOUR BOOKSTORE

THE LITTLE, BROWN HANDBOOK SERIES